Toxicological Effects of Veterinary Medicinal Products
in Humans
Volume 1

Issues in Toxicology

Series Editors:
Professor Diana Anderson, *University of Bradford, UK*
Dr Michael D Waters, *Integrated Laboratory Systems, Inc., N Carolina, USA*
Dr Martin F Wilks, *University of Basel, Switzerland*
Dr Timothy C Marrs, *Edentox Associates, Kent, UK*

How to obtain future titles on publication:
A standing order plan is available for this series. A standing order will bring delivery of each new volume immediately on publication.

For further information please contact:
Book Sales Department, Royal Society of Chemistry, Thomas Graham House, Science Park, Milton Road, Cambridge, CB4 0WF, UK
Telephone: +44 (0)1223 420066, Fax: +44 (0)1223 420247
Email: booksales@rsc.org
Visit our website at www.rsc.org/books

Toxicological Effects of Veterinary Medicinal Products in Humans

Volume 1

Kevin N. Woodward

TSGE, Concordia House, St James Business Park, Grimbald Crag Court, Knaresborough, North Yorkshire, HG5 8QB, UK
Email: Kevin.Woodward@TSGEurope.com

RSCPublishing

Issues in Toxicology No. 14

ISBN: 978-1-84973-417-2
ISSN: 1757-7179

A catalogue record for this book is available from the British Library

Published by The Royal Society of Chemistry,
Thomas Graham House, Science Park, Milton Road,
Cambridge CB4 0WF, UK

Registered Charity Number 207890

For further information see our website at www.rsc.org

Printed in the United Kingdom by CPI Group (UK) Ltd, Croydon, CR0 4YY, UK

Preface

The term "veterinary medicinal product" describes those medicines developed specifically for use in animals. The development of these products involves an enormous amount of intellectual effort and physical labour as well as a considerable amount of financial investment in order to ensure that animals have available products that are of the appropriate quality and with the correct degree of effectiveness. These products also need to be safe for the animal patient as well as for the user, for the consumer of edible animal products and for the environment. On the other hand, the term "veterinary drug" is misleading, as the majority of drugs used in veterinary medicine, with very few exceptions, either are used in human medicine or have been used in the past in human medicine. As a consequence, we tend to know a considerable amount about the toxicity of veterinary drugs from their use in human medicine. We only know a little regarding the safety of veterinary medicinal products in humans from their use in animals.

This books attempts to bring together some of this knowledge and experience to assess the safety of veterinary medicinal products. As described in the pages that follow, this involves user safety and safety of those who consume products derived from animals treated with veterinary medicines, and for the most part this means examining their toxicological and pharmacological properties. However, some veterinary drugs are also microbiologically active, and this presents certain hazards that also need to be taken into account. Finally, like human drugs, these products also eventually find their way into the environment. As a result, to examine the potential hazards arising from veterinary medicine, we need to evaluate their toxicological and pharmacological properties, *and* we need to consider their microbiological properties and their eventual fate in the natural environment. This latter aspect is of concern not only because organisms might encounter the remnants of veterinary medicines as a result of environmental contamination, but also because of the potential effects for human health from the contamination of land and drinking

Issues in Toxicology No. 14
Toxicological Effects of Veterinary Medicinal Products in Humans: Volume 1
By Kevin N. Woodward
© The Royal Society of Chemistry 2013
Published by the Royal Society of Chemistry, www.rsc.org

water. I have tried to reach a balance, and review the main issues that might impact on human safety arising from the use of veterinary medicinal products. It is not possible to cover every product or drug in a work of this nature, and I have made no attempt to do so. Some products are used infrequently, and some are only used in certain countries. Many others are human drugs that are used off-label in animals. I have attempted to cover the major drug classes as well as some individual drugs of interest. Some of these are now of historical interest as many have fallen out of use or have been replaced with more effective and safer alternatives. Nevertheless, it would be remiss to avoid discussion of these where they may have impacted human safety in the past, so I have included them here.

I would like to thank the authors who have invested significant efforts by providing chapters for this book – Dr Tim Marrs, Derek Renshaw and Professor Peter Silley. I would also like to thank my family – and dogs – for their forbearance and patience while I have been working on this project.

Kevin Woodward
Surrey

Contents

Issues in Toxicology No. 14
Toxicological Effects of Veterinary Medicinal Products in Humans: Volume 1
By Kevin N. Woodward
© The Royal Society of Chemistry 2013
Published by the Royal Society of Chemistry, www.rsc.org

Volume 2

CHAPTER 1

Occupational Health and Safety Among Veterinarians and Veterinary Workers

1.1 Introduction

Many people use, and are therefore potentially exposed to, veterinary medicinal products. These include the pet-owning public, farmers, animal breeders and keepers, and, of course, veterinarians and other veterinary staff such as veterinary nurses and practice receptionists. The public may be intermittently exposed to veterinary medicinal products, apart from those with animals with chronic conditions such as epilepsy and diabetes where exposures may be more frequent. Farmers may be responsible for the administration of a wide variety of drugs and, occasionally, exposures have the potential to be significant, for example when dipping sheep and mixing or administering in-feed antimicrobial agents. Veterinarians and veterinary nurses are potentially exposed to a wide range of veterinary drugs including anaesthetics, euthanasia agents, antineoplastic agents and non-steroidal anti-inflammatory drugs. It is thus tempting to assume that these professionals are assailed on a daily basis by the combined actions of a number of pharmacologically and toxicologically active agents, and if these could be removed from veterinary practice, the world, or at least the veterinary world, would be a better place in which to live and work.

However, just as it would be wrong to assume that the industrial workplace is a chemophobe's nightmare, or a toxicologists dream, it is equally incorrect to think of the veterinary surgery or clinic as a toxicological playground. Although industry, especially the chemical industry, has had its fair share of chemical disasters, such as those involving asbestos, benzene, vinyl chloride

Issues in Toxicology No. 14
Toxicological Effects of Veterinary Medicinal Products in Humans: Volume 1
By Kevin N. Woodward
© The Royal Society of Chemistry 2013
Published by the Royal Society of Chemistry, www.rsc.org

monomer and a number of halogenated hydrocarbons to name but a few, the vast majority of mortalities and morbidities in industry arise from accidents including those involving machinery, explosions and fires. Similarly, it would be incorrect to assume that veterinary workers are immersed in toxic soups of pharmacologically active materials. Even if they were, there are numerous other hazards, with associated risks, which may pose greater dangers than the majority of pharmaceutical or biological agents encountered in veterinary practice.

The main topic of this book is the potential for veterinary pharmaceutical products to cause harm to human beings, especially through toxicological modes of action. However, just as with industry, this must be seen in perspective with all other potential hazards and this chapter attempts to review this perspective.

1.2   Physical Injuries

1.2.1   Accidents and Related Incidents

In a study reported in 1988 of a survey of members of the American Veterinary Medical Association where 995 people responded, nearly 65% had suffered a major animal-related injury.[1] Of these, 17% were hospitalised and 25% required surgical intervention. The main body regions affected were the hand (53%), arms (28%), head (21%), thorax (8%), genitals (4%) and abdomen (3%).

Injuries arose from kicks (36%), bites (3%), crush (12%) and scratches (4%). Other causes of injury involved goring, head butting, pushing and animals falling onto the veterinarian. Cattle (47%), dogs (24%) and horses were the animals most frequently involved in incidents. Car crashes arising from work-related activities were also common.

Ten years later in 1998, of 1797 companion animal veterinarians approached in another survey, 735 (41%) responded.[2] From these respondents, 55% reported that they had had at least one incident. These included dog and cat bites, lifting injuries and slips, trips and falls. Exposure to potentially hazardous substances formed a small category. In this study, professional assistants, veterinary technicians and lay people were affected as well as veterinarians.

In 2010, in a study of veterinarians in the Kampala region of Uganda, the incidence of animal-related injuries was 72%, a surprisingly high figure.[3] The majority of these were accounted for by cattle (72%), followed by cats (25%), dogs (23%) and birds (13%). Injuries caused by poultry did not require hospital treatments, unlike those caused by the other animals encountered. The upper limb was the most frequently injured part of the body (68%), while vaccination was the major activity associated with injury.

In fact several studies have demonstrated the dangers to veterinarians of working with animals including dogs, cats, pigs, cattle and horses, and as already described these include bites, kicks and crushing injuries. Horse-associated injuries, especially kicks, may result in fractures, which, in one survey, were the most common cause of horse-inflicted injury with the head, face and lower limbs being the most affected parts.[4–14] In an unusual case, a veterinarian suffered a dissection to the internal carotid artery resulting in cerebral ischaemia with cranial nerve involvement, because of the exertions involved in the caesarean delivery of a calf.[15]

These occupational hazards may be exacerbated when the animals are even larger than cattle and horses, particularly when those animals are wild. Deaths of handlers and veterinarians have been associated with elephants and tigers, and following attacks by venomous animals.[16–18] Working with exotic species in zoos is associated with major animal-related injuries, back injuries, injuries incurred during necropsies, formalin exposures, animal allergy, zoonotic infection and insect allergies.[19]

Some effects of working with animals are less obvious in their origins. An orthopaedic surgeon in Canada encountered a few cases where large-animal veterinarians who had regularly carried out rectal examinations on farm animals reported right shoulder and neck pain, associated with neurological deficit in the median, ulnar and radial nerves. He subsequently organised a survey of large animal practitioners to investigate the extent of this problem. It became clear that these symptoms were relatively common in large animal practitioners, at least in Canada, but they could be ameliorated by periods of rest and by adopting correct postures during the examination procedures.[18]

In fact, lifting patients, handling patients using awkward grip and hand movements, surgery, rectal examinations and repetitive movements result in or contribute to shoulder injuries, back pain and other musculoskeletal disorders in veterinarians.[19–25]

Perhaps the most bizarre, if somewhat untypical, accident involving a veterinarian occurred in Antarctica when a young female veterinarian involved in field work with Adélie penguins, fell into a crevasse while driving a quad bike, and was crushed between the vehicle and the crevasse wall six metres below the surface. She developed hypothermia and abdominal injuries and underwent two emergency surgical procedures before being evacuated by helicopter and ship and eventually making a recovery.[26]

Certain areas of animal production, notably those involving intensive farming methods, offer significant opportunities for occupational health problems to arise. Aquaculture is an obvious example. Aquaculture enterprises are often based in relatively hostile environments or at least in environments that have the capacity to become hostile because of seasonal influences or changes in the weather. In the United Kingdom, salmon production is based in northerly locations in Scotland, and in Scandinavian countries at even more northerly locations. Fish farming may be conducted in isolated areas in Scottish sea lochs and in some fjords. In all cases, these areas are subject to wide variations in climatic conditions with cold and heat at the extremes, and with rain, snow, ice, winds and gales among the weather conditions for aquaculture workers to contend with.

Farmed fish, like all farmed animals, are susceptible to various viral, bacterial, fungal and parasitic conditions and an armoury of prophylactic products, mainly vaccines, and chemotherapeutants, including antimicrobial drugs and antiparasitic agents, have been developed to combat or treat the various conditions and to ensure the viability of the industry. The diseases are diagnosed by veterinarians and others involved in animal health and welfare, and, similarly, the drugs and vaccines are administered by fish farm employees, usually under the direction of a veterinarian. Hence, the environments where fish farms are frequently located, or more specifically the environments where salmon (and other cold water fish) are located, offer particular challenges in terms of occupational safety.

Musculoskeletal disorders are common from lifting nets within cages where the fish are reared and the feedstuffs used in aquaculture may attract rats, which create a risk for leptospirosis. Other hazards include exposure to hydrogen sulfide that arises from anaerobic reactions in the bottom of fishponds, drowning, hypothermia, electricity, sunburn, fire and explosions from oxygen exposure and ice-related accidents.[27–29]

1.2.2 Needlestick Injuries

Needlestick injuries are a specific and common type of accident among veterinarians, veterinary nurses, physicians and nurses. In general, they involve "dry" needles *i.e.* needles with little or no pharmaceutical product on their surface or contained within them and they therefore represent a physical hazard rather than a chemical one as the dose of any drug will be minute. However, it must be recognised that some needlestick injuries with some potent pharmacological acting agents might represent a pharmacological or even toxicological hazard. Similarly, with live vaccines containing zoonotic organisms there is a risk of an adverse outcome. Nevertheless, the usual result is a physical injury rather than a biological or pharmacological insult.

In the UK, the agency responsible for regulating veterinary medicinal products, the Veterinary Medicines Directorate (VMD), reports the results of its pharmacovigilance scheme, the Suspected Adverse Reactions Surveillance Scheme, annually in the *Veterinary Record*, the journal of the British Veterinary Association. In the report for 1990, the VMD first noted that some of the reports involving adverse reactions to veterinary medicinal products in humans involved simple needlestick injuries.[30] This was barely mentioned thereafter until ten years later when it was noted that 28 reports submitted to the agency concerned needlestick injuries.[31] Since that time, the occurrence of needlestick injuries has featured regularly in the VMD's reports.[32–39] These are illustrated in Table 1.1.

It is evident from Table 1.1 that needlestick injuries in the UK are a common feature of the VMD's reports. However, even allowing for the under-reporting that is a frequent feature of all adverse reaction reporting schemes, whether for human or veterinary adverse reaction reporting schemes, the actual incidence is very low when compared with the vast numbers of injectable products administered daily to both companion and farm animals. The UK's expert body, the

Table 1.1 Needlestick injuries reported to the VMD.

	2003	2004	2005	2006	2007	2008	2009	2010
Total human adverse reactions	90	70	104	126	138	145	107	94
Needlestick injuries	19	24	−[a]	−[b]	−[c]	−[d]	−[e]	36

[a]90% of human reactions involving vaccines or other injectable products were needlestick injuries.
[b]91% of human reactions involving vaccines or other injectable products were needlestick injuries.
[c]84% of human reactions involving vaccines or other injectable products were needlestick injuries.
[d]88% of human reactions involving vaccines or other injectable products were needlestick injuries.
[e]86% of human reactions involving vaccines or other injectable products were needlestick injuries.

Veterinary Products Committee, has made various recommendations for improving the UK scheme, one of which addresses the under-reporting of needlestick injuries.[40]

These injuries are by no means restricted to UK veterinarians and similar reports have been made elsewhere.[19,41–46] Although needlestick injuries tend to be associated with treatment of terrestrial animals, they have also been reported in operators vaccinating fish.[27,28,47]

Although needlestick injuries are frequently considered to be "simple" physical injuries, they carry with them the risk of inflammatory reactions, infection and transmission of zoonotic agents from vaccines.[27,28,42,44,46,48–50] Thus, needlestick injuries in veterinary practice and animal care and production have much in common with needlestick injuries in human medicine where similar concerns exist.[51–75]

1.2.3 Zoonotic Diseases

Veterinarians and others involved in animal health and welfare are exposed to zoonotic agents not only through the use of live vaccines, but also through exposure to animals themselves and to their environments. For some diseases, veterinarians are recognised as being at high risk. These include rabies, avian and swine influenza, brucellosis, toxoplasmosis, salmonellosis, leptospirosis, Lyme disease, echinococcosis, Q fever, psittacosis, Rift Valley fever, cat scratch disease (*Bartonella henselae*), cutaneous larva migrans, anthrax, bovine tuberculosis, yersiniosis, blastomycosis, listeriosis and methicillin-resistant *Staphylococcus aureus* (MRSA).[76–125] Where possible, the risks associated with these biological hazards should be mitigated by preventive measures such as vaccination, personal hygiene and containment measures.

1.2.4 Dermatoses

Non-infectious dermatoses are common among veterinarians. For example, among a survey of veterinarians in Kansas, some 60% responded and, of these, 24 reported non-infectious recurrent or persistent dermatoses of the forearm, of which 66% were related to work.[126] In a European study, dermatologists were questioned about their experiences with dermatoses in veterinarians. Seven dermatologists had experiences with dermatoses in a total of 58 veterinarians and, of these, 12 cases were infectious disease. The remaining 46 cases could be classified as contact urticarial, irritant or allergic contact dermatitis.[127] Similar results have been seen in other studies[128–132] Responsible agents included animal protein fluids during obstetric procedures, antiseptic agents, canine milk and canine seminal fluid.[133–138]

1.2.5   Allergies

In addition to the allergic dermatoses (see Section 1.2.4), veterinarians and others who work with animals are susceptible by the nature of their work to other conditions with an allergic basis. These include animal-related allergic rhinitis, asthma, cough, chest tightness, sneezing and reductions in lung function and may be due to exposure to animal fur, feathers and other sources of animal protein, including urinary proteins. Companion animals (mainly cats and dogs) and farm animals (cattle, pigs and horses) have been implicated in the aetiology of these conditions.[139–150]

1.2.6   Neoplastic Diseases

Veterinarians are exposed to a range of agents, some of which may be carcinogenic. These include pesticides, solar radiation, ionising radiation for diagnostic and therapeutic purposes and pathogens. There have been a number of studies undertaken to determine if veterinarians are at risk from particular types of cancer.

A study of the health status of veterinarians in Illinois in 1981 suggested that the incidence of cancer was low (1%).[151] However, this study examined what may have been an unusually healthy population of currently working individuals. A separate study of US veterinarians suggested a higher incidence of some forms of cancer, notably leukaemia and Hodgkin's lymphoma, and cancers of the skin and brain for the period 1966–1977.[152] When this was expanded to cover the period 1947–1977, there were elevated numbers of lymphatic and haematopoietic neoplasms as well as cancers of the colon, brain and skin and it was postulated that for the excess incidence of leukaemias, there may have been an association with the early uses of diagnostic radiation.[153] There is also some evidence to suggest that veterinarians, along with other occupational groups, may be at risk from multiple myeloma,[154] while another study suggested an increased incidence of cancer of the large bowel, specifically in those with more than 30 years in the veterinary profession in the US and malignant melanoma for those with more than 20 years.[155] In Sweden, a study of cancer incidence among male veterinarians suggested increased risks from cancers of the oesophagus, colon, pancreas and brain as well as an increased risk of malignant melanoma.[156]

When studies of cancer in veterinarians are taken together, and notably cohort studies, the main conclusions are that veterinarians probably have an increased risk from lymphomas, leukaemia, melanoma and colon cancer although the latter is marginal.[157] The excess of melanoma is almost certainly due to exposure to the sun, which may not be surprising as veterinarians, or at least large-animal practitioners, spend a considerable proportion of their time outdoors. There is no convincing explanation for the excess risk of lympho-haematopoietic cancers, although exposure to ionising radiation is thought to play a role. However, there are excess risks of these types of cancer in agricultural workers who are unlikely to be exposed to radiation.[158,159] It has been suggested that zoonotic viruses may play a part in the aetiology of these neoplasms. Unfortunately for this hypothesis, the zoonotic diseases encountered by veterinarians and agricultural workers are not thought to be carcinogenic, while the oncogenic viruses encountered in animals, such as feline and bovine leukaemia viruses, are not known to cause disease in humans.

The use of X-ray units, including that of portable units, is not thought to contribute a major radiation hazard to operators, especially with modern equipment and better understanding of its safe use, and the precautions that veterinarians and veterinary technical staff take to reduce unnecessary and inadvertent exposures.[160–168]

1.2.7 Specific Risks for Women

The effects described so far may affect male and female veterinary workers equally. However, pregnant veterinary workers may be vulnerable to other hazards that in general are not relevant, or are less relevant, to men or to non-pregnant women. These include ionising radiation, physical trauma and lifting injuries and exposure to agents causing zoonotic disease such as toxoplasmosis and listeriosis, all of which may have adverse effects on pregnancy.[169,170] Exposure to anaesthetic gases also poses a risk for pregnancy outcome and this is discussed further in a separate chapter.

A number of studies suggest that female veterinarians are at risk from spontaneous abortion, and possibly, for "small for gestational age" births, although the incidence of malformations does not appear to be affected.[171–177] The reasons for these findings are unclear but exposure to high doses of radiation (more than 5 to 10 X-ray films per week) carried an increased risk.[172,174] If anything, these findings emphasise the need for hygiene and protective measures from biological, physical and chemical hazards, not only in female veterinarians, veterinary staff and animal handlers, but also in their male counterparts,[169,173,178] particularly as some research suggests that the children from both male and female veterinarians may be at elevated risk of developing some cancers.[179]

1.2.8 Mental Health

There is evidence that veterinary surgeons, across a number of countries, suffer from depressive symptoms and anxiety. For example, in the UK, veterinarians have a much higher degree of these conditions than the general population.[180] Some of these effects appear to arise from working conditions, with good relationships with colleagues producing a good outcome, and anxiety and depressive symptoms being associated with poor working conditions.[181] Other contributing factors include time pressures due to workload, long working hours, dealing with difficult clients and inadequate periods of free time.[182,183] Stress associated with euthanizing animals was also a major factor.[184–187] Similar findings have been made in other countries.[10,23,153,182,183,188,189] These stresses can lead to alcohol, tobacco and drug abuse as well as to accidents.[182,189–192]

The effects described above may eventually lead to suicidal thoughts and suicidal behaviour.[185,193] Moreover, the suicide rate among professionals, including veterinarians and physicians, is higher than that of the general population in several countries, including the UK, USA and Australia.[194–200] There may be some influence on suicide rates in veterinarians and healthcare workers by the fact that they have ready access to suitable means. For veterinarians this means both drugs and fire arms.[194,197] This latter phenomenon is common in specific groups with access to the means of suicide. For example, patients with diabetes, and occasionally their physicians, may use insulin overdose as a means of suicide.[201–205]

1.3   Conclusions

Veterinarians and veterinary workers in general face many hazards and their associated risks in the course of their daily lives. These hazards may be faced in the veterinary clinic, on farms, in zoos or even while travelling between workplace locations. They may be physical, biological or psychological. However, and returning to the theme of this book, veterinarians, veterinary nurses and their assistants, and indeed veterinary students, use veterinary pharmaceuticals and biologics in the course of their normal working day, and the hazards and associated risks must be considered. Nevertheless, they must be seen in the context of the other occupational hazards already described in the preceding paragraphs, as many of these are far more significant in terms of health impact, well-being and even lethality than is exposure to the majority of veterinary drugs and vaccines.

It is also important to recognise that in addition to veterinarians, veterinary medicinal products are also handled and administered by a variety of other groups including farmers, fish farm workers and members of the pet-owning public. In addition, consumers may be potentially exposed to residues of veterinary drugs and the other components of the product when they eat food of animal origin, such as meat, offal, meat products, milk and dairy products, fish, eggs and honey. These issues will be addressed in this work.

References

1. J. Landercasper, T. H. Cogbill, P. J. Strutt and B. O. Landercasper, Trauma and the veterinarian, *J. Trauma*, 1988, **28**, 1255–1259.
2. A. G. Poole, S. M. Shane, M. T. Kearney and W. Rehn, Survey of occupational hazards in companion animal practices, *J. Am. Vet. Med. Assoc.*, 1998, **212**, 1386–1388.

3. R. M. Kabuusu, E. O. Keku, R. Kiyini and T. J. McCann, Prevalence and patterns of self-reported animal-related injury among veterinarians in metropolitan Kenya, *J. Vet. Sci.*, 2011, **11**, 363–365.
4. M. Lucas, L. Day and L. Fritschi, Injuries to Australian veterinarians working with horses, *Vet. Rec.*, 2009, **164**, 207–209.
5. M. J. Wilkins, P. C. Bartlett, L. J. Judge, R. J. Erskine, M. L. Boulton and J. B. Kaneene, Veterinarian injuries associated with bovine TB testing livestock in Michigan, 2001, *Prev. Vet. Med.*, 2009, **89**, 185–190.
6. M. Lucas, L. Day, A. Shirangi and L. Fritschi, Significant injuries in Australian veterinarians and use of safety precautions, *Occup. Med.*, 2009, **59**, 327–333.
7. K. A. Houpt, Why horse behaviour is important to the equine clinician, *Equine Vet. J.*, 2006, **38**, 386–387.
8. L. Fritschi, L. Day, A. Shirangi, I. Robertson, M. Lucas and A. Vizard, Injury in Australian veterinarians, *Occup. Med.*, 2006, **56**, 199–203.
9. A. Nienhaus, C. Skudlik and A. Seidler, Work-related accidents and occupational diseases in veterinarians and their staff, *Int. Arch. Occup. Environ. Health*, 2005, **78**, 230–238.
10. J. Jeyaretnam and H. Jones, Physical, chemical and biological hazards in veterinary practice, *Aust. Vet. J.*, 2000, **78**, 751–758.
11. J. Jeyaretnam, H. Jones and M. Phillips, Disease and injury among veterinarians, *Aust. Vet. J.*, 2000, **78**, 625–629.
12. D. J. Mattey, Occupational risks from cattle, *Vet. Rec.*, 1996, **139**, 631.
13. O. Svoboda and M. Cupak, Occupational diseases and accidents among veterinarians, *Prac. Lek.*, 1962, **14**, 284–288.
14. R. L. Gordon and S. Rhodes, Injuries in a swine confinement facility, *J. Occup. Med.*, 1993, **35**, 518–521.
15. P. Berlit and C. Klötzsch, Case report: a veterinarian who collapsed after the delivery of a calf by caesarean section, *J. Neurol. Sci.*, 1998, **154**, 89–90.
16. R. Langley, Physical hazards of animal handlers, *Occup. Med.*, 1999, **14**, 181–194.
17. R. L. Langley and J. L. Hunter, Occupational fatalities due to animal-related events, *Wilderness Environ. Med.*, 2001, **12**, 168–174.
18. M. bin Zakaria, N. W. Lerche, B. B. Chomel and P. H. Kass, Accidental injuries associated with nonhuman primates exposure at two regional primate research centers (USA): 1988–1993, *Lab. Anim. Sci.*, 1996, **46**, 298–304.
19. D. J. Hill, R. L. Langley and W. M. Morrow, Occupational injuries and illnesses reported by zoo veterinarians in the United States, *J. Zoo Wildl. Med.*, 1998, **29**, 371–385.
20. R. L. Ailsby, Occupational arm, shoulder, and neck syndrome affecting large animal practitioners, *Can. Vet. J.*, 1996, **37**, 411.
21. A. M. Scuffham, E. C. Firth, M. A. Stevenson and S. J. Legg, Tasks considered by veterinarians to cause them musculoskeletal discomfort, and suggested solutions, *N. Z. Vet. J.*, 2010, **58**, 37–44.

22. A. M. Scuffham, S. J. Legg, E. C. Firth and M. A. Stevenson, Prevalence and risk factors associated with musculoskeletal discomfort in New Zealand veterinarians, *Appl. Ergon.*, 2010, **41**, 444–453.
23. D. R. Smith, P. A. Leggat and R. Speare, Musculoskeletal disorders and psychosocial risk factors among veterinarians in Queensland, Australia, *Aust. Vet. J.*, 2009, **87**, 260–265.
24. G. Singleton, Shoulder injuries in veterinary surgeons, *Vet. Rec.*, 2005, **157**, 491–492.
25. C. L. Gabel and S. G. Gerberich, Risk factors for injury among veterinarians, *Epidemiology*, 2002, **13**, 80–86.
26. R. K. Plowright, Crevasse fall in the Antarctic: a patient's perspective, *Med. J. Aust.*, 2000, **173**, 576–578.
27. J. D. M. Douglas, Salmon farming: occupational health in a new rural industry, *Occup. Med. (London)*, 1995, **45**, 89–92.
28. R. M. Duborrow, Health and safety concerns in fisheries and aquaculture, *Occup. Med.*, 1999, **14**, 373–406.
29. T. J. Ogunsanya, R. M. Duborrow, M. L. Myers, H. P. Cole and S. L. Thompson, Safety on North Carolina and Kentucky trout farms, *J. Agric. Saf. Health*, 2011, **17**, 33–61.
30. A. Gray, Suspected Adverse Reaction Scheme (SARRS): 1990 report, *Vet. Rec.*, 1991, **129**, 62–65.
31. A. Gray and S. Knivett, Suspect adverse reactions, 2001, *Vet. Rec.*, 2002, **151**, 749–752.
32. F. Dyer, R. Mulugeta, C. Evans and A. Tait, Suspected adverse reactions, 2003, *Vet. Rec.*, 2004, **154**, 806–808.
33. F. Dyer, R. Mulugeta, M. Spagnuolo-Weaver and A. Tait, Suspected adverse reactions, 2004, *Vet. Rec.*, 2005, **156**, 561–563.
34. F. Dyer, M. Spagnuolo-Weaver and A. Tait, Suspected adverse reactions, 2005, *Vet. Rec.*, 2006, **158**, 464–466.
35. F. Dyer, M. Spagnuolo-Weaver, S. Cooles and A. Tait, Suspected adverse reactions, 2006, *Vet. Rec.*, 2007, **160**, 748–750.
36. F. Dyer, M. Spagnuolo-Weaver, S. Cooles and A. Tait, Suspected adverse reactions, 2007, *Vet. Rec.*, 2008, **163**, 69–72.
37. F. Dyer, E. Brown, S. Cooles and A. Tait, Suspected adverse reactions, 2008, *Vet. Rec.*, 2009, **165**, 162–164.
38. F. Dyer, G. Diesel, S. Cooles and A. Tait, Suspected adverse reactions, 2009, *Vet. Rec.*, 2010, **167**, 118–121.
39. F. Dyer, G. Diesel, S. Cooles and A. Tait, Suspected adverse reactions, 2010, *Vet. Rec.*, 2011, **168**, 610–643.
40. Veterinary Products Committee Working Group, *The Suspected Adverse Reactions Surveillance Scheme*, Report (2004) available from the Veterinary Medicines Directorate, Addlestone, Surrey, UK.
41. J. S. Weese and M. Faires, A survey of needle handling practices and needlestick injuries in veterinary technicians, *Can. Vet. J.*, 2009, **50**, 37–44.
42. J. S. Weese and D. C. Jack, Needlestick injuries in veterinary medicine, *Can. Vet. J.*, 2008, **49**, 780–784.

43. K. L. Stewart, Handling needles properly minimizes hazards, *J. Am. Vet. Med. Assoc.*, 2009, **235**, 1272.
44. P. A. Leggat, D. R. Smith and R. Speare, Exposure rate of needlestick injuries among Australian veterinarians, *J. Occup Med. Toxicol.*, 2009, **4**, 25.
45. M. Sillis, Disposal of veterinary sharps, *Vet. Rec.*, 2003, **152**, 116.
46. J. R. Wilkins and M. E. Bowman, Needlestick injuries among female veterinarians: frequency, syringe contents and side-effects, *Occup. Med.*, 1997, **47**, 451–457.
47. H. L. Leira and K. J. Baalsrud, Operator safety during injection vaccination of fish, *Dev. Biol. Stand.*, 1997, **90**, 383–387.
48. C. Jennissen, C. Wallace, K. Donham, D. Rendell and S. Brumby, Unintentional needlestick injuries in livestock production: a case series and review, *J. Agromedicine*, 2011, **16**, 58–71.
49. A. M. Oliveira, R. G. Maggi, C. W. Woods and E. B. Breitschweerdt, Suspected needlestick transmission of *Bartonella vinsonii* subspecies *berkhoffii* to a veterinarian, *J. Vet. Intern. Med.*, 2010, **24**, 1229–1232.
50. E. A. Whitney, E. Ailes, L. M. Myers, J. T. Saliki and R. L. Berkelman, Prevalence of and risk factors for serum antibodies against Leptospira serovars in US veterinarians, *J. Am. Vet. Med. Assoc.*, 2009, **234**, 938–944.
51. W. L. Sibbit, P. A. Band, L. G. Kettwich, C. R. Sibbitt, L. J. Sibbitt and A. D. Bankhurst, Safety syringes and anti-needlestick devices in orthopaedic surgery, *J. Bone Joint Surg. Am.*, 2011, **93**, 1641–1649.
52. M. Kakizaki, N. Ikeda, M. Ali, B. Enkhtuya, M. Tsolmon, K. Shibuya and C. Kuroiwa, Needlestick injury among healthcare workers at public tertiary hospitals in an urban community in Mongolia, *BMC Res. Notes*, 2011, **4**, 184.
53. P. A. Patrician, E. Pryor, M. Fridman and L. Loan, Needlestick injuries among nursing staff: association with shift level staffing, *Am. J. Infect. Control*, 2011, **39**, 477–482.
54. D. M. Vandijck, S. O. Labeau and S. I. Blot, Prevention of needlestick injuries among healthcare workers, *Am. J. Infect. Control.*, 2011, **39**, 347–348.
55. K. M. Alghamdi and R. A. Alkhodair, Practical techniques to enhance the safety of health care workers in office-based surgery, *J. Cutan. Med. Surg.*, 2011, **15**, 48–54.
56. S. Al-Benna, Needlestick and sharps injuries among theatre care professionals, *J. Periop. Pract.*, 2010, **20**, 440–445.
57. C. Colombo, V. Masserey and C. Ruef, Incidence of needlestick injuries and other sharps exposures in Swiss acute care hospitals: results of a sentinel surveillance study, *J. Hosp. Infect.*, 2011, **77**, 181–183.
58. T. Duff, Needlestick injuries, *Anaesthesia*, 2010, **65**, 1225–1226.
59. K. Cheung, S. C. Ho, S. S. Ching and K. K. Chang, Analysis of needlestick injuries among nursing students in Hong Kong, *Accid. Anal. Prev.*, 2010, **42**, 1744–1750.

60. J. K. Leiss, Management practices and risk of occupational blood exposure in U.S. paramedics: Needlesticks, *Am. J. Ind. Med.*, 2010, **53**, 866–874.

61. R. Bali, P. Sharma and A. Garg, Incidence and patterns of needlestick injuries during intermaxillary fixation, *Br. J. Oral Maxillofac. Surg.*, 2011, **49**, 221–224.

62. S. Dorevitch, S. E. Lacey, A. Abelmann and J. Zautcke, Occupational needlestick injuries in a U.S. airport, *J. Occup. Environ. Med.*, 2010, **52**, 551–554.

63. M. Chakravarthy, Enhanced risk of needlestick injuries and exposure to blood and body fluids to cardiac anesthesiologists: need for serious introspection, *Ann. Card. Anaesth.*, 2010, **13**, 1–2.

64. S. Adams, S. G. Stoikovic and S. H. Leveson, Needlestick injuries during surgical procedures: a multidisciplinary online study, *Occup. Med. (London)*, 2010, **60**, 139–144.

65. G. K. Sharma, M. M. Gilson, H. Nathan and M. A. Makary, Needlestick injuries among medical students: incidence and implications, *Acad. Med.*, 2009, **84**, 1815–1821.

66. M. M. Quinn, P. K. Markkanen, C. J. Galligan, D. Kriebel, S. M. Chalupka, H. Kim, S. R. Sama, A. K. Laramie and L. Davis, Sharps injuries and other blood and body fluid exposures among home health care nurses ad aides, *Am. J. Public Health*, 2009, **99**(3), S710–S717.

67. O. Varsou, J. S. Lemon and F. D. Dick, Sharps injuries among medical students, *Occup. Med. (London)*, 2009, **59**, 509–511.

68. D. R. Smith, P. A. Leggat and L. J. Walsh, Workplace hazards among Australian dental students, *Aust. Dent. J.*, 2009, **54**, 186–188.

69. R. Bali, P. Sharma, S. Angi and Shruti, Needlestick injuries in health care providers, *Nurs. J. India*, 2008, **99**, 251–254.

70. G. K. Joardar, C. Chatterjee, S. K. Sadhukhan, M. Chakraborty, P. Dass and A. Mandal, Needle sticks injury among nurses involved in patient care: a study in two medical college hospitals of West Bengal, *Indian J. Public Health*, 2008, **52**, 150–152.

71. B. Peng, P. J. Tully, K. Boss and J. E. Hiller, Sharps injury and body fluid exposure among health care workers in an Australian tertiary hospital, *Asia Pac. J. Public Health*, 2008, **20**, 139–147.

72. P. Trueman, M. Taylor, N. Tweena and B. Chubb, The cost of injuries associated with insulin administration, *Br. J. Community Nurs.*, 2008, **13**, 413–417.

73. D. Myers, C. Epling, J. Dement and D. Hunt, Risk of sharp device-related blood and body fluid exposure in operating rooms, *Infect. Control Hosp. Epidemiol.*, 2008, **29**, 1139–1148.

74. W. J. Thomas and J. R. Murray, The incidence and reporting rates of needle-stick injury among UK surgeons, *Ann. R. Coll. Surg. Engl.*, 2009, **91**, 12–17.

75. S. Wicker, A. M. Ludwig, R. Gottschalk and H. F. Rabenau, Needlestick injuries among health care workers: occupational hazard or avoidable hazard? *Wien. Klin. Wochenschr.*, 2008, **120**, 486–492.

76. B. A. Hanselman, S. A. Kruth, J. Roussea, D. E. Low, B. M. Willey, A. McGeer and J. S. Weese, Methicillin-resistant *Staphylococcus aureus* colonization in veterinary personnel, *Emerg. Infect. Dis.*, 2006, **12**, 1933–1938.

77. A. J. Reid, Brucellosis – a persistent occupational hazard in Ireland, *Int. J. Occup. Environ. Health*, 2005, **97**, 302–304.

78. C. A. Johnson-Delaney, Safety issues in exotic pet practice, *Vet. Clin. North Am. Exot. Anim. Pract.*, 2005, **8**, 515–524.

79. E. J. Regan, G. A. Harrison, S. Butler, J. McLauchlin, M. Thomas and S. Mitchell, Primary cutaneous listeriosis in a veterinarian, *Vet. Rec.*, 2005, **157**, 207.

80. M. M. Cooke, A. J. Gear, A. Naidoo and D. M. Collins, Accidental *Mycobacterium bovis* infection in a veterinarian, *N. Z. Vet. J.*, 2002, **50**, 36–38.

81. A. G. Kalamas, Anthrax, *Anesthesiol. Clin. North America*, 2004, **22**, 533–540.

82. B. Gummow, A survey of zoonotic diseases contracted by South African veterinarians, *J. S. Afr. Vet. Assoc.*, 2003, **74**, 72–76.

83. F. van Kolfschooten, Dutch veterinarian becomes the first victim of avian influenza, *Lancet*, 2003, **361**, 1444.

84. T. Abe, K. Yamaki, T. Hayakawa, H. Fukuda, Y. Ito, H. Kume, T. Komiya, K. Ishihara and K. Hirai, A seroepidemiological study of the risks of Q fever infection in Japanese veterinarians, *Eur. J. Epidemiol.*, 2001, **17**, 1029–1032.

85. D. J. Weber and W. A. Rutala, Zoonotic infections, *Occup. Med.*, 1999, **14**, 247–284.

86. D. T. Ramsey, Blastomycosis in a veterinarian, *J. Am. Vet. Med. Assoc.*, 1994, **205**, 968.

87. A. Fanning, S. Edwards and G. Hauer, *Mycobacterium bovis* infection in humans exposed to elk in Alberta, *Can. Dis. Wkly Rep.*, 1991, **17**, 239–240.

88. Anon., Transmission of salmonellae to veterinarians, *Vet. Rec.*, 1991, **129**, 415.

89. I. J. Visser, Cutaneous salmonellosis in veterinarians, *Vet. Rec.*, 1991, **129**, 364.

90. J. G. Fox and N. S. Lipman, Infections transmitted by large and small laboratory animals, *Infect. Dis. Clin. North Am.*, 1991, **5**, 131–163.

91. T. Nesbakken, G. Kapperud, J. Lassen and E. Skjerve, *Yersinia enterocolitica* O:3 antibodies in slaughter house employees, veterinarians and military recruits. Occupational exposure to pigs as a risk factor for yersiniosis, *Contrib. Microbiol. Immunol.*, 1991, **12**, 32–39.

92. R. F. DiGiacomo, N. V. Harris, N. L. Huber and M. K. Cooney, Animal exposures and antibodies to *Toxocara gondii* in a university population, *Am. J. Epidemiol.*, 1990, **131**, 729–733.

93. J. R. August and T. M. Chase, Toxoplasmosis, *Vet. Clin. North Am. Small Anim. Pract.*, 1987, **17**, 55–71.

 94. B. F. Kingscote, Leptospirosis: an occupational hazard to veterinarians, *Can. Vet. J.*, 1986, **27**, 78–81.
 95. M. I. Okolo, Studies on anthrax in food animals and persons occupationally exposed to the zoonoses in Eastern Nigeria, *Int. J. Zoonoses*, 1985, **12**, 276–282.
 96. B. F. Kingscote, Leptospirosis in two veterinarians, *CMAJ*, 1985, **133**, 879–880.
 97. R. J. Martin, P. R. Schnurrenberger and J. F. Walker, Exposure to rabies – an occupational hazard for veterinarians, *Can. Vet. J.*, 1982, **23**, 317–322.
 98. P. J. Constable and J. M. Harrington, Risks of zoonoses in a veterinary service, *Br. Med. J.*, 1982, **284**, 246–248.
 99. G. T. Woods, P. R. Schnurrenberger, R. J. Martin and W. A. Tomkins, Swine influenza virus in swine and man in Illinois, *J. Occup. Med.*, 1981, **23**, 263–267.
100. R. Bentley, M. Daly and T. Harris, Toxocara infection among veterinarians, *Vet. Rec.*, 1980, **106**, 277–278.
101. P. R. Schnurrenberger, J. K. Grigor, J. F. Walker and R. J. Martin, The zoonosis prone veterinarian, *J. Am. Vet. Med. Assoc.*, 1978, **173**, 373–376.
102. L. T. Glickman and R. H. Cypress, Toxocara infection in animal hospital employees, *Am. J. Public Health*, 1977, **67**, 1193–1195.
103. I. E. Roeckel and E. T. Lyons, Cutaneous larva migrans. An occupational disease, *Ann. Clin. Lab. Sci.*, 1977, **7**, 405–410.
104. R. A. Robinson and R. V. Metcalf, Zoonotic infections in veterinarians, *N. Z. Vet J.*, 1976, **24**, 24–25.
105. P. R. Schnurrenberger, J. F. Walker and R. J. Martin, Brucella infections in Illinois veterinarians, *J. Am. Vet. Med. Assoc. J.*, 1975, **167**, 1084–1088.
106. H. Kronberger, H. Treckmann, M. Hagert and F. Schüpei, Psittacosis of the examining veterinarian due to parrots, *Z. Gesamte Inn Med.*, 1974, **29**, 945–949.
107. K. L. Hughes, Brucellosis in veterinarians, *Aust. Vet. J.*, 1972, **48**, 527–528.
108. H. Pivnick, H. Worton, D. L. Smith and D. Barnum, Infection of veterinarians in Ontario by *Brucella abortus* strain 19, *Can. J. Public Health*, 1966, **57**, 225–231.
109. E. V. Morse, V. Allen and G. Worley, Brucellosis and leptospirosis serological test results on serums of Wisconsin veterinarians, *J. Am. Vet. Med. Assoc.*, 1955, **126**, 59.
110. B. N. Archer, J. Weyer, J. Paweska, D. Nkosi, P. Leman, K. S. Tint and L. Blumberg, Outbreak of Rift Valley fever affecting veterinarians and farmers in South Africa, *S. Afr. Med. J.*, 2011, **10**, 263–266.
111. A. J. Stewardson and M. L. Grayson, Psittacosis, *Infect. Dis. Clin. North Am.*, 2010, **24**, 7–25.
112. R. Monno, L. Fumarolo, P. Trerotoli, D. Cavone, G. Giannelli, C. Rizzo, L. Cicerone and M. Musti, Seroprevalence of Q fever, brucellosis and leptospirosis in farmers and agriculture workers in Bari, Southern Italy, *Ann. Agric. Environ. Med.*, 2009, **16**, 205–209.

113. C. C. Chang, P. S. Lin, M. Y. Hou, C. C. Lin, M. N. Hung, T. M. Wu, P. Y. Shu, W. Y. Shih, J. H. Lin, W. C. Chen, H. S. Wu and L. J. Lin, Identification of risk factors of *Coxiella burnetti* (Q fever) infection in veterinary associated populations in southern Taiwan, *Zoonoses Public Health*, 2010, **57**, 955–101.

114. E. Bosnak, A. M. Hvass, S. Villumsen and H. Nielsen, Emerging evidence for Q fever in humans in Denmark: role of contact with dairy cattle, *Clin. Microbiol. Infect.*, 2010, **16**, 1285–1288.

115. T. F. Rasso, A. O. Carrasco, J. C. Silva, M. F. Marvulo and A. A. Pinto, Seroprevalence of antibodies to *Chlamydophila psittaci* in zoo workers in Brazil, *Zoonoses Public Health*, 2010, **57**, 411–416.

116. W. S. Baker and G. C. Gray, A review of published reports regarding zoonotic pathogen infection in veterinarians, *J. Am. Vet. Med. Assoc.*, 2009, **234**, 1271–1278.

117. E. A. Whitney, R. F. Massung, A. J. Candee, E. C. Ailes, L. M. Myers, N. E. Patterson and R. L. Berkelman, Seroepidemiological and occupational risk survey for *Coxiella burnetti* antibodies among US veterinarians, *Clin. Infect. Dis.*, 2009, **48**, 550–557.

118. M. Lierz, A. Jansen and H. M. Hafez, Avian *Mycoplasma lipofaciens* transmission to veterinarian, *Emerg. Infect. Dis.*, 2008, **14**, 1161–1163.

119. D. Cieri, C. Turchi and G. Torzi, Occupational brucellosis in the veterinary service of the Local Health Service in the Abruzzo Region (Italy), *G. Ital. Med. Lav. Ergon.*, 2007, **29**(3), 817–819.

120. K. Lee, H. S. Lin, W. W. Park, S. H. Kim, D. Y. Lee, M. Y. Park and Y. Hur, Seroprevalence of brucellosis among risk population in Gyeongsangbuk-do, 2006, *J. Prev. Med. Public Health*, 2007, **40**, 285–290.

121. S. Kiliç, F. D. Al, B. Celebi and C. Babür, The investigation of seroprevalence of cystic echinococcus in veterinary surgeons, *Turkiye Parazitol. Derg.*, 2007, **31**, 109–111.

122. K. P. Myers, S. F. Setterquist, A. W. Capuano and G. C. Gray, Infection due to 3 avian influenza subtypes in United States veterinarians, *Clin. Infect. Dis.*, 2007, **45**, 4–9.

123. A. S. Agasthya, S. Isloor and K. Prabhudas, Brucellosis in high risk individuals, *Indian J. Med. Microbiol.*, 2007, **25**, 28–31.

124. P. M. Rabinowitz, Z. Gordon and L. Odofin, Pet-related infections, *Am. Fam. Phys.*, 2007, **76**, 1314–1322.

125. L. H. Kahn, Confronting zoonoses, linking human and veterinary medicine, *Emerg. Infect. Dis.*, 2006, **12**, 556–561.

126. A. E. Tauscher and D. V. Belsito, Frequency and etiology of hand and forearm dermatoses among veterinarians, *Am. J. Contact Dermat.*, 2002, **13**, 116–124.

127. D. M. Bulcke and S. A. Devos, Hand and forearm dermatoses among veterinarians, *J. Eur. Acad. Dermatol. Venereol.*, 2007, **21**, 360–363.

128. P. Susitaival, J. Kirk and M. B. Schenker, Self-reported hand dermatitis in California veterinarians, *Am. J. Contact Dermat.*, 2001, **12**, 103–108.

129. P. Susitaival, J. Kirk and M. B. Schenker, Atopic symptoms among California veterinarians, *Am. J. Ind. Med.*, 2003, **44**, 166–171.

130. E. Rudzki, P. Rebandel, Z. Grzwa, Z. Pomorski, B. Jakiminska and E. Zawisza, Occupational dermatitis in veterinarians, *Contact Dermatitis*, 1982, **8**, 72–73.

131. R. Valsecchi, P. Leghissa and R. Continovis, Occupational contact dermatitis and contact urticaria in veterinarians, *Contact Dermatitis*, 2003, **49**, 167–168.

132. A. van Gelder, A. Spierenburg and L. J. Lipman, Occupational contact dermatitis in veterinarians, *Tijdschr. Diergeneeskd.*, 2008, **133**, 26–27.

133. M.-S. Doutre, Occupational contact urticarial and protein contact dermatitis, *Eur. J. Dermatol.*, 2005, **15**, 419–424.

134. C. Foti, A. Antelmi, G. Mistrello, F. Guarneri and R. Filotico, Occupational contact urticaria and rhinoconjunctivitis from dog's milk in a veterinarian, *Contact Dermatitis*, 2007, **56**, 169–171.

135. A. Krakowiak, M. Kowalczyk and C. Palczyñski, Occupational contact urticaria and rhinoconjunctivitis in a veterinarian from bull terrier's seminal fluid, *Contact Dermatitis*, 2004, **50**, 385.

136. A. Roger, R. Guspi, V. Garcia-Patos, A. Barriga, N. Rubira, C. Nogueiras, A. Catells and A. Cadahia, Occupational protein dermatitis in a veterinary surgeon, *Contact Dermatitis*, 1995, **32**, 248–249.

137. P. A. Leggat, D. R. Smith and R. Speare, Hand dermatitis among veterinarians from Queensland, Australia, *Contact Dermatitis*, 2009, **60**, 336–338.

138. I. J. Visser, Pustular dermatitis in veterinarians following delivery in farm animals: an occupational disease, *Tijdschr. Diergeneeskd.*, 1998, **123**, 114–117.

139. C. I. Andersen, S. G. Von Essen, L. M. Smith, J. Spencer, R. Jolie and K. J. Donham, Respiratory symptoms and airway obstruction in swine veterinarians: a persistent problem, *Am. J. Ind. Med.*, 2004, **46**, 386–392.

140. S. Samadi, D. J. Heederik, E. J. Kropp, A. R. Jamshidifard, T. Willemse and I. M. Wouters, Allergen and endotoxin exposure in a companion animal hospital, *Occup. Environ. Med.*, 2010, **67**, 486–492.

141. S. Samadi, J. Spitohoven, A. R. Jamshidifard, B. R. Berend, L. Lipman, D. J. Heederik and I. M. Wouters, Allergy among veterinary medicine students in The Netherlands, *Occup. Environ. Med.*, 2012, **69**, 48–55.

142. J. P. Seward, Occupational allergy to animals, *Occup. Med.*, 1999, **14**, 285–304.

143. A. Krakowiak, C. Palczyñski, J. Walusiak, T. Wittczak, U. Ruta, W. Dudek and B. Szuic, Allergy to animal fur and feathers among zoo workers, *Int. Arch. Occup. Environ. Health*, 2002, **75**(suppl.), S113–S116.

144. A. Krakowiak, P. Krawczyk, B. Szuic, M. Wiszniewska, M. Kowalczyk, J. Walusiak and C. Palczyñski, Prevalence and host determinants of occupational asthma in animal shelter workers, *Int. Arch. Occup. Environ. Health*, 2007, **80**, 423–432.

145. A. Krakowiak, M. Wiszniewska, P. Krawczyk, B. Szulc, T. Wittczak, J. Walusiak and C. Palczyñski, Risk factors associated with airway allergic diseases from exposure to laboratory animal allergens among veterinarians, *Int. Arch. Occup. Environ. Health*, 2007, **80**, 465–475.

146. A. R. Elbers, P. J. Blaauw, M. de Vries, P. J. van Gulick, O. L. Smithuis, R. P. Gerrits and M. J. Tielen, Veterinary practice and occupational health. An epidemiological study of several professional groups of Dutch veterinarians. I. General physical examination and prevalence of allergy, lung function disorders, and bronchial hyperactivity, *Vet. Q.*, 1996, **18**, 127–131.

147. A. R. Elbers, M. de Vries, P. J. van Gulick, R. P. Gerrits, O. L. Smithuis, P. J. Blaauw and M. J. Tielen, Veterinary practice and occupational health. An epidemiological study of several professional groups of Dutch veterinarians. II. Peak expiratory flow variability, dust and endotoxin measurements, use of respiratory protection devices, and time distribution of professional activities, *Vet. Q.*, 1996, **18**, 132–136.

148. S. Von Essen, G. Moore, S. Gibbs and K. L. Larson, Respiratory issues in beef and pork production: recommendations from a expert panel, *J. Agromedicine*, 2010, **15**, 216–225.

149. I. Lutsky, G. L. Baum, H. Teichtahl, A. Mazar, F. Aizer and S. Bar-Sela, Occupational respiratory disease in veterinarians, *Ann. Allergy*, 1985, **55**, 153–156.

150. L. A. Will, E. G. Nassif, R. L. Engen, R. A. Patterson and D. Zimmerman, Allergy and pulmonary impairment in Iowa veterinarians, *N. Engl. Reg. Allergy Proc.*, 1987, **8**, 173–177.

151. R. J. Martin, T. Habtemariam and P. R. Schnurrenberger, The health characteristics of veterinarians in Illinois, *Int. J. Zoonoses*, 1981, **8**, 63–71.

152. A. Blair and H. M. Hayes, Cancer and other causes of death in U.S. veterinarians, 1966–1977, *Int. J. Cancer*, 1980, **25**, 181–185.

153. A. Blair and H. M. Hayes, Mortality patterns among US veterinarians, 1947–1977: an expanded study, *Int. J. Epidemiol.*, 1982, **11**, 391–397.

154. L. W. Figgs, M. Dosemeci and A. Blair, Risk of multiple myeloma by occupation and industry among men and women: a 24-state death certificate study, *J. Occup. Med.*, 1994, **36**, 1210–1221.

155. J. M. Miller and J. J. Beaumont, Suicide, cancer, and other causes of death among California veterinarians, 1960–1992, *Am. J. Ind. Med.*, 1995, **27**, 37–49.

156. N. Travier, G. Gridley, A. Blair, M. Dosemeci and P. Boffetta, Cancer incidence among male Swedish veterinarians and other workers of the veterinary industry: a record-linkage study, *Cancer Causes Control*, 2003, **14**, 587–593.

157. L. Fritschi, Cancer in veterinarians, *Occup. Environ. Med.*, 2000, **57**, 289–297.

158. A. Blair, Cancer risks associated with agriculture: epidemiologic evidence, *Basic Life Sci.*, 1982, **21**, 93–111.

159. N. Pearce and J. S. Reif, Epidemiologic studies of cancer in agricultural workers, *Am. J. Ind. Hyg.*, 1990, **18**, 133–148.

160. L. Fritschi, A. Shirangi, I. D. Robertson and L. M. Day, Trends in exposure of veterinarians to physical and chemical hazards and use of protection practices, *Int. Arch. Occup. Environ. Health*, 2008, **81**, 371–378.
161. R. Tyson, D. C. Smiley, R. S. Pleasant and G. B. Daniel, Estimated operator exposure for hand holding portable x-ray units during imaging of the equine distal extremity, *Vet. Radiol. Ultrasound*, 2011, **52**, 121–124.
162. A. Shirangi, L. Fritschi and C. D. Holman, Prevalence of occupational exposures and protective practices in Australian female veterinarians, *Aust. Vet. J.*, 2007, **85**, 32–38.
163. R. Langley, Physical hazards of animal handlers, *Occup. Med.*, 1999, **14**, 181–194.
164. R. G. Whitelock, Radiation hazards from horses undergoing scintigraphy using technetium-99m, *Equine Vet. J.*, 1997, **29**, 26–30.
165. K. Hartung, Radiation exposure of the hands and feet during x-ray studies in small animals, *Tierarztl. Prax.*, 1992, **20**, 187–193.
166. S. A. Moritz, W. D. Hueston and J. R. Wilins, Patterns of ionizing radiation exposure among female veterinarians, *J. Am. Vet. Med. Assoc.*, 1989, **195**, 737–739.
167. P. Wiggins, M. B. Schenker, R. Green and S. Samuels, Prevalence of hazardous exposures in veterinary practice, *Am. J. Ind. Med.*, 1989, **16**, 55–66.
168. K. Hartung and B. Münzer, Possibilities for reducing radiation exposures during radiography of small animals, *Tierarztl. Prax.*, 1984, **12**, 505–510.
169. R. M. Moore, Y. M. Davies and R. G. Kaczmarek, An overview of occupational hazards among veterinarians, with particular reference to pregnant women, *Am. J. Ind. Hyg.*, 1993, **54**, 113–120.
170. S. Shuhaiber, G. Koren, R. Boskovic, T. R. Einarson, O. Porrat Soldin and A. Einarson, Seroprevalence of *Toxoplasma gondii* infection among veterinary staff in Ontario, Canada (2002): Implications for teratogenic risk, *BMC Infect. Dis.*, 2003, **3**, 8.
171. J. R. Wilkins and L. L. Steele, Occupational factors and reproductive outcome among a cohort of female veterinarians, *J. Am. Vet. Med. Assoc.*, 1998, **213**, 61–67.
172. A. Shirangi, L. Fritschi, C. D. Holman and C. Bower, Birth defects in offspring of female veterinarians, *J. Occup. Environ. Med.*, 2009, **51**, 525–533.
173. T. Epp and C. Waldner, Occupational health hazards in veterinary medicine: zoonoses and other biological hazards, *Can. Vet. J.*, 2012, **53**, 144–150.
174. A. Shirangi, L. Fritschi and C. D. Holman, Maternal occupational exposures and risk of spontaneous abortion in veterinary practice, *Occup. Environ. Med.*, 2008, **65**, 719–725.
175. M. B. Schenker, S. J. Samuels, R. S. Green and P. Wiggins, Adverse reproductive outcomes among female veterinarians, *Am. J. Epidemiol.*, 1990, **132**, 960–106.

176. S. Shuhaiber and G. Koren, Occupational exposure to inhaled anesthetic. Is it a concern for pregnant women? *Can. Fam. Physician*, 2000, **46**, 2391–2392.

177. A. Shirangi, L. Fritschi and C. D. Holman, Association of unscavenged anesthetic gases and long working hours with preterm delivery in female veterinarians, *Obstet. Gynecol.*, 2009, **113**, 1008–1017.

178. W. F. Crimmins, Practices should take precautions to protect workers, *J. Am. Vet. Med. Assoc.*, 2001, **218**, 1251–1252.

179. J. H. Olsen, P. de Nully Brown, G. Schulgen and O. M. Jensen, Parental employment at time of conception and risk of cancer in offspring, *Eur. J. Cancer*, 1991, **27**, 958–965.

180. D. J. Bartram, G. Yadegarfar, J. M. Sinclair and D. S. Baldwin, Validation of the Warwick-Edinburgh Mental Well-being Scale (WEMWBS) as an overall indicator of population mental health and well-being in the UK veterinary profession, *Vet. J.*, 2011, **187**, 397–398.

181. D. J. Bartram, G. Yadegarfar and D. S. Baldwin, Psychosocial working conditions and work-related stressors among UK veterinary surgeons, *Occup. Med. (London)*, 2009, **59**, 334–341.

182. M. Harling, P. Strehmel, A. Schablon and A. Nienhaus, Psychosocial stress, demoralization and the consumption of tobacco, alcohol and medical drugs by veterinarians, *J. Occup. Med. Toxicol.*, 2009, **4**, 4.

183. D. R. Smith, P. A. Leggat, R. Speare and M. Townley-Jones, Examining the dimensions and correlates of workplace stress among Australian veterinarians, *J. Occup. Med. Toxicol.*, 2009, **4**, 32.

184. V. Rohlf and P. Bennett, Perpetration-induced traumatic stress in persons who euthanize nonhuman animals in surgeries, animal shelters, and laboratories, *Soc. Anim.*, 2005, **13**, 201–209.

185. B. Platt, K. Hawton, S. Simkin and R. J. Mellanby, Suicidal behaviour and psychosocial problems in veterinary surgeons: a systematic review, *Soc. Psychiatry Pyschiatr. Epidemiol.*, 2012, **47**, 223–240.

186. D. J. Platt and D. S. Baldwin, Veterinary surgeons and suicide: a structured review of possible influences on increased risk, *Vet. Rec.*, 2010, **166**, 388–397.

187. D. J. White and R. Shawan, Emotional responses of animal shelter workers to euthanasia, *J. Am. Vet. Med. Assoc.*, 1996, **208**, 846–849.

188. L. Fritschi, D. Morrison, A. Shirangi and L. Day, Psychological well-being of Australian veterinarians, *Aust. Vet. J.*, 2009, **87**, 76–81.

189. R. Trimpop, B. Kirkaldy, J. Athanasou and C. Cooper, Individual differences in working hours, work perception and accident rates in veterinary surgeons, *Work Stress*, 2000, **14**, 181–188.

190. D. J. Bartram, J. M. Sinclair and D. S. Baldwin, Alcohol consumption among veterinary surgeons in the UK, *Occup. Med. (London)*, 2009, **59**, 323–326.

191. D. R. Smith, P. A. Leggat and R. Speare, The latest endangered species in Australia: a tobacco-smoking veterinarian, *Aust. Vet. J.*, 2010, **88**, 369–370.

192. R. J. Mellanby, B. Platt, S. Simkin and K. Hawton, Incidence of alcohol-related deaths in the veterinary profession in England and Wales, 1993–2005, *Vet. J.*, 2009, **181**, 332–335.

193. D. J. Bartram, G. Yadegarfar and D. S. Baldwin, A cross-sectional study of mental health and well-being and their associations in the UK veterinary profession, *Soc. Psychiatry Pyschiatr. Epidemiol.*, 2009, **44**, 1075–1085.

194. K. Skegg, H. Firth, A. Gray and B. Cox, Suicide by occupation: does access to means increase the risk? *Aust. N. Z. J. Psychiatry*, 2010, **44**, 429–434.

195. D. J. Bartram, J. M. Sinclair and D. S. Baldwin, Interventions with potential to improve the mental health and wellbeing of UK veterinary surgeons, *Vet. Rec.*, 2010, **166**, 518–523.

196. D. J. Bartram and D. S. Baldwin, Veterinary surgeons and suicide: influence, opportunities and research directions, *Vet. Rec.*, 2008, **162**, 36–40.

197. B. Platt, K. Hawton, S. Simkin and R. J. Mellanby, Systematic review of the prevalence of suicide in veterinary surgeons, *Occup. Med. (London)*, 2010, **60**, 436–446.

198. K. Hawton, E. Agerbo, S. Simkin, B. Platt and R. J. Mellanby, Risk of suicide in medical and related occupational groups: A national study based on Danish case population-based registers, *J. Affect. Disord.*, 2011, **134**, 320–326.

199. H. Meitzner, C. Griffiths, A. Brock, C. Rooney and R. Jenkins, Patterns of suicide by occupation in England and Wales: 2001–2005, *Br. J. Psychiatry.*, 2008, **193**, 73–76.

200. H. Jones-Fairnie, P. Ferroni, S. Silburn and D. Lawrence, Suicide in Australian veterinarians, *Aust. Vet. J.*, 2008, **86**, 114–116.

201. K. S. Russell, J. R. Stevens and T. A. Stern, Insulin overdose among patients with diabetes: a readily available means of suicide, *Prim. Care Companion J. Clin. Psychiatry*, 2009, **11**, 258–262.

202. D. B. Jefferys and G. N. Volans, Self poisoning in diabetic patients, *Hum. Toxicol.*, 1983, **2**, 345–348.

203. D. B. Golston, M. Kovacs, V. Y. Hoy, P. L. Parrone and L. Stiffler, Suicidal ideation and suicide attempts among youth with insulin-dependent diabetes mellitus, *J. Am. Acad. Child Adolesc. Psychiatry*, 1994, **33**, 240–246.

204. M. Guclu, C. Ersoy and S. Imamoglu, Suicide attempt of a physician with 3600 units of insulin and rapid onset acute hepatitis, *Intern. Med. J.*, 2009, **39**, e5–e7.

205. Y. Thewjitcharoen, N. Lekpittaya and T. Himathongkam, Attempted suicide by massive insulin injection: a case report and review of the literature, *J. Med. Assoc. Thai.*, 2008, **91**, 1920–1924.

CHAPTER 2

Regulation of Veterinary Medicines

2.1 Introduction

Disasters frequently precipitate legislation, and medicines are no exception to this observation.[1,2] Thalidomide was introduced in the late 1950s to treat morning sickness during pregnancy but it was soon discovered to be teratogenic, producing limb defects (phocomelia) and other abnormalities in the children of women who had taken the drug.[3-8] In 1937 in the USA, Elixir of Sulfanilamide was given to 353 patients over the course of one week. This resulted in what was estimated to be 105 deaths including those of 34 children. It was due to the use of diethylene glycol as the solvent in this product. Diethylene glycol is nephrotoxic and it results in acute renal failure due to cortical tubular degeneration and proximal tubular necrosis.[9-12] This has been shown to be due to the metabolite diglycolic acid.[13]

These events led directly to the regulation of human and veterinary medicines in the UK and the USA, and, ultimately, in most other developed countries.[11,14] In the UK, the thalidomide disaster resulted in the establishment of the Committee on Safety of Drugs, often referred to as the Dunlop Committee after its chairman Sir Derek Dunlop. Oddly, at least by modern standards, this committee had no regulatory powers but worked with the pharmaceutical industry in a voluntary manner. In a similar way, veterinary medicines had also been dealt with on a voluntary basis. Many veterinary drugs were similar to their human drug counterparts and so were handled in a similar manner on the advice of the Veterinary Products Committee (VPC). Others had more in common with pesticides or at least their active ingredients were also

Issues in Toxicology No. 14
Toxicological Effects of Veterinary Medicinal Products in Humans: Volume 1
By Kevin N. Woodward
© The Royal Society of Chemistry 2013
Published by the Royal Society of Chemistry, www.rsc.org

used in pesticide products, and the Advisory Committee on Pesticides and Other Toxic Chemicals provided advice on these. However, following the introduction of the Medicines Act 1968, human and veterinary medicines succumbed to statutory control and government ministers responsible for these activities (the Licensing Authority) were advised by the Committee on the Safety of Medicines (CSM) for human drugs and the VPC for veterinary drugs. These committees were statutory bodies constituted under the terms of Section 4 of the Medicines Act 1968.[15–18]

Applications for marketing authorisations (MAs) in the UK are now made to the Veterinary Medicines Directorate (VMD) for veterinary medicinal products and to the Medicines and Healthcare products Regulatory Agency (MHRA) for human medicinal products. Each is advised by a number of expert committees, with the principal ones being the VPC and Commission on Human Medicines, respectively.

In the United States, human medicines are regulated by the Food and Drug Administration (FDA), while conventional veterinary drugs (pharmaceuticals) such as antibiotics, anti-inflammatory agents and anaesthetics are controlled by the FDA's Center for Veterinary Medicine (CVM). However, there are separate agencies for the control of vaccines and other biologics, and for ecto-parasiticides. The former are regulated by the United States Department of Agriculture (USDA) and the latter by the Environmental Protection Agency (EPA). In contrast, in Europe, and in many other territories, these two groups of products are regarded as veterinary medicines and are dealt with by veterinary medicine regulatory agencies. The notable exception to this is Germany. Here, veterinary pharmaceuticals and ectoparasiticides are regulated by the Bundesampt für Verbraucherschutz und Lebensmittelsicherheit (BVL; Federal Office of Consumer Protection) and veterinary biologics by the Paul-Erlich-Institute (PEI).[18–22]

2.2 Criteria for Evaluation and Authorisation of Veterinary Medicinal Products

In almost all jurisdictions, veterinary (and human) medicinal products are assessed using three criteria: quality, efficacy and safety. Quality in this context refers to pharmaceutical quality and aspects surrounding synthesis of the active ingredient(s) and other components of the formulation, manufacturing and product stability. Efficacy refers to the performance of the drug for its intended purpose. Specifically this means not so much "does it work?" but does it do what its sponsor claims it should do. The term "safety" might appear to be self-explanatory and for human medicines this primarily means "safety for the patient". However, for veterinary drugs this term is broader. It includes not only patient safety, but also safety for the environment, for the user and, for products intended for use in food producing animals, safety for consumers. These criteria are shown in more detail in Table 2.1.[20]

Table 2.1 Major aspects of quality, safety and efficacy.

Quality
Manufacturing methods and dosage form/presentation
Composition
Analysis
Control of starting materials
Control of finished product
Stability and shelf-life
Labelling and product literature
Packaging
Quality related to safety (toxic degradation products or contaminants, microbiological contaminants, leaching of potentially toxic materials from packaging *e.g.* from plastic containers)
Sterility

Efficacy
Pharmacodynamics
Pharmacokinetics
Laboratory studies *e.g. in vitro* studies of mode of action or studies using artificial infection/infestation
Clinical trials

Safety
Consumer safety (food animals only)
User safety
Environmental safety
Target animal (patient) safety
Residues (food animals only)
Pharmacokinetics
Residues depletion (using either/both radiolabelled and unlabelled material)
Residues analysis
Routine analytical method for residues surveillance

For companion animal products (cats, dogs, ornamental fish, mice, rats, guinea-pigs, hamsters and other pet animals), safety data usually comprise a package of toxicology data that is primarily used to assess user safety. Hence, the major issue being addressed is what might the consequences be of human exposure during use, misuse or abuse. For food-producing animals, this is still a very important aspect of product assessment although the user safety elements become more important as there may be more animals to treat, even possibly a flock or herd, and those animals may be larger and more difficult to control, which may exacerbate user safety concerns not only from the use of the drug, but also from the behaviour of the animals (see Chapter 1).

User safety data usually take two forms. Firstly, a package of toxicity data with which to assess the inherent biological hazards of the formulation and data on physico-chemical properties, particularly those related to user safety, for example vapour pressure (and so likelihood of respiratory exposure), particle size (for similar reasons), pH, flammability and explosivity. Secondly, a package of data relating to exposure or possibilities for exposure (respiratory, ocular, self-injection, dermal) during use, and an appraisal of the risks in view of the known hazards.[19,20,23] This is discussed further in Chapter 4.

Consumer safety also requires a package of toxicity data. This is used in the elaboration of maximum residue limits (MRLs) in the European Union (Chapter 3). In the US, there is a similar approach but unlike the EU, which has separate legislation for authorisation of veterinary medicinal products and for establishing MRLs, here the approval process and the evaluation of residues is integrated. Moreover, the MRL approach is not employed in the US but a similar parameter, the safe concentration, is used instead.

2.3   European Union Legislation

The European Union (EU) began its life as the European Economic Community in 1958 when it had just six members – Belgium, (West) Germany, Italy, Luxembourg, France and the Netherlands. Since then, it has expanded considerably, with Romania and Bulgaria being the last countries to join what is now the EU in January of 2007. In addition to the now 27 members of the EU, there are also three countries that comprise the European Free Trade Area block, Iceland, Norway and Liechtenstein, which have agreed to enact legislation in certain areas including social policy but which are not members of the EU. These countries enjoy the "four freedoms" available to full members – free movement of goods, free movement of persons, free movement of services and free movement of capital – but have no decision-making roles and do not receive any funding from the EU. Much of EU legislation concerns these four freedoms, especially by removing barriers to trade. As certain aspects of sovereign legislation in pharmaceuticals could constitute barriers to trade and hence compromise at least one of the four freedoms, free movement of goods, then one of the driving forces behind EU pharmaceuticals legislation is the removal of barriers to trade through the harmonisation of requirements, labelling and establishment of pan-EU MRLs.[19,20,24]

The 27 EU countries may later be joined by a number of states waiting accession. These comprise Turkey, Croatia and the former Yugoslav Republic of Macedonia. The existing EU countries are shown in Table 2.2.

In the US and many other countries, there is a single route to obtaining an approval or licence for a veterinary medicinal product. An application is made to the regulatory authority in that country and an approval or licence is issued to sell the product, again in that country. It is not quite so straightforward in the EU. EU legislation is complex and it has evolved over time with various amendments being added on. In the early 2000s it was revised substantially, and this process continues. The essential elements of EU veterinary legislation are shown in Table 2.3. The various EU procedures are discussed below.

Table 2.2 European Union Member States in 2012.

Country	Symbol	Accession Date
Belgium	BE	1958
France	FR	1958
Germany[a]	DE	1958
Italy	IT	1958
Luxembourg	LU	1958
Netherlands	NL	1958
Denmark	DK	1973
Ireland	EI	1973
United Kingdom	UK	1973
Greece	EL	1981
Spain	ES	1986
Portugal	PT	1986
Austria	AT	1995
Finland	FI	1995
Sweden	SE	1995
Cyprus	CY	2004
Czech Republic	CZ	2004
Estonia	EE	2004
Hungary	HU	2004
Latvia	LV	2004
Lithuania	LI	2004
Malta	MT	2004
Poland	PO	2004
Slovakia	SK	2004
Slovenia	SI	2004
Bulgaria	BG	2007
Romania	RO	2007

[a]Germany acceded originally as West Germany but the name now applies to the reunified country derived from West and East Germany.

2.3.1 The National Procedure

The national procedure is essentially what most EU countries had in place prior to joining the EU. The system provides for a marketing authorisation in a single EU member state, authorised in accordance with the requirements of EU legislation. If the sponsor wishes for the product to be authorised in two or more EU countries, then the national route cannot be used.

2.3.2 The Mutual Recognition Procedure

This was originally allowed for under Article 17 of Directive 81/851/EEC but is now a provision of Directive 2001/82/EC (as amended). The procedure can be initiated either by a member state or by the applicant, the latter being the predominant approach. In the mutual recognition procedure, the applicant first obtains a national authorisation as described in Section 2.3.1. Next, the applicant identifies those member states where a marketing authorisation is

Table 2.3   Major elements of EU veterinary legislation, 1965 to 2010.[a]

Legislation	Main Provisions
Directive 65/65/EEC	1965: Formed basis for future legislation for human and veterinary medicines
Directive 81/851/EEC	1981: Regulatory framework and requirements for authorisation of veterinary medicinal products in what are now EU countries
Directive 81/852/EEC	1981: Sets out testing and scientific requirements for quality, efficacy and safety for authorisation of veterinary medicinal products in what are now EU countries
Regulation (EEC) No. 2377/90	1990: Establishment of MRLs for pharmacologically active substances
Regulation (EEC) No. 2309/93	1993: European Medicines Evaluation Agency (EMEA) opens in 1995, centralised and mutual recognition procedures commence
–	2000: Review of the veterinary legislation begins
Directive 2001/82/EC	Consolidates much of existing veterinary legislation, in part to facilitate its review
Directive 2004/28/EC	2004: Introduces numerous amendments to 2001/82/EC and adds new procedure for authorisation of veterinary medicinal products, the decentralised procedure
Regulation (EC) No. 726/2004	2004: Also introduces numerous changes and renames EMEA the European Medicines Agency (EMA) in recognition of its wider remit
Directive 2009/9/EC	2009: Amends Directive 2001/82/EC as "Annex 1". Sets out updated requirements for testing and scientific data for quality, efficacy and safety required to support marketing authorisation applications
Regulation (EC) No. 470/2009	2009: New requirements for the establishment of MRLs
Regulation (EU) No. 37/2010	2010: Tables of consolidated MRLs and related classifications published

[a]Note: this table omits many amending Directives, and legislation on peripheral issues *e.g.* fees payable to the EMA and variations.

desired, and it then informs the original member state, who now becomes the Reference Member State (RMS), while the others, which might be just two or three, or the entire trading block of 27 EU countries plus the EEA states, become the Concerned Member States (CMSs). The original application made to the RMS is updated and resubmitted, and submitted to all CMSs. The procedure can be complex, and may frequently result in a relatively long list of scientific questions arising from the newly involved member states. However, once all of the issues have been resolved, the procedure concludes and marketing authorisations can be issued. It is important to recognise that the outcome of this procedure is the issuance of individual albeit harmonised marketing authorisations by national regulatory authorities. If 15 countries are involved, 15 marketing authorisations are issued; if 27, then 27 marketing authorisations are issued.

2.3.3 The Decentralised Procedure

The decentralised procedure shares many of the elements of the mutual recognition procedure and, like the mutual recognition procedure, it is also a provision of Directive 2001/82/EC (as amended). The main difference is that there is no initial application for a single national marketing authorisation. A simultaneous application is made to the RMS and to the CMSs. The benefit of this procedure is that, in theory, it is more rapid than the mutual recognition procedure precisely because it omits that initial national step. In practice, one of the main benefits of the national procedure is the useful feedback from the national regulatory authority. This can be consolidated into the dossier intended for mutual recognition prior to submission to the CMSs. There is no scope for this during the Decentralised Procedure and so the applicant must have high confidence in the content and standard of the dossier before choosing this route. However, the end result of this procedure is the same as that for the mutual recognition procedure: two or more harmonised marketing authorisations issued by the national regulatory authorities in the countries concerned by the application.

2.3.4 The Centralised Procedure

The Centralised Procedure was originally provided for under Regulation (EEC) No. 2309/93 but is now governed by Regulation (EC) No. 726/2004. Applications are made to the European Medicines Agency, where a rapporteur and co-rapporteur are appointed from the membership of the Committee for Medicinal Products for Veterinary Use (CVMP, previously the Committee for Veterinary Medicinal Products), which is established under the regulation. The rapporteur and co-rapporteur work together to assess the scientific content of the application dossier and present this to the CVMP. The CVMP may ask questions of the applicant and at the end of the procedure it can issue either a negative or a positive opinion. If the opinion is positive, it is transmitted to the European Commission in Brussels, which then issues an EU-wide marketing authorisation valid in all EU and EEA countries. The Centralised Procedure is mandatory for some types of product including those derived from biotechnology and recombinant DNA technologies and optional for so-called novel products including those that employ novel means of administration, contain new active ingredients or are intended for new indications. It is popular with the veterinary pharmaceutical industry because it involves a single list of questions from a single body, the CVMP, and hence has a higher degree of predictability than the Mutual Recognition or Decentralised procedures.

The CVMP also plays a role in both the Mutual Recognition and Decentralised Procedures. If a dispute occurs between national regulatory authorities involved in one of these procedures over the assessment of a dossier, or there is a difference of scientific interpretation, then a scientific deadlock might result that cannot be resolved. The legislation makes provision for this and it is possible for the problem to be referred to the Co-ordination Group for Mutual Recognition and Decentralised Procedures (veterinary) or CMDv. This group, established under Directive 2001/82/EC, is made up from representatives of the national authorities and it attempts to resolve these outstanding issues. It has had considerable success in its interventions. However, not all such disputes can be resolved through the CMDv and these are then referred to the CVMP. The CVMP can take the side of one of the proponents in the dispute, or it can reach a compromise position. The outcome, as with the Centralised Procedure, is a negative or a positive opinion on the issue at stake. This opinion is again transmitted to the European Commission and it eventually becomes a point of European law that is binding on all member states.

2.3.5   Maximum Residue Limits

MRLs, as already noted, are the subject of a separate chapter. However, it should be noted that the procedures underlying the establishment of MRLs mirror those of the Centralised Procedure. Applications are made to the EMA and a rapporteur and co-rapporteur are appointed. Their assessment is then considered by the CVMP and a negative or positive opinion is issued, usually after a list of questions has been transmitted to the applicant and a satisfactory response has been despatched.[19,20,25,26] The positive opinion is then transmitted to the European Commission and the MRLs are adopted and eventually published in the *Official Journal of the European Union*. Summary reports that provide the scientific basis for the establishment of each MRL can be found on the EMA's website (http://www.ema.europa.eu/).

In 1990, Regulation (EEC) No. 2377/90 entered into force. This first introduced the concept of the MRL to the veterinary area (it had been used previously for pesticide residues) and it required that all pharmacologically active ingredients intended for use in food animals be entered into Annexes I–III of the regulation before a marketing authorisation could be granted in the EU. It was applied retrospectively to all existing pharmacologically active ingredients and any not entered into Annexes I–III were lost for use in food animals. The term "pharmacologically active ingredient" is not synonymous with "active ingredient". It includes any ingredient used in a veterinary medicinal product, including vaccines, which has pharmacological activity or more specifically pharmacodynamic activity. Thus, solvents, antioxidants, stabilisers and colouring agents are also subject to the requirements of the regulation. The applications to the EMA are supported by a package of safety (mainly toxicology) and residues depletion data generated in the food animal or commodity (*e.g.* milk, eggs or honey) concerned. The overall intention is to ensure that consumers of food of animal origin are protected from potentially harmful drug residues. This is achieved by establishing withdrawal periods, the time that must elapse between drug administration and slaughter of the animal or the collection of food of animal origin (milk, eggs, honey). Withdrawal periods form part of the terms of marketing authorisations for food animal medicines and appear in the product literature and on labels.

The three Annexes were:

- Annex I – full MRLs (examples include the major active ingredients; MRLs are usually cited as micrograms of substance per kilogram of edible tissue – muscle, fat, liver, milk *etc.*)
- Annex II – no MRLs required on public health grounds (examples include biologically inert materials or substances that are rapidly metabolised by the animal to innocuous metabolites, substances not absorbed from the animal's gastrointestinal tract and substances of plant origin such as vegetable oils and sugars)
- Annex III – provisional MRLs (a temporary position, usually because of some minor deficiency in the data package. Once resolved, Annex III substances are usually transferred to Annex I)

There was one further Annex, Annex IV. This was the destination of substances, ten in total, considered unsafe on consumer safety grounds. These substances, and substances where the CVMP was unable to reach a positive opinion, may not be used in veterinary medicinal products intended for use in food animals. Similarly, substances for which no applications have been made and which have not been considered by the CVMP may not be used in food-producing animals. For the purposes of this Regulation specifically, and EU veterinary legislation generally, food producing animals include cattle, pigs, sheep, goats, horses, poultry and other farmed or kept game birds, rabbits, reindeer, deer, farmed fish and bees.

In 2009, Regulation (EEC) No. 2377/90 was replaced and repealed by Regulation (EC) No. 470/2009, which introduced a number of improvements and modifications to the original regulation. It also removed the four annexes referred to above. The consolidated list of MRLs now appears in Regulation (EU) No. 37/2010 and the four annexes are replaced by two tables. Table 1 lists all those substances that were originally in Annexes I to III as "allowed substances" with the terms of the entry set out in six columns, while Table 2, "prohibited substances", lists the previous occupants of Annex IV.

2.3.6 Pharmacovigilance

Pharmacovigilance is a term used to describe the gathering of information on adverse drug reactions. It is an integral part of the regulatory environment for both human and veterinary medicines in the EU, the US and elsewhere.[20,27–29]

In the EU, pharmacovigilance requirements for veterinary medicinal products are set out in Directive 2001/82/EC (as amended) and, for the operation of the centralised procedure, in Regulation (EC) No. 726/524.

Veterinary pharmacovigilance at the EU level had already operated in some countries for some time, as it was originally required by Directive 81/851/EEC as amended by Directive 93/40/EEC and Directive 540/95/EEC. At the national level in the EU Member States, pharmacovigilance requirements were implemented to varying degrees ranging from almost non-existent in some countries, to the more complex systems that existed in France, Germany and the Netherlands. In the UK, the VMD's Suspected Adverse Reactions Reporting Scheme (SARRS) has operated successfully since 1987. Following the creation of the EMA, the introduction of the Centralised Procedure and the effective functioning of the mutual recognition and the decentralised procedures, and particularly since the review of the legislation already described, there has been an increased impetus behind veterinary pharmacovigilance in the EU.

2.3.6.1 *Pharmacovigilance Requirements for Veterinary Medicines in the EU*

The scope for pharmacovigilance parallels the regulatory requirements for medicines. That is to say that wherever there is a need to show some scientific aspect for the properties of a medicine, there is a need to monitor that requirement as part of pharmacovigilance activities. For example, and very simply, applicants for MAs for human or veterinary medicinal products must conduct studies to demonstrate that those products are safe for use in patients, and they must make use of pharmacovigilance activities to monitor patient safety once those products are marketed. As mentioned earlier, medicinal products must meet strict criteria of quality, efficacy and safety and they are therefore subject to post-marketing surveillance, pharmacovigilance, to ensure that these carry forward into clinical use in humans and animals.

Clearly for veterinary medicinal products, like their counterparts intended for use in humans, safety to the patient is crucial. Indeed, to help to ensure this, veterinary medicinal products are tested in the intended patients at the therapeutic dose and at multiples of the therapeutic dose, and for the intended duration of use, and with multiples of the duration of use, in what are known as target animal safety (TAS) studies. These studies form part of the submission dossier and underpin the terms of the eventual MA. Taken together with data obtained from preclinical studies in laboratory animals, and information gained from clinical trials, it is possible to use these TAS studies to evaluate safety during clinical veterinary use. Of course other more specialist studies may also be needed. For example, investigations in juvenile animals and studies during pregnancy and in lactation may also be required (or contraindications included in the product literature).

Medicines given to companion animals pose minimal environmental risks. However, this may not be true of medicines used to treat food-producing animals. Food animals are usually reared on a herd or flock basis, and if animals are treated on a herd or flock basis then there may be potential for environmental exposure, albeit local in many circumstances (*e.g.* the farm where they are kept), from excreta in particular. The excreta are usually applied to the land as manure, often to arable land, and so there is a potential risk of environmental contamination. In some circumstances, this potential may be even greater. For example, sheep suffer from various ectoparasites and one of the ways of treating these is to dip the animals in a solution of ecto-parasiticide. These dip baths are often situated near to watercourses to provide a ready source of solvent *i.e.* water, for their constitution. This also means that they can easily contaminate the same watercourses either through run-off from dipped sheep or from surrounding land or by accidental or deliberate discharge of the dip contents. As these dips contain substances that could potentially harm the environment, such as synthetic pyrethroids or organo-phosphorus compounds, then this is an obvious cause for concern. Drugs used in aquaculture to treat fish (usually salmon or trout in the UK and northern Europe but other species such as cod are being introduced) appear to pose an even greater potential problem as they are usually administered directly into the aquatic environment. For all these reasons, veterinary medicinal products in the EU are subject to what is known as a Phase I environmental risk assessment. This uses predictors of environmental contamination and concentration, along with data on stability, solubility, chemical and biodegradability and other physico-chemical properties, to examine (among other things) the possible degree of environmental penetration and persistence. Based on the outcome of this Phase I assessment, Phase II studies may be required. These may include, but are not restricted to, studies of the toxicity of the product to aquatic organisms, effects on the food web and phytotoxicity. Marketing authorisations will only be granted once regulatory authorities are assured that the product in question does not pose an unacceptable environmental risk. Environmental risk assessment in other countries such as the USA follows a similar approach.

There must also be confidence that the veterinary medicinal product does not offer an unacceptable risk to users and to others potentially exposed. This might mean veterinarians, veterinary nurses, kennel or cattery employees, farmers and farm workers (including fish farms), and members of the pet-owning public. In addition, for medicines applied dermally to companion animals, exposure might also occur on stroking or carrying. Applicants for marketing authorisations for veterinary medicinal products must assess user safety under European user safety guidelines, and make judgments of the degree and extent of potential user exposure, and evaluate the risks from such exposures based on the hazards identified in preclinical studies such as acute or repeat dose toxicity, skin or eye irritation or dermal sensitisation, or from physico-chemical properties.

2.3.6.2 Specific Pharmacovigilance Requirements

Essentially, any breaches of any of the aspects of safety described above, and any suspected lack of efficacy, are reportable adverse reactions to veterinary medicinal products. For purposes of illustration, some examples of the safety areas covered by veterinary pharmacovigilance are given in Table 2.4.

Any such events should be reported to the relevant competent authorities within the EU. Serious adverse reactions are subject to expedited reporting (see later), and reactions should be classified where possible as to whether or not

Table 2.4   Examples of safety aspects of EU veterinary pharmacovigilance.

Safety area	Examples
Animal (patient)	Adverse idiosyncratic or expected toxic or exaggerated pharmacological effects *e.g.* hepatic necrosis, cardiomyopathy, central nervous system effects, hypersensitivity reactions
Human (users)	Adverse skin or ocular effects following contamination, toxic effects *e.g.* following inadvertent oral exposure (hand-to-mouth contamination of food or smoking materials), systemic effects following use of medical gases/gaseous anaesthetics, accidental self-injection, needlestick injuries
Environmental	Environmental contamination incidents; ecotoxicity following such incidents *e.g.* poisoning of fish, invertebrates, birds; phytotoxicity
Consumer	Violation of MRL values, discovery of residues of substances in Table 2 of Regulation (EU) No. 37/2010 or substances prohibited by other EU legislation *e.g.* growth-promoting hormones, or substances not entered into Table 1 of Regulation No. (EU) 470/2009, and either not considered under the Regulation, or with the CVMP unable to give a positive opinion. Toxicity following ingestion of residues[a]

[a]Except in exceptional circumstances, it is highly unlikely that residues in food of animal origin would elicit a toxic response in a consumer. It is equally unlikely that an association would be made if such an event did occur.

they were expected (cited on the label and product literature) or unexpected. Moreover, adverse reactions should be classified in terms of their causality using the ABON notation. Briefly, this requires the investigator to allocate a coding (A, B, O or N) depending on the degree of association of the adverse reaction with the veterinary medicinal product administered.

The ABON coding criteria are briefly summarised below:

A   Reasonable association temporally between administration and onset of adverse reaction, clinical plausibility (*e.g.* based on toxicology and pharmacology, no other equally plausible explanation)

B   Causality associated with drug is one possible cause but does not meet criteria of A

O   Evidence suggests beyond doubt that drug was not responsible

N   No reliable or adequate evidence to make a causality assessment

Prior to the review of the legislation mentioned earlier, one of the major aspects of the old legislation was the system of renewals. All marketing authorisations were issued for a period of five years, after which, and every five years for the life-span of the product, they were subject to an application for renewal. The system was applied in an inconsistent manner across the EU with some countries requiring merely an application form, while others demanded updates to the dossier to include new safety, quality and efficacy data, frequently merely to comply with EU Guidelines adopted since the granting of the marketing authorisation or the last renewal. Needless to say, the veterinary pharmaceutical industry had a severe dislike of this system and during the review of the legislation it campaigned vigorously against it. It was successful in this and the renewals system was replaced with what has been described as an "enhanced" system of pharmacovigilance.

These requirements are now set out in Directive 2001/82/EC as amended by 2004/28/EC. Briefly, they can be summarised as follows:

- Member States to encourage reporting of suspected adverse reactions (SARs) and may impose specific requirements on veterinarians and others to report
- Member States shall establish a pharmacovigilance system, and notably for adverse reactions in animals and in humans exposed to veterinary medicinal products. Relevant information to be collated and sent to other Member States and to the EMA
- The marketing authorisation shall have a Qualified Person for Pharmacovigilance responsible for establishment and maintenance of a database for SARs and providing information and responses to regulatory authorities
- Marketing authorisation holder shall maintain detailed records of all SARs
- Except in exceptional circumstances these shall be sent electronically to the authorities
- All serious and human adverse reactions must be reported within 15 days to Member State on which they occurred
- All serious *unexpected* adverse reactions, all adverse reactions in humans, or transmission of an infectious agent *via* a veterinary medicinal product occurring in a third country, must also be reported within 15 days to the EU Member States and to the EMA
- Provision of Periodic Safety Update Reports (PSURs) at 6, 12, 18, 24 and 36 months, then at 3-year intervals
- The EMA, Member States and the Commission to establish a data processing network for pharmacovigilance
- European Commission, with the EMA, Member States and interested parties, will draw up Guidelines on collection, verification and presentation of SARs, and on electronic reporting
- Member States may vary, suspend or withdraw marketing authorisations in response to pharmacovigilance data and, where required, take urgent action

Regulation (EC) No. 726/2004 reflects much of the content of the Directive but it focuses on the operation and the regulatory requirements affecting the Centralised Procedure, and the roles of the EMA and the CVMP. For example, all relevant pharmacovigilance data for products authorised under the Centralised Procedure must be reported to the EMA. Similarly, the frequency of PSURs became 6, 12, 18, 24 and 36 months and then every 3 years, this being one of the aspects of the enhanced pharmacovigilance referred to earlier. Under the previous provisions of the legislation, where the emphasis was placed on renewals, the timing of PSURs was 6, 12 and 18 months, and 2, 3 and 5 years and then every 5 years. Under the new system, renewals are restricted to one after 5 years and the products are then subject to the more frequent PSUR regime. However, less frequent PSURs can be requested by the marketing authorisation holder, and more frequent ones demanded by the CVMP and EMA, on the basis and justification of the available evidence.

2.3.6.3   Events to be Reported

All suspected adverse reactions should be reported but only those that are serious or that occur in exposed humans, usually after occupational exposure, need to be reported within 15 days – the so-called expedited reports. In addition, and as mentioned above, serious unexpected adverse reactions occurring in third countries should be reported in an expedited manner. Neither the Directive nor the Regulation define or provide any clear detail as to what constitutes a suspected adverse reaction. However, guidance is provided in Volume 9B of the Rules Governing Medicinal Products in the European Union, Guidelines on Pharmacovigilance for Medicinal Products for Veterinary Use. The human medicines version was published as Volume 9A in September 2008 but the veterinary equivalent was only published in late 2011. These documents are available from the European Commissions Eudralex website at http://ec.europa.eu/health/documents/eudralex/index.

Volume 9B defines a SAR as *a reaction which is harmful and unintended and which occurs at doses normally used in animals for the prophylaxis, diagnosis or treatment of disease or modification of physiological function.* A serious SAR is one that results in death, is life-threatening, produces significant disability or incapacity, is a congenital anomaly or birth defect or one that results in permanent or prolonged signs in treated animals. However, even this leaves room for interpretation. For example, undoubtedly, the death of a dog or a horse following treatment with a veterinary medicinal product is "serious", but Volume 9B makes it clear that for animals that are intensively reared, such as poultry, fish or bees, then death of a certain number of animals might be expected or considered normal, and thus the term "serious" might not apply. Death of course is not a serious SAR (for veterinary medicinal products) when it is the intended outcome of the treatment *i.e.* for euthanasia products, although failure to induce death is an example of lack of efficacy.

In addition, PSURs should also include details of all adverse reactions, serious and non-serious, information on any adverse environmental effects, reports of lack of efficacy and, with reference to the final item described in the Introduction, any violations of MRLs that might be suggestive of misuse of the product (*e.g.* overdosing), failure to observe the correct withdrawal period or that the withdrawal period is inadequate.

2.3.6.4   Guidelines and Guidance

Volume 9B provides a wealth of information on matters relating to veterinary pharmacovigilance. However, there are also several Guidelines available in the veterinary section of the EMA's website under *Pharmacovigilance*. A number of these guidelines, which have been drafted by the CVMP's Pharmacovigilance Working Party, are intended for the industry, while others are aimed at practising veterinarians or competent authority regulators. There are a number of adopted guidelines, draft guidelines or points to consider documents, in addition to the EMA's Crisis Management Plan for centrally authorised products. Of the adopted guidelines the most important from the point of view of marketing authorisation holders are:

- Note for Guidance on pharmacovigilance of veterinary medicinal products – Guidance on procedures for MAHs, EMEA/CVMP/183/96 – the essential guide for the industry on the major matters relating to veterinary pharmacovigilance
- Guideline on harmonising the approach to causality assessment for adverse reactions to veterinary medicinal products, EMEA/CVMP/552/03 – an essential guideline for assigning causality, which provides a systematic approach
- Veterinary pharmacovigilance in the EU – a simple guide to reporting adverse reactions, EMEA/CVMP/PhVWP/110607/2005
- Procedures for competent authorities for pharmacovigilance information for veterinary medicinal products, EMEA/CVMP/98-Rev.1-FINAL
- Strategy for triggering pharmacovigilance investigations preceding regulatory actions by EU competent authorities, EMEA/CVMP/900/03-FINAL
- Recommendation for the basic surveillance of EudraVigilance veterinary data, EMA/CVMP/PhVWP/471721/2006

The International Cooperation on Harmonisation of Technical Requirements for Registration of Veterinary Medicinal Products, VICH, the veterinary counterpart of the perhaps better known ICH, which covers human pharmaceuticals, has also been developing a range of guidelines, some of them in the area of pharmacovigilance. Three VICH pharmacovigilance guidelines have been finalised or are near to finalisation – management of adverse event reports (GL 24), management of PSURs (GL 29) and a controlled list of terms (GL 30) – and others are in development including GL35 (electronic standards for transfer of data and GL42 (data elements for submission of adverse events reports. For further details see http://www.vichsec.org/. The European industry representative body IFAH-Europe, which represents the interests of the animal health industry, has also provided guidance in the form of a Good Veterinary Pharmacovigilance Practice Guide. This is an excellent document that succinctly describes the regulatory requirements and expectations.

2.3.6.5   *Pharmacovigilance Inspections*

Directive 2001/82/EC as amended by Directive 2004/28/EC and Regulation (EC) 726/2004 require that EU Member State competent authorities and EMEA monitor pharmacovigilance activities in the EU and ensure the compliance with a number of principles including "pharmacovigilance obligations". One way of carrying out these duties is to conduct pharmacovigilance inspections. As the pharmaceutical industry has the major responsibility for product stewardship and pharmacovigilance reporting, it is the industry that is inspected.

The legal basis for pharmacovigilance inspections is Article 80 of the amended Directive. This allows the competent authorities to make both announced and unannounced inspections in a number of areas including pharmacovigilance. Article 44(1) of the Regulation places the onus on Member States to ensure that the requirements of the Regulation, including pharmacovigilance requirements, are verified and enforced. Several EU Member States now have functioning pharmacovigilance inspection units that cover veterinary medicinal products.

Pharmacovigilance inspections are intended to ensure that companies have functioning veterinary pharmacovigilance systems that comply with the requirements of the EU and national legislative requirements. These include the presence of a qualified person, a system for pharmacovigilance activities – usually a computer database – compliance with reporting requirements, follow-up of initial adverse reaction reports, continuous monitoring of the safety profiles of marketed products and timely preparation and submission of PSURs. Training records are also likely to be subject to scrutiny as are organisational charts and reporting responsibilities. Any shortcomings noted by the inspectorates will require remedial attention.

2.4   Conclusions

Veterinary medicinal products are subject to extensive control in the EU and in most of the world's other countries. One of the cornerstones of those controls is the consideration of quality, efficacy and safety, and the data that support these. Only when regulatory authorities are content with these aspects will a marketing authorisation, licence or approval be granted. The assessment of human safety, especially from the vantage points of user and consumer safety, is based on a number of key data sets and, of these, one of the most important is a set of toxicity data.

Assessment does not finish once a product is marketed. As part of the continuous assessment of quality, efficacy and safety, most regulatory authorities, including those in the EU, are responsible for a complex collection of pharmacovigilance requirements. This will help to ensure that safety, including safety to humans exposed to veterinary medicinal products, is constantly monitored. Toxicological responses in humans, if detected, must be reported under these pharmacovigilance provisions.

The veterinary legislation is once again the subject of review in the EU. The likely outcome of this exercise is still unclear although there are initiatives to ensure that the operation of the legislation and the regulatory procedures can by streamlined and made much more efficient.[30-33] Regardless, the emphasis on safety is likely to remain.

References

1. H. P. A. Illing, Toxicology and disasters in *General and Applied Toxicology*, ed. B. Ballantyne, T. Marrs and T. Syversen, Macmillan, Basingstoke, 2nd edn, 2000, pp. 1811–1839.
2. H. P. A. Illing, Introduction in *Toxicity and Risk: Context, Principles and Practice*, Taylor and Francis, London, 2001, pp. 1–10.
3. W. G. McBride, Thalidomide and congenital abnormalities, *Lancet*, 1961, **2**, 1358.
4. W. Lenz and K. Knapp, Thalidomide and embryopathy, *Arch. Environ. Health*, 1962, **5**, 100–105.
5. A. E. Rodin, L. A. Koller and J. D. Taylor, Association of thalidomide (Kevadon) with congenital anomalies, *CMAJ*, 1962, **86**, 744–746.
6. P. A. Lancaster, Causes of birth defects: lessons from history, *Congenit. Anom. (Kyoto)*, 2011, **51**, 2–5.
7. A. A. Mitchell, Adverse drug reactions *in utero*: perspectives on teratogens and strategies for the future, *Clin. Pharmacol. Ther.*, 2011, **89**, 781–783.
8. N. Vargesson, Thalidomide-induced limb defects: resolving a 50-year-old puzzle, *Bioessays*, 2009, **31**, 1327–1336.
9. E. M. K. Gelling and P. R. Cannon, Pathological effects of elixir of sulphanilamide (diethylene glycol) poisoning, *JAMA*, 1938, **111**, 919–926.
10. M. D. B. Stephens, Introduction in *Detection of New Adverse Drug Reactions*, ed. M. D. B. Stephens, J. C. C. Talbot and P. A. Routledge, Macmillan Reference, Ltd, London, 4th edn, 1999, pp. 1–57.
11. P. M. Wax, Elixirs, diluents, and the passage of the 1938 Federal Food, Drug and Cosmetic Act, *Ann. Intern. Med.*, 1995, **122**, 456–461.
12. A. Gupta and L. K. Waldhauser, Adverse drug reactions from birth to early childhood, *Pediatr. Clin. North Am.*, 1997, **44**, 79–92.
13. G. M. Landrey, S. Martin and K. E. McMartin, Diglycolic acid is the nephrotoxic metabolite in diethylene glycol poisoning inducing necrosis in human proximal tubule cells *in vitro*, *Toxicol. Sci.*, 2011, **124**, 35–44.
14. P. F. D'Arcy, Pharmaceutical toxicity in *General and Applied Toxicology*, ed. B. Ballantyne, T. Marrs and T. Syversen, Macmillan, Basingstoke, 2nd edn, 2000, pp. 1425–1441.
15. M. F. Cuthbert, J. P. Griffin and W. H. W. Inman, The United Kingdom in *Controlling the Therapeutic Use of Drugs: An International Comparison*, ed.

W. M. Wardell, American Institute for Public Policy Research, Washington DC, 1978, pp. 99–134.

16. I. H. Harrison, Historical background and introduction in *The Law on Medicines. A Comprehensive Guide*, MTP Press, Lancaster, 1986, vol. 1, pp. 17–31.

17. W. J. Brinley Morgan, Legislation covering the licensing of veterinary medicines in the United Kingdom, *Vet. Rec.*, 1983, **113**, 310–313.

18. K. N. Woodward, Regulation of veterinary drugs in Europe, including the UK in *General and Applied Toxicology*, ed. B. Ballantyne, T. Marrs and P. Turner, Macmillan, Basingstoke, 1st edn, 1993, pp. 1105–1128.

19. K. N. Woodward, Regulation of veterinary drugs in *General and Applied Toxicology*, ed. B. Ballantyne, T. Marrs and T. Syversen, Macmillan, Basingstoke, 2nd edn, 2000, pp. 1633–1652.

20. K. N. Woodward, Veterinary pharmacovigilance. Part 1. The legal basis in the European Union, *J. Vet. Pharmacol. Ther.*, 2005, **28**, 131–147.

21. C. Ibrahim and A. Wilke, Pharmacovigilance in Germany in *Veterinary Pharmacovigilance. Adverse Reactions to Veterinary Medicinal Products*, ed. K. N. Woodward, Wiley-Blackwell, Chichester, 2009, pp. 65–90.

22. A. C. Cartwright, Introduction and history of pharmaceutical regulation in *Pharmaceutical Product Licensing. Requirements for Europe*, ed. A. C. Cartwright and B. R. Matthews, Ellis Horwood, New York, pp. 29–45.

23. K. N. Woodward, Assessment of user safety, exposure and risk to veterinary medicinal products in the European Union, *Regul. Toxicol. Pharmacol.*, 2008, **50**, 114–128.

24. K. N. Woodward, Elements of veterinary pharmacovigilance in *Veterinary Pharmacovigilance. Adverse Reactions to Veterinary Medicinal Products*, ed. K. N. Woodward, Wiley-Blackwell, Chichester, 2009, pp. 9–17.

25. K. N. Woodward, Progress with the establishment of maximum residue limits for veterinary drugs in the European Union, *Toxicol. Environ. News*, 1997, **4**, 46–54.

26. K. N. Woodward, Assessing the safety of veterinary drug residues in *Pesticide, Veterinary and Other Residues in Food*, ed. D. H. Watson, CRC Press/Woodhead Publishing, Cambridge, 2004, pp. 157–174.

27. K. N. Woodward, Veterinary pharmacovigilance in the European Union in *Veterinary Pharmacovigilance. Adverse Reactions to Veterinary Medicinal Products*, ed. K. N. Woodward, Wiley-Blackwell, Chichester, 2009, pp. 19–46.

28. K. N. Woodward, Veterinary pharmacovigilance. Part 2. Veterinary pharmacovigilance in practice – the operation of a spontaneous reporting scheme in a European Union country – the UK, and schemes in other countries, *J. Vet. Pharmacol. Ther.*, 2005, **28**, 149–170.

29. T. M. Hodge, Pharmacovigilance in the US – an industry perspective in *Veterinary Pharmacovigilance. Adverse Reactions to Veterinary Medicinal Products*, ed. K. N. Woodward, Wiley-Blackwell, Chichester, 2009, pp. 231–285.

30. K. N. Woodward and C. W. Evans, Pharmacovigilance inspections in the European Union in *Veterinary Pharmacovigilance. Adverse Reactions to*

Veterinary Medicinal Products, ed. K. N. Woodward, Wiley-Blackwell, Chichester, 2009, pp. 163–175.
31. R. Clayton, Veterinary medicines legislative review – the big debate, *Regulatory Rapporteur*, 2011, **8**, 29–31.
32. European Policy Evaluation Consortium (EPEC). Assessment of the impact of the revision of Veterinary Pharmaceutical Legislation, 2011 at http://www.ec.europa.eu/health/files/veterinary/11-07-2011_final_report_.pdf
33. B. Boenisch, Review of the veterinary medicines legislation: contribution from industry. Presentation at the 6th TOPRA Annual Veterinary Symposium, Rome, 17 October 2011.

CHAPTER 3

Consumer Safety – Maximum Residue Limits

3.1 Introduction

In the European Union (EU), the prime purpose of maximum residue limits (MRLs) for veterinary drugs is to protect the health of those who consume food of animal origin. Thus, these MRLs, as will become clear later, are based firmly on safety data, and primarily on the results of toxicity testing.

Directive 2001/82/EC as amended by Directive 2004/28/EC stipulates that pharmacologically active substances intended for use in food animals must have MRLs, or an MRL is not required, on public health grounds, before marketing authorisations can be granted in the EU. Until the recent past this meant that pharmacologically active substances must be entered into one of the Annexes I to III of Council Regulation No. (EEC) 2377/90, the so-called MRL Regulation.[1–5] The purpose of this legislation was to ensure that substances intended for use in food animals are adequately assessed for their harmful potential, and notably their toxicity, and that consumers of food of animal origin are adequately protected. However, toxicity was not the only concern. Pharmacologic properties, especially pharmacodynamic properties, which may be highly desirable for sick animals, may not be at all desirable if they occur in the consumer who has eaten animal products. This sentiment applies not only to pharmacodynamic effects of drugs expressed in the animal (*e.g.* β-adrenergic effects, various hormonal effects, anaesthesia, analgesia), but it is also true of other effects such as microbiological properties, as will become evident later in this chapter. The presence of a drug residue in an edible product is not in itself problematic. What is critical is how much of the drug is present, and how long it persists. Veterinary drug residues may be composed of the original substance,

Issues in Toxicology No. 14
Toxicological Effects of Veterinary Medicinal Products in Humans: Volume 1
By Kevin N. Woodward
© The Royal Society of Chemistry 2013
Published by the Royal Society of Chemistry, www.rsc.org

the parent drug and, frequently, various metabolites, or a combination of parent drug and metabolites. Some of these may be present as residues that are covalently bound to macromolecules such as proteins or nucleic acids.[6–9] These bound residues are subject to various metabolic processes including eventual conversion to non-toxic metabolic products including water and carbon dioxide and other physiological substances, and excretion in the urine, expired air or bile. In other words, they will eventually decrease in concentration as time passes, as a result of the animal's metabolism. This is known as residues depletion or depuration. Consequently, the risks posed by residues of a veterinary drug depend not only on its toxic, pharmacological and micro-biological activities, and those of its metabolites, but also on its rate of disappearance from the animal.

3.2 Establishment of MRLs in the EU

As already described briefly in Chapter 2, MRLs are established in the EU by the Committee for Medicinal Products for Veterinary Use (CVMP), following applications made to the European Medicines Agency (EMA). Specifically, the CVMP issues an opinion after consideration of the available toxicological and residues depletion data and the information on the proposed analytical method, provided by the applicant. This opinion used to take the form of an entry into one of the four Annexes of Regulation (EEC) No. 2377/90. The actual decision, in legal terms, was taken by the European Commission, and the Annex entries were published in the *Official Journal of the European Union*. The nature of the Annexes is shown below:

- Annex I: Full MRLs; the data supplied are adequate to address safety and residues concerns
- Annex II: On public health grounds, MRLs are not necessary. These entries include those for simple salts, innocuous substances and compounds that are rapidly converted in the animal to non-toxic metabolites
- Annex III: Provisional MRLs. The majority of data in the supporting dossiers are satisfactory but some relatively minor points need addressing. Satisfactory resolution leads to Annex I (or possibly Annex II) entry
- Annex IV: Substances not considered safe on public health grounds. Annex IV entries include the nitrofurans, nitroimidazoles, chloramphenicol and dapsone

However, Regulation (EEC) No. 2377/90 has now been replaced and repealed by Regulation (EC) No. 470/2009. This made some changes and amendments to the requirements for MRLs and also dispensed with the Annex format. Substances are now entered into one of two tables. Table 1, "allowed substances", lists those drugs that previously would have been included in Annexes I to III while Table 2, "prohibited substances", lists the ten substances that used to be listed in Annex IV. Regulation (EU) No. 37/2010 provides a consolidated list of all the substances, in Tables 1 and 2, which were previously included in Annexes I to IV of Regulation (EEC) No. 2377/90. The general requirements and provisions of the original regulation still apply under the new regulation, Regulation (EC) No. 470/2009.

Companies wishing to market a veterinary medicinal product for use in food-producing animals must therefore supply sufficient data to satisfy the CVMP that the pharmacologically active agent is safe for consumers and that MRLs can be established or are not required. The major components of these data are toxicological, pharmacological and microbiological, along with data on residues depletion and analytical methodologies. In fact, the two major components of an MRL application are termed the safety file and the residues file, and the outline contents of these are shown in Tables 3.1 and 3.2.

From the studies outlined in the safety file, the critical areas of toxicology, microbiology and pharmacology can be identified and a toxicological profile, or perhaps more appropriately a biological profile, can be constructed. From these data no-observed effect levels (NOELs) can be identified and, from the point of view of hazard assessment, the lowest NOEL is usually chosen unless there is good reason for it not to be chosen (*e.g.* because the toxicity noted is species-specific to the animal used in the test system or the effect is discountable on mechanistic or dose-response considerations).

The NOEL is a key component of the MRL because it forms the basis of the calculation of the acceptable daily intake or ADI. The ADI concept was developed in 1957 by the Joint FAO/WHO Expert Committee on Food Additives (JECFA),[10] and its use described by the World Health Organization's *Environmental Health Criteria 70.*[11] This concept was largely based on the ideas

Table 3.1   Major contents of the safety file.

- Safety Expert Report
- Characterisation (*e.g.* name, structure, impurities, molecular weight)
- Physico-chemical properties (*e.g.* melting and boiling points, vapour pressure, solubility in water and organic solvents, pH, density)
- Pharmacology
  - Pharmacodynamics – major effects, especially those related to its therapeutic mode of action *e.g.* anaesthesia, analgesia, hormonal effects
  - Pharmacokinetics – absorption, biotransformation, tissue distribution and excretion
- Toxicological studies
  - Single dose (acute toxicity)
  - Repeat dose (at least 90 days' duration)
  - Reproductive toxicity
    - Study of effects on reproduction
    - Embryotoxicity/teratology
  - Genotoxicity
  - Carcinogenicity
- Microbiological effects on human gut flora
- Pharmacological, microbiological and toxicological observations in humans (where available)
- Effects on food processing *e.g.* microbiological effects on starter cultures used in yoghurt production

Table 3.2 Major contents of the residues file.

- Residue Expert Report
- Characterisation (*e.g.* name, structure, impurities, molecular weight)
- Physico-chemical properties (*e.g.* melting and boiling points, vapour pressure, solubility in water and organic solvents, pH, density)
- Pharmacokinetics in target animals (sheep, pigs, cattle, fish *etc.*)
- Residues studies
  - Residues depletion studies in each target species
    - Studies with radiolabelled drug
    - Studies with unlabelled drug
- Elaboration of MRLs
- Routine Analytical Methods
  - Description of the method
  - Validation of the method (*e.g.* precision, accuracy, limit of detection, limit of quantification, susceptibility and interference, practicability and applicability)

of René Truhaut.[12,13] In the ADI calculation, the NOEL is divided by a suitable safety factor, usually 100, to give the ADI value. The 100-fold safety factor concept is empirical and arises from the contention that there is a10-fold human variability in susceptibility, and a 10-fold animal-human variability, giving the overall safety factor of 100. It is therefore logical that in those few examples where the NOEL is derived from human studies, the safety factor used to calculate the ADI is usually 10.[3,14–20] However, higher safety factors may also be used, for instance where there are minor flaws in the data package such as too few animals surviving in a particular study, or because of the nature of the toxicity observed. As an example, irreversible effects such as teratogenicity may sometimes attract a higher (and somewhat arbitrary) safety factor. As the NOEL is usually expressed as mg of substance per kg body weight, mg/kg body weight/day, the ADI is based on the same units:

$$ADI = \frac{NOEL}{100} \, mg/kg \, body \, weight$$

It is often considered useful to factor in the average human body weight, taken by several regulatory authorities including the EU as 60 kg, to give the ADI in terms of mg per person:

$$ADI = \frac{NOEL \times 60}{100} \, mg \, per \, person$$

The ADI has received critical attention over the years, not least because of the arbitrary nature of the safety factor and the lack of scientific justification for its 10-by-10-fold nature. It has been suggested that increased scientific knowledge of pharmacokinetics and pharmacodynamics for specific molecules could be used to determine safety factors that are more scientifically sound. Thus, rather than a factor of 10 for species differences, and a further factor of 10 for human differences, there would be subfactors for species differences in kinetics and dynamics, and human differences in kinetics and dynamics for specific substances,[21] and so differences in absorption, first pass metabolism, renal plasma flow and plasma half-life could be taken into account.[22] However, the major drawback to such an approach is the lack of relevant data, particularly from human exposure, that would leave part of the safety factor incomplete, and would require more animal data to contribute to other aspects of the calculation. There are few examples where all of the necessary data are available.[23] Other approaches, including graphical representation of data[24] and the fitting of dose response models to toxicological data,[25] suffer from other drawbacks, but, as with the pharmacokinetic and pharmacodynamic approach, they require more data than are currently provided by routine laboratory testing. Although the ADI concept and the magnitude of the safety factor used to derive it have been addressed and refined by Renwick and others in recent years,[21,26–28] the considerations have yet to be extended to ADI calculations for veterinary drugs. What is more, there is now a large catalogue of drugs that would need to be re-evaluated if the approach to the calculation of the ADI was altered and it is still questionable if, even then, it would have any effect on the dimensions of the MRL. More importantly, it should be recognised that the ADI can change if new studies become available and, in any case, the value is a regulatory standard, not a scientific fact.[29]

The ADI is defined as the quantity of a substance or, in the context of this chapter, residues of a veterinary drug that can be ingested by humans over the course of a lifetime without causing adverse effects.[30] Clearly this definition too presents some problems, although these could be considered semantic in most cases. Consider a drug that is otherwise non-toxic, but causes some degree of foetotoxicity. The NOEL is then established on the basis of foetotoxicity, and the ADI calculated accordingly. It is likely that this ADI is applicable to only a limited part of the population, namely pregnant women, and probably only for a limited period of gestation (the sensitive stage of organogenesis). As it is the lowest NOEL that has been employed, then it can be argued that the entire population is protected. However, it does call into question the ADI definition and its concept of lifetime exposure. There is also concern about the ADI's ability to protect groups who might be more sensitive to the adverse effects of a substance such as the elderly, pregnant women and the very young.[31,32] While this is probably addressed by the current very large safety factors used in the ADI calculation, and further assumptions made in the elaboration of MRLs, it cannot be answered with any degree of certainty.

The microbiological safety of residues is also considered in the identification of NOELs. The issues here are not toxicological, but arise from several areas of concern on the possible adverse effects of residues of antimicrobial drugs.[33–37] These can be summarised as follows:

They might:

- Perturb the bacterial ecology of the gastrointestinal tract, particularly that of the colon
- Weaken the barrier effect of the gastrointestinal flora allowing the ingress and growth of pathogens

- As a result, thus increase the susceptibility and vulnerability of the consumer to pathogenic bacteria and, significantly, to bacteria pathogenic to the gastrointestinal tract
- Provide conditions that could lead to the colonisation of the gastrointestinal tract by other organisms, although not necessarily pathogens, including bacteria and fungi
- Provide conditions that could be conducive to the development of antimicrobial resistance.

Many of these concerns arise from the use of antimicrobial drugs in humans as therapeutic doses may lead to some of these effects. Indeed, sometimes the perturbations in colonic flora can be dramatic following the therapeutic use of antibiotics in humans and some antibiotics are used to sterilise the contents of the gastrointestinal tract prior to surgery. However, there is no firm evidence that minute quantities of residues present in food of animal origin can have such effects in humans and, as the concentrations of residues in food to which humans are exposed are extremely low, it seems highly unlikely that major adverse effects would occur. Nevertheless, it is considered prudent to investigate the potential of residues of antimicrobial drugs to adversely affect the human gastrointestinal flora. Unfortunately, there are no well-validated or even widely accepted experimental models for this, but several approaches are available:

Studies in humans – These involve human volunteers given doses of the test compound. The faeces are then examined for population changes in species of bacteria.

Studies in gnotobiotic animals – Gnotobiotic animals are animals whose own gut flora is absent. They are implanted with human gut flora and treated with antibiotic drugs to determine whether there are any adverse effects on the adopted bacteria. These studies are notoriously difficult to interpret, not least because the effects of the host animal on the implanted gut flora may be greater than those of the administered drug. Nevertheless, a recent study with germ-free mice investigated the effects of ciprofloxacin on the implanted human gut flora. The drug significantly decreased the populations of anaerobic bacteria, and notably the population of *Enterobacteriacae*. In mice challenged with a strain of *Salmonella* the bacteria were found in the faeces, suggesting a breakdown of the barrier effect. The NOEL in this study was found to be less than 0.125 mg/kg bw, the lowest dose used.[38] The study demonstrates the potential utility of this type of experiment in investigating the effects of antimicrobial substances on the human gut flora.

In vitro **studies** – These *in vitro* studies may examine a number of endpoints, including the development of antimicrobial drug resistance.[39–41] They generally involve determination of the so-called minimum inhibitory concentrations (MIC_{50} values) or some similar measurement, either through serial dilution or using continuous culture methodologies that aim to model microflora interactions, the ecology of the human colon and the effects of pH and anaerobiosis. It seems likely that a more systematic approach, using both *in vitro* and *in vivo* models, is likely to be employed in the future along with harmonised guidelines and approaches to hazard assessment.[39,42–44]

Many antimicrobial drugs have the capacity to disrupt fermentation due to toxic effects on the microorganisms involved. This is important if the drug is intended for use in lactating animals, where the milk may be employed to produce cheese or yoghurt. Under these circumstances it is necessary to conduct studies with dairy starter cultures to determine the likely inhibitive effect of the antimicrobial in question, and to identify the inhibitive concentration (Table 3.1). As these tests are very sensitive, this value usually plays a leading role in establishing the MRL and it may take precedence over the ADI value, especially if it is significantly lower.

Occasionally, the main biological effects of a drug may be pharmacological rather than toxicological, and again these may involve animal studies or investigations in humans. Such effects may be more significant with some substances such as anaesthetics, analgesics and β-agonists, as noted earlier with clenbuterol, than classical toxicological effects, and in those circumstances the NOEL, and the subsequent ADI, may be based on the pharmacological properties. Nevertheless, the important issue is to identify the residue of toxicological concern (or where relevant of microbiological or pharmacological concern) and to understand their pharmacokinetic and biological behaviours *in vivo*.[45–47]

The major requirements for EU MRLs are set out in a number of Guidelines issued by the CVMP through the EMEA, as well as in the *Rules Governing Medicinal Products in the European Union, Volume 8*. Together, these provide a major source of advice and guidance on all aspects relating to MRLs in the EU including such aspects as minor species, injection site residues and acceptable daily intakes. They are shown in Table 3.3.

3.3   MRLs – Other Considerations

Elaboration of MRLs is far more problematic in many ways than the calculation of ADI values. This is because a number of factors have to be taken into account. Fundamentally, the magnitude of the MRLs has to be such that consumers of food of animal origin do not exceed the ADI. In addition to this, the MRL values established for different tissues have to be practicable; there is little point in setting the MRL for muscle at an order of magnitude higher than that for liver for a particular species if pharmacokinetics and residues depletion data show that in reality the values are likely to be the other way around. Consequently, patterns of residues depletion across a limited range of tissues must also be considered and there is no simple equation to determine MRL values.

Some information on the distribution and metabolism of a specific drug in a particular animal species is provided by pharmacokinetic studies in that animal. However, the main information is provided by determination of specific

Table 3.3 Major EU Guidelines relevant to the establishment of MRLs.

Guideline	Content
Rules Governing Medicinal Products in the European Union. Volume 8. Notice to Applicants and Note for Guidance. Establishment of maximum residue limits (MRLs) for residues of veterinary medicinal products in foodstuffs of animal origin.	Covers all requirements for contents of the Safety file and Residues file, and provides advice on studies, methodology and legal requirements.
EMEA/CVMP/SWP/66781/2005 Safety and resides data requirements for veterinary medicinal products intended for minor uses or species.	Provides extensive advice on approach to be taken when developing data to support MRLs intended for a minor veterinary use or in a minor species.
EMEA/CVMP/153a/97-FINAL Note for guidance on the establishment of maximum residue limits for minor animal species.	General guidance on the approach to minor species and MRLs.
EMEA/CVMP/153b/97-FINAL Note for guidance on the establishment of maximum residue limits for *Salmonidae* and other fin fish.	Establishes criteria and procedures for determining MRLs for fish, notably for salmon.
EMEA/CVMP/SWP/139646/2005-CONSULTATION Concept paper on guidance on the approach to demonstrate whether a substance is capable of pharmacological activity.	Sets out ideas for developing a guideline to demonstrate pharmacological activity (or lack of it). Especially intended for use where sponsor attempts to demonstrate lack of pharmacological activity and hence exemption from MRL requirements.
EMEA/CVMP/542/03-FINAL Guideline on injection site residues.	Provides advice on scientific, procedural and regulatory aspects of injection site residues, including how to address the injection site from the sampling and analytical chemistry viewpoints.
EMEA/CVMP/SWP/122154/2005-CONSULTATION Concept paper on a guideline on the assessment of pharmacological/ pharmacodynamic data to establish a pharmacological ADI.	Establishes ideas to determine where appropriate pharmacological ADI on the basis of pharmacodynamic data.
EMEA/CVMP/276/99-FINAL Note for guidance for the assessment of the effect of antimicrobial substances on dairy starter cultures.	Provides guidance for the conduct and interpretation of studies designed to investigate inhibitory effects of anti-microbials *e.g.* on yogurt and cheese starter cultures.
EMEA/CVMP/187/00-FINAL Note for guidance on risk analysis approach for residues of veterinary medicinal products in food of animal origin.	Discusses extrapolation of MRLs from major to minor species or from several species to "all food species" based on risk analysis approach (see also EMEA/CVMP/069/02, Implementation of note for guidance on risk analysis approach for residues of veterinary medicinal products in food of animal origin).

Table 3.4   Daily food intake factors (grams) used in the EU in the elaboration of MRLs.

Large animals		Poultry		Fish/bees	
Muscle	300	Muscle	300	Muscle + skin	300
Liver	100	Liver	100	Honey	20
Kidney	50	Kidney	10		
Fat	50	Fat + skin	90		
Milk	1500	Eggs	100		

residues depletion profiles. Groups of the intended target species, cattle, sheep, pigs or fish for example, are given the drug at the therapeutic dose, sometimes in the intended market formulation, and subgroups of animals are then serially slaughtered (or milk and eggs collected at sequential time points) and tissues (or milk or eggs) collected for chemical or radiochemical analysis. In practice, the major tissues designated for analysis are muscle, liver, kidney and fat except for pigs, fish and poultry where skin, which is also eaten, is additionally analysed.

The amount of residue consumed by humans depends not only on how much is present in tissues and organs, but also on how much food containing the residue is eaten. Consequently, a "market basket" approach to food intake has been adopted. This makes use of food intakes that are certainly in excess of what might be considered normal but, in doing so, it does take into account individuals who might be considered to be extreme consumers. The values used in the EU are given in *Rules Governing Medicinal Products in the European Union, Volume 8* and are shown in Table 3.4. This approach could be improved by a more accurate knowledge of actual dietary intake and better information on dietary food and food commodity consumption.[48–50]

Thus, MRLs are elaborated rather than calculated by considering the practical aspects of pharmacokinetic factors and residues time-depletion profiles, particularly the depletion of the marker residue while bearing in mind the ADI, and ensuring that in considering the magnitude of the MRLs, the ADI values will not be exceeded. Under the requirements of Regulation No. (EC) 470/2009, MRLs must be practicable, and that is taken to mean, in part, that there is an adequate analytical method with which to determine the drug or its metabolites. Indeed, there is a direct requirement for the provision of an analytical method suitable for use in residues surveillance (Table 3.2).

Similar requirements for toxicity and residues depletion data exist under legislation in the United States.[4,51–55] Many of the issues surrounding the calculations of ADI values, the types of toxicity and residues studies to be conducted, the use of microbiological safety studies, to name but a few, apply here also.[56–59] In the US, there is no separate MRL legislation as such, and in fact the approach to determining safety limits is subtly different from that of the EU. Having calculated an ADI, the next step is to calculate a safe concentration for a particular tissue, for example for liver. Using an ADI value of 0.1 μg per kg per day, the safe concentration calculation (SC) is:

$$SC = \frac{ADI \times human\ weight}{Daily\ Tissue\ Intake}$$

$$SC = \frac{0.1\ \mu g/kg\ per\ day \times 60\ kg}{0.1\ kg/day} = 60\ \mu g/kg = 60\ ppb$$

Using this value, and data from total residues depletion studies, a tolerance for liver can be established for the drug. The same process can then be conducted for other tissues and for milk.[51,56] Food consumption values used in the United States are essentially similar to those used in the EU and are shown in Table 3.4. The tolerance is essentially equivalent to the MRL although the use of simple arithmetic to derive it makes it somewhat easier to understand. A different approach is used for carcinogenic veterinary drugs. The Federal Food, Drug and Cosmetic Act prohibits the use of carcinogenic drugs in food animals unless it can be shown that no residues are present as a result of drug treatment. Clearly, this is almost impossible as modern methods of analysis are capable of detecting minute amounts of compound. To ensure food safety, a model is used to estimate an upper limit of low-dose risk based on a lifetime risk of one per million as an "insignificant risk" for cancer. Due to uncertainties, including the uncertainties of animal to human extrapolation and those concerned with the magnitude of the risk, the model has numerous conservative elements in-built, thus ensuring consumer safety.[60]

The MRL and tolerance values are employed to derive withdrawal periods for marketed veterinary medicines.[61] The withdrawal period is the time from administration of the medicine, or last administration in a multidose regime, to the point where residues have depleted to below the MRL or tolerance. This is done by conducting studies where animals are treated with the medicine in question, as the formulation to be marketed, and then slaughtering the animals at intervals and analysing the key tissues of muscle, fat, liver and kidney. Similar studies are conducted with dairy cattle for milk and with poultry for eggs. A withdrawal period can be then derived by examining the time-dependent issue depletion (or depletion in milk or eggs) against the MRL or tolerance values. In practice, use is made of various statistical models in calculating the withdrawal period. The withdrawal period, or milk/egg withhold time, then becomes part of the terms of the marketing authorisation, and appears as such in the product literature and on the product label.[4,56] Farmers are then required to observe these withdrawal times after their animals have been treated with veterinary medicines to ensure that any residues present are below the relevant MRL or tolerance values.

The MRL process in the EU applied not only to new pharmacological substances, but also to existing ones used in food-animal products. From 1990 onwards, the CVMP undertook a major programme of work reviewing these older substances while at the same time dealing with applications for new chemical entities. Perhaps inevitably, some of these fell by the wayside and found their way into the prohibited list for safety reasons. Others were withdrawn by the sponsor either because of the costs of providing data packages, often for off-patent materials, or because the CVMP was unable to reach a conclusion on safety on the basis of the available data. The consequences for all of these materials are exactly the same – they cannot be used in veterinary medicinal products intended for food animals. Over the period 1992 to the present, a whole range of therapeutic substances was entered into one of the Annexes I to III of Council Regulation (EEC) No. 2377/90.[62,63] The majority of the substances entered into Annex I are antimicrobial drugs and antiparasitic agents including ectoparasiticides and endectocides. Similarly, a range of substances, mainly excipients, was entered into Annex II. These include salts, vitamins, medical gases, solvents, polymers and substances approved for use in foodstuffs. These substances are now listed in Table 1 of Regulation (EU) No. 37/2010.

3.4 The Joint FAO/WHO Expert Committee on Food Additives (JECFA)

JECFA began evaluating the toxicity and residues data on veterinary drugs in the mid-1980s, with a view to establishing MRL values.[64] The MRLs developed are subsequently used by the Codex Alimentarius system, which, like JECFA, is a joint FAO and WHO body, as part of its food standards programme, through the Codex Committee on Residues of Veterinary Drugs in Food.[15,16,65–68] In practice this means that veterinary drug assessments and MRL values are available to developing countries that might not have the means to conduct scientific assessments themselves, and that scientific monographs on toxicity and residues characteristics are readily available in the public domain. It also means that the deliberations and decisions of the JECFA are transparent as these are published in a separate report series.

Occasionally, the MRLs set by JECFA are different from those set by the EU or from US tolerances. Or JECFA might set an MRL whereas other bodies felt unable to do so. For example, the EU has not published an MRL for the anabolic steroid trenbolone acetate, whereas JECFA established an MRL.[69] This raises the spectre of trade disputes between the EU and countries that adopt the JECFA MRL, or at least its scientific approach, or those that develop and use their own national standards. Differences in scientific opinions can differ for a number of reasons including scientific approaches, attitudes to risk assessment, different risk-benefit conclusions or even from political influence.[70–73] However, some of the variations in MRLs that arise from various national, multinational (*e.g.* the EU) and international bodies (*e.g.* JECFA and Codex) arise not because of differences in the interpretation of toxicity data, but because different food intake values are used in their elaboration. Approaches to resolve this problem, which could lead to disputes between various trading blocks, would be either to harmonise food intake values across regulatory authorities and international bodies, or to determine the equivalence of MRLs to reveal whether or not the ADI values in each country are being exceeded.[74,75] However, the development of international food standards should not only help to protect consumers at the global level, but should also eventually prevent the erection of barriers to trade and ensuing international trade disputes,[17,76,77] in the same way that EU MRLs facilitate inter-community trade.

The risks involved in exceeding the ADI are dependent on the biological properties of individual drugs. The nature and magnitude of these risks can only be evaluated through knowledge of the extent of human consumer exposure and the dose response of the drug in the studies from which the NOEL (and hence the ADI value) were derived.[78] As violative residues form a part of veterinary pharmacovigilance in the EU, it is important that not only is there adequate residues surveillance, but also that any ensuing risks are seen in perspective. The MRL has a number of in-built conservatisms including the safety factors used in the calculation of the ADI and the magnitude of the food intake values. Exceeding the MRL by no means suggests that the ADI will be exceeded and, if it is, individual scientific analysis is required to determine if this presents a consumer safety issue. This may have specific implications if the concept of hormesis, adverse effects induced by very low levels of potentially toxic agents, is shown to have foundation.[79–84]

3.5   Practical Uses of MRLs

The major use of MRLs is in the determination of withdrawal periods. The withdrawal period, as already described, the period between treatment or last treatment in a multidose regimen and when the animal may be slaughtered for human consumption, is derived from the point when residues deplete to below the MRL in all target tissues in all the animals in a group. Similar concepts apply for milk and eggs, although here of course residues do not deplete and the commodity has to be discarded until residues fall below the MRL values for milk or eggs.[1,85] Honey often presents a particular problem as bees, which are treated on a hive basis, often need medication during the period of maximum honey flow. If this results in residues of honey above the MRL, it will mean that the honey produced is not suitable for human consumption, as the residues do not deplete. Consequently, drugs for the treatment of diseases in bees need to be formulated so that MRLs for honey are not exceeded in the first instance. Fish are poikilothermic animals but possess extensive drug-metabolising capacities.[86–91] Their rates of metabolism and indeed the nature of their metabolic processes can vary with the ambient water temperature, depending on the species of fish, as well as season, sex and prior exposure to inducers of cytochrome P-450.[2,86,88,92–102] Hence, whereas withdrawal periods for mammals and avian species are quoted in days, those for fish are quoted in degree days to take account of the dual effects of time and temperature.[2]

Withdrawal periods are legal requirements in the EU and in several other countries and are established during the authorisation process. In the EU, the withdrawal period, even if it is zero, must appear in the product literature and on the label for veterinary medicines intended for food-producing animals. However, it is futile imposing withdrawal periods if these are not observed in practice. Withdrawal periods and MRLs must be monitored and enforced through surveillance for residues of veterinary drugs in food of animal origin.

A number of problems can arise with MRLs and their practical application. One issue that can cause problems is the persistence of residues at the intramuscular or subcutaneous injection site.[85,103–111] This is particularly noticeable in the case of irritant drugs, which may cause inflammation, necrosis, fibrosis and encapsulation of the injection site leading to enhanced drug persistence. It is particularly significant as some products are designed to act in this way to provide a convenient depot effect. These can lead to long withdrawal periods, which experience suggests are more likely to be ignored, and they can result in violative residues as a consequence. There is now growing regulatory opposition in some parts of the EU and elsewhere to the authorisation of such formulations.

Injection site residues are usually taken into account by basing the withdrawal period on depuration of residues at that injection site that is treated as normal muscle. This generally results in long withdrawal times, which not only may result in the affected veterinary product being regarded as less commercially attractive, but also may mean that the withdrawal period is ignored, with the consequence of violative residues occurring. One solution is to discount the injection site either in the establishment of MRLs or in the setting of withdrawal periods. This would mean that residues at the injection site were evaluated toxicologically to ensure consumer safety without having a formal MRL value in place. These issues need to be resolved, not only to assure consumer safety, but also to prevent disruption of international trade in meat and meat products.[112] In the EU, the CVMP has developed a guideline on this issue (Table 3.3).

Problems can also arise when drugs are used off-label.[113] The MRL is based on the residues depletion and hence pharmacokinetic behaviour in the target animal. If used in another species, residues problems could occur, although this is probably unlikely. One way around this problem is to have very long withdrawal periods. This approach is used in the EU where standard withdrawal periods are employed. These are greatly in excess of any withdrawal period that is likely to have been arrived at through the conventional use of residue depletion studies. Another approach is used in the US through establishing safe concentrations for off-label use. Other proposals employ provisional acceptable intakes to assess safety and establish withdrawal periods and risk-based approaches.[114,115]

As already alluded to, generating the safety and residues data to support MRL applications is extremely expensive. Not surprisingly, manufacturers prefer not to make this investment for either minor therapeutic uses (*e.g.* rare diseases) or for minor species (*e.g.* rabbits, goats, deer, reindeer, ducks, turkeys and fish) and generating the data required to support MRL applications may result in a fall in innovation in the pharmaceutical sector and a concomitant rise in innovation in the biologics area. Even when toxicity data are available to establish MRLs for major species it still leaves a significant cost to generate residues depletion and pharmacokinetic data in the minor species, to develop a validated analytical assay and then to generate depletion data post-MRL to determine withdrawal periods. In view of this, the CVMP has drawn up guidance and advice for establishing MRLs for minor species. Historically, MRLs have been established on a species-specific basis but the CVMP has used a risk-based approach to extrapolate MRLs from major species to minor or from major species to "all food species" or "all ruminant species", depending on the available data. This has served to make MRLs "available" to food species that would otherwise have been left without and, consequently, deprived of appropriate medications.

However, even with this provision, the costs of generating species-specific data for post-MRL withdrawal period depletion studies can be significant. This often means that sponsors are deterred from investments in minor species products. This is particularly important with fish for although it might be economic to generate data for a major fish species such as Atlantic salmon, it might prove less attractive to go on further and to generate data packages for other species, even related ones like rainbow trout. Faced with a range of chemotherapeutic products for use in aquaculture, and a number of species,[116–120] this obviously raises major issues for therapeutic treatment and animal welfare. This has led to the concept of crop grouping where a surrogate species represents a number of species or even many species. In addition to water temperature, a number of factors affect drug metabolism, distribution and excretion in fish including gill ventilation volumes and rate, gill anatomy, intestinal anatomy and motility and cardiac output and oxygen consumption rate. Taking these factors into account along with phylogenetic considerations and typical habitat temperatures, it should be possible to group types or species of fish together and generate regulatory data in one to satisfy requirements for all.[121,122] The US authorities have expressed an interest in this approach, providing the concept of crop grouping stands up to scientific scrutiny.[123] However, there currently appears to be no enthusiasm for this approach outside of the US and the CVMP has instead embarked on the route of extrapolating MRLs from major species to minor species based on a minimal data set.

3.6 Residues Surveillance

The EU and the United States have in place extensive systems for residues surveillance so that residues can be monitored and violations of statutory limits such as MRLs can be detected.[3,4,58,63,124–127] This not only provides significant confidence for consumers, but also allows offenders who have permitted violations to occur to be prosecuted. The results of residues monitoring are published in many countries including the US and the UK. These results demonstrate that residues of veterinary medicines are indeed generally very low in food of animal origin, and that MRL and tolerance violations are extremely rare.[58,126,128,129]

Violative residues may occur because withdrawal periods have not been observed (or are inadequate), because higher doses or longer periods of administration than those authorised and specified in product literature have been used or because illegal or unauthorised drugs have been given. The purpose of residues surveillance is to monitor the levels of compliance in a country or geopolitical area.

However, regulatory systems of any type depend on two main factors as a measure of success – compliance by those they are aimed at and public confidence by those they aim to protect. If lack of compliance comes to be regarded as the norm, then public confidence may collapse. Once that collapse has occurred, it is extremely difficult, and occasionally virtually impossible, to regain the trust that has been lost. Establishing the safety and residue depletion profiles of veterinary drugs, and elaborating MRLs and subsequently determining withdrawal periods for food of animal origin, is an interesting (and expensive) but ultimately futile exercise, if those withdrawal periods are then ignored or rendered useless by overdosing or by dosing for periods longer than those recommended. Similarly, the system will fall into disrepute, and again may be seen as failing, if drugs prohibited on the basis of potential human health risks are used to treat food-producing animals. Even if these abuses fail to materialise, through consumption of food from third countries, where different MRLs are employed, or where MRLs have not been established for some or all veterinary drugs used in food animals, consumers may be exposed, at worst, to potentially hazardous residues and, at best, to residues arising from drugs that have not been fully evaluated.

It is clearly in the interests of government institutions to ensure that legislation is enforced and is seen to be enforced effectively, particularly on issues related to food safety. In the United States too, food safety lobbying is a reality and consumer-based advocacy groups lobby Congress in attempts to strengthen legislation and enforcement.[124]

Concerns over the safety of residues, particularly their potential toxic effects, have been expressed over the last 30 years.[31,49,50,53,55,65,82,112,124–127,130] Some of these issues have been addressed elsewhere in this chapter. However, it is concerns such as these that have initially led to and later refined legislation relating to the registration of veterinary drugs, the establishment of MRLs and surveillance of residues of veterinary drugs in food of animal origin.

3.6.1 Residues and Residues Studies

Residues are the metabolites of veterinary drugs, and their associated parent compounds, that remain in the animal or its produce (eggs, milk and honey) after treatment. Their behaviour depends on the nature of the drug and its metabolites and on the pharmacokinetics of the drug in the animal concerned. Those that are metabolised and excreted rapidly also rapidly deplete in the treated animal. Those that are slowly metabolised may also deplete rapidly if their excretion is not dependent on metabolism. Others may be subject to slow excretion, especially those that bind to macromolecules and are thus not available for metabolism and/or excretion. The majority of animals that are now farmed, including fish and shellfish, are susceptible to arrays of bacterial, fungal or parasitic disease and there are ranges of drugs available for the treatment of these conditions as indeed there are for a variety of non-infectious diseases. Some drugs may be metabolised largely to physiological substances such as water, bicarbonate and carbon dioxide, and be excreted relatively rapidly. Others may be converted to a variety of metabolites, which together with any remaining parent drug may depurate over shorter or longer periods of time.

Residues may be found in all edible tissues. Although the behaviour of drugs in animals may be examined through residues depletion studies, a more comprehensive understanding may be gleaned through well-conducted pharmacokinetic studies so that metabolism, distribution and excretion can be investigated, along with some of the determining factors.[128] This also assists in demonstrating species differences, if any, between animal species and, together with results from similar studies in laboratory species, provides a better picture of the processes involved, the nature of the metabolites and the rates of clearance and excretion. A good understanding of the pharmacokinetic behaviour of drugs, especially in the food animals to be treated, can underpin the design of formal residues studies and help to reduce costs and the need to repeat work. Furthermore, targeted analytical chemistry and other physico-chemical methods of analysis for residues can only be attempted if the likely metabolites, or more appropriately analytes, are known and understood.[1,95,59,63,129–135]

Milk and fish are frequently regarded as "healthy" foods of high nutritional value. The presence of drug residues in these foods, and particularly the presence of antibiotic residues, is regarded by consumers as especially troublesome (if not hazardous) because of this perception. However, residues of veterinary drugs can and do find their ways into these commodities.[136–149] Similarly, the presence of residues in eggs and poultry products also gives rise to consumer concerns,[150–154] while residues of almost any substance regarded as a pesticide, despite their veterinary use, can lead to consumer concerns and such substances are found in food of animal origin.[135,137,141,155,156]

In the EU, the hormonal growth promoters such as testosterone and trenbolone acetate were banned from use in food animals in 1988 (although they are still authorised in some non-EU countries; see Chapter 13). This was partly on consumer health grounds, although this was not considered at the time to be a critical issue and socioeconomic and trade issues played a major part in the story,[69,157–160] largely because residues of these drugs are low in concentration and for natural hormones, generally within normal physiological limits. Directive 96/22/EC confirmed this prohibition and added other substances such as thyrostatic compounds, drugs with oestrogenic, androgenic or gestagenic activity and some β-agonists. Some of these substances, for example testosterone, zeranol, trenbolone acetate and allyl trenbolone, had previously been used, some quite legally, as growth promoters or production enhancers, particularly in cattle.[161–172] A number of these possess potent endocrine activity[173,174] but a recent report by the UK's Veterinary Products Committee recognises some potential hazards and associated risks arising from the use of these hormonal substances, but fails to give a firm endorsement of the EU-wide ban.[175] Other drugs, such as the β-agonists salbutamol and clenbuterol, had been authorised for therapeutic purposes including tocolysis in cattle, but not for performance enhancement purposes. These drugs have repartitioning effects, reducing body fat while increasing lean tissue deposition.[176] Under Directive 96/22/EC the uses of many of these agents were restricted to therapeutic uses (*e.g.* testosterone and some β-agonist drugs) or prohibited altogether for use in food animals (*e.g.* trenbolone and its derivatives and zeranol). The milk production enhancer bovine somatotropin (BST) was also prohibited in the EU but this was largely for socioeconomic reasons although animal welfare concerns were cited at the time.[177] Regardless, BST has been used for several years in the US and in other countries without any major animal health problems.

To ensure regulatory compliance, residues surveillance is conducted in all EU countries.[1,4,63,178–180] Under Directive 96/23/EC, the competent authorities of EU member states are required to submit each year to the European Commission for approval an annual plan for sample collection and residues analyses to be conducted the following year. The numbers in each plan, and the analytes to be determined, are largely based on the results of previous years and on risk assessments.[1] Applicants for MRLs are required to submit an analytical method suitable for determining reasons with their submission. This may be used, with or without adaptation, for residues surveillance for the drug in question. In addition, EU control and reference laboratories develop their own methods for products of interest while there is a bewildering array available in the literature or in specialised texts.[1,77,181–187] The analytical methods used must comply with the requirements of Commission Directive 2002/657/EC, which establishes performance characteristics for these methods.

3.6.2   Residues Surveillance for Veterinary Drugs in the UK

As already described, veterinary drug residue surveillance in the United Kingdom is part of a broader European Union exercise that is permanently in place. The competent authority for drug residue surveillance in the UK is the Veterinary Medicines Directorate (VMD), which has been responsible for the scheme for many years and which since 2001 has devolved parts of that task, including the provision of guidance and advice to the Veterinary Residues Committee (VRC), which has recently been reconstituted as a committee of experts. The VRC is an independent committee that "provides oversight into how the UK's surveillance for residues is carried out". The reports of veterinary surveillance in the UK are published annually and provide a detailed source of data, one of the main reasons why the UK model was chosen to exemplify residues surveillance activities.[129,188–201]

In the UK, the exercise conducted under the EU legislation is known as the Statutory Surveillance Scheme. In addition to this there is a Non-Statutory Surveillance Scheme funded by UK government that is based on UK rather than on EU priorities. It is a more limited programme, which examines residues in foods eaten by average consumers or of foods consumed by susceptible groups such as infants.

In the Statutory Scheme the numbers of MRL violations were low in 2001. Most of these were related to tetracycline and sulfonamide residues in pig kidney but these occurred in 2–8 samples out of over 1000 tested. Similarly, only a small number of samples of hen kidney and turkey kidney appeared to have residues of antimicrobial drugs above the MRL. One sample of cattle liver from 331 tested had residues of avermectin drugs above the MRL. Only one sheep sample, of 746 tested, had residues of organophosphorus compounds above the MRL. This might appear surprising in view of the numbers of sheep dipped in organophosphorus formulations each year. However, various surveys of organophosphorus residues in a number of food commodities have shown that concentrations of these compounds are generally very low.[135] Several unauthorised or prohibited drugs were detected, but the numbers in all cases were low.

In 2006, the overall numbers were again very low and only small numbers of samples from each category proved positive by exceeding the reference point. The major finding of note was nicarbazin residues in 26 of 305 samples of broiled liver and 17 cattle with progesterone concentrations in excess of the reference point in 17 of 373 samples. In the latter case, the majority of the 17 samples only marginally exceeded the reference point of 0.5 µg/kg and it remains likely that the material was of endogenous, rather than exogenous, origin.

The Non-Statutory Scheme looked at a number of areas. Again, the numbers of residues violations were low. For 2001, there were 1320 samples included in the plan and 7726 analyses intended while in 2006 there were 1483 samples and 5030 analyses. In this latter scheme in 2006, some 34 residues were detected at concentrations above the action limits and of particular interest and concern were residues of nitrofurans found in warm-water crustacean samples, a finding that will undoubtedly promote further research and regulatory action.

For the latest year for which results are available, 2010, residue concentrations were usually below the MRL or other limits in most of the samples examined.[201] The notable findings were nicarbazin in chicken liver in 29 out of 639 samples analysed and low positive rates for all of the antimicrobial drugs in cattle tissue (Table 3.5). A small number of cattle and sheep urine samples gave positive results for the prohibited steroid hormones boldenone and nortestosterone.

Similar findings were made in the scheme for the 2002 to 2009 period.[193–200] These results provide significant reassurance on the safety of food of animal origin available in the UK. They are similar to the results obtained in previous years.[175–192] Although some of the MRL violations almost certainly arose from failure to observe withdrawal periods, there is probably also a significant contribution from contamination of unmedicated feed with components of medicated feed at feed mills. Here, MRL violations may occur as a result of the contamination (or carryover) of unmedicated feed with sulfonamide, chlortetracycline, penicillins and ionophore antimicrobials such as monensin,[202–211]

Table 3.5 Occurrence of unauthorised or prohibited drugs in the Statutory Surveillance Scheme, 2010.

Commodity	Analyte	Number of samples	Number with drug above reference point
Egg	Nicarbazin	465	2
Trout muscle	Malachite green/ leucomalachite green	101	1
Milk	Nitroxynil	498	6[a]
	Triclabendazole sulfone		1
Broiler liver	Ionophores and nicarbazin	639	
	Diclazuril		3
	Maduramycin		1[a]
	Nicarbazin		29[a]
Calf kidney	Oxytetracycline	185	3[a]
	Sulfadiazine		1[a]
Cattle kidney	Florfenicol	101	3[a]
Cattle kidney	Dihydrostreptomycin	1318	2[a]
Cattle kidney	Nitrofurans	158	1
Cattle kidney	Ibuprofen	735	3
Cattle serum	Testosterone	567	1
Cattle urine	Steroids	2178	
	Boldenone		11
	Nortestosterone		6
Cattle urine	Thiouracil	409	3
Cattle urine	Zeranol	314	3
Horse kidney	Phenylbutazone	60	5
Pig kidney	Chlortetracycline	840	2[a]
	Sulfadiazine		2[a]
Sheep kidney	Dihydrostreptomycin	2780	1[a]
Sheep liver	Oxfendazole	961	1[a]
Sheep urine	Steroids	450	
	Alpha-boldenone		7
	Alpha-nortestosterone		10

[a]In excess of EU MRL; remainder in excess of other limit such as limit of quantitation of the analytical assay.

which is of concern because of the implications for monitoring and control and as other contaminants, particularly microbiological varieties, might also be present.[212] An ADI approach has been suggested to evaluate the impact of this problem.[213] The surveillance results are similar to those found for residues surveillance in the United States, although here penicillin and streptomycin are major contributors. Failure to observe withdrawal periods was a major factor in the origin of violative residues in the US.[58,127]

Residue violations in fish tissue might occur from environmental exposure to veterinary medicines. However, far more likely is contamination arising from other environmental pollutants.[214,215] For example, a recent survey of residues in farmed salmon from around the world has revealed polychlorinated dibenzo-p-dioxins, dibenzofurans, DDT, chlordane and heptachlor epoxide.[216] Nevertheless, environmental contamination with veterinary drugs has given rise to concern over the eventual occurrence of residues in food of animal origin,[205] particularly from farmyard slurry.[217] Concern has also been expressed over contamination of surface waters in the USA by the anabolic growth promoter trenbolone, a constituent of feedlot effluent,[218] and whether oestrogenic growth promoters in the environment might evoke adverse events.[173] Some of these issues are discussed in more detail in Chapter 16.

Although reports of adverse effects in humans from residues of veterinary drugs in food are rare, they have occurred following ingestion of veal liver containing residues of the β-agonist drug clenbuterol,[219–221] and, in 2003, 39 people in Liaoyang, China, were affected by pork containing clenbuterol residues with 29 requiring hospital treatment for symptoms including involuntary twitching and acute thirst.[222] In general, however, it is difficult to associate human health problems with residues of veterinary drugs. Any adverse effects are likely to be acute rather than chronic, as illustrated by the example of clenbuterol.[56,58,124,125,223] The determination of NOELs involves laboratory animal studies and relatively high doses of test compounds, while the calculation of ADI values makes use of large safety factors, and so the elaboration of MRLs errs on the side of consumer safety. Hence, it is extremely unlikely that minor violations have any significant public health implications.[184]

Residues surveillance indicates that residues concentrations, particularly those of antimicrobial drugs, are low in milk, but there are reports of so-called bulk tank failures.[223,224] These occur not because of violation of any MRL by specific substances, but because the tests used by the dairy producers are inherently more sensitive and these are used as industry standards rather than as regulatory or consumer safety limits.[225–228] The Delvotest SP, a specific test used widely by the dairy industry, can detect several antibiotics used in cattle, including cloxacillin, framycetin, neomycin, penicillin G and sulfonamides, at concentrations below the MRL.[229] Such tests can therefore cause major problems for farmers. Although they may have observed the requirements of the product literature, including the withdrawal period, and although the concentration of the antibiotic may be well below the MRL, the milk may still fail the "standard" imposed by the dairy industry and the farmer is then faced with a financial penalty.[229–231] This is complicated by the fact that some of the available tests are sensitive to natural inhibitory substances found in milk, such as those produced soon after calving.[229] Although failure in these tests can often carry a financial penalty, they are not a pharmacovigilance issue unless confirmatory methods of analysis demonstrate that there has been a violation of the MRL.

3.7 Residues Avoidance

Clearly, the most appropriate way of avoiding residues in food of animal origin is to use only those veterinary medicines authorised for the specific use in the species concerned at the recommended doses, for the recommended dosing periods and subsequently observing the recommended withdrawal periods. However, clinical necessity occasionally requires that animals, including food-producing animals, be treated with non-authorised drugs when there is no suitable alternative available and this is foreseen and permitted under certain circumstances by EU legislation. Directive 2001/82/EC, as amended by Directive 2004/28/EC, requires EU Member States to permit a veterinarian, under "his direct personal responsibility", and specifically in the interests of animal welfare, to make some exceptions to the use of authorised products, where there is no suitable authorised product in the Member State concerned. These are:

- To use a product authorised in the Member State for another species, or for the treatment of another condition in the same species
- If no product exists, to use a product authorised for human use in the Member State concerned or
- To use a product authorised in another EU Member State for use in the same species or in another food-producing species for the condition or for another condition or
- To use a product prepared extemporaneously by a person authorised to do this under national legislation in the Member State concerned.

If any of these alternatives, widely known as the cascade, are followed, then prolonged withdrawal periods, commonly referred to as standard withdrawal periods, must be applied in accordance with the Directive. These are:

- Eggs – 7 days
- Milk – 7 days
- Meat from poultry and mammals – 28 days
- Fish – 500 degree days

Use of these extended withdrawal periods for off-label use should ensure that residues have depleted to safe and non-violative concentrations in the commodity concerned and any risk must be seen as being restricted to produce from individual animals as the cascade is not envisaged for use in large numbers – for the majority of diseases of livestock and other food animals, authorised medicinal products are available. Further reassurance can be obtained where necessary using a withdrawal estimator algorithm.[232]

Withdrawal periods are established in the EU and in other countries using statistical methods that are the subject of EU Guidelines. Readers should be aware that other methods of determination are available.[232–236] Suitable withdrawal periods, the awareness of the responsibilities placed on them by farmers and veterinarians, adequate record keeping and ensuring Good Agricultural (and Veterinary) Practice should together serve to ensure that the chances of obtaining violative residues are minimised.[237–244] Some product formulations, especially those intentionally formulated for depot effects, can prolong residues depletion.[245,246] This is particularly true for products intended for intramuscular or subcutaneous injection, as discussed earlier, where prolonged absorption can be both a therapeutic benefit and a residues risk, especially at the site of the injection itself. Persistence of residues at the injection site is a major problem with injectable formulations.[85,104–107,109–111,247] As a result of inter-animal variations, these products do not easily lend themselves to the use of statistical methods for withdrawal period calculation and, under these circumstances, risk management techniques, including basing withdrawal periods on the basis of the temporal depuration of residues at the injection site to below the MRL for muscle, may be the only practical resort, even though this may result in exceptionally long withdrawal periods.[11,85,245,105,248] This brings with it the problem of observance of withdrawal periods – they may well be ignored by farmers if there are what are considered to be overriding economic or animal husbandry considerations, even though the risk of an individual eating an injection site is low and the hazard presented is an acute one rather than the long-term option embodied in the MRL concept through the use of the ADI. Consequently, it is in the interests of sound science to establish practicable withdrawal periods where injection sites are involved on the basis of residues depletion focussed on an acute factor rather than on the MRL.[11,85]

The effects of cooking have been examined for a limited range of products to determine if this could reduce residue concentrations. Some cooking procedures can lead to reductions in residue content although the mechanisms involved are obscure as only small amounts of drug appear to be leached into the cooking liquids (which themselves may be used for culinary purposes). For example, some cooking methods significantly reduced concentrations of residues of nicarbazin in some food commodities whereas other methods had little effect.[249] Cooking had minimal or no effects on concentrations of chloramphenicol, oxytetracycline, streptomycin, sulfadimidine (sulfamethazine) or ampicillin in beef.[250] Benzylpenicillin was stable at 65 °C but not at higher temperatures. Up to 50% of residues present in meat passed into cooking fluids.[251] Oxytetracycline and tetracycline residue concentrations were significantly reduced by cooking,[252,253] while sulfadimidine was found to be thermally stable.[254] Oxfendazole residues were seemingly reduced at high temperatures for prolonged periods, but this resulted in the formation of an amine derivative, formed from hydrolysis of the carbamate moiety,[255] which then raises questions over the safety of this material. The quinolone drugs oxolinic acid and flumequine were stable during cooking of fish.[256] Levamisole and clenbuterol were stable in boiling water but unstable at 260 °C in cooking oil.[257,258] Ivermectin was also stable, although up to 50% of total residue was leached by the cooking liquids.[259] Ronidazole was converted to a 2-hydroxy derivative in aqueous conditions, whereas dimetridazole was seemingly stable.[260] With most of these substances, the relevance to human food safety is unclear as the identities and biological properties of the degradation products are unknown.[261] Some sulfonamide drugs appear to degrade on prolonged frozen storage but were seemingly stable for up to 3 months.[255,262] Sulfadimidine may be converted to the N^4-glucopyranosyl derivative on prolonged storage in pig liver[263] but, once again, the implications of this for consumer safety are unknown.

All of this demonstrates that reliance on cooking and food processing to reduce residue concentrations in food is unwise. While processing may have some beneficial effects in diluting residue concentrations, too little is known about the fate of these residues and the safety of any degradation products to place any reliance on cooking, freezing or any other form of processing in ensuring consumer safety.

3.8   Conclusions

Residue violations usually occur because animals have been overdosed with drug or because the withdrawal period has not been observed. As MRLs are intended to protect consumer health from any potential harmful effects of residues in food of animal origin, then clearly violation of MRLs may constitute a public health risk. However, the consumer is only likely to be at risk if the ADI value is also exceeded and, even then, there are a number of conservatisms built into the ADI and the MRL to ensure that, in most cases, there will be no significant health risk. Nevertheless, policing of concentrations of residues of authorised drugs, and indeed policing of residues of illegal or prohibited drugs is of importance to prevent veterinary drug misuse and abuse and to ensure sound public health practices are maintained. It is clearly in the interests of international trade to ensure that MRLs are harmonised, and that food commodities are not the subjects of violative residues or of trade disputes (see Chapter 13).

The MRL concept is a more practical approach to the evaluation of the safety of veterinary drug residues in food of animal origin than any of the possible contenders, including zero tolerance and widespread application of the precautionary principle,[264,265] and they are likely to be around, in one form or another, for some time to come, despite the fact that they can be regarded by some as counter-productive and contrary to the use of scientific principles in safety assessment.[266,267]

Violative residues are problematic in that infringements are generally "invisible". A veterinarian, milk processor, farmer or butcher cannot know if an animal has violative residues, unlike the situation with adverse drug reactions where an obvious and reportable event usually occurs. In general, violative residues are only detected by government agencies in pursuit of surveillance schemes of the types described here. However, other agencies do examine food for residues. These include milk suppliers and processors and food retailers and the onus is very much with them to report any residue violations that they detect to the responsible authorities. Under these restricted circumstances, reporting of residues violations are analogous to other areas of reporting in pharmacovigilance activities. Failure to observe withdrawal periods may lead to violative residues and subsequent recalls of affected food commodities as happened recently in the UK with residues, including residues of doramectin in lamb where breeding animals were inadvertently sent to slaughter.[268,269] However, with doramectin at least, residues may deplete at different rates in parasitised and non-parasitised sheep[270] and this may be representative, or at least indicative, of residue depletion in other animals with other drugs and diseases.

Together, the MRL approach, which is primarily based on consumer safety considerations, and the residues surveillance systems in place across most of the globe, offers a valuable service in providing consumers of animal produce with a large measure of reassurance.

References

1. S. N. Dixon, Veterinary drug residues in *Food Chemical Safety*, ed. D. H. Watson, CRC Press/Woodhead Publishing, Cambridge, 2001, vol. 1, pp. 109–147.
2. R. Ancuceanu, Maximum residue limits of veterinary medicinal products and their regulation in European Community law, *Eur. Law J.*, 2003, **9**, 215–240.
3. K. N. Woodward, Progress with the establishment of maximum residue limits for veterinary drugs in the European Union, *Toxicol. Environ. News*, 1997, **4**, 46–54.
4. K. N. Woodward, Regulation of veterinary drugs in *General and Applied Toxicology*, ed. B. Ballantyne, T. Marrs and T. Syversen, Macmillan Reference Ltd, Basingstoke, 2nd edn, 2000, pp. 1633–1652.
5. K. N. Woodward, Elements of veterinary pharmacovigilance in *Veterinary Pharmacovigilance. Adverse Reactions to Veterinary Medicinal Products*, Wiley-Blackwell, Chichester, 2009, pp. 9–17.
6. J. E. Baer, T. A. Jacob and F. J. Wolf, Cambendazole and nondrug macromolecules in tissue residues, *J. Toxicol. Environ. Health*, 1977, **2**, 895–903.
7. T. M. Farber, Problems in the evaluation of tissue residues, *J. Environ. Pathol. Toxicol.*, 1980, **3**, 73–79.
8. S. S. Thorgeirsson and P. J. Wirth, Covalent binding of foreign chemicals to tissue macromolecules, *J. Toxicol. Environ. Health*, 1977, **2**, 873–881.
9. N. E. Weber, Overview of bound residue chemistry, *Drug Metab. Rev.*, 1990, **22**, 611–615.
10. JECFA, *Procedures for the Testing of Intentional Food Additives to Establish their Safety for Use*, Second Report of the Joint FAO/WHO Expert Committee on Food Additives, WHO Technical report Series 144, WHO, Geneva, 1957.
11. World Health Organization, *Principles for the Safety Evaluation of Food Additives and Contaminants in Food, Environmental Health Criteria 70*, World Health Organization, Geneva, 1987.
12. D. Benson, *The Acceptable Daily Intake. A Tool for Ensuring Food Safety*, International Life Sciences Institute (ILSI) Monograph, ILSI, 2000, Brussels.
13. E. Poulsen, René Truhaut and the acceptable daily intake: A personal note, *Teratog. Carcinog. Mutagen.*, 1995, **15**, 273–275.
14. World Health Organization, *Principles and Methods for Risk Assessment of Chemicals in Food*, Chapter 8, Maximum residue limits for pesticides

and veterinary drugs, Environmental Health Criteria 240, World Health Organization, Geneva, 2009, pp. 8-2–8-53.

15. J. L. Herrman and M. Younes, Background to the ADI/TDI/PTWI, *Regul. Toxicol. Pharmacol.*, 1999, **30**, S109–S113.
16. J. Herrman, The role of the World Health Organisation in the evaluation of pesticides, *Regul. Toxicol. Pharmacol.*, 1993, **17**, 282–286.
17. K. N. Woodward, Choice of safety factor in setting acceptable daily intakes, *Reg. Affairs J.*, 1991, **2**, 787–790.
18. K. N. Woodward, Assessing the safety of veterinary drug residues in *Pesticide, Veterinary and Other Residues in Food*, ed. D. H. Watson, CRC Press/Woodhead Publishing, Cambridge, 2004, pp. 157–174.
19. K. N. Woodward, The evolution of safety assessments for veterinary medicinal products in the European Union, *Vet. Hum. Toxicol.*, 2004, **46**, 199–205.
20. J. A. Zarn, B. E. Engeli and J. R. Schlatter, Study parameters influencing NOAEL and LOAEL in toxicity feeding studies for pesticides: Exposure duration versus dose decrement, dose spacing, group size and chemical class, *Regul. Toxicol. Pharmacol.*, 2011, **61**, 243–250.
21. A. G. Renwick, Safety factors and establishment of acceptable daily intakes, *Food Add. Contam.*, 1991, **8**, 135–150.
22. A. G. Renwick, Data-derived safety factors for the evaluation of food additives and environmental contaminants, *Food Add. Contam.*, 1993, **10**, 275–305.
23. R. Kroes, I. Munro and E. Poulsen, Workshop on the scientific evaluation of the safety factor for the acceptable daily intake (ADI): editorial summary, *Food Add. Contam.*, 1993, **10**, 269–273.
24. M. L. Dourson, R. C. Hertzberg, R. Hartung and K. Blackburn, Novel methods for the estimation of acceptable daily intake, *Toxicol. Ind. Health*, 1985, **1**, 23–33.
25. K. S. Crump, A new method for determining allowable daily intakes, *Fundam. Appl. Toxicol.*, 1984, **4**, 854–871.
26. International Programme on Chemical Safety, *Chemical-Specific Adjustment Factors for Interspecies Differences and Human Variability. Guidance Document for Use of Data in Dose/Concentration-Response Assessment*, World Health Organization, 2005, Geneva.
27. A. G. Renwick, Structure-based thresholds of toxicological concern – guidance for application to substances present at low levels in the diet, *Toxicol. Appl. Pharmacol.*, 2005, **207**(2), 585–591.
28. E. D. Rubery, S. M. Barlow and J. H. Steadman, Criteria for setting quantitative estimates of intakes of chemicals in food in the U.K., *Food Add. Contam.*, 1990, **7**, 287–302.
29. C. D. Carrington and P. M. Bolger, The limits of regulatory toxicology, *Toxicol. Appl. Pharmacol.*, 2010, **243**, 191–197.
30. J. A. Zarn, E. Hänggi, A. Kuchen and J. R. Schlatter, The significance of the subchronic toxicity in the dietary risk assessment of pesticides, *Regul. Toxicol. Pharmacol.*, 2010, **58**, 72–78.

31. A. Somogyi, Residues of carcinogenic animal drugs in food: difficulties in evaluation of human safety in *Carcinogenic Risks. Strategies for Intervention*, International Agency for Research on Cancer (IARC) Scientific Publication No. 25, IARC, Lyon, France, 1979.
32. A. B. Gebara, C. H. Ciscato, S. H. Monteiro and G. S. Souza, Pesticide residues in some commodities: dietary risk for children, *Bull. Environ. Contam. Toxicol.*, 2011, **86**, 506–510.
33. J. Boisseau, Basis for the evaluation of the microbiological risks due to veterinary drug residues in food, *Vet. Microbiol.*, 1993, **35**, 187–192.
34. D. E. Corpet, An evaluation of the methods to assess the effect of anti-microbial residues on human gut flora, *Vet. Microbiol.*, 1992, **35**, 199–212.
35. D. E. Corpet, Current models for testing antibiotic residues, *Vet. Hum. Toxicol.*, 1993, **35**(1), 37–46.
36. S. L. Gorbach, Perturbation of the intestinal microflora, *Vet. Hum. Toxicol.*, 1993, **35**, 15–23.
37. A. R. M. Kidd, *The Potential Risk of Effects of Antimicrobial Residues on Human Gastro-Intestinal Microflora*, Report prepared at the invitation of Federation European de la Santé Animale (FEDESA), FEDESA, Brussels, Belgium, 1994.
38. A. Perrin-Guyomard, M. P. Poul, D. E. Corpet, P. Sanders, H. Fernández and M. Bartholomew, Impact of residual and therapeutic doses of ciprofloxacin in the human-flora associated mice model, *Regul. Toxicol. Pharmacol.*, 2005, **42**, 151–160.
39. C. E. Cerniglia and S. Kotarski, Evaluation of veterinary drug residues in food for their potential to affect human intestinal microflora, *Regul. Toxicol. Pharmacol.*, 1999, **29**, 238–261.
40. C. J. Rumney and I. R. Rowland, *In vivo* and *in vitro* models of the human colonic flora, *Crit. Rev. Food Sci. Nutr.*, 1992, **31**, 299–331.
41. K. N. Woodward, The use of microbiological end-points in the safety evaluation and elaboration of maximum residue limits for veterinary drugs intended for use in food producing animals, *J. Vet. Pharmacol. Ther.*, 1998, **21**, 47–53.
42. C. E. Cerniglia and S. Kotarski, Approaches in the safety evaluation of antimicrobial agents in food to determine the effects on the human intestinal microflora, *J. Vet. Pharmacol. Ther.*, 2005, **28**, 3–20.
43. S. H. Jeong, Y. K. Song and J. H. Cho, Risk assessment of ciprofloxacin, flavomycin, olaquindox and colistin sulphate based on microbiological impact on human gut biota, *Regul. Toxicol. Pharmacol.*, 2009, **53**, 209–216.
44. P. Silley, Impact of antimicrobial residues on gut communities: are the new regulations effective?, *J. Appl. Microbiol.*, 2007, **102**, 1220–1226.
45. S. C. Fitzpatrick, Identifying the "residue of toxicological concern" – exposure assessments, *Drug Metab. Rev.*, 1995, **27**, 557–561.
46. A. MacDonald, Identifying the "residue of toxicological concern" – bioavailability and bioactivity testing, *Drug Metab. Rev.*, 1995, **27**, 549–556.

47. L. T. Mulligan, New toxicological testing approaches based upon exposure/activity/availability assessments, *Drug Metab. Rev.*, 1995, **27**, 573–579.
48. R. Kroes, D. Müller, J. Lambe, M. R. H. Löwik, J. van Klaveren, J. Kleiner, R. Massey, S. Mayer, I. Urieta, P. Verger and A. Visconti, Assessment of intake from the diet, *Food Chem. Toxicol.*, 2002, **40**, 327–385.
49. J. R. Tomerlin, M. R. Berry, N. L. Tran, S.-B. Chew, B. J. Petersen, K. D. Tucker and K. H. Fleming, Development of a dietary exposure potential model for evaluating dietary exposure to chemical substances in food, *J. Expos. Anal. Environ. Epidemiol.*, 1997, **7**, 81–101.
50. D. R. Tennant, Risk analysis in *Food Chemical Safety*. ed. D. H. Watson, CRC Press/Woodhead Publishing, Cambridge, 2001, vol. 1, pp. 15–36.
51. P. Frank and J. H. Schafer, Animal health products in *Regulatory Toxicology*, ed. S. C. Gad, Taylor and Francis, London, 2001, pp. 70–84.
52. G. B. Guest, Veterinary drug registration in the United States in *Veterinary Pharmacology. Toxicology and Therapy in Food Producing Animals*. ed. F. Simon, P. Lees and G. Semjen, University of Veterinary Science, Budapest, 1990, pp. 269–272.
53. M. A. Miller and W. T. Flynn, Regulation of antibiotic use in animals in *Antimicrobial Therapy in Veterinary Medicine*, ed. J. Prescott, J. D. Baggott and R. D. Walker, Iowa State University Press, Ames, 2000, pp. 760–771.
54. S. F. Sundlof, Legal controls of veterinary drugs in *Veterinary Pharmacology and Therapeutics*, ed. H. R. Adams, Iowa State Press, Ames, 8th edn, 2001, pp. 1149–1156.
55. R. H. Teske, Chemical residues in food, *J. Am. Vet. Med. Assoc.*, 1992, **201**, 253–256.
56. L. G. Friedlander, S. D. Brynes and A. H. Fernández, The human food evaluation of new animal drugs, *Vet. Clin. North Am. Food Anim. Pract.*, 1999, **15**, 1–11.
57. D. Kobylka, Safety assessment of animal drugs, *Regul. Toxicol. Pharmacol.*, 1982, **2**, 146–152.
58. J. C. Paige, M. H. Chaudry and F. M. Pell, Federal surveillance of veterinary drugs and chemical residues (with recent data), *Vet. Clin. North Am.*, 1999, **15**, 45–61.
59. M. K. Perez, Human safety data collection and evaluation for the approval of new animal drugs, *J. Toxicol. Environ. Health*, 1977, **3**, 837–857.
60. D. W. Gaylor, J. A. Axelrad, R. P. Brown, J. A. Cavagnaro, W. H. Cyr, K. L. Hulebak, R. J. Lorentzen, M. A. Miller, L. T. Mulligan and B. A. Schwetz, Health risk assessment practices in the U.S. Food and Drug Administration, *Regul. Toxicol. Pharmacol.*, 1997, **26**, 307–321.
61. R. C. Parker, Determination of withdrawal periods for pharmaceutical products used in food animals in *Veterinary Pharmacovigilance. Adverse Reactions to Veterinary Medicinal Products*, ed. K. N. Woodward, Wiley-Blackwell, Chichester, 2009, pp. 569–585.
62. European Medicines Agency, Status of MRL Procedures, MRL assessments in the context of Council Regulation (EEC) No. 2377/90, EMEA/CVMP/765/99-Rev. 1, 2007.

63. K. N. Woodward, Maximum residue limits in *Veterinary Pharmacovigilance. Adverse Reactions to Veterinary Medicinal Products*, ed. K. N. Woodward, Wiley-Blackwell, Chichester, 2009, pp. 547–567.

64. Food and Agriculture Organization, Report of a Joint FAO/WHO Expert Consultation, Rome, 29 October–5 November 1984, FAO Food and Nutrition Paper 32, 1985, FAO, Rome.

65. T. Berg, The international regulation of chemical contaminants in food. Risk analysis in *Food Chemical Safety*, ed. D. H. Watson, CRC Press/Woodhead Publishing, Cambridge, vol. 1, pp. 263–294.

66. J.-S. Chen, The role of science in Codex standards, *Biomed. Environ. Sci.*, 2001, **14**, 145–148.

67. L. Crawford and E. G. Kugler, Codex Committee on Veterinary Drug Residues, *Regul. Toxicol. Pharmacol.*, 1986, **6**, 381–384.

68. M. Luetzow, Harmonisation of exposure assessment for food chemicals; the international perspective, *Toxicol. Lett.*, 2003, **140–141**, 419–425.

69. F. X. Van Leeuwen, The approach taken and conclusions reached by the Joint FAO-WHO Expert Committee on Food Additives, *Ann. Rech. Vet.*, 1991, **22**, 253–256.

70. H. P. A. Illing, Possible risk considerations for toxic risk assessment, *Hum. Exp. Toxicol.*, 1991, **10**, 215–219.

71. H. P. A. Illing, Are societal judgments being incorporated into the uncertainty factors used in toxicological risk assessment?, *Regul. Toxicol. Pharmacol.*, 1999, **29**, 300–308.

72. P. Illing, The importance of risk perception and risk communication for toxicological risk assessment in *Toxicity and Risk. Context, Principles and Practice*, Taylor and Francis, London, 2001, pp. 43–56.

73. R. Nilsson, M. Tasheva and B. Jaeger, Why different regulatory decisions when the scientific information base is similar? – Human risk assessment, *Regul. Toxicol. Pharmacol.*, 1993, **17**, 292–332.

74. S. C. Fitzpatrick, S. D. Brynes and G. B. Guest, Dietary intake values as a means to harmonization of maximum residue levels for veterinary drugs. I. Concept, *J. Vet. Pharmacol. Ther.*, 1995, **18**, 325–327.

75. S. C. Fitzpatrick, A. Vilim, G. Lambert, M. S. Yong and S. D. Brynes, Dietary intake estimates as a means to harmonization of maximum residue levels for veterinary drugs. II. Proposed application to the Free Trade Agreement between the United States and Canada, *Regul. Toxicol. Pharmacol.*, 1996, **24**, 177–183.

76. K. N. Woodward, Maximum residue limits – the impact of UK and EC legislation in *Recent Advances in Animal Nutrition*, ed. P. C. Garnsworthy and D. J. A. Cole, Nottingham University Press, Nottingham, 1993, pp. 165–172.

77. K. N. Woodward and G. Shearer, Antibiotic use in the European Union – Regulation and current methods of detection in *Chemical Analysis for Antibiotics Used in Agriculture*, ed. H. Oka, H. Nakazawa, K. Harada and J. D. MacNeil, Association of Official Analytical Chemists International, Arlington, 1995, pp. 47–76.

78. A. G. Renwick and R. Walker, An analysis of the risk of exceeding the acceptable daily intake, *Regul. Toxicol. Pharmacol.*, 1993, **18**, 463–480.

79. E. J. Calabrese, Overcompensation stimulation: a mechanism for the hormetic effect, *Crit. Rev. Toxicol.*, 2001, **31**, 425–470.

80. E. H. Calabrese and L. A. Baldwin, Hormesis: a generalizable and unifying hypothesis, *Crit. Rev. Toxicol.*, 2001, **31**, 353–424.

81. E. J. Calabrese and L. A. Baldwin, Chemotherapeutics and hormesis, *Crit. Rev. Toxicol.*, 2003, **33**, 305–353.

82. J. McEvoy, Safe limits for veterinary drug residues: what do they mean?, *Northern Ireland Veterinary Today*, Spring Edition, 2001, 37–40.

83. K. K. Rozman and J. Doull, Scientific foundations of hormesis. Part 2. Maturation, strengths, limitations, and possible applications in toxicology, pharmacology and epidemiology, *Crit. Rev. Toxicol.*, 2003, **33**, 451–462.

84. A. R. D. Stebbing, A mechanism for hormesis – a problem in the wrong discipline, *Crit. Rev. Toxicol.*, 2003, **33**, 463–467.

85. A. Sanquer, G. Wackowiez and B. Havrileck, Critical review on the withdrawal period calculation for injection site residues, *J. Vet. Pharmacol. Ther.*, 2001, **29**, 355–364.

86. B. F. Droy, T. Tate, J. J. Lech and K. M. Kleinhow, Influence of ormetoprim on the bioavailability, distribution, and pharmacokinetics of sulfadimethoxine in rainbow trout (*Oncorhynchus mykiss*), *Comp. Biochem. Physiol.*, 1989, **94C**, 303–307.

87. B. F. Droy, M. S. Goodrich, J. J. Lech and K. M. Kleinhow, Bioavailability, disposition and pharmacokinetics of ^{14}C-ormetoprim in rainbow trout (*Salmo gairdneri*), *Xenobiotica*, 1990, **20**, 147–157.

88. K. M. Kleinhow, M. J. Melancon and J. J. Lech, Biotransformation and induction: implications for toxicity, bioaccumulation and monitoring of environmental xenobiotics in fish, *Environ. Health Perspect.*, 1987, **71**, 105–119.

89. K. M. Kleinhow and J. J. Lech, A review of the pharmacokinetics and metabolisms of sulfadimethoxine in the rainbow trout (*Salmo gairdneri*), *Vet. Hum. Toxicol.*, 1988, **30**(1), 26–30.

90. J. W. Nichols, J. M. McKim, M. E. Andersen, M. L. Gargas, H. J. Clewell and R. J. Erickson, A physiologically based toxicokinetic model for the uptake and disposition of waterborne organic chemicals in fish, *Toxicol. Appl. Pharmacol.*, 1990, **106**, 433–447.

91. H. Segner and J.-P. Cravedi, Metabolic activity in primary cultures of fish hepatocytes, *Alt. Lab. Anim.*, 2001, **29**, 251–257.

92. J. L. Allen and J. B. Hunn, Fate and distribution of some drugs used in aquaculture, *Vet. Hum. Toxicol.*, 1986, **28**(1), 21–24.

93. M. G. Barron, B. D. Tarr and W. L. Hayton, Temperature dependence of di-2-ethylhexyl phthalate (DEHP) pharmacokinetics in rainbow trout, *Toxicol. Appl. Pharmacol.*, 1987, **88**, 305–312.

94. R. L. Binder, M. J. Melancon and J. J. Lech, Factors influencing the persistence and metabolism of chemicals in fish, *Drug Metab. Rev.*, 1984, **15**, 697–724.

95. J. P. Cravedi, Role of biotransformation in the fate and toxicity of chemicals: consequences for the assessment of residues in fish, *Rev. Méd. Vét.*, 2002, **153**, 419–424.
96. A. M. Guarino and J. J. Lech, Metabolism, disposition, and toxicity of drugs and other xenobiotics in aquatic species, *Vet. Hum. Toxicol.*, 1986, **28**(1), 38–44.
97. A. M. Guarino, Regulatory and scientific roles for biodistribution studies in aquatic species, *Vet. Hum. Toxicol.*, 1991, **33**(1), 54–59.
98. M. O. James, Overview of *in vitro* metabolism of drugs by aquatic species, *Vet. Hum. Toxicol.*, 1986, **28**(1), 2–8.
99. J. J. Lech and M. J. Vodicnik, Biotransformation of chemicals by fish: an overview, *J. Natl Cancer Inst.*, 1984, **65**, 355–358.
100. D. R. Livingstone, The fate of organic xenobiotics in aquatic ecosystems: quantitative and qualitative differences in biotransformation by invertebrates and fish, *Comp. Biochem. Physiol.*, 1998, **120A**, 43–49.
101. A. J. Niimi, Biological half-lives of chemicals in fishes, *Rev. Environ. Contam. Toxicol.*, 1987, **99**, 1–46.
102. C. Sarasquete and H. Segner, Cytochrome P4501A (CYP1A) in teleostean fishes. A review of immunohistochemical studies, *Sci. Total Environ.*, 2000, **247**, 313–332.
103. A. L. Banting and J. D. Baggot, Comparison of the pharmacokinetics and local tolerance of three injectable oxytetracycline formulations in pigs, *J. Vet. Pharmacol. Ther.*, 1996, **19**, 50–55.
104. J. G. Beechinor, T. Buckley and F. J. Bloomfield, Prevalence and public health significance of blemishes in cuts of Irish beef, *Vet. Rec.*, 2001, **149**, 43–44.
105. J. G. Beechinor and F. J. Bloomfield, Variability in residues of tilmicosin in cattle muscle, *Vet. Rec.*, 2001, **149**, 182–183.
106. S. A. Brown, Challenges in development of sustained release parenteral formulations, *J. Vet. Pharmacol. Ther.*, 2000, **23**(1), Q1.
107. D. M. Gaylor and A. M. Monro, The safety assessment of drug residues at injection sites, *J. Vet. Pharmacol. Ther.*, 1996, **19**, 312.
108. H. Mawhinney, S. M. Oakenfull and T. J. Nicholls, Residues from long-acting antimicrobial preparations in injection sites in cattle, *Aust. Vet. J.*, 1996, **74**, 140–142.
109. J. F. M. Nouws, Injection sites and withdrawal times, *Ann. Rech. Vet.*, 1990, **21**, 145s–150s.
110. J. F. M. Nouws, A. Smulder and M. Rappalini, A comparative study on irritation and residue aspects of five oxytetracycline formulations administered intramuscularly to calves, pigs and sheep, *Vet. Quart.*, 1990, **12**, 129–138.
111. A. Sanquer, G. Wackowiez and B. Havrileck, Qualitative assessment of human exposure to consumption of injection site residues, *J. Vet. Pharmacol. Ther.*, 2001, **29**, 345–353.
112. P. T. Reeves, Residues of veterinary drugs at injection sites, *J. Vet. Pharmacol. Ther.*, 2007, **30**, 1–17.

113. M. A. Payne, R. E. Barnes, S. E. Sundlof, A. Craigmill, A. I. Webb and J. E. Riviere, Drugs prohibited for extra label use in food animals, *J. Am. Vet. Med. Assoc.*, 1999, **215**, 28–32.
114. R. E. Baynes, T. Martín-Jiménez, A. L. Craigmill and J. E. Riviere, Estimating provisional acceptable residues for extralabel drug use in livestock, *Regul. Toxicol. Pharmacol.*, 1999, **29**, 287–299.
115. R. Gehring, R. E. Baynes and J. E. Riviere, Application of risk assessment and management principles to the extralabel use of drugs in food-producing animals, *J. Vet. Pharmacol. Ther.*, 2006, **29**, 5–14.
116. T. A. Bell, New animal drug approvals and the United States aquaculture industry: a partnership for growth, *Vet. Hum. Toxicol.*, 1995, **26**, 679–685.
117. J. H. Brown, Antibiotics: their use and abuse in aquaculture, *World Aquaculture*, 1989, **20**, 34–43.
118. J. F. Burka, K. L. Hammel, T. E. Horsberg, G. R. Johnson, D. J. Rainnie and D. J. Speare, Drugs in salmonid aquaculture – a review, *J. Vet. Pharmacol. Ther.*, 1997, **20**, 333–349.
119. M. Roth, R. H. Richards and C. Sommerville, Current practices in the chemotherapeutic control of sea lice infestations in aquaculture, *J. Fish Dis.*, 1993, **16**, 1–26.
120. J. Stone, I. H. Sutherland, C. S. Sommerville, R. H. Richards and K. J. Varma, The efficacy of emamectin benzoate as an oral treatment of sea lice, *Lepeophtheirus salmonis* (Krøyer), infestations in Atlantic salmon, *Salmo salar* L, *J. Fish Dis.*, 1999, **22**, 269–270.
121. W. H. Gingerich, G. R. Stehly, K. J. Clark and W. L. Hayton, Crop grouping: a proposal for public aquaculture, *Vet. Hum. Toxicol.*, 1998, **40**(2), 24–31.
122. W. Hayton, Experimental approach to test the crop grouping concept in fish, Presented at Crop Grouping Program Review, National Fisheries Research Center-La Crosse, US National Biologic Service, 1995, La Crosse, Wisconsin, USA.
123. K. J. Greenlees and T. A. Bell, Aquaculture crop grouping and new animal drug approvals: a CVM perspective, *Vet. Hum. Toxicol.*, 1998, **40**(2), 19–23.
124. J. C. Paige, L. Tollefson and M. Miller, Public health impact on drug residues in animal tissues, *Vet. Hum. Toxicol.*, 1997, **39**, 162–169.
125. J. C. Paige, L. Tollefson and M. A. Miller, Health implications of residues of veterinary drugs and chemicals in animal tissues, *Vet. Clin. North Am.*, 1999, **15**, 31–43.
126. S. F. Sundlof, A. H. Fernandez and J. C. Paige, Antimicrobial drug residues in food-producing animals in *Antimicrobial Therapy in Veterinary Medicine*, ed. J. Prescott, J. D. Baggott and R. D. Walker, Iowa State University Press, Ames, 2000, pp. 744–759.
127. W. R. Van Dresser and J. R. Wilcke, Drug residues in food animals, *J. Am. Vet. Med. Assoc.*, 1989, **194**, 1700–1710.
128. M. M. Pullen, Residues in *Meat and Health. Advances in Meat Research*, ed. A. M. Pearson and T. R. Dutson, Elsevier, London, 1990, pp. 135–156.

129. Veterinary Residues Committee, *Annual Report on Surveillance for Veterinary Residues in 2001*, 2002. Available at: http://www.vmd. defra.gov.uk/vrc/.

130. S. D. Brynes, Demystifying 21 CFR Part 556 – Tolerances for residues of new animal drugs in food, *Regul. Toxicol. Pharmacol.*, 2005, **42**, 324–327.

131. B. Ludwig, Use of pharmacokinetics when dealing with residue problems in food-producing animals, *Dtsch. Tierärztl. Wochenschr.*, 1989, **96**, 243–248.

132. H. D. Mercer, J. D. Baggot and R. A. Sams, Application of pharmaco-kinetic methods to the drug residue profile, *J. Toxicol. Environ. Health*, 1977, **2**, 787–801.

133. D. M. Morton, The toxicological evaluation of drug residues, *J. Toxicol. Environ. Health*, 1977, **3**, 65–72.

134. G. Shearer, Testing for residues and results of current programmes, *Pig Vet. J.*, 1990, **24**, 80–87.

135. K. N. Woodward, Residues of anticholinesterases in foodstuffs in *Clinical & Experimental Toxicology of Organophosphates and Carbamates*, ed. B. Ballantyne and T. C. Marrs, Butterworth Heinemann, Oxford, 1992, pp. 364–372.

136. J. M. Booth and F. Harding, Testing for antibiotic residues in milk, *Vet. Rec.*, 1986, **119**, 565–569.

137. H. E. Braun, R. Frank and L. A. Miller, Residues of cypermethrin in milk from cows wearing impregnated ear tags, *Bull. Environ. Contam. Toxicol.*, 1985, **35**, 61–64.

138. S. Chinabut, T. Somsiri, C. Limsuwan and S. Lewis, Problems associated with shellfish farming, *Sci. Tech. Rev.*, 2006, **25**, 627–635.

139. A. Esposito, L. Fabrizi, D. Luchetti, L. Marvasi, E. Coni and E. Guadalini, Orally administered erythromycin in rainbow trout (*Oncorhynchus mykiss*): residues in edible tissues and withdrawal time, *Antimicrob. Chemother.*, 2007, **51**, 1043–1047.

140. J. T. Feagan, The detection of antibiotic residues in milk. Part I. The use of microbiological assay techniques. Part II. Dye-marking of antibiotics, *Dairy Sci. Abstr.*, 1966, **28**, 53–60.

141. T. E. Horsberg, T. Høy and O. Ringstad, Residues of dichlorvos in Atlantic salmon (*Salmo salar*) after delousing, *J. Agric. Food Chem.*, 1990, **38**, 1403–1406.

142. A. Ibach, M. Petz, A. Heer, N. Mencke and R. Krebber, Oxacillin residues in milk after drying off with Stapenor® Retard TS, *Analyst*, 1998, **123**, 2763–2765.

143. L. Intorre, G. Castells, C. Cristòfol, S. Bertini, G. Soldani and M. Arboix, Residue depletion of thiamphenicol in the sea-bass, *J. Vet. Pharmacol. Ther.*, 2002, **25**, 59–63.

144. J. C. Olson and A. C. Sanders, Penicillin in milk and milk products: some regulatory and public health considerations, *J. Milk Food Technol.*, 1975, **38**, 630–633.

145. B. Shaikh, N. Rummel, C. Gieseker, S. Serfling and R. Reimschuessel, Metabolism and residue depletion of albendazole and its metabolites in rainbow trout, tilapia and Atlantic salmon after oral administration, *J. Vet. Pharmacol. Ther.*, 2003, **26**, 421–427.

146. K. Šinigoj-Gačnik, V. Cerkvenik-Flajs and S. Vadnjal, Evidence of veterinary drug residues in Slovenian freshwater fish, *Bull. Environ. Contam. Toxicol.*, 2005, **75**, 109–114.

147. R. V. Sudershan and R. V. Bhat, A survey of veterinary drug use and residues in milk in Hyderabad, *Food Add. Contam.*, 1995, **12**, 645–650.

148. M. R. Talley, The National Milk Safety Program and drug residues in milk, *Vet. Clin. North Am. Food Anim. Pract.*, 1999, **15**, 63–73.

149. V. Unnikrishnan, M. K. Bhavadasan, B. Surendra Nath and C. Ram, Chemical residues and contaminants in milk: a review, *Indian J. Anim. Sci.*, 2005, **75**, 592–598.

150. A. Anadón, M. R. Martínez-Larrañaga, M. J. Díaz, P. Bringas, M. A. Martínez, M. L. Fernández-Cruz, M. C. Fernández and R. Fernández, Pharmacokinetics and residues of enrofloxacin in chickens, *Am. J. Vet. Res.*, 1995, **56**, 501–506.

151. K. De Wasch, L. Okerman, S. Croubels, H. De Brabander, J. Van Hoof and P. De Backer, Detection of residues of tetracycline antibiotics in pork and chicken meat: correlation between results of screening and confirmatory tests, *Analyst*, 1998, **123**, 2737–2741.

152. C. A. Kan and M. Petz, Residues of veterinary drugs in eggs and their distribution between yolk and white, *J. Agric. Food Chem.*, 2000, **48**, 6397–6403.

153. L. D. Lashev and R. Mihailov, Pharmacokinetics of sulphamethoxazole and trimethoprim administered intravenously and orally to Japanese quail, *J. Vet. Pharmacol. Ther.*, 1994, **17**, 327–330.

154. L. Mortier, A. C. Huet, C. Charlier, E. Daeseleire, P. Delahaut and C. Van Peteghem, Incidence of residues of nine anticoccidials in eggs, *Food Add. Contam.*, 2005, **22**, 1120–1125.

155. R. E. Baynes, A. L. Craigmill and J. E. Riviere, Residue avoidance after topical application of veterinary drugs and parasiticides, *J. Am. Vet. Med. Assoc.*, 1997, **210**, 1288–1289.

156. M. Szerletics-Túri, K. Soós and E. Végh, Determination of residues of pyrethroids and organophosphorus ectoparasiticides in food of animal origin, *Acta Vet. Hung.*, 2000, **48**, 139–149.

157. T. M. Farber, Anabolics: the approach taken in the USA, *Ann. Rech. Vet.*, 1991, **22**, 295–298.

158. G. E. Lamming, G. Ballarini, E. E. Baulieu, P. Brookes, P. S. Elias, R. Ferrando, C. L. Galli, R. J. Heitzman, B. Hoffman, H. Karg, H. H. D. Meyer, G. Michel, E. Poulsen, A. Rico, F. X. R. van Leeuwen and D. S. White, Scientific report on anabolic agents in animal production, *Vet. Rec.*, 1987, **121**, 389–392.

159. J. K. Leighton, Center for Veterinary Medicine's perspective on the beef hormone case, *Vet. Clin. North Am. Food Anim. Pract.*, 1999, **15**, 167–180.

160. M. A. Miller and J. K. Leighton, Risk assessment strategies for hormones and hormone-like substances, *Scientific Conference on Growth Promotion in Meat Production*, Proceedings of a Conference, European Commission, Brussels, 1996, pp. 383–399.

161. A. M. Baker and H. W. Gonyou, Effects of Zeranol implantation and late castration on sexual, agonistic and handling behaviour in male feedlot cattle, *J. Anim. Sci.*, 1986, **62**, 1224–1232.

162. C. D. Cranwell, J. A. Unruh, J. R. Brethour, D. D. Simms and R. E. Campbell, Influence of steroid implants and concentrate feeding on performance and carcass composition of cull beef cows, *J. Anim. Sci.*, 1996, **74**, 1770–1776.

163. D. G. Gray, J. A. Unruh, M. E. Dikeman and J. S. Stevenson, Implanting young bulls with Zeranol from birth to flour four slaughter ages: III. Growth performance and endocrine aspects, *J. Anim. Sci.*, 1986, **63**, 747–782.

164. J. M. Hayden, W. G. Bergen and R. A. Merkel, Skeletal muscle, protein metabolism and serum growth hormone, insulin and cortisone concentrations in growing steers implanted with estradiol-17β , trenbolone acetate, estradiol-17β plus trenbolone acetate, *J. Anim. Sci.*, 1992, **70**, 2109–2119.

165. R. C. Herschler, A. W. Olmstead, A. J. Edwards, R. L. Hale, T. Montgomery, R. L. Preston, S. J. Bartle and J. J. Sheldon, Production responses to various doses and ratios of estradiol and trenbolone acetate implants in steers and heifers, *J. Anim. Sci.*, 1995, **73**, 2873–2881.

166. D. W. Hunt, D. M. Henricks, G. C. Skelley and L. W. Grimes, Use of trenbolone acetate and estradiol in intact and castrate male cattle: effects on growth, serum hormones, and carcass characteristics, *J. Anim. Sci.*, 1991, **69**, 2452–2462.

167. S. J. Jones, R. D. Johnson, C. R. Calkins and M. F. Dikeman, Effects of trenbolone acetate on carcass characteristics and serum testosterone and cortisol concentrations in bulls and steers on different management and implant schemes, *J. Anim. Sci.*, 1991, **69**, 1363–1369.

168. R. R. Massart, A. Prandi, U. Fazzini, M. Sindic, L. Nicolay, M. Falaki, A. Burny and D. Portetelle, Aspects of the use of anabolic steroids in animal production, *Scientific Conference on Growth Promotion in Meat Production*, Proceedings of a Conference, European Commission, Brussels, 1996, pp. 63–85.

169. H. H. D. Meyer, Biochemistry and physiology of anabolic hormones used for improvement of meat production, *APMIS*, 2001, **109**, 1–8.

170. R. L. Patterson, S. J. Bartle, T. R. Kasser, J. W. Day, J. J. Veenhuizen and C. A. Baile, Anabolic agents and meat quality: a review, *Meat Sci.*, 1985, **14**, 191–220.

171. A. R. Peters, Endocrine manipulation – toxicological frontiers, *J. Reprod. Fertil.*, 1992, **45**(Suppl.), 193–201.

172. A. Zarkawi, H. Galbraith and J. S. M. Hutchinson, Influence of trenbolone acetate, zeranol and oestradiol-17β implantation on growth performance and reproductive functions in beef heifers, *Anim. Product.*, 1991, **52**, 249–253.

173. R. Le Guevel and F. Pakdel, Assessment of oestrogenic potency of chemicals used as growth promoter by *in-vitro* methods, *Hum. Reprod.*, 2001, **16**, 1030–1036.

174. A. Mantovani and A. Macri, Endocrine effects in the hazard assessment of drugs used in animal production, *J. Exper. Clin. Cancer Res.*, 2002, **21**, 445–456.

175. Veterinary Products Committee, *Risks Associated with the Use of Hormonal Substances in Food Producing Animals*, 2006. Available at: http://www.vpc.gov.uk.

176. P. J. Buttery and J. M. Dawson, The mode of action of beta-agonists as manipulators of carcass composition in *Beta-Agonists and Their Effects on Animal Growth and Carcass Quality*, ed. J. P. Hanrahan, Elsevier, London, 1987, pp. 29–43.

177. D. Waltner-Toews and S. A. McEwen, Residues of hormonal substances in foods of animal origin: a risk assessment, *Prev. Vet. Med.*, 2004, **20**, 235–247.

178. A. Macri and P. Marabelli, Veterinary drug surveillance, *Annali dell'Istituto Superiore di Sanita*, 1992, **28**, 421–424.

179. K. N. Woodward, Regulation of veterinary products in Europe, including the UK in *General and Applied Toxicology*, ed. B. Ballantyne, T. Marrs and P. Turner, Macmillan, Basingstoke, 1993, pp. 1105–1128.

180. K. N. Woodward, Veterinary pharmacovigilance. Part 2. Veterinary pharmacovigilance in practice – the operation of a spontaneous reporting scheme in a European Union country – the UK, and schemes in other countries, *J. Vet. Pharmacol. Ther.*, 2005, **28**, 149–170.

181. R. L. Ellis, Validation and harmonisation of analytical methods for residue detection at the international level in *Residues of Veterinary Drugs and Mycotoxins in Animal Products*, ed. G. Enne, H. A. Kuiper and A. Valentini, Wageningen Press, Wageningen, 1996, pp. 52–62.

182. R. J. Heitzman (ed.), *Veterinary Drug Residues. Residues in Food Producing Animals and their Products. Reference Materials and Methods*, Commission of the European Communities, Report Eur 15127-EN, Blackwell Scientific Publications, Oxford, 1994.

183. H. A. Kuiper and J. R. Andersen (ed.), In vitro *Toxicological Studies and Real Time Analysis of Residues in Food,* FLAIR-Concerted Action No. 8, RIKILT-DMO/DMRI, Wageningen, 1994.

184. J. D. MacNeil, Drug residues in animal tissues, *J. AOAC Int.*, 2003, **86**, 116–127.

185. H. Oka, H. Nakazawa, K.-I. Harada and J. MacNeil (ed.), *Chemical Analysis for Antibiotics Used in Agriculture*, AOAC International, Arlington, 1995.

186. M. Tuomola and T. Lövgren, The rapid detection of coccidiostat drug residues in farm animals in *Pesticide, Veterinary and Other Residues in Food*, ed. D. H. Watson, CRC Press/Woodhead Publishing, Cambridge, 2004, pp. 262–274.

187. N. van Hoof, K. de Wasch, H. Noppe, P. Poelmans and H. F. de Brabender, The rapid detection of veterinary drug residues in *Pesticide, Veterinary and Other Residues in Food*, ed. D. H. Watson, CRC Press/Woodhead Publishing, Cambridge, 2004, pp. 224–248.

188. Veterinary Medicines Directorate, *The Veterinary Medicines Directorate Annual Report on Surveillance for Veterinary Residues in 1995*, VMD, Addlestone, 1996.

189. Veterinary Medicines Directorate, *The Veterinary Medicines Directorate Annual Report on Surveillance for Veterinary Residues in 1996*, VMD, Addlestone, 1997.

190. Veterinary Medicines Directorate, *The Veterinary Medicines Directorate Annual Report on Surveillance for Veterinary Residues in 1997*, VMD, Addlestone, 1998.

191. Veterinary Medicines Directorate, *The Veterinary Medicines Directorate Annual Report on Surveillance for Veterinary Residues in 1998*, VMD, Addlestone, 1999.

192. Veterinary Medicines Directorate, *The Veterinary Medicines Directorate Annual Report on Surveillance for Veterinary Residues in 1999*, VMD, Addlestone, 2000.

193. Veterinary Medicines Directorate, *The Veterinary Medicines Directorate Annual Report on Surveillance for Veterinary Residues in 2000*, VMD, Addlestone, 2001.

194. Veterinary Residues Committee, *Annual Report on Surveillance for Veterinary Residues in Food in the UK, 2003*, 2004. Available at: http://www.vmd.defra.gov.uk/vrc/.

195. Veterinary Residues Committee, *Annual Report on Surveillance for Veterinary Residues in Food in the UK, 2004*, 2005. Available at: http://www.vmd.defra.gov.uk/vrc/.

196. Veterinary Residues Committee, *Annual Report on Surveillance for Veterinary Residues in Food in the UK, 2005*, 2006. Available at: http://www.vmd.defra.gov.uk/vrc/.

197. Veterinary Residues Committee, *Annual Report on Surveillance for Veterinary Residues in Food in the UK, 2006*, 2007. Available at: http://www.vmd.defra.gov.uk/vrc/.

198. Veterinary Residues Committee, *Annual Report on Surveillance for Veterinary Residues in Food in the UK, 2007*, 2008. Available at: http://www.vmd.defra.gov.uk/vrc/.

199. Veterinary Residues Committee, *Annual Report on Surveillance for Veterinary Residues in Food in the UK, 2008*, 2009. Available at: http://www.vmd.defra.gov.uk/vrc/.

200. Veterinary Residues Committee, *Annual Report on Surveillance for Veterinary Residues in Food in the UK, 2009*, 2010. Available at: http://www.vmd.defra.gov.uk/vrc/.

201. Veterinary Residues Committee, *Annual Report on Surveillance for Veterinary Residues in Food in the UK, 2010*, 2011. Available at: http://www.vmd.defra.gov.uk/vrc/.

202. C. T. Elliott, W. J. McCaughey, S. R. H. Crooks and J. D. G. McEvoy, Effects of short term exposure of unmedicated pigs to sulphadimidine contaminated housing, *Vet. Rec.*, 1994, **134**, 450–451.

203. D. G. Kennedy, P. J. Hughes and W. J. Blanchflower, Ionophore residues in eggs in Northern Ireland: incidence and cause, *Food Add. Contam.*, 1998, **15**, 535–541.

204. D. G. Kennedy, W. G. Smyth, S. A. Hewitt and J. D. G. McEvoy, Monensin carry-over into unmedicated broiler feeds, *Analyst*, 1998, **123**, 2529–2533.

205. D. G. Kennedy, A. Cannavan and R. J. McCracken, Regulatory problems caused by contamination, a frequently overlooked cause of veterinary drug residues, *J. Chromatogr., A*, 2000, **882**, 37–52.

206. W. J. McCaughey, C. T. Elliott, J. N. Campbell, W. J. Blanchflower and D. A. Rice, Tissue residues in pigs fed meal contaminated with sulphadimidine during mixing, *Ir. Vet. J.*, 1990, **43**, 127–130.

207. W. J. McCaughey, C. T. Campbell and C. T. Elliott, Reduction of sulphadimidine in pig feeding stuffs, *Vet. Rec.*, 1990, **126**, 113.

208. J. D. G. McEvoy, S. R. H. Crooks, C. T. Elliott, W. J. McCaughey and D. G. Kennedy, Origin of chlortetracycline in pig tissue, *Analyst*, 1994, **119**, 2603–2606.

209. J. D. G. McEvoy, C. S. Mayne, H. C. Higgins and D. G. Kennedy, Transfer of sulfamethazine from contaminated dairy feed to cows' milk, *Vet. Rec.*, 1999, **144**, 470–475.

210. J. D. G. McEvoy, C. S. Mayne, H. C. Higgins and D. G. Kennedy, Transfer of chlortetracycline from contaminated dairy feed to cows' milk, *Vet. Rec.*, 2000, **146**, 102–106.

211. J. D. G. McEvoy, Contamination of animal feedingstuffs as a cause of residues in food: a review of regulatory aspects, incidence and control, *Anal. Chim. Acta*, 2002, **473**, 3–26.

212. J. Moreno-Lopez, Contaminants in feed for food-producing animals, *Pol. J. Vet. Sci.*, 2002, **5**, 123–125.

213. E. R. Nestmann and B. S. Lynch, Method for calculating ADI-derived guidance for drug carryover levels in medicated feed, *Regul. Toxicol. Pharmacol.*, 2007, **47**, 232–239.

214. M. Easa, M. Shereif, A. Shaaban and K. Mancy, Public health implications of waste water reuse for fish production, *Water Sci. Technol.*, 1995, **32**, 145–152.

215. G. L. Jensen and K. J. Greenlees, Public health issues in aquaculture, *Rev. Sci. Tech.*, 1997, **16**, 641–651.

216. R. A. Hites, J. A. Foran, D. O. Carpenter, M. C. Hamilton, B. A. Knuth and S. J. Schwager, Global assessment of organic contaminants in farmed salmon, *Science*, 2004, **303**, 226–229.

217. K. Berger, B. Petersen and H. Büning-Pfaue, Persistence of drug residues from slurry in the food chain, *Arch. Lebensmittel.*, 1987, **37**, 85–108.

218. V. S. Wilson, C. Lambright, J. Ostby and L. E. Gray, *In vitro* and *in vivo* effects of 17β-trenbolone: a feedlot effluent contaminant, *Toxicol. Sci.*, 2002, **70**, 202–211.
219. C. Pulce, D. Lamaison, G. Keck, C. Bostvironnois, J. Nicolas and J. Descotes, Collective human food poisonings by clenbuterol residues in veal liver, *Vet. Hum. Toxicol.*, 1991, **33**, 480–481.
220. G. Brambilla, Health aspects of the use of beta-2 adrenergic drugs in animal production, *Annali dell'Istituto Superiore di Sanita*, 1992, **28**, 437–439.
221. Anon, Poisoned pork, *The Times (London)*, October 22, 2003, 15.
222. J. C. Paige, The issues of residues and human health, *J. Am. Vet. Med. Assoc.*, 1998, **213**, 1735–1736.
223. A. Q. M. Biggs, Avoiding milk antibiotic residues – how the practitioner can help and advise, *Cattle Pract.*, 2000, **8**, 283–285.
224. D. H. Black and J. G. Cook, Bulk tank milk failures, *Vet. Rec.*, 2001, **148**, 91–92.
225. J. S. Cullor, Testing the tests intended to detect antibiotic residues in milk, *Vet. Med.*, 1994, **87**, 462–472.
226. J. S. Cullor, Risks and prevention of contamination of dairy products, *Rev. Sci. Tech.*, 1997, **16**, 472–481.
227. J. S. Cullor, A. van Eenennaam, I. Gardner, L. Perani, J. Dellinger, W. L. Smit, M. A. Payne, L. Jensen and W. M. Guterbock, Performance of various tests used to screen antibiotic residues in milk samples from individual animals, *J. AOAC. Int.*, 1994, **77**, 862–870.
228. P. W. Edmonson, Bulk tank milk failures, *Vet. Rec.*, 2001, **148**, 122–123.
229. M. Pott, Antibiotics in milk – residue levels and bulk tank failures, *Cattle Pract.*, 1993, **1**, 261–271.
230. M. Pott, Milk "antibiotic" residues – a pharmaceutical company view, *Cattle Pract.*, 2000, **8**, 287–292.
231. M. Hurst, Milk antibiotic residues – a milk industry perspective, *Cattle Pract.*, 2000, **8**, 279–282.
232. T. Martínez-Jiménez, R. E. Baynes, A. Craigmill and J. E. Riviere, Extrapolated withdrawal-interval estimator (EWE) algorithm: a qualitative approach to establishing extralabel withdrawal times, *Regul. Toxicol. Pharmacol.*, 2002, **36**, 131–137.
233. J. Buur, R. Baynes, G. Smith and J. Riviere, Use of probabilistic modeling within a physiologically based pharmacokinetic model to predict sulfamethazine residue withdrawal times in edible tissues in swine, *Antimicrob. Chemother.*, 2006, **50**, 2344–2351.
234. D. Concordet and P. L. Toutain, The withdrawal time estimation of veterinary drugs: a non-parametric approach, *J. Vet. Pharmacol. Ther.*, 1997, **20**, 374–379.
235. D. Concordet and P. L. Toutain, The withdrawal time estimation of veterinary drugs revisited, *J. Vet. Pharmacol. Ther.*, 1997, **20**, 380–386.

236. R. D. Fisch, Withdrawal time estimation of veterinary drugs: extending the range of statistical methods, *J. Vet. Pharmacol. Ther.*, 2000, **23**, 159–162.
237. Anon, Keeping out of trouble: what you need to know about withholding periods, *Aust. Vet. J.*, 2002, **80**, 456–457.
238. R. Early, Good Agricultural practice and HACCP systems in the management of pesticides and veterinary residues on the farm in *Pesticide, Veterinary and Other Residues in Food*, ed. D. H. Watson, Woodhead Publishing/CRC Press, Cambridge, 2004, pp. 119–154.
239. P. S. Gaunt, Veterinarians' role in the use of veterinary feed directive drugs in aquaculture, *J. Am. Vet. Med. Assoc.*, 2006, **229**, 362–364.
240. R. Gehring, R. E. Baynes and J. E. Riviere, Application of risk assessment and management principles to the extralabel use of drugs in food-producing animals, *J. Vet. Pharmacol. Ther.*, 2006, **29**, 5–14.
241. N. T. Kavanagh, Preventing tissue residues in fattening pigs, *Pig Vet. J.*, 1990, **24**, 72–79.
242. M. A. Payne, A. Craigmill, J. E. Riviere and A. I. Webb, Extralabel use of penicillin in food animals, *J. Am. Vet. Med. Assoc.*, 2006, **229**, 1401–1403.
243. H. Price, Residues and records: "I know what I've treated my animals with", *Northern Ireland Today*, 2006. Available at: www.afbini.gov.uk/cattle-nivt-residues.pdf.
244. A. S. J. P. A. M. Van Miert, Efficacy of drugs and good veterinary practice in *Residues of Veterinary Drugs and Mycotoxins in Animal Products*, ed. G. Enne, H. A. Kuiper and A. Valentini, Wageningen Press, Wageningen, 1996, pp. 87–94.
245. B. KuKanich, R. Gehring, A. I. Webb, A. L. Craigmill and J. E. Riviere, Effect of formulation and route of administration on tissue residues and withdrawal times, *J. Am. Vet. Med. Assoc.*, 2005, **227**, 1574–1577.
246. H. Mawhinney, S. M. Oakenfull and T. J. Nicholls, Residues from long-acting antimicrobial preparations in injection sites in cattle, *Aust. Vet. J.*, 1996, **74**, 140–142.
247. A. L. Banting and J. D. Baggot, Comparison of the pharmacokinetics and local tolerance of three injectable oxytetracycline formulations in pigs, *J. Vet. Pharmacol. Ther.*, 1996, **19**, 50–55.
248. G. O. Korsrud, J. O. Boison, M. G. Papich, W. D. G. Yates, J. D. McNeil, E. D. Janzen, J. J. McKinnon, D. A. Landry, G. Lambert, M. S. Yong and L. Ritter, Depletion of penicillin G residues in tissues and injection sites of yearling beef steers dosed with benzathine penicillin alone or in combination with procaine penicillin G, *Food Add. Contam.*, 1994, **11**, 1–6.
249. J. A. Tarbin, J. Bygrave, T. Bigwood, D. Hardy, M. Rose and M. Sharman, The effect of cooking on veterinary drug residues in food: Nicarbazin (dinitrocarbanilamide component), *Food Add. Contam.*, 2005, **22**, 1126–1131.
250. J. J. O'Brien, N. Campbell and T. Conaghan, Effect of cooking and cold storage on biologically active antibiotic residues in meat, *J. Hyg.*, 1981, **87**, 511–523.

251. M. D. Rose, J. Bygrave, W. H. H. Farrington and G. Shearer, The effect of cooking on veterinary drug residues in food. Part 8. Benzylpenicillin, *Analyst*, 1997, **122**, 1095–1099.

252. M. Kühne, U. Körner and S. Wenzel, Tetracycline residues in meat and bone meals. Part 2. The effect of heat treatments on bound tetracycline residues, *Food Add. Contam.*, 2001, **18**, 593–600.

253. M. D. Rose, J. Bygrave, W. H. H. Farrington and G. Shearer, The effect of cooking on veterinary drug residues in food. 4. Oxytetracycline, *Food Add. Contam.*, 1996, **13**, 275–286.

254. M. D. Rose, W. H. H. Farrington and G. Shearer, The effect of cooking on veterinary drug residues in food. 3. Sulphamethazine (sulphadimidine), *Food Add. Contam.*, 1995, **12**, 739–750.

255. M. D. Rose, G. Shearer and W. H. H. Farrington, The effect of cooking on veterinary drug residues in food. 5. Oxfendazole, *Food Add. Contam.*, 1997, **14**, 15–26.

256. L. Steffenak, V. Hormazabal and M. Yndestad, Effect of cooking on residues of the quinolones oxolinic acid and flumequine in fish, *Acta Vet. Scand.*, 1994, **35**, 299–301.

257. M. D. Rose, G. Shearer and W. H. H. Farrington, The effect of cooking on veterinary drug residues in food. 1. Clenbuterol, *Food Add. Contam.*, 1995, **12**, 67–76.

258. M. D. Rose, L. C. Argent, G. Shearer and W. H. H. Farrington, The effect of cooking on veterinary drug residues in food. 2, Levamisole, *Food Add. Contam.*, 1995, **12**, 184–194.

259. M. D. Rose, W. H. H. Farrington and G. Shearer, The effect of cooking on veterinary drug residues in food. 7. Ivermectin, *Food Add. Contam.*, 1998, **15**, 157–161.

260. M. D. Rose, J. Bygrave and M. Sharman, The effect of cooking on veterinary drug residues in food. Part 9. Nitroimidazoles, *Analyst*, 1998, **124**, 289–294.

261. W. A. Moats, The effect of food processing on veterinary residues in foods *Impact of Food Processing on Food Safety*, ed. L. S. Jackson, M. G. Knize and J. N. Morgan, *Advances in Experimental Medicine and Biology*, Kluwer Academic/Plenum Publishers, New York, 1999, vol. 459, pp. 233–241.

262. G. Alfredsson and A. Ohlson, Stability of sulphonamide drugs in meat during storage, *Food Add. Contam.*, 1998, **15**, 302–306.

263. O. W. Parks, Evidence for transformation of sulfamethazine to its N^4-glucopyranosyl derivative in swine liver during storage, *J. AOAC*, 1984, **67**, 566–569.

264. T. Heberer, M. Lahrssen-Wideerholt, H. Schafft, K. Abraham, H. Pzyrembel, K. J. Henning, M. Schauzu, J. Braunig, M. Goetz, L. Niemann, U. Gundert-Remy, A. Luch, B. Appel, U. Banasiak, G. F. Böl, A. Lampen, R. Wittowski and A. Hensel, Zero tolerances in food and animal feed – are there any scientific alternatives? A European point of view on an international controversy, *Toxicol. Lett.*, 2007, **175**, 118–135.

265. T. Jostmann, Precautionary principle for toxic chemicals – no alternative to safeguard societal benefits, *Hum. Exp. Toxicol.*, 2007, **26**, 847–849.
266. J. C. Hanekamp and J. Kwakman, Beyond zero tolerance: a new approach to food safety and residues of pharmacologically active substances in foodstuffs of animal origin, *Env. Liability*, 2004, **1**, 33–39.
267. I. Forrester and J. C. Hanekamp, Precaution, science and jurisprudence: a test case, *J. Risk. Res.*, 2006, **9**, 297–311.
268. Anon, Drug residue fears prompt lamb recall in UK, *AnimalPharm*, 2007, No. 624, 2.
269. T. Foster, Letter from UK Food Standards Agency, 23 October 2007. Available at: http://www.foodstandards.gov.uk.
270. R. Pérez, C. Palma, M. J. Nuñez and I. Cabezas, Patterns of doramectin tissue residue depletion in parasitized vs nonparasitized lambs, *Parasitol. Res.*, 2008, **102**, 1051–1057.

CHAPTER 4

The Assessment of User Safety

4.1 Introduction

In assessing the safety of medicinal products, whether for human or for veterinary use, safety for the patient is of paramount importance. However, many veterinary medicines offer unique opportunities for exposure of those involved in administering the drug and they too must be protected from any harmful effects. This is particularly important for those products that are given under circumstances not normally associated with the conventional administration of medicines, for example those given on the farm or in the aquaculture industry.

Many veterinary medicines contain the same active ingredients as their human drug counterparts. These include many antimicrobial drugs, anaesthetics, anti-inflammatory agents, antineoplastic drugs and some anthelmintic products. On the other hand, some are different. Furthermore, some veterinary drugs are formulated or used in such a way that there is greater opportunity for user exposure than with the majority of human medicines. Some examples of these are given in Table 4.1. Veterinary vaccines are generally species-specific and are used to prevent diseases in the animal concerned. Vaccines are available for the prophylaxis of disease in most common species including cats, dogs, sheep, cattle, pigs, horses, goats and poultry and are usually given by injection although some poultry vaccines, and notably those for the prevention of coccidiosis, are given orally. Vaccines used in fish, generally those encountered in aquaculture operations, may be given by injection or by bath treatments.

Regulatory authorities in most jurisdictions now assess user safety aspects of veterinary medicinal products prior to granting a marketing authorisation or approval. In the European Union this process has been formalised through the implementation of specific guidelines on user safety.[1,2] Applicants for marketing authorisations are required to conduct a user safety risk assessment,

Issues in Toxicology No. 14
Toxicological Effects of Veterinary Medicinal Products in Humans: Volume 1
By Kevin N. Woodward
© The Royal Society of Chemistry 2013
Published by the Royal Society of Chemistry, www.rsc.org

Table 4.1   Some veterinary medicinal products and possible routes of exposure.

Type of product	Examples of drug type	Route of exposure
In-feed	Antimicrobial drugs, antiparasitic drugs	Dermal, inhalation
Drinking water	Antimicrobial drugs, coccidiostats	Dermal
Dips and spray applications	Organophosphorus compounds, synthetic pyrethroids	Dermal (including contact with treated animals); inhalation from aerosols
Pour-on formulations; spot-on products	Organophosphorus compounds, synthetic pyrethroids, anthelmintics	Dermal (including contact with treated animals)
Administered by drench	Anthelmintics	Dermal
Vaccines	Numerous types	Percutaneous, particularly when using pressurised automatic vaccination equipment
Volatile anaesthetics	Halothane, isoflurane	Inhalation, notably when used in poorly ventilated areas and without suitable gas scavenging equipment
Euthanasia drugs	Barbiturates	Self-injection

which takes into account the hazards, including toxicological hazards, associated with the active ingredient and the formulation, and to interpret these hazards in terms of risk and the communication of any risks through the product literature. There are two guidelines available, both of which have been developed by the Committee for Medicinal Products for Veterinary Use (CVMP) working within the European Medicines Agency (EMA). One set of guidelines covers pharmaceuticals (including ectoparasiticides) and the other covers biological products including vaccines.[3,4] The purpose of both guidelines is clear. They are intended to provide guidance for drug sponsors to assess the hazards and risks associated with a medicinal product, taking into account its intended use, its mode and extent of use, its physico-chemical, toxicological and other biological properties, the possible degree of user exposure and any risk mitigating factors, and then to convey information about the hazards and risks to the end users including veterinarians, veterinary staff, farmers and the animal-owning public, so that recommended precautionary measures can be followed. The legal basis is enshrined in Directive 2001/82/EC as amended by Directive 2004/28/EC and Directive 2009/9/EC.

The current versions of both the pharmaceutical guideline and the immunological guideline provide comprehensive guidance and advice on the hazard and risk assessment processes. However, this has not always been the case. The CVMP originally produced a user safety guideline for veterinary pharmaceuticals which came into effect in 2003.[5] This provided an extensive commentary on many of the aspects involved in user safety assessment but, unfortunately, it failed to provide any substantive advice on the processes involved.[6,7]

Following a consultation exercise, the CVMP revised the guideline and produced the more practicable version that is currently in use and referred to above. This chapter will examine the provisions of the guidelines from the practical viewpoint of having to write a user risk assessment.

4.2 The Assessment Process

As described above, the major aim of the user safety risk assessment is to identify hazards and risks associated with the intended use of a veterinary medicinal product, and then to determine how the risks might be minimised or otherwise mitigated, and then to communicate that information to users, and recommend measures that should be taken to minimise risks. This process is summarised in Figure 4.1.

Depending on the type of product, the main hazards may be toxicological, microbiological, flammability, explosivity (pharmaceuticals) or immunological, including potential exposure to zoonotic organisms used as antigens in vaccines. Thus, drawing on the advice set out in the guidelines, and as set out in Figure 4.1, the major aspects may be regarded as:

- An assessment of the toxicity, pharmacological properties, physico-chemical properties or potential for zoonotic infection (vaccines)
- An assessment of how and when the user will be exposed to the product
- Conclusions on the hazards and potential exposures that may lead to risks to the user and how these risks might be characterised and quantified
- Information to pass to the user to reduce risks.

4.2.1 Hazard Identification and Assessment

Pharmaceutical active ingredients used in veterinary medicinal products are subject to an extensive array of testing to provide data to regulatory authorities as part of the pre-authorisation process. The same is true of components used in veterinary vaccines and other biological products. These tests may include:

- Pharmacological studies to identify and quantify therapeutic effects and pharmacokinetic behaviour in laboratory and target animal (the patient)
- Safety pharmacology studies
- Range of toxicological studies
- Range of microbiological studies *e.g.* to investigate effects on the human gut flora
- For vaccines, reversion to virulence and potential for zoonotic infection *e.g.* brucellosis and rabies vaccines
- Target animal safety (tolerance) studies at the intended dose and at multiples of the intended dose.

The majority of the studies described above will already be available for other purposes within the dossier. For example, for food animals, safety

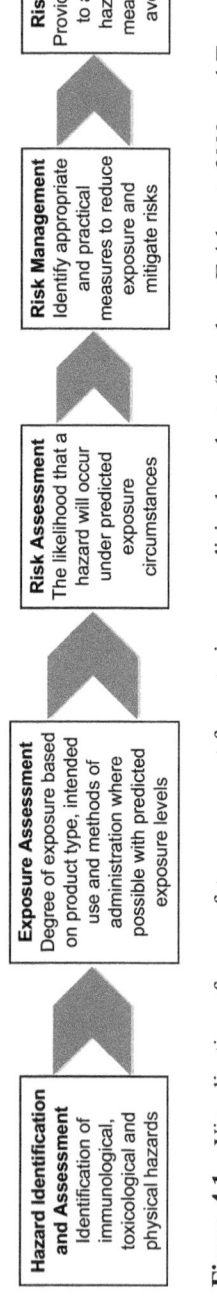

Figure 4.1 Visualisation of user safety assessment for veterinary medicinal products (based on Fairhurst, 2000, and Tennant, 2001[8,9]).

Table 4.2 Toxicity studies generally required to support applications for marketing authorisations for veterinary medicinal products in the EU.

Study	Comments
Safety pharmacology	May be available if the drug is also used in human medicine
Pharmacological studies	Often available for drugs to support mode of action *e.g.* analgesic effects, anaesthetic effects, hormonal effects
Acute toxicity	For older drugs, LD_{50} studies are usually available. For drugs developed in recent years, studies designed to reduce the numbers of animals and to look at end-points other then death may have been conducted[9,10]
Repeat dose studies	To examine organ specific toxicity, dose response effects and no-observed effect level (NOEL) values
Reproductive effects	Examine effects on reproductive performance and fertility, and embryotoxicity, foetotoxicity and teratogenicity. These effects are important in the context of women of child-bearing age working with veterinary medicinal products
Genotoxicity	Studies for the ability of drugs/formulations to induce mutations and clastogenic effects
Carcinogenicity	These studies are usually only required if genotoxicity studies are positive or if the drug or formulation is related to known carcinogens[11,12]
Studies of other effects	Studies of specific toxic (*e.g.* immunotoxic) or pharmacologic (*e.g.* hormonal) effects or mechanistic studies underlying particular aspects of toxicity

pharmacology and toxicology studies will have been generated to provide data for establishing maximum residues, while reversion to virulence studies for vaccines are required to support the general safety of vaccines. Safety information may also be available from the use of the drug in human medicine, including data derived from pharmacovigilance activities. In general, the studies set out in Table 4.2 are required to identify the pharmacological and toxicological profiles of the molecule and to identify no-observed effect level (NOELs) and dose-response relationships. However, it may also be necessary to conduct studies with the formulation to identify particular safety issues associated with the formulation, and constituents of the formulation such as solvents. These generally include skin and eye irritation and skin sensitisation, but they may also include oral and dermal toxicity studies. For gaseous, aerosol, volatile or dusty formulations, inhalation toxicity studies may be required. If the drug or components of the formulation are known to cause hypersensitivity reactions other than skin sensitisation, then this aspect may need further investigation.[13,14] A number of drugs used topically in human medicine are known sensitisers and some of these are also used in veterinary medicine where they are suspected of causing occupational dermatitis.[15–20] The identification of skin sensitisers has for many years relied on tests in the guinea pig, and notably the guinea pig maximisation test, which occasionally provides disparate results.[21–24] The development and validation of newer tests such as the local lymph node assay or studies of the responses to lymphocytes may ease this problem and facilitate the classification of more substances and formulations, including those used in veterinary medicines, as skin sensitisers.[25–28]

Vaccines usually contain innocuous materials such as bacteria- or virus-derived proteinaceous materials, which act as antigens for prophylaxis of the disease caused by the pathogens from which they were derived (or from bacteria or viruses closely related to such pathogens). In most circumstances, the excipients in vaccine formulations such as solvents, adjuvants and other materials, some derived from the manufacturing process, are also innocuous. However, some vaccines contain mineral oils as adjuvants and these have been associated with adverse effects, notably following user self-injection when administered by high-pressure equipment. These accidents are medical emergencies, which, if left untreated, may result in tissue damage and, when injected into the confined anatomical space of a digit or the hand, damage may arise from a combination of the kinetic energy of the delivered material and the pressure with which it is delivered (see Chapter 14).[29–41]

Some veterinary drug formulations contain organic solvents that may be flammable, as may some aerosol-forming products, and these may even pose hazards and risks of explosions. Gaseous and volatile products, if toxicologically or pharmacologically active, may offer the possibility of systemic exposure, and subsequent adverse effects. Assessment of occupational aerosol exposure can be problematic.[42,43]

4.2.2 Exposure Assessment

The probability of an adverse effect to a veterinary drug occurring in a user such as a veterinarian or member of the pet-owning public following exposure is a function not only of the product's innate hazards, but also of the type and extent of exposure. Hence, exposure assessment is a crucial part of user safety risk assessment. The degree to which a user is exposed may depend on a number of factors including the nature of the product, its method of application, the type of animal it is intended for and the ability of the user to administer the product. The scope for user exposure, except from deliberate consumption, may be illustrated by the following examples:

- Low potential for user exposure: tablets, capsules, boluses and sustained-release devices, flavoured medicated chews
- Medium potential for user exposure: topical creams and liquids for manual application, spot-on products for application to companion animals (including exposure to the product on the animal following treatment), pharmaceutical liquid formulations and vaccines intended for conventional (*i.e.* manual) injection
- High potential for user exposure: Pour-on liquid formulations for large animal treatments, high-volume injectable products including poultry and fish vaccines, especially if given by high-pressure injection, products given in feed or drinking water to production animals, ectoparasiticide products administered by dipping, spraying or showering.

However, it is not sufficient to concentrate on administration of the product to the animal, important though this may be, and especially for recalcitrant animals whose behaviour could affect human exposure to the product. Some other tasks involving veterinary medicinal products may lead to exposure. These include:

- Diluting and mixing concentrated liquid products such as organo-phosphorus sheep dip formulations, antimicrobial drugs for addition to drinking water on farms and some vaccines given orally (poultry) or using bath treatments (fish)
- Removing dipped, showered or sprayed sheep from the dipping area
- On-farm mixing of antibiotic premixes with unmedicated feed
- Connecting containers containing large volumes of vaccine for mass administration to the administration device
- Charging an anaesthetic delivery device with liquid anaesthetic
- Administering some drugs used in aquaculture (due to climatic conditions and notably ice (falling and self-contamination with formulation) and wind (product dispensed into sea cages blowing back onto operator)
- Opening product packs.

Physical injuries may also arise from lifting and carrying heavy containers or bags of products, while needlestick injuries, as with human medical practice, are relatively common (Chapter 1).

The major question that needs to be addressed is not "will exposure occur?" but "if exposure is likely to occur, how often will it happen, to what extent and what will be the duration of exposure?". There is a large difference between spilling a liquid formulation onto the hands, and subsequently washing to remove any material, and spilling material onto clothing, which is then worn for a substantial period of time. Equally important is the duration between repeated exposures. If exposure does occur, the degree of absorption needs to be estimated. This is particularly difficult for dermal exposures as frequently there is a lack of information about the degree of absorption and systemic exposure *e.g.* from toxicokinetics studies, and estimates are replaced by educated guesses or, worse, by assumptions. This is problematic because the most frequent exposures tend to be dermal because of spills, drips, leaks and breakages. Syringes may part company from needles during injections and result in contamination of the hands and face. If data are available from absorption studies, then these can be used to make estimates of possible systemic exposures but in the absence of such information, other approaches will need to be taken.

4.2.2.1 Dermal Exposure

A number of models have been developed to predict the degree of percutaneous absorption but, unfortunately, access to these is not always guaranteed.[44–50] Many of these have some aspects in common such as the use of physico-chemical properties and values (viscosity, volatility) and factors for determining the degree and likely extent of dermal exposure including the chances of a spillage occurring, and the number of events likely. Information derived from questionnaires such as known splashing rates and worker cleansing habits may also be included and, together, the information can be used to make some estimates of the degree and extent of dermal exposure.[50–52]

If dermal exposure is predicted, then knowledge of pharmacokinetics (*e.g.* from percutaneous absorption studies in animal models or possibly even in humans) can be used to estimate the fraction of the dose likely to be absorbed. Other data can be used to support the results of these studies or they can be used in mathematical models of percutaneous absorption. These data would include physico-chemical properties that might allow some predictions on passage of the material through skin (polarity, solubility in lipophilic solvents, octanol-water partition coefficients).[53–56] Sometimes, exposure is not to the drug itself, but to the animal that has been treated. Ectoparasiticides, anti-inflammatory drugs and some antimicrobial drugs may be topically applied and there is then a risk of user or owner contamination through contact such as handling or stroking the treated animal or animals. This might lead to dermal contamination and subsequently, through hand-to mouth transfer, to oral exposure producing risks, especially to children who handle companion animals. Adverse reactions have been reported in companion animal owners through this route of exposure.[57] Estimates of potential exposures through this route may be made by using absorbent pads or gloves to stroke treated animals, followed by solvent extraction and determination of the amounts of drug removed.[58]

Both the Organisation for Economic Co-operation and Development (OECD) and the European Commission have produced helpful guidelines on dermal exposure and dermal absorption.[59,60] The former considers chemicals in general while the latter focuses on plant protection products. However, both documents examine various aspects of absorption and factors that affect it such as the nature of the chemical, the nature of the vehicle, dermal metabolism and models of percutaneous absorption. The European Commission document is currently under review by the European Food Safety Authority and a revised draft is available.[61,62] These documents can be usefully employed to consider dermal absorption in the context of veterinary medicinal products. Supplemental information and advice can be found in the International Programme on Chemical Safety's Environmental Health Criteria 235 (dermal absorption).[56]

In the past, several predictive models for dermal (and inhalation) exposure to pesticides have been used for registration purposes.[63–65] A specific model has been developed in the EU to handle exposures to biocides and other chemicals. This is the European Union System for the Evaluation of Substances (EUSES), which is available for download at the European Chemicals Bureau (ECB).[66] This is designed to evaluate exposures and effects, including environmental exposures, but it also addresses occupational exposure through the incorporation of the EASE (Estimation and Assessment of Substance Exposure) model. This makes use of physico-chemical properties, toxicological data and containment measures such as ventilation or full containment to predict dermal and inhalation exposures.[67–69] The EASE model has been validated for a number of exposure scenarios.[69–71] This has an enormous potential for use in user exposure to veterinary medicinal products and, indeed, it has been employed to effect by this author for estimation of dermal and inhalation exposures. Other models have been developed for exposure to ectoparasiticides during shearing of sheep.[72] A separate and earlier model, the European Predictive Operator Exposure Model (EURO POEM), appears to be less developed and is seemingly no longer being actively pursued.[73–75]

4.2.2.2 *Accidental Self-injection*

Needlestick injuries and actual self-injection of veterinary medicinal products are potentially hazardous accidents. Needlestick injuries generally have a benign outcome as the amount of formulation involved is minimal; it usually amounts to a wet needle (see Chapter 1). However, actual self-injection may lead to the systemic exposure to the active constituent and its excipients. These may be toxicologically or pharmacologically active *e.g.* the prostaglandins, steroid hormones, analgesics, injectable anaesthetics and the euthanasia agents. There have been incidents including fatalities with the immobilising drug etorphine and with the antimicrobial drug tilmicosin, again including fatalities.[40,76–83]

However, it must be stressed that such instances are rare. The two examples mentioned above depended on unusual circumstances. Etorphine is an exceptionally potent opiate (see Chapter 13) and humans are exquisitely sensitive to its effects, while tilmicosin is a cardiac toxicant that is more toxic when given intravenously. Thus, in most circumstances, the extreme effects noted with these two drugs will not be expected or, indeed, predicted.

For needlestick injuries with a wet needle *i.e.* a needle contaminated with the liquid formulation under review, it is reasonable to assume that the maximum amount transferred due to the injury is 0.1 ml. Where self-injection may be forecast as a reasonable exposure scenario, it must be assumed that some fraction of the syringe contents will be injected. It is extremely difficult to predict what this dose may be as it will depend on the size of the syringe, which in turn may depend on the size of the animal being injected. The most realistic approach is to assume that a fraction of the syringe contents of around 10 to 50%, dependent on the syringe size and the viscosity of the formulation (and therefore, ease of delivery), may be injected. Automated, high-pressure injection equipment is normally used to deliver vaccines, usually for the mass vaccination of poultry. With this equipment, the desired dose volume is usually pre-set and in these circumstances it must be assumed that the entire intended or recommended dose will be delivered. However, here the hazards are mainly physical and are associated with high-pressure injuries rather than toxicological or pharmacological hazards (see Section 4.2.1). Nevertheless, self-injection of a veterinary vaccine containing hydrocarbon material as the adjuvant has resulted in an autoimmune response while self-injection with Johne's disease (*Mycobacterium paratuberculosis*; paratuberculosis), a product that also contained Freund's complete adjuvant, resulted in tissue damage at the injection site in veterinarians using the products. This was similar to the effects that have been reported after injections with Freund's adjuvant (a preparation containing inactivated and dried mycobacteria, mineral oil and water) alone and with other formulations containing Freund's adjuvant.[37,38,84–88] Self-injection injuries are discussed in Chapters 1 and 14.

4.2.2.3   Inhalation Exposure

It is often difficult to obtain data on the possible extent of inhalation exposure to dusty medicated feeds, volatile liquids and gaseous products. Nevertheless, the potential for inhalation exposure must be addressed if there is any likelihood that inhalable material will be encountered during use. Consequently, the sponsor of the veterinary medicinal product or the author of the user risk assessment needs to consider suitable approaches that may prove to be acceptable to regulatory authorities.

It is possible to argue that inhalation is unlikely or of low importance based on scientific considerations such as low volatility, use of ventilation or exhaust systems where the product will be used, use of scavenging systems, use of dust suppressants in dusty medicated feed formulations or that any particles of dust that are in the product are not in the respirable range. Alternatively, it may be possible to state that the product is intended for outdoor use only and that any vapours or gases produced will dissipate. Finally, it may be possible to suggest that as the product is of low toxicity by the inhalation route (and by other routes leading to systemic absorption), inhalation exposure will offer no undue risks for human health.

Some products used in veterinary medicine offer scope for inhalation exposure. Among them is the volatile anaesthetic halothane (see Chapter 5). A small number of human patients given the drug develop severe and potentially fatal hepatic injuries, which are thought to arise from the action of reactive metabolites formed in the liver with proteins, the products of which then elicit an immune response.[89,90] For this reason, and because of other health concerns such as neurotoxicity, occupational exposure to halothane in human medicine is recognised as a health problem.[89–105] As a result, extensive efforts have been made to reduce workplace exposure.[106–121] This has led to major concerns over the safety of veterinarians and veterinary workers exposed to halothane and other volatile anaesthetics during surgical procedures.[122–137] However, these concerns have led in turn to recommendations for safer use and for better occupational hygiene measures (see Chapter 5).[138–141]

For any product where there is a possibility that atmospheric contamination with dust, gas or vapour may occur, the practical option may be to attempt to determine occupational concentrations during typical operations such as emptying containers, mixing, provision or administration to animals and disposal. These studies are often complex and are best left to individuals or organisations that have experience with their conduct. However, a few points are worth making. Exposure studies should model the actual use of the veterinary medicinal product under realistic conditions similar to those that will occur during normal use. This may mean that such studies will have to be carried out on-farm or in circumstances that replicate on-farm conditions, using equipment that would normally be used *e.g.* feed mixers. Sampling may need to be conducted at various points, including those where the containers or bottles are opened, those where mixing (*e.g.* of medicated feed with premix) occurs and those points at which product is provided or administered to the animals (*e.g.* feed-lot or during veterinary surgery). Sampling can then be carried out using automated equipment or using personal sampling devices, preferably placed at lapel level to measure concentrations in the breathing zone.[142–147]

It is not practicable to suggest advice on the numbers of samples to be taken or on the positioning of samplers other than those designed for personal use. In fact the numbers will depend on the workplace environment (*e.g.* veterinary clinic, dairy farm or pig production unit). Other factors such as temperature, particle size, sample stability and the extent of ventilation, as well as statistical considerations, will need to be taken into account.[147–150]

The types of samplers will depend on the nature of the veterinary medicinal product being studied *e.g.* whether it is a gas, a volatile liquid, an aerosol or a dusty formulation. In sampling dusty materials, particle size must also be taken into account.[151–153] Other considerations include air movement conditions, the re-suspension of dust from clothing and the entrapment of dust in areas of the sampler other than the filter as this may introduce measurement bias.[154–156] It is also essential to identify the components of the dust collected if this is at all possible. Specifically, the pharmaceutical content needs to be distinguished from inert materials such as feed, minerals and inorganic carriers such as limestone, and the particle sizes determined as only those in the respirable range will have any repercussions for toxicological risk assessment.[157–159]

If experimental procedures and simulated exposures are impractical for scientific or economic reasons, then modelling may be a realistic alternative. The EASE model referred to earlier, as part of the EUSES suite, is an ideal candidate that can incorporate physico-chemical, toxicological and other measurements or models such as those dealing with particle size and pulmonary deposition.[160–162]

4.2.2.4 Oral Exposure

The major route for oral exposure to veterinary medicines is likely to be hand to mouth. This may arise from direct contact with contaminated hands or by transfer through food and smoking materials. It is extremely difficult to predict the likely doses arising in these circumstances and, as with self-injection, the only practical solution is to consider fractions of the intended dose for the animal, based on the likelihood and degree of exposure, which to some extent will be based on physical properties of the product (dustiness, viscosity, volatility).

Oral exposure may also arise as a result of inhalation exposure. Particulate material may adhere to the tongue and buccal cavity or they may be retrieved from the respiratory system where they have lodged or as a result of expulsion from the lungs. The total exposure must then be assumed to be the total of the inhaled fraction and the oral fraction.

In this respect the particle size is important. In fact, it is essential to take into account the aerodynamic diameter of the particle that is related to its physical diameter and its density.[163]

$$\text{Aerodynamic diameter} = \text{physical diameter} \times (\text{density})^2$$

As an illustration, a particle of physical diameter 2 µm and density of 4 g cm^{-3} will behave identically to a particle of 4 µm and a density of 1 g cm^{-3}. Hence, when considering respirable particles and the overall respirable fraction, the aerodynamic diameter is the measurement of interest, and not purely the physical diameter.

Oral exposure may also occur as a result of deliberate misuse or abuse, and the possibility that children may consume veterinary medicinal products also has to be considered. The latter appears to be rare but it needs to form part of a user risk assessment, especially as children may be more sensitive to the pharmacological or toxicological effects of the formulation.[164,165]

4.3   Biological Monitoring

Biological monitoring can be used to confirm and quantify exposure or to determine if adverse effects are occurring. The data can be generated prior to drafting a user risk assessment and the results included, or they can be produced post-authorisation to confirm the results of safety, including user safety assessments. Biological monitoring implies either a prior knowledge of possible adverse effects that can be readily detected, or of pharmacokinetic behaviour, either in animals or in humans, so that specific metabolites or markers of exposure can be identified and quantified as appropriate and specific biomarkers selected.[8,166–173] In turn, this may involve development of indices of exposure, possibly including physiologically based pharmacokinetic modelling.[169,174–180] However, as the majority of exposures to veterinary medicinal products is usually likely to be low, such measures will normally only be required under exceptional circumstances and then only for more toxic substances or formulations such as organophosphorus compounds of the type used in sheep dips.[181,182]

Biomonitoring may also be conducted by examining biological adverse effects in exposed individuals, for example by investigating genetic damage in workers and other populations exposed to benzene, pesticides, other chemicals and environmental pollutants.[183–197] These techniques have been employed in the biomonitoring of healthcare workers including nurses and pharmacists handling and administering cytotoxic drugs such as cyclophosphamide, ifosfamide and 5-fluorouracil and some of these studies have confirmed a higher occurrence of genetic damage indicated by increases in micronuclei, sister chromatid exchanges, chromosome and DNA damage, as well as mutagenic activity in the urine, in exposed personnel.[198–232] There are no comparable studies for veterinary personnel, possibly because cancer treatments generally take place in general clinics as there are relatively few facilities dedicated to veterinary oncology when compared with human medicine. Nevertheless, concern has been expressed about the exposure of veterinary personnel to cytotoxic drugs, and the UK regulatory authority, the Veterinary Medicines Directorate, has in the past published advice about their safe use.[233–235] Exposure to cytotoxic drugs is considered to be possible not only through direct contact, but also with the urine and other fluids of treated animals (see Chapter 7).[236–239]

4.4 Risk Assessment

Risk is the probability that a hazard will be realised or expressed. Consequently, when considering veterinary medicines and user risk assessments the issue under consideration is whether the hazards identified (pharmacological, toxicological, physico-chemical) earlier in the process of assessment will be expressed during use and, if so, what probability does this carry? However, there is usually insufficient information to make this quantitative assessment.[240] Consequently, the process of risk assessment in these circumstances is really one of risk estimation. The toxicology and pharmacology may well be characterised and NOELs identified but the question arises as to whether any effects might be expressed in exposed workers or other users.

Nevertheless, an attempt has to be made to try to determine, even if in only semi-quantitative terms, what risks users of the product might expect. To do this in a meaningful way, it is often helpful to assume that users will be totally unprotected so that the effects of exposure might be predicted and then, in the next phase of the assessment, identify specific ways of mitigating any risks. The most convenient way of doing this is to compare likely exposure levels and assumed doses with NOEL values or, if these are not available, with lowest observed effect levels (LOELs), taking into account the likely routes of exposure that are most realistic and comparing these with the results of toxicology studies and the routes of exposure used in these. Where appropriate, the duration of exposure expected from use should be compared with the results from the corresponding toxicity studies. For example, single or intermittent and infrequent exposure should be compared with the results of acute toxicity studies, while prolonged exposure needs to be viewed in light of the results of repeat dose toxicity studies. If the major route of occupational exposure is inhalation, then the results of acute inhalation and repeat dose inhalation toxicity studies will become relevant. However, if the major route of exposure is dermal then not only are the results of percutaneous toxicity studies and skin absorption of interest, but so are those from skin irritation and dermal sensitisation studies. If skin absorption is likely to occur, then the likely or estimated degree of absorption is important.

The potential for local effects must be considered if skin or eye contact is likely or possible, so knowledge of the irritant and sensitising potential of the drug and the formulation is crucial. Dermal effects are important because skin contamination may be the major route of exposure as it is for many chemicals and other products. Adverse effects have been reported in users with several veterinary drugs following skin contamination. For example, the antimicrobial drug olaquindox has been reported to cause allergic and photoallergic effects, notably in pig farmers, while the macrolide antibiotic spiramycin has resulted in contact dermatitis and bronchial asthma.[241–247]

Qualitative risk and quantitative risk are terms that are often used in risk assessment. These terms may be regarded as unhelpful as risk implies a quantitative assessment. In producing a user risk assessment, the terms are possibly even more misleading as neither the drug sponsor nor the author of the user risk assessment are trying to calculate the probability of an adverse event occurring. They are in fact attempting to assess what might happen if exposure occurs under normal conditions of use. As a result, and in general, abuse and misuse, freak accidents and extreme user conditions are not normally considered. Indeed, the user safety guidelines make it clear that the exposure scenarios should be realistic and that the degree of exposure or contamination should be related to the toxicology of the compound or formulation.

This can be exemplified by reference to oral exposure. In this case, the likely dose, or an estimated dose can be compared with the NOEL (or NOELs) identified in toxicity studies. However, it is also valid to compare the exposures with the acceptable daily intake, the ADI (see Chapter 3), as this value is based on oral consumption and is derived by dividing a suitable NOEL, frequently the lowest identified, by an appropriate safety factor. If the product is used only in companion animals, and there is no ADI available for consumer safety purposes, there is no reason why the investigator cannot calculate a value using the usual criteria[2,248–254] (see also Chapter 3).

The degree of exposure expected can then be compared with the NOEL or the ADI to determine the margin of exposure (MOE). A number of factors need to be considered when calculating the MOE, including the likely degree of systemic absorption, the severity of the adverse effect, the numbers of people likely to be exposed, the differences between routes of exposure in animal models and the dose-response relationship. If the MOE is low, then risk management measures may not be required. However, if the MOE is large, then suitable measures and recommendations will be needed to protect human health.

For substances that may be inhaled, occupational exposure limits for use in the industrial setting may be available. Examples of these include the threshold limit value, or TLV, developed by several regulatory organisations but notably by the American Conference of Governmental Industrial Hygienists.[255–258] Unfortunately, the entries for pharmaceuticals or for substances that can be used as pharmaceuticals in the UK exposure limit list are limited to enflurane, halothane, isoflurane, nitrous oxide, paracetamol (acetaminophen) dust, nitrous oxide and carbon dioxide[259] (see also Chapter 5). However, occupational exposure limits can be derived *de novo* using toxicology and pharmacology data, assumptions on pulmonary absorption and suitable safety factors to allow for intra- and inter-species variability and other variables.[260–265] Some of these are based on industrial and manufacturing environments but that does not limit their utility and all of these methods can be supplemented, where relevant, with physiologically based pharmacokinetic models.[266–268]

4.5 Risk Management

Risk management can be defined in a number of ways. The Royal Society in the UK defined it as "the making of decisions concerning risk and their subsequent implementation", while the World Health Organization described it as "the managerial, decision making and active hazard control process to deal with those environmental agents for which the risk evaluation has indicated the risk is too high".[269] Risk management, or risk reduction, sets out the measures to reduce exposure and hence to mitigate risk. This implies that any precautions made are practical and any specialist equipment or protective clothing is practicable and readily available. There must be a reasonable expectation that, in practice, any precautionary measures will be followed. If these measures are not practical, almost certainly users of veterinary medicinal products will ignore them.

There are a number of measures available to regulatory authorities to control exposure to veterinary formulations and one of these is to restrict the availability of the product, for example to classify the product as "prescription only". However, the veterinarian may still prescribe the product for use on pets at home meaning that untrained professionals will be required to administer it, while, on the other hand, there is no guarantee that trained professionals like veterinarians will use the product safely. Nevertheless, many potentially hazardous products will be used on farms or in the veterinary clinic by trained professionals. Examples of products include anaesthetics, sedatives, vaccines containing attenuated zoonotic organisms and euthanasia agents. Closed delivery systems can be used or recommended for some potentially hazardous materials, while dusty medicated feeds may (and usually do) have some method of dust suppression such as the admixture with vegetable oil or propylene glycol.

Packaging and containers can be designed to reduce potential exposures and methods of administration modified such as the use of pour-on formulations rather than sprays. It may also be appropriate to limit the size of packs to reduce the amount of material available for use and minimise the quantities left over as waste. Personal protective equipment (PPE) may also be recommended and this may include the use of impervious gloves, masks, goggles, and protective clothing including impervious aprons and boots, as appropriate. However, as already described, these should only be recommended if they are practicable for administration of the product. The recommendations for protective clothing and equipment are more likely to be observed in practice if these are practical under normal conditions of use. For example, it is of little utility recommending the use of impregnable gloves and aprons, heavy boots, respirators and goggles for heavy manual work such as dipping sheep. Almost certainly these recommendations will be ignored. The EU user safety guideline recommends that "PPE must be readily available to the user and measures should not hamper the use of the product...".

Measures recommended should therefore be appropriate, proportional and adequate to provide the necessary degree of protection and should be suitable for the intended use. For example, recommending the use of gloves may be inadequate if the gloves that are likely to be used, frequently household gloves, are permeable to a solvent in the formulation or if the gloves are likely to be damaged by components of the formulation. Respirators must be suitable for the protection intended as those designed for use with solvents may be unsuitable for dusts. They should be selected for use with the hazard in questions such as fine dusts, coarse dusts, vapours, aerosols as appropriate.[270,271] They must also have the correct workplace protection factor (WPF) for the use intended. This is defined as the ratio of the concentration of dust or aerosol outside the respirator with that inside the respirator, while the device is worn in the work environment.[272,273] There is, however, a wide within-wearer variability of WPF across respirator users and this has led in turn to the development of assigned protection factors (APFs) to reduce the effects of these variations and to facilitate equipment choice.[273,274]

4.6 Risk Communication

In the context of veterinary medicinal products, the purpose of risk communication is to convey information about risks to the end user of the product. That is, to disseminate information on hazards and risks associated with a product, and the measures necessary under risk management to reduce exposure and mitigate risks. For veterinary medicinal products this generally means information, warnings and recommendations for safe use provided in the product literature or on the label, or for posters and warning notices displayed in the workplace. In the EU, this also means in the Summary of Product Characteristics (SPC) that forms the basis for the subsequent label. The purposes of risk communication are four-fold: to provide information on the risks involved; to provide information on specific exposures to avoid; to suggest how these can be avoided or reduced; and to provide information on what should happen if exposure occurs. An example is given below:

> *Avoid skin, eye or mucosal contact.*
> *Immediately after exposure wash the exposed skin with large amounts of fresh water.*
> *Remove contaminated clothes that are in direct contact with skin.*
> *If symptoms occur, seek the advice of a doctor.*

> *In the case of accidental oral intake or self-injection, seek medical advice*
> *immediately and show the package leaflet to the doctor.*

Unfortunately, risk communication has its own problems ranging from complacency on behalf of the audience for which it is intended, overburdening that audience with messages about risks and hazards and people's individual perceptions of risk.[275–283] Moreover, extensive information on product labels or package inserts is liable to go unread, especially where the label is small and the font size even smaller. Nevertheless, education accompanied by attitude changes on behalf of users of veterinary medicines and the provision of clear messages that are commensurate with the risks involved should help to ease these problems.[277,281] After all, the benefits of this hazard and risk assessment process will only be realised if the target audience actually reads the advice.

Finally, it has to be recognised that if it is not possible to achieve a suitable risk assessment, for example if any necessary advice is likely to be ignored or if there is evidence that the product has inherent properties that mean that it cannot be used safely, then the only viable option for the regulator is either not to grant a marketing authorisation or approval or, if it is already being marketed, to suspend or revoke authorisations or approvals.

To facilitate user compliance, in addition to avoiding cramming warnings and recommendations on to labels, labels should be designed to be clear and uncluttered and safety precautions should be concise and unambiguous.

4.7 Conclusions

The approaches described here, although largely based on the EU model, are applicable anywhere. The evaluation of user safety, with or without complex guidelines, follows the same model in almost all regulatory jurisdictions and is essentially that depicted in Figure 4.1. It is a logical process that considers the hazards of a substance coupled with the risks to human health that those hazards are associated with in the preparation and administration of the product.

The major aim of this process, indeed perhaps the only aim, is to ensure that instructions and recommendations regarding safe use actually reach the user regardless of whether that user is a veterinarian, another veterinary professional, a farmer, a fish farmer or a pet owner. Many of the judgments made in the review process are cautious or even precautious. That is, the assessment process tends to build worst case on to worst case (*e.g.* the lowest NOEL from toxicity studies, the highest degree of exposure during exposure assessment, the worst possible outcome if exposure does occur and the repeated asking of "what if" – what if he/she falls into it, drinks the whole container of it, is uniquely sensitive to its effects, is working on a remote farm miles away from a doctor, and so on). As already described, the outcome of risk assessment may be not to authorise a product or to take one off of the market. However, this has to be seen in terms of benefits and not just risks, and those benefits can be societal as well as therapeutic. For example, the risks associated with using a cytostatic anticancer drug in dogs and cats must be weighed against the benefits to the animals and with the needs of the owner, the latter often being solely emotional. In such circumstances, authorisation must be considered, but carefully controlled conditions of use implemented.[284–286]

It must also be remembered that authorisation is not the end of the story. Most countries now have modern and efficient pharmacovigilance systems in place to detect adverse drug reactions, not only in treated animals but also in exposed humans including those occupationally exposed.[39,40,287–289] Findings from pharmacovigilance programmes (see Chapter 2), especially adverse events in exposed users, can be used to refine risk assessments and to amend product label warnings and recommendations.

The process of user safety risk assessment is not difficult but it is rarely straightforward except for the simplest of products. It may be complicated with toxicological issues such as defining NOELs and agreeing ADI values. In the EU the process is facilitated by the now clear and helpful guidelines for pharmaceuticals and vaccines. The overall aim of the assessment must be to balance the hazards and the associated user risks, along with other risks (environmental and patient) with the benefits of treating the animal and with those for its owner and the public in general. Balancing benefits and risks is never easy even in human medicine where the risks are frequently borne by the patient – the individual who stands to gain most from treatment.[290–293] This becomes more difficult with veterinary drugs where the risks are borne not only by the patient but also by those treating them (and often eating them). A well-considered user risk assessment facilitates the regulatory process and focuses major safety issues.

References

1. K. N. Woodward, User safety assessment of veterinary medicinal products in *Veterinary Pharmacovigilance. Adverse Reactions to Veterinary Medicinal Products*, ed. K. N. Woodward, Wiley-Blackwell, Chichester, 2009, pp. 529–545.
2. K. N. Woodward, The evolution of safety assessments for veterinary medicinal products in the European Union, *Vet. Hum. Toxicol.*, 2004, **46**, 199–205.
3. Committee for Medicinal Products for Veterinary Use (CVMP), Guideline on user safety for pharmaceutical veterinary medicinal products, March 2010, EMA/CVMP/543/03-Rev.1.
4. Committee for Medicinal Products for Veterinary Use (CVMP), Guideline on user safety for immunological veterinary medicinal products, April 2007, EMEA/CVMP/IWP/54533/2006.
5. Committee for Veterinary Medicinal Products (CVMP), Guideline on user safety for pharmaceutical veterinary medicinal products, EMA/CVMP/543/03-FINAL.
6. K. N. Woodward, The European veterinary user safety guidelines for pharmaceuticals, *Regul. Affairs. J.*, 2007, **18**, 535–540.

7. K. N. Woodward, Assessment of user safety exposure and risk to veterinary medicinal products in the European Union, *Regul. Pharmacol. Toxicol.*, 2008, **50**, 114–128.
8. S. Fairhurst, Industrial toxicology and hygiene in *General and Applied Toxicology*, ed. B. Ballantyne, T. C. Marrs and T. Syversen, Macmillan, London, 2nd edn, 2000, pp. 1473–1488.
9. D. R. Tennant, Risk analysis in *Food Chemical Safety*, CRC Press/ Woodhead Publishing Ltd, Cambridge, 2001, vol. 1, *Contaminants*, pp. 15–36.
10. C. R. Rhodes, Principles of testing for acute effects in *General and Applied Toxicology*, ed. B. Ballantyne, T. C. Marrs and T. Syversen, Macmillan, London, 2nd edn, 2000, pp. 33–54.
11. M. J. van den Heuvel, D. G. Clark, R. J. Fielder, P. P. Koundakjian, G. J. Oliver, D. Pelling, N. J. Tomlinson and A. P. Walker, The international validation of a fixed-dose procedure as an alternative to the classical LD_{50} test, *Food Chem. Toxicol.*, 1990, **28**, 469–482.
12. D. M. Galer and A. M. Monro, Veterinary drugs no longer need testing for carcinogenicity in rodent bioassays, *Regul. Toxicol. Pharmacol.*, 1998, **28**, 115–123.
13. A. D. Dayan, Allergy to antimicrobial residues in food: an assessment of the risk to man, *Vet. Microbiol.*, 1993, **35**, 213–226.
14. K. N. Woodward, Hypersensitivity in humans and exposure to veterinary drugs, *Vet. Hum. Toxicol.*, 1991, **33**, 168–172.
15. Anon, Cutaneous drug reaction reports, *Am. J. Clin. Dermatol.*, 2002, **3**, 223–227.
16. C. A. Menezes de Pádua, W. Uter and A. Schnuck, Contact allergy to topical drugs: prevalence in a clinical setting and estimation of frequency at the population level, *Pharmacoepidemiol. Drug Saf.*, 2007, **16**, 377–384.
17. C. Pétavy-Catala, L. Machet and L. Vaillant, Consort contact urticarial due to amoxicillin, *Contact Dermatitis*, 2001, **44**, 246.
18. A. Rodrígues-Morales, A. A. Llamazares, R. P. Benito and C. M. Cóchera, Fixed drug eruption from quinolones with a positive lesional patch test to ciprofloxacin, *Contact Dermatitis*, 2001, **44**, 246.
19. N. K. Veien, Systemic contact dermatitis, *Int. J. Dermatol.*, 2011, **50**, 1445–1456.
20. E. Rudzki and P. Rebandel, Airborne contact dermatitis due to ethacridine lactate in a veterinary surgeon, *Contact Dermatitis*, 2001, **45**, 234.
21. E. D. Schlede and R. Eppler, Testing for skin sensitisation according to the notification procedure for new chemicals: the Magnusson and Kligman test, *Contact Dermatitis*, 1995, **32**, 1–4.
22. T. Maurer, P. Thomann, E. G. Weinrich and R. Hess, Predictive evaluation in animals of the contact allergic potential of medically important substances. I. Comparison of different methods of inducing and measuring cutaneous sensitization, *Contact Dermatitis*, 1978, **4**, 321–333.
23. B. Magnusson and A. M. Kligman, The identification of contact allergens by animal assay. The guinea pig maximization test, *J. Invest. Dermatol.*, 1969, **52**, 268–275.

24. D. Basketter, N. Ball, S. Cagen, J. C. Carillo, H. Certa, D. Eigler, C. Garcia, H. Esch, C. Graham, C. Haux, R. Kreiling and A. Mehling, Application of a weight of evidence approach to assessing discordant sensitisation datasets: implications for REACH, *Regul. Toxicol. Pharmacol.*, 2009, **55**, 90–96.

25. K. M. Jung, W. H. Jang, Y. K. Lee, Y. N. Yum, S. Sohn, B. H. Kim, J. H. Chung, Y. H. Park and K. M. Lim, B cell increases and *ex vivo* IL-2 production as secondary endpoints for the detection of sensitizers in non-radioisotopic local lymph node assay using flow cytometry, *Toxicol. Lett.*, 2012, **209**, 255–263.

26. R. J. Dearman, D. A. Basketter and I. Kimber, Local lymph node assay: use in hazard and risk assessment, *J. Appl. Toxicol.*, 1999, **19**, 299–306.

27. G. F. Gerberick, C. A. Ryan, I. Kimber, R. J. Dearman, L. J. Lea and D. A. Basketter, Local lymph node assay: validation assessment for regulatory purposes, *Am. J. Contact Derm.*, 2000, **11**, 3–18.

28. I. Kimber, G. Maxwell, N. Gilmour, R. J. Dearman, P. S. Friedmann and S. F. Martin, Allergic contact dermatitis: A commentary on the relationship between T lymphocytes and skin sensitising potency, *Toxicology*, 2012, **29**, 18–24.

29. F. D. Burke and O. Brady, Veterinary and industrial high pressure injection injuries, *Br. Med. J.*, 1996, **312**, 1436.

30. G. Couzens and F. D. Burke, Veterinary high pressure injuries with inoculation in larger animals, *J. Hand Surg.*, 1995, **20**, 497–499.

31. D. P. Gwynne-Jones, Accidental self-injection with oil-based veterinary vaccines, *N. Z. Med. J.*, 1996, **109**, 363–365.

32. D. P. Jones, Accidental self inoculation with oil based veterinary vaccines, *N. Z. Med. J.*, 1996, **109**, 363–365.

33. N. C. Neal and F. D. Burke, High pressure injection injuries, *Injury*, 1996, **22**, 467–470.

34. I. Utrobicić, Z. Pogorelić and N. Druzijanić, High-pressure injection injuries of the hand – report of two cases, *Acta Chir. Belg.*, 2011, **111**, 46–50.

35. J. K. O'Neill, S. W. Richards, D. M. Ricketts and M. H. Patterson, The effects of injection of bovine vaccine into a human digit.: a case report, *Environ. Health*, 2005, **4**, 21.

36. S. T. O'Sullivan, J. M. O'Donoghue and T. P. F. O'Connor, Occupational high-pressure injection injury to the hand, *Dermatology*, 1997, **194**, 311.

37. P. A. Windsor, R. Bush, I. Links and J. Eppleston, Injury caused by self-inoculation with a vaccine of a complete Freund's adjuvant nature (Gudair) used for control of paratuberculosis, *Austr. Vet. J.*, 2005, **83**, 216–220.

38. G. D. Richardson, I. I. Links and P. A. Windsor, Gudair (OJD) vaccine self-inoculation: a case for early debridement, *Med. J. Austr.*, 2005, **183**, 151–152.

39. K. N. Woodward, Veterinary pharmacovigilance. Part 4. Adverse reactions in humans to veterinary medicinal products, *J. Vet. Pharmacol. Ther.*, 2005, **28**, 185–201.

40. K. N. Woodward, Adverse reactions in humans following exposure to veterinary drugs in *Veterinary Pharmacovigilance. Adverse Reactions to Veterinary Medicinal Products*, ed. K. N. Woodward, Wiley-Blackwell, Chichester, 2009, pp. 475–515.

41. D. M. Bourget and J. Perrone, High pressure decisions: recognition and management of uncommon hand injuries, *J. Med. Toxicol.*, 2011, **7**, 162–163.

42. J. H. Vincent, Occupational and environmental aerosol exposure assessment: a scientific journey from the past, through the present and into the future, *J. Environ. Monit.*, 2012, **14**, 340–347.

43. W. Eduard, D. Hederik, C. Duchaine and B. J. Green, Bioaerosol exposure assessment in the workplace: the past, present and recent advances, *J. Environ. Monit*, 2012, **14**, 334–349.

44. D. Fitzpatrick, J. Corish and B. Hayes, Modelling of skin permeability in risk assessment – the future, *Chemosphere*, 2004, **55**, 1309–1314.

45. P. G. Georgopoulos and P. G. Lioy, Conceptual and theoretical aspects of human exposure and dose assessment, *J. Expos. Anal. Environ. Epidemiol.*, 1994, **4**, 253–285.

46. R. Oppl, F. Kalberlah, P. G. Evans and J. J. Van Hemmen, A toolkit for dermal risk assessment and management: an overview, *Ann. Occup. Hyg.*, 2003, **47**, 629–640.

47. J. Marquart, D. H. Brouwer, J. H. J. Gijsbers, I. H. M. Kinks, N. Warren and J. J. Van Hemmen, Determinants of dermal exposure relevant for exposure modeling in regulatory risk assessment, *Ann. Occup. Hyg.*, 2003, **47**, 599–607.

48. T. Schneider, R. Vermeulen, D. H. Brouwer, J. K. Cherrie, H. Kromhout and C. L. Fogh, Conceptual model for assessment of dermal exposure, *Occup. Environ. Med.*, 1999, **56**, 765–773.

49. J. J. Van Hemmen, J. Aufarth, P. G. Evans, B. Rajan-Sithanparanadarajah, H. Marquart and R. Oppl, RISKOFDERM: risk assessment of occupational dermal exposure to chemicals. An introduction to a series of papers on the development of a toolkit, *Ann. Occup. Hyg.*, 2003, **47**, 595–598.

50. B. Van-Wendel-de-Joode, D. H. Brouwer, R. Vermeulen, J. J. Van Hemmen, D. Heederik and H. Kromhout, DREAM: a method for semi-quantitative dermal exposure assessment, *Ann. Occup. Hyg.*, 2003, **47**, 71–87.

51. M. Cattani, K. Cena, J. Edwards and D. Pisaniello, Potential dermal and inhalation exposure to chlorpyrifos in Austrian pesticide workers, *Ann. Occup. Hyg.*, 2001, **45**, 299–308.

52. European Centre for Ecotoxicology and Toxicology of Chemicals (ECETOC), Percutaneous absorption, Monograph No. 20, ECETOC, Brussels, 1993.

53. R. O. Potts and R. H. Guy, Predicting skin permeability, *Pharm. Res.*, 1992, **9**, 663–669.

54. A. Wilschut, W. F. ten Berge, P. J. Robinson and T. E. McKone, Estimating skin permeation. The validation of five mathematical skin permeation models, *Chemosphere*, 1995, **30**, 1275–1296.

55. M. B. Reddy, R. H. Guy and A. L. Bunge, Does epidermal turnover reduce percutaneous penetration? *Pharm. Res.*, 2000, **17**, 1414–1419.
56. International Programme on Chemical Safety, Dermal Absorption, Environmental Health Criteria 235, IPCS, WHO, Geneva, 2006.
57. R. G. Ames, S. K. Brown, J. Rosenberg, R. J. Jackson, J. W. Stratton and S. G. Quenon, Health symptoms and occupational exposure to flea control products among California pet handlers, *Am. Ind. Hyg. Assoc.*, 1989, **50**, 466–472.
58. United States Environmental Protection Agency, Occupational and Residential Exposure Guidelines, OPPTS 875.1200 Dermal Exposure – Indoor, EPA 712-C-96-209, 1996.
59. Organisation for Economic Co-operation and Development, OECD Environment, Health and Safety Publications, Series on Testing and Assessment, No. 156, Guidance Notes on Dermal Absorption, ENV/JM/MONO (2011) 36, OECD, 2011. Available at: http://www.oecd.org.
60. European Commission, Guidance Document on Dermal Absorption, Sanco/222/2000 rev. 7, 19 March 2004.
61. European Food Safety Authority, Guidance on Dermal Absorption, EFSA Panel on Plant Protection Products and their Residues (PPR), EFSA, 2011. Available at: http://www.efsa.europa.eu/en/.
62. European Food Safety Authority, Technical Report of EFSA, Outcome of the public consultation on the draft guidance on dermal absorption and the draft scientific opinion on the science behind the revision of the guidance document on dermal absorption, EFSA, 2011. Available at: http://www.efsa.europa.eu/en/.
63. W. Luo, S. Medrek, J. Misra and G. J. Nohynek, Predicting human skin absorption of chemicals: development of a novel quantitative structure activity relationship, *Toxicol. Ind. Health*, 2007, **23**, 39–45.
64. T. Søeborg, L. H. Basse and B. Halling-Sørensen, Risk assessment of topically applied products, *Toxicology*, 2007, **236**, 140–148.
65. J. J. van Hemmen, Predictive exposure modelling for pesticide registration purposes, *Ann. Occup. Hyg.*, 1993, **37**, 541–564.
66. Institute for Health and Consumer Protection/Joint Research Centre, The new EUSES 2.1.2 version (2012) is an update of EUSES 2.1, containing all emission scenario documents for biocides, 2012. Available at: http://ihcp.jrc.europa.eu.
67. C. Northage, EASEing into the future, *Ann. Occup. Hyg.*, 2005, **49**, 99–101.
68. J. Tickner, J. Friar, K. S. Creely, J. W. Cherie, D. E. Pryde and J. Kingston, The development of the EASE model, *Ann. Occup. Hyg.*, 2005, **49**, 103–110.
69. J. W. Cherie, J. Tickner, J. Friar, K. S. Creely, J. Soutar, G. Hughson, R. Rae, N. D. Warren and D. E. Pryde, Evaluation and further development of the EASE model 2.0, Health and Safety Executive, Bootle, 2003. Available at: http://www.hse.gov.uk.
70. J. W. Cherie and G. W. Hughson, The validity of the EASE Expert System for inhalation exposures, *Ann. Occup. Hyg.*, 2005, **49**, 125–134.

71. K. S. Creely, J. Tickner, A. J. Soutar, G. W. Hughson, D. E. Pryde, N. D. Warren, R. Rae, C. Money, A. Phillips and J. W. Cherie, Evaluation and further development of EASE model 2.0, *Ann. Occup. Hyg.*, 2005, **49**, 135–145.

72. V. Villière, An Australian experience of using work practices to establish an exposure model for shearers, *Ann. Occup. Hyg.*, 2001, **45**, S103–S105.

73. K. Machera, M. Goumeno, E. Kapetanakis, A. Kalamarakis and C. R. Glass, Determination of potential dermal and inhalation exposure of operators, following application of the fungicide penconazole in vineyards and greenhouses, *Fresenius Environ. Bull.*, 2001, **10**, 464–469.

74. K. Machera, M. Goumeno, E. Kapetanakis, A. Kalamarakis and C. R. Glass, Determination of potential dermal and inhalation operator exposure to malathion in greenhouses with whole body dosimetry, *Ann. Occup. Hyg.*, 2003, **47**, 61–70.

75. J. J. Van Hemmen, EUROPOEM, a predictive occupational exposure database for registration purposes of pesticides, *Appl. Occup. Environ. Hyg*, 2001, **16**, 246–250.

76. Anon, Immobilon: why the VPC suspended the licence, *Vet. Rec.*, 1976, **99**, 156.

77. S. Firn, Accidental poisoning by an animal-immobilising agent, *Lancet*, 1973, **ii**, 95–96.

78. P. G. E. Goodrich, Accidental self-injection, *Vet. Rec.*, 1977, **100**, 458–459.

79. J. C. Vaudrey, Accidental injection with Immobilon, *Vet. Rec.*, 1974, **94**, 52.

80. L. A. Crown and R. B. Smith, Accidental veterinary antibiotic injection into a farm worker, *Tenn. Med.*, 1999, **92**, 339–340.

81. E. K. Kuffner and R. C. Dart, Death following intravenous injection of Micotil® 300, *J. Toxicol. Clin. Toxicol.*, 1996, **34**, 574.

82. M. F. Veerhuizen, T. J. Wright, R. F. McManus and J. G. Owens, Analysis of reports of human exposure to Micotil 300 (tilmicosin injection), *J. Am. Vet. Med. Assoc.*, 2006, **229**, 1737–1742.

83. S. Von Essen, J. Spencer, B. Haas, P. List and S. A. Seifert, Unintentional human exposure to tilmicosin (Micotil® 300), *J. Toxicol. Clin. Toxicol.*, 2003, **41**, 229–233.

84. Y. Kuroda, D. C. Nacionales, J. Akaogi, W. H. Reeves and M. Satoh, Autoimmunity induced by adjuvant hydrocarbon oil components of vaccines, *Biomed. Pharmacother.*, 2004, **58**, 325–337.

85. G. Lippi, G. Targher and M. Franchini, Vaccination, squalene and anti-squalene antibodies: facts or fiction? *Eur. J. Intern. Med.*, 2010, **21**, 70–73.

86. C. J. Patterson, M. LaVenture, S. S. Hurley and J. P. Davis, Accidental self-inoculation with *Mycobacterium paratuberculosis* bacterin (Johne's bacterin) by veterinarians in Wisconsin, *J. Am. Vet. Med. Assoc.*, 1988, **192**, 1197–1199.

87. N. M. Shah, G. K. Mangat, C. Balakrishnan, V. I. Buch and V. R. Joshi, Accidental self-injection with Freund's complete adjuvant, *J. Assoc. Phys. India*, 2001, **49**, 366–368.

88. H. M. Chapel and P. J. August, Report of nine cases of adjuvant injury to man with Freund's complete adjuvant, *Clin. Exp. Immunol.*, 1976, **24**, 538–541.

89. H. M. Mehendale, R. A. Roth, A. J. Gandolfi, J. E. Klaunig, J. J. Lemasters and L. R. Curtis, Novel mechanisms in chemically induced hepatotoxicity, *FASEB J.*, 1994, **8**, 1285–1295.

90. J. Neuberger and R. Williams, Halothane hepatitis, *Digest. Dis.*, 1988, **61**, 52–64.

91. G. L. Bird and R. Williams, Anaesthesia-induced liver disease, *Monogr. Allergy*, 1992, **30**, 174–191.

92. E. D. Kharasch, Adverse drug reactions with halogenated anesthetics, *Clin. Pharmacol. Ther.*, 2008, **84**, 158–162.

93. J. Neuberger, Halothane hepatitis, *Eur. J. Gastroenterol. Hepatol.*, 1998, **10**, 631–633.

94. J. K. Aronson (ed.), Inhalational anaesthetics – halogenated, in *Meyler's Side Effects of Drugs Used in Anaesthesia*, Elsevier, Oxford, 2009, pp. 15–41.

95. E. Björnsson, P. Jerlstad, A. Bergqvist and R. Olsson, Fulminant drug-induced failure leading to death or liver transplantation in Sweden, *Scand. J. Gastroenterol.*, 2005, **40**, 1095–1101.

96. S. Belfrage, I. Ahlgren and S. Axelson, Halothane hepatitis in an anaesthetist, *Lancet*, 1966, **ii**, 1466–1467.

97. T. H. Corbett, R.G. Cornell, J. L. Endres and K. Lieding, Birth defects among the children of nurse-anesthetists, *Anesthesiol.*, 1974, **41**, 341–345.

98. J. M. Duvaldestin, R. I. Mazze, Y. Nivoche and J. M. Desmonts, Occupational exposure to halothane results in enzyme induction in anesthetists, *Anesthesiol.*, 1981, **54**, 57–61.

99. G. Franco, Occupational exposure to anesthetics: liver injury, microsomal enzyme induction and preventive aspects, *G. Ital. Med. Lav.*, 1989, **11**, 205–208.

100. H. Grimmeisen, Chronic exposure to halothane: liver damage in anaesthetists, *Anaesthetist*, 1973, **22**, 41–46.

101. S. Keiding, M. Dossing and F. Hardt, A nurse with liver injury associated with occupational exposure to halothane in a recovery unit, *Dan. Med. Bull.*, 1984, **31**, 255–256.

102. G. Klatskin and D. V. Kimberg, Recurrent hepatitis attributable to halothane sensitization in an anesthetist, *N. Engl. J. Med.*, 1969, **280**, 515–522.

103. S. Lings, Halothane related liver affection in an anaesthetist, *Br. J. Ind. Med.*, 1988, **45**, 716–717.

104. R. Luchini, D. Placidi, F. Toffoletto and L. Alessio, Neurotoxicity in operating room personnel working with gaseous and nongaseous anesthesia, *Int. Arch. Occup. Environ. Med.*, 1996, **68**, 188–192.

105. S. Popova, A. Krüsteva and P. Traĭkova, Toxic hepatitis and spontaneous abortion in female anesthesiologists, *Khirurgiia*, 1980, **33**, 118–120.

106. K. Homishak, S. Widmer and R. Stauffer, Scavenging anesthetic gas from a membrane oxygenator during cardiopulmonary bypass, *J. Extra Corpor. Technol.*, 1996, **28**, 88–90.
107. S. Merdl, C. Byhahn, U. Abdel-Rahman, G. Mattheis and K. Westphal, Occupational exposure to inhalational anesthetics during cardiac surgery on cardiopulmonary bypass, *Ann. Thorac. Surg.*, 2003, **75**, 1924–1927.
108. H. W. Linde and D. L. Bruce, Occupational exposure of anaesthetists to halothane, nitrous oxide and radiation, *Anaesthesiol.*, 1969, **30**, 363–368.
109. T. H. Cohen, B. W. Brown, D. L. Bruce, H. F. Sascorbi, T. H. Corbett, T. W. Jones and C. E. Whichter, A survey of anesthetic health hazards among dentists, *J. Amer. Dent. Assoc.*, 1975, **90**, 1291–1296.
110. L. Hunter, An occupational health approach to anaesthetic air pollution, *Med. J. Aust.*, 1976, **1**, 465–468.
111. C. Whitcher and R. Piziali, Monitoring occupational exposure to inhalation anesthetics, *Anesth. Analg.*, 1977, **56**, 778–785.
112. K. Korttila, P. Pfaffli, M. Linnoila, E. Blomgren, H. Hanninen and S. Hakkinen, Operating nurses' psychomotor and driving skills after occupational exposure to halothane and nitrous oxide, *Acta Anesthesiol. Scand.*, 1978, **22**, 33–39.
113. H. T. Davenport, M. J. Halsey, B. Wardley-Smith and P. E. Bateman, Occupational exposure to anaesthetics in 20 hospitals, *Anaesthesia*, 1980, **35**, 354–359.
114. R. Harrison, Medical surveillance for workplace hepatotoxins, *Occup. Med.*, 1990, **5**, 515–530.
115. T. E. Kole, Environmental and occupational hazards of the anesthesia workplace, *Am. Assoc. Nurse Anesth. J.*, 1990, **58**, 327–331.
116. K. A. Henderson and I. P. Matthews, Staff exposure to anaesthetic gases in theatre and non theatre areas, *Eur. J. Anaesthesiol.*, 2000, **17**, 149–151.
117. K. Sitarek, W. Wesolowski, M. Kucharska and G. Celichowski, Concentrations of anaesthetic gases in hospital operating theatres, *Int. J. Occup. Med. Environ. Health*, 2000, **13**, 61–66.
118. C. Byhahn, H. J. Wilke and K. Westphal, Occupational exposure to volatile anaesthetics: epidemiology approaches to reducing the problem, *CNS Drugs*, 2001, **15**, 197–215.
119. J. Stachnik, Inhaled anaesthetic agents, *Am. J. Health Syst. Pharm.*, 2006, **63**, 623–634.
120. S. Babich and R. P. Burakoff, Occupational hazards of dentistry. A review of literature from 1990, *N. Y. State Dent. J.*, 1997, **63**, 26–31.
121. D. J. Culley, Z. Xie and G. Crosby, General anaesthetic-induced neuro-toxicity: an emerging problem for young and old? *Curr. Opin. Anaesthesiol.*, 2007, **20**, 408–413.
122. J. E. Burkhart and T. J. Stobbe, Real-time measurement and control of waste gases during veterinary surgeries, *Am. Ind. Hyg. Assoc. J.*, 1990, **51**, 640–645.

123. D. W. Dreesen, G. L. Jones, J. Brown and J. L. Rawlings, Monitoring for trace anesthetic gases in a veterinary hospital, *J. Am. Vet. Med. Assoc. J.*, 1981, **179**, 797–799.
124. R. J. Gardner, J. Hampton and J. S. Causton, Inhalation anaesthetics – exposure and control during veterinary surgery, *Ann. Occup. Hyg.*, 1991, **35**, 377–388.
125. C. J. Green, Anaesthetic gases and health risks to laboratory personnel: a review, *Lab. Anim.*, 1981, **15**, 397–403.
126. R. E. Korczynski, Anaesthetic gas exposure in veterinary clinics, *Appl. Occup. Environ. Hyg.*, 1999, **14**, 384–390.
127. J. E. Milligan, J. L. Sablan and C. E. Short, A survey of waste anesthetic gas concentrations in the U.S. Air Force veterinary surgeries, *J. Am. Vet. Med. Assoc.*, 1980, **177**, 1021–1022.
128. R. M. Moore, Y. M. Davis and R. G. Kaczmarek, An overview of occupational hazards among veterinarians with particular reference to pregnant women, *Am. Ind. Hyg. Assoc. J.*, 1993, **54**, 113–120.
129. D. L. Potts and B. F. Craft, Occupational exposure of veterinarians to waste anesthetic gases, *Appl. Ind. Hyg.*, 1988, **3**, 132–138.
130. S. M. Schuchman, F. L. Frye and R. P. Barrett, Toxicities and hazards for clinicians in small animal practice, *Vet. Clin. North Am.*, 1975, **5**, 727–735.
131. T. M. Stimpfel and E. L. Gershey, Selecting anaesthetic agents for human safety and animal recovery after surgery, *FASEB J.*, 1991, **5**, 2099–2104.
132. G. S. Ward and R. R. Byland, Concentrations of halothane in veterinary operating and treatment rooms, *J. Am. Vet. Med. Assoc.*, 1982, **180**, 174–177.
133. G. S. Ward and R. R. Byland, Concentrations of methoxyfluorane and nitrous oxide in veterinary operating rooms, *Am. J. Vet. Res.*, 1982, **43**, 360–362.
134. W. E. Wingfield, D. L. Ruby, R. M. Buchan and B. J. Gunther, Waste anesthetic gas exposure to veterinarians and animal technicians, *J. Am. Vet. Med. Assoc.*, 1981, **178**, 399–402.
135. C. E. Short, Thoughts on studies linking occupational exposure to anesthetic waste gases, *J. Am. Vet. Med. Assoc.*, 2009, **235**, 660–661.
136. J. A. Smith, Anesthetic pollution and waste anesthetic gas scavenging, *Semin. Vet. Med. Surg.*, 1993, **8**, 90–103.
137. R. E. Meyer, Anesthesia hazards to animal workers, *Occup. Med.*, 1999, **14**, 225–234.
138. C. E. Short and R. C. Harvey, Anesthetic waste gases in veterinary medicine: analysis of the problem and suggested guidelines for reducing personnel exposures, *Cornell Vet.*, 1983, **73**, 363–374.
139. L. Fritschi, A. Shirangi, I. D. Robertson and L. M. Day, Trends in exposure of veterinarians to physical and chemical hazards and use of protection practices, *Int. Arch. Occup. Environ. Med.*, 2008, **81**, 371–378.
140. A. Shirangi, L. Fritschi and C. D. Holman, Prevalence of occupational exposures and protective practices in Australian female veterinarians, *Aust. Vet. J.*, 2007, **85**, 32–38.

141. D. L. Ruby, R. M. Buchan and B. J. Gunter, Waste anesthetic gas and vapour exposures in veterinary hospitals and clinics, *Am. Ind. Hyg. Assoc. J.*, 1980, **41**, 229–231.

142. S. E. Lacey, L. M. Conroy, J. E. Franke, R. A. Wadden, D. R. Hedeker and L. S. Forst, Personal dust exposures at a food processing facility, *J. Agromed.*, 2006, **11**, 49–58.

143. C. Peretz, N. de Pater, J. de Monchy, J. Oosterbrink and D. Heederik, Assessment to exposure to wheat flour and the shape of its relationship with specific sensitization, *Scand. J. Work Environ. Health*, 2005, **31**(1), 65–74.

144. T. A. Kuhibusch, C. Asbach, H. Fissan, D. Göhler and M. Stinz, Nanoparticle exposure at nanotechnology workplaces: a review, *Part. Fibre Toxicol.*, 2011, **8**, 22.

145. J. J. Schauer, B. J. Majestic, R. J. Sheesley, M. M. Shafer, J. T. Deminter and M. Mieritz, Improved source apportionment and speciation of low-volume particulate matter samples, *Res. Resp. Health Eff. Inst.*, 2010, **153**, 3–75.

146. V. L. Tatum, A. E. Ray and D. C. Rovell-Rixx, The performance of personal inhalable dust samplers in wood-products industry facilities, *Appl. Occup. Environ. Hyg*, 2001, **16**, 763–769.

147. A. Thorpe, Assessment of personal direct-reading dust monitors for the measurement of airborne inhalable dust, *Ann. Occup. Hyg.*, 2007, **51**, 97–112.

148. R. H. Brown, Sampling and analysis of industrial air in *IARC Scientific Publications*, 85, International Agency for Research on Cancer, Lyon, 1988, pp. 149–163.

149. M. Harper and L. V. Guild, Experience in the use of the NIOSH diffusive sampler evaluation protocol, *Am. Ind. Hyg. Assoc. J.*, 1996, **57**, 1115–1123.

150. M. Harper and B. S. Muller, An evaluation of the total and inhalable samplers for the collection of wood dust in three wood products industries, *J. Environ. Monit.*, 2002, **4**, 648–656.

151. R. S. Coombes and D. A. Warren, Characterizing and controlling industrial dust: a case study in small particle measurement, *Environ. Monit. Assess.*, 2005, **106**, 43–58.

152. M. Harper, B. S. Muller and A. Bartolucci, Determining particle size distributions in the inhalable range for wood dust collected by air samplers, *J. Environ. Monit.*, 2002, **4**, 642–647.

153. T. Schneider, V. Schlüssen, P. S. Vinzents and J. Kildesø, Passive sampler used for simultaneous measurement of breathing zone size, distribution, inhalable dust concentration and other size fractions involving large particles, *Ann. Occup. Hyg.*, 2002, **46**, 187–195.

154. B. S. Cohen, N. H. Hartley and M. Lippmann, Bias in air sampling techniques used to measure inhalation exposure, *Am. Ind. Hyg. Assoc. J.*, 1984, **45**, 187–192.

155. O. Witschger, S. A. Grinshpun, S. Fauvel and G. Basso, Performance of personal inhalable aerosol samplers in very slowly moving air when facing the aerosol source, *Ann. Occup. Hyg.*, 2004, **48**, 351–368.

156. M. A. Puskar, J. M. Harkins, J. D. Moomey and L. H. Hecker, Internal wall losses of pharmaceutical dusts during closed-face, 37-mm polystyrene cassette sampling, *Am. Ind. Hyg. J*, 1991, **52**, 280–286.

157. F. J. Hearl, Industrial hygiene sampling and applications to ambient silica modelling, *J. Expo. Anal. Environ. Epidemiol.*, 1997, **7**, 279–289.

158. H. Notø, K. Halgard, H. L. Daae, R. K. Bentsen and W. Eduard, Comparative study of an inhalable and a total dust sampler for personal sampling of dust and polycyclic aromatic hydrocarbons and particulate phase, *Analyst*, 1996, **121**, 1191–1196.

159. C. A. Soutar, B. G. Millere, N. Gregg, A. D. Jones, R. T. Cullen and R. T. Bolton, Assessment of human risks from exposure to low toxicity occupational dusts, *Ann. Occup. Hyg.*, 1997, **41**, 123–133.

160. J.-I. Choi and C. S. Kim, Mathematical analysis of particle deposition in human lungs: an improved single path transport model, *Inhal. Toxicol.*, 2007, **19**, 925–939.

161. P. A. Jaques and C. S. Kim, Measurement of total lung deposition of inhaled ultrafine particles in healthy men and women, *Inhal. Toxicol.*, 2000, **12**, 715–731.

162. J. Löndahl, A. Massling, J. Pagels, E. Swietlicki, E. Vaclavik and S. Loft, Size resolved respiratory tract deposition of fine and ultrafine hydrophobic and hygroscopic aerosol particles during rest and exercise, *Inhal. Toxicol.*, 2007, **19**, 116.

163. P. M. Hext, Inhalation toxicity in *General and Applied Toxicology*, ed. B. Ballantyne, T. C. Marrs and T. Syversen, Macmillan, London, 2000, pp. 587–601.

164. M. Dourson, G. Charnley and R. Scheuplein, Differential sensitivity of children and adults to chemical toxicity. I. Biological basis, *Regul. Toxicol. Pharmacol.*, 2002, **35**, 429–447.

165. M. Dourson, G. Charnley and R. Scheuplein, Differential sensitivity of children and adults to chemical toxicity. II. Risk and regulation, *Regul. Toxicol. Pharmacol.*, 2002, **35**, 448–467.

166. C. J. Waterfield and J. A. Timbrell, Biomarkers: an overview in *General and Applied Toxicology*, ed. B. Ballantyne, T. C. Marrs and T. Syversen, Macmillan, London, 2000, pp. 1841–1854.

167. E. J. Olajos and H. Salem, Occupational toxicology in *General and Applied Toxicology*, ed. B. Ballantyne, T. C. Marrs and T. Syversen, Macmillan, London, 2000, pp. 1453–1471.

168. H.-W. Leung and D. J. Paustenbach, Application of pharmacokinetics to derive biological exposure indexes from threshold limit values, *Am. Ind. Hyg. Assoc. J.*, 1988, **49**, 445–450.

169. H.-W. Leung, Use of physiologically based pharmacokinetic models to establish biological exposure indices, *Am. Ind. Hyg. Assoc. J.*, 1992, **53**, 369–374.

170. International Programme on Chemical Safety, Biomarkers in risk assessment: validity and validation, Environmental Health Criteria 222, IPCS, WHO, Geneva, 2001.

171. R. F. Henderson, W. E. Bechtold, J. A. Bond and J. D. Sun, The use of biological markers in toxicology, *Crit. Rev. Toxicol.*, 1989, **20**, 65–82.

172. P. O. Droz, M. M. Wu, W. G. Cumberland and M. Berode, Variability in biological monitoring of solvent exposure. I. Development of a population model, *Br. J. Ind. Med.*, 1989, **46**, 447–460.

173. A. Duggan, G. Charnley, W. Chen, A. Chukwudede, R. Hawk, R. I. Krieger, J. Ross and C. Yarborough, Di-allyl phosphate biomonitoring data: assessing cumulative exposure to organophosphate pesticides, *Regul. Toxicol. Pharmacol.*, 2003, **37**, 282–395.

174. V. Fiserova-Bergerova, Development of biological exposure indices (BEIs) and their implementation, *Appl. Ind. Hyg.*, 1987, **2**, 87–92.

175. V. Fiserova-Bergerova, Applications of toxicokinetics models to establish biological exposure indicators, *Ann. Occup. Hyg.*, 1990, **34**, 639–651.

176. S. M. Hays, R. A. Becker, H. W. Leung, L. L. Aylward and D. W. Pyatt, Biomonitoring equivalents: a screening approach for interpreting biomonitoring results from a public health perspective, *Regul. Toxicol. Pharmacol.*, 2007, **47**, 96–109.

177. C. R. Kirman, L. M. Sweeney, M. E. Mek and M. L. Gargas, Assessing the low dose-dependency of allometric scaling performance using physiologically based pharmacokinetic modelling, *Regul. Toxicol. Pharmacol.*, 2003, **38**, 345–367.

178. M. L. Rigas, M. S. Okino and J. J. Quackenboss, Use of a pharmacokinetic model to assess chlorpyriphos exposure and dose in children, based on urinary biomarker measurements, *Toxicol. Sci.*, 2001, **61**, 374–381.

179. R. S. Thomas, P. L. Bigelow, T. J. Keefe and R. S. H. Yang, Variability in biological exposure indices using physiologically based pharmacokinetic modeling and Monte Carlo simulation, *Am. Ind. Hyg. Assoc. J.*, 1996, **57**, 23–32.

180. G. Truchon, R. Tardif, P.-O. Droz, G. Charest-Tardif and G. Pierrehumbert, Biological exposure indicators: quantification of biological variability using toxicokinetics modeling, *J. Occup. Environ. Med.*, 2006, **3**, 137–143.

181. J. H. Kim, R. C. Stevens, M. J. MacCoss, D. R. Goodlet, A. Scherl, R. J. Richter, S. M. Suzuki and C. E. Furlong, Identification of biomarkers of organophosphorus exposures in humans, *Adv. Exp. Med. Biol.*, 2010, **660**, 61–71.

182. C. Lu, T. Rodríguez, A. Funez, R. S. Irish and R. A. Fenske, Assessment of occupational exposure to diazinon in Nicaraguan plantation workers using saliva Biomonitoring, *Ann. N. Y. Acad. Sci.*, 2006, **1076**, 355–356.

183. Y. M. Tan, J. Sobus, D. Chang, R. Tornero-Velez, M. Goldsmith, J. Pleil and C. Dary, Reconstructing human exposures using biomarker and other "clues", *J. Toxicol. Environ. Health B. Crit. Rev.*, 2012, **15**, 22–38.

184. M. Valverde and E. Rojas, Environmental and occupational biomonitoring using the Comet assay, *Mutat. Res.*, 2009, **681**, 93–109.

185. L. A. McCauley, M. Lasarey, J. Muniz, V. Nazar Stewart and G. Kisby, Analysis of pesticide exposure and DNA damage in immigrant farmworkers, *J. Agromedicine*, 2008, **13**, 237–246.
186. G. M. Bortoli, M. B. Azevedo and L. B. Silva, Cytogenetic monitoring of Brazilian workers exposed to pesticides: micronucleus analysis on buccal epithelial cells of soybean growers, *Mutat. Res.*, 2009, **675**, 1–4.
187. M. V. Coronas, T. S. Pereira, J. A. Rocha, A. T. Lemos, J. M. Fachel, D. M. Salvadori and V. M. Vargas, Genetic Biomonitoring of an urban population exposed to mutagenic airborne pollutants, *Environ. Int.*, 2009, **35**, 1023–1029.
188. R. J. Preston, J. A. Skare and M. J. Aardema, A review of biomonitoring studies measuring genotoxicity in humans exposed to hair dyes, *Mutagenesis*, 2010, **25**, 17–23.
189. A. Izzotti, A. Pulliero, R. Puntoni, M. Peluso, R. Filiberti, A. Munnia, G. Assennato, G. Ferri and D. F. Merlo, Duration of exposure to environmental carcinogens affects DNA-adduct level in human lymphocytes, *Biomarkers*, 2010, **15**, 575–582.
190. P. J. Boogaard, L. L. Aylward and S. M. Hays, Application of human biomonitoring in the characterisation of health risks under REACH, *Int. J. Hyg. Environ. Health*, 2012, **215**, 238–241.
191. P. A. Schulte and J. E. Hauser, The use of biomarkers in occupational health research, practice, and policy, *Toxicol. Lett.*, 2012, **213**, 91–99.
192. S. Angelini, F. Maffei, J. L. Bermejo, G. Ravegnini, G. D. L'insalata, F. S. Cantelli-Forti, Violante and P. Hrelia, Environmental exposure to benzene, micronucleus formation and polymorphisms in DNA-repair genes: A pilot study, *Mutat. Res.*, 2012, **743**, 99–104.
193. L. Palanikumar and N. Panneerselvam, Micronuclei assay: a potential biomonitoring protocol in occupational exposure studies, *Genetika*, 2011, **47**, 1169–1174.
194. L. T. Budnik and X. Baur, The assessment of environmental and occupational exposure to hazardous substances by biomonitoring, *Dtsch. Arztebl. Int.*, 2009, **106**, 91–97.
195. S. Bull, K. Fletcher, A. R. Boobis and J. M. Battershill, Evidence for genotoxicity of pesticides in pesticide applicators: a review, *Mutagenesis*, 2006, **21**, 93–103.
196. C. Bolognesis, A. Crues, P. Ostrosky-Wegman and R. Marcos, Micronuclei and pesticide exposure, *Mutagenesis*, 2011, **26**, 19–26.
197. W. A. Anwar, Monitoring of human populations at risk by different cytogenetic end points, *Environ. Health Perspect.*, 1994, **102**(4), 131–134.
198. P. Møller, L. E. Knudsen, S. Loft and H. Wallin, The comet assay as a rapid test in biomonitoring occupational exposure to DNA-damaging agents and the effect of confounding factors, *Cancer Epidemiol. Biomarkers Prev.*, 2000, **9**, 1005–1015.
199. N. Kopjar and V. Garaj-Vrhovac, Application of the alkaline comet assay in human biomonitoring for genotoxicity: a study on Croatian medical personnel handling antineoplastic drugs, *Mutagenesis*, 2001, **16**, 71–78.

200. T. Cornetta, L. Padua, A. Testa, E. Levoli, F. Festa, G. Tranfo, L. Baccelliere and R. Cozzi, Molecular biomonitoring of nurses handling antineoplastic drugs, *Mutat. Res.*, 2008, **638**, 75–82.

201. R. Turci, C. Sottani, A. Ronchi and C. Minoia, Biological monitoring of hospital personnel occupationally exposed to antineoplastic agents, *Toxicol. Lett.*, 2002, **134**, 57–64.

202. C. L. Ursini, D. Cavallo, A. Colombi, M. Giglio, A. Marinaccio and S. Iavicoli, Evaluation of early DNA damage in healthcare workers handling antineoplastic drugs, *Int. Arch. Occup. Environ. Health*, 2006, **80**, 134–140.

203. P. J. Sessink and R. P. Bos, Drugs hazardous to healthcare workers. Evaluation of methods for monitoring occupational exposure to cytostatic drugs, *Drug Saf.*, 1999, **20**, 347–359.

204. M. Sorsa, K. Hemminki and H. Vainio, Occupational exposure to anticancer drugs – potential and real hazards, *Mutat. Res.*, 1985, **154**, 135–149.

205. M. Sorsa, L. Pyy, S. Salomaa, L. Nylund and J. W. Yager, Biological and environmental monitoring of occupational exposure to cyclophosphamide in industry and hospitals, *Mutat. Res.*, 1988, **204**, 465–479.

206. R. Barale, G. Sozzi, P. Toniolo, O. Borghi, D. Reali, N. Loprieno and G. Della Porta, Sister-chromatid exchanges in lymphocytes and mutagenicity in urine of nurses handling cytostatic drugs, *Mutat. Res.*, 1985, **157**, 235–240.

205. D. Cavallo, C. L. Ursini, B. Perniconi, A. D. Francesco, M. Giglio, F. M. Rubino, A. Marinaccio and S. Iavicoli, Evaluation of genotoxic effects induced by exposure to antineoplastic drugs in lymphocytes and exfoliated buccal cells of oncology nurses and pharmacy employees, *Mutat. Res.*, 2005, **587**, 45–51.

207. D. Cavallo, C. L. Ursini, E. Omodeo-Santé and S. Iavicoli, Micronucleus induction and FISH analysis in buccal cells and lymphocytes of nurses administering antineoplastic drugs, *Mutat. Res.*, 2007, **628**, 11–18.

208. D. Cavallo, C. L. Ursini, B. Rondinone and S. Iavicoli, Evaluation of a suitable DNA damage biomarker for human biomonitoring of exposed workers, *Environ. Mol. Mutagen.*, 2009, **50**, 781–790.

209. N. Kopjar, D. Zeljezić, V. Kasuba and R. Rozgaj, Antineoplastic drugs as a potential risk factor in occupational settings: mechanisms of action at the cell level, genotoxic effects, and their detection using different biomarkers, *Arh. Hig. Rada. Toksikol.*, 2010, **61**, 121–146.

210. V. Kasuba, R. Rozgaj and V. Garaj-Vrhovac, Analysis of sister chromatid exchanges and micronuclei in peripheral blood lymphocytes of nurses handling cytostatic drugs, *J. Appl. Toxicol.*, 1999, **19**, 401–404.

211. G. Thiringer, G. Granung, A Holmén, B. Högstedt, B. Järvholm, D. Jönnson, L. Persson, J. Wahlström and J. Westin, Comparison of methods for the biomonitoring of nurses handling antitumor drugs, *Scand. J. Environ. Health*, 1991, **17**, 133–138.

212. G. M. Machado-Santelli, E. M. Cerqueira, C. T. Oliveira and C. A. Pereira, Biomonitoring of nurses handling antineoplastic drugs, *Mutat. Res.*, 1994, **322**, 203–208.

213. F. Oesch, J. G. Hengstler, M. Arand and J. Fuchs, Detection of primary DNA damage: application to biomonitoring of genotoxic occupational exposure and in clinical therapy, *Pharmacogenetics*, 1995, **5**(Special No.), S118–S122.
214. R. P. Bos and P. J. Sessink, Biomonitoring of occupational exposures to cytostatic anticancer drugs, *Rev. Environ. Health*, 1997, **12**, 43–58.
215. F. Fucic, A. Jazbec, A. Mijic, Đ. Šešo-Šimic and R. Tomec, Cytogenetic consequences after occupational exposure to antineoplastic drugs, *Mutat. Res.*, 1998, **416**, 59–66.
216. A. Suspiro and J. Prista, Biomarkers of occupational health exposure to anticancer drugs: a minreview, *Toxicol. Lett.*, 2011, **207**, 42–52.
217. A. A. El-Ebiary, A. A. Abuelfadi and N. I. Sarhan, Evaluation of genotoxicity induced by exposure to antineoplastic drugs in lymphocytes of oncology nurses and pharmacists, *J. Appl. Toxicol.*, 2011, epub ahead of print.
218. A. B. Boughattas, S. Bouraoui, F. Debbabi, H. El Ghazel, A. Saad and N. Mrizak, Genotoxic risk assessment of nurses handling antineoplastic drugs, *Ann. Biol. Clin (Paris)*, 2010, **68**, 545–553.
219. P. V. Rekhadevi, N. Sailaja, M. Chandrasekhar, M. Mahboob, M. F. Rahman and P. Grover, Genotoxicity assessment in oncology nurses handling anti-neoplastic drugs, *Mutagenesis*, 2007, **22**, 395–401.
220. H. Waksvik, O. Klepp and A. Brøgger, Chromosome analyses of nurses handling cytostatic drugs, *Cancer Treat. Rep.*, 1981, **65**, 607–610.
221. A. Testa, M. Giachelia, S. Palma, M. Appolloni, L. Padua, G. Tranfo, M. Spagnoli, D. Trindelli and R. Cozzi, Occupational exposure to anti-neoplastic agents induces a high level of chromosome damage. Lack of an effect of GST polymorphisms, *Toxicol. Appl. Pharmacol.*, 2007, **223**, 46–55.
222. J. Rubeš, S. Kucharová, M. Vozdová, P. Musilová and Z. Zudová, Cytogenetic analysis of peripheral lymphocytes in medical personnel by means of FISH, *Mutat. Res.*, 1998, **412**, 293–298.
223. H. Pohlová, M. Černá and P. Rössner, Chromosomal aberrations, SCE and urine mutagenicity in workers occupationally exposed to cytostatic drugs, *Mutat. Res.*, 1986, **174**, 213–217.
224. A. Pilger, I. Köhler, H. Stettner, R. M. Mader, B. Rizowski, R. Terkola, E. Diem, E. Franz-Hainzi, C. Konnaris, E. Valic and H. W. Rüdiger, Long-term monitoring of sister-chromatid exchanges and micronucleus frequencies in pharmacy personnel occupationally exposed to cytostatic drugs, *Int. Arch. Occup. Environ. Health*, 2000, **73**, 442–448.
225. U. Oestreicher, G. Stephan and M. Glatzel, Chromosome and SCE analysis in peripheral lymphocytes of persons occupationally exposed to cytostatic drugs handled with and without use of safety covers, *Mutat. Res.*, 1990, **242**, 271–277.
226. H. Norppa, M. Sorsa, H. Vainio, P. Gröhn, E. Heinonen, L. Hosti and E. Nordman, Increased sister chromatid exchange frequencies in lymphocytes of nurses handling cytostatic drugs, *Scand. J. Work Environ. Health*, 1980, **6**, 299–301.

227. E. Nikula, K. Kiviniitty, J. Leisti and P. J. Taskinen, Chromosome aberrations in lymphocytes of nurses handling cytostatic agents, *Scand. J. Work Environ. Health*, 1984, **10**, 71–74.
228. S. Milković-Kraus and D. Horvat, Chromosomal abnormalities among nurses occupationally exposed to antineoplastic drugs, *Am. J. Ind. Med.*, 1991, **19**, 771–774.
229. J. J. McDevitt, P. S. J. Lees and M. A. McDiarmid, Exposure of hospital pharmacists and nurses to antineoplastic agents, *J. Occup. Med.*, 1993, **35**, 57–60.
230. S. Izdes, S. Sardas, E. Kadioglu, C. Kaymak and E. Ozcagli, Assessment of genotoxic damage in nurses occupationally exposed to anaesthetic gases or antineoplastic drugs by the comet assay, *J. Occup. Health*, 2009, **51**, 283–286.
231. E. M. Goloni-Bertollo, E. H. Tajara, A. J. Manzato and M. Varella-Garcia, Sister chromatid exchanges and chromosome aberrations in lymphocytes of nurses handling antineoplastic drugs, *Int. J. Cancer*, 1992, **50**, 341–344.
232. W. A. Anwar, S. I. Salama, M. M. El Serafy, S. A. Hemida and A. S. Hafez, Chromosomal aberrations and micronucleus frequency in nurses occupationally exposed to cytotoxic drugs, *Mutagenesis*, 1994, **9**, 315–317.
233. C. Pellicaan and E. Teske, Risks of using cytostatic drugs in veterinary medical practice, *Tidschr. Diergeneeskd.*, 1999, **124**, 210–215.
234. C. Pellicaan, E. Teske, H. Vaarkamp and T. Willemse, Use of carcinogenic veterinary drugs in the veterinary clinic. An unacceptable risk for people? *Tidschr. Diergeneeskd.*, 2002, **127**, 734–734.
235. Veterinary Medicines Directorate, Handling cytotoxic drugs under veterinary practice conditions, MAVIS (Medicines Act Veterinary Information Service), edn 43, July, 2002. Available at: http://www.vmd.defra.gov.uk/pdf/mavis/mavis43.pdf.
236. A. Knobloch, S. A. Mohring, N. Eberle, I. Nolte, G. Hamscher and D. Simon, Drug residues in serum of dogs receiving anticancer chemotherapy, *J. Vet. Intern. Med.*, 2010, **24**, 379–383.
237. T. A. Cave, P. Norman and D. Mellor, Cytotoxic drug use in treatment of dogs and cats with cancer by UK veterinary practices (2003 to 2004), *J. Small Anim. Pract.*, 2007, **48**, 371–377.
238. S. Takada, Principles of chemotherapy safety procedures, *Clin. Tech. Small Anim. Pract.*, 2003, **18**, 73–74.
239. G. Hamscher, S. A. Mohring, A. Knobloch, N. Eberle, H. Nau, I. Nolte and D. Simon, Determination of drug residues in urine of dogs receiving anti-cancer chemotherapy by liquid chromatography-electrospray ionisation-tandem mass spectroscopy: is there an environmental or occupational risk? *J. Anal. Toxicol.*, 2010, **34**, 142–148.
240. British Medical Association, The measurement of risk in *Living With Risk*, John Wiley & Sons, Chichester, 1987, pp. 19–28.
241. P. G. Bedello, M. Goitre, D. Cane and G. Roncarolo, Allergic contact dermatitis to Bayo-N-OX-1, *Contact Dermatitis*, 1985, **12**, 284.

242. H. Belhadjali, M. C. Maguerray, F. Journe, F. Giordano-Labardie, H. Lefevre and J. Bazex, Allergic and photoallergic contact dermatitis in a pig breeder with prolonged photosensitivity, *Photodermatol. Photoimmunol. Photomed.*, 2002, **18**, 52–53.

243. R. J. Davies and J. Pepys, Asthma due to inhaled chemical agents – the macrolide antibiotic spiramycin, *Clin. Allergy*, 1975, **1**, 99–107.

244. M. Francalanci, M. Gola, S. Giorgini, A. Muccinelli and A. Sertoli, Occupational photocontact dermatitis from olaquindox, *Contact Dermatitis*, 1986, **15**, 112–114.

245. N. Hjorth and K. Weismann, Occupational dermatitis among veterinary surgeons caused by spiramycin, tylosin and penethamate, *Acta. Derm. Venereol.*, 1973, **53**, 229–232.

246. P. L. Paggiaro, A. M. Loi and G. Toma, Bronchial asthma and dermatitis in a chick breeder, *Clin. Allergy*, 1979, **9**, 571–574.

247. J. Sanchez-Perez, M. P. Lopez and A. Garcia-Diez, Airborne allergic dermatitis from olaquindox in a rabbit breeder, *Contact Dermatitis*, 2002, **46**, 185.

248. K. N. Woodward, Maximum residue limits in *Veterinary Pharmacovigilance. Adverse Reactions to Veterinary Medicinal Products*, ed. K. N. Woodward, Wiley-Blackwell, Chichester, 2009, pp. 547–567.

249. J. Herrman and M. Younes, Background to the ADI/TDI/PTWI, *Regul. Toxicol. Pharmacol.*, 1999, **30**, S109–S113.

250. F. C. Lu, Acceptable daily intake: inception, evolution and application, *Regul. Toxicol. Pharmacol.*, 1988, **8**, 45–60.

251. A. G. Renwick, Safety factors and establishment of acceptable daily intakes, *Food Addit. Contam.*, 1991, **8**, 135–150.

252. E. Dybing, J. Doe, J. O'Brien, A. G. Renwick, J. Schlatter, P. Steinberg, A. Tritsscher, R. Walker and M. Younes, Hazard characterisation of chemicals in food and diet, dose-response, mechanisms and extrapolation, *Food Chem. Toxicol.*, 2002, **40**, 237–282.

253. Joint FAO/WHO Expert Committee on Food Additives, Procedures for Testing of Intentional Additives to Establish their Safety for Use, Second report of the Joint FAO/WHO Expert Committee on Food Additives, WHO Technical Report Series 144, WHO, Geneva, 1957.

254. Joint FAO/WHO Expert Committee on Food Additives, Principles for the Safety Assessment of Food Additives and Contaminants in Food, Environmental Health Criteria 70, International Programme on Chemical Safety, WHO, Geneva, 1987.

255. ACGIH, Threshold limit values for 1950, *Am. Med. Assoc. Arch. Ind. Hyg. Occup. Med.*, 1950, **2**, 98–100.

256. J. M. Pauli, The origin and basis of threshold limit values, *Am. J. Ind. Med.*, 1984, **5**, 227–238.

257. G. E. Ziem and B. I. Castleman, Threshold limit values: historical perspective and current practice, *J. Occup. Med.*, 1989, **31**, 910–918.

258. B. D. Culver, Stokinger Award lecture 2005 – innovation for the TLV process, *J. Occup. Environ. Hyg.*, 2005, **2**, D70–D73.

259. Health and Safety Executive, *EH40/2005 Workplace Exposure Limits*, 2nd edn, Health and Safety Executive, Bootle, 2011. Available at: http://www.hse.gov.uk/pubns/priced/EH40.pdf.

260. H. P. A. Illing, Extrapolation from toxicity data to occupational exposure limits: some considerations, *Ann. Occup. Hyg.*, 1991, **35**, 569–580.

261. H. P. A. Illing, Possible considerations for toxic risk assessment, *Hum. Exp. Toxicol.*, 1991, **10**, 215–219.

262. R. L. Zielhuis, P. C. Noordan, C. L. Maas, J. J. Kolk and H. P. A. Illing, Harmonisation of criteria documents for standard setting in occupational health: report of a meeting, *Regul. Toxicol. Pharmacol.*, 1991, **13**, 241–262.

263. R. L. Zielhuis and F. W. van der Kreek, The use of a safety factor in setting health based permissible levels for occupational exposures, *Int. Arch. Occup. Environ. Health*, 1979, **42**, 191–201.

264. S. Fairhurst, The uncertainty factor in setting of occupational exposure standards, *Ann. Occup. Hyg.*, 1995, **39**, 375–385.

265. International Programme on Chemical Safety, Assessing Human Health Risks of Chemicals: Derivation of Guidance Values for Health-Based Exposure Limits, Environmental Health Criteria 170, IPCS, WHO, Geneva, 1994.

266. G. V. McHattie, M. Rackham and E. L. Teasdale, The derivation of occupational exposure limits in the pharmaceutical industry, *J. Soc. Occup. Med.*, 1988, **38**, 105–108.

267. B. D. Naumann, E. V. Sargent, B. S. Sharkman, W. J. Fraser, G. T. Becker and G. D. Kirk, Performance-based occupational exposure limits for pharmaceutical active ingredients, *Am. Ind. Hyg. Assoc. J.*, 1996, **57**, 33–42.

268. W. A. Chiu, H. A. Barton, R. S. DeWoskin, P. Schlosser, C. M. Thompson, B. Sonawane, J. C. Lipscomb and K. Krishnan, Evaluation of physiologically based pharmacokinetic models for use in risk assessment, *J. Appl. Toxicol.*, 2007, **27**, 218–237.

269. P. P. Koundakjian and H. P. A. Illing, Introduction in *Risk Management of Chemicals*, ed. M. L. Richardson, Royal Society of Chemistry, Cambridge, 1992, pp. 3–13.

270. R. C. Brown, Protection against dust by respirators, *Int. J. Occup. Saf. Ergonom.*, 1995, **1**, 14–28.

271. R. M. Howie, Respiratory protective equipment, *Occup. Environ. Med.*, 2005, **62**, 423–428.

272. K. S. Crump, Statistical issues with respect to workplace protection factors for respirators, *J. Occup. Environ. Hyg.*, 2007, **4**, 208–214.

273. M. Nicas and J. Neuhaus, Variability in respiratory protection and the assigned protection factor, *J. Occup. Environ. Hyg.*, 2004, **1**, 99–109.

274. N. Vaughan and B. Rajan-Sithamparanadarajah, Meaningful workplace protection factor measurement: experimental protocols and data treatment, *Ann. Occup. Hyg.*, 2005, **49**, 549–561.

275. H. Sugimori and T. Orii, Pharmaceutical safety and risk communication, *Yakugaku Zaashi*, 2012, **132**, 531.

276. E. R. Stone, J. F. Yates and A. M. Parker, Risk communication: absolute versus relative expressions of low probability risks, *Organiz. Behav. Hum. Decis. Process.*, 1994, **60**, 387–408.

277. L. Frewer, The public and effective risk communication, *Toxicol. Lett.*, 2004, **149**, 391–397.

278. M. M. Schapira, A. B. Nattinger and C. A. McHorney, Frequency or probability? A qualitative study of risk communication formats used in health care, *Med. Decis. Making*, 2001, **21**, 459–467.

279. K. M. Thompson, Variability and uncertainty meet risk management and risk communication, *Risk Anal.*, 2002, **22**, 647–654.

280. G. M. Breakwell, Risk communication: factors affecting impact, *Br. Med. Bull.*, 2000, **56**, 110–120.

281. O. Renn, Risk communication: Towards a rational discourse with the public, *J. Hazard. Mater.*, 1992, **29**, 465–519.

282. A. Edwards, Communicating risks, *Br. Med. J.*, 2003, **327**, 691–692.

283. E. Kurz-Milcke, G. Gigerenzer and L. Martignan, Transparency in risk communication: graphical and analog tools, *Ann. N. Y. Acad. Sci.*, 2008, **1128**, 18–28.

284. H. P. A. Illing, Are societal judgments being incorporated into uncertainty factors used in toxicological risk assessment? *Regul. Toxicol. Pharmacol.*, 1999, **29**, 300–308.

285. H. P. A. Illing, The importance of risk perception and risk communication for toxicological risk assessment in *Toxicity and Risk. Context, Principles and Practice*, Taylor and Francis, London, 2001, pp. 43–56.

286. M. D. Rogers, Risk analysis under uncertainty, the precautionary principle, and the new EU chemicals strategy, *Regul. Toxicol. Pharmacol.*, 2003, **37**, 370–381.

287. G. Keck and C. Ibrahim, Veterinary pharmacovigilance: between regulation and science, *J. Vet. Pharmacol. Ther.*, 2001, **24**, 22–27.

288. W. C. Keller, N. Battaller and D. S. Oeller, Processing and evaluation of adverse drug reaction reports at the Food and Drug Administration Center for Veterinary Medicine, *J. Am. Vet. Med. Assoc.*, 1998, **213**, 208–211.

289. K. N. Woodward, Veterinary pharmacovigilance. Part 1. The legal basis in Europe, *J. Vet. Pharmacol. Ther.*, 2005, **28**, 131–147.

290. A. Breckenridge, For the good of the patient: risks and benefits of medicines, *Pharmacol. Drug Saf.*, 2003, **12**, 145–150.

291. W. L. Holden, Benefit-risk analysis. A brief review and proposed quantitative approaches, *Drug Saf.*, 2003, **26**, 853–862.

292. R. H. B. Meyboom and A. C. G. Egberts, Comparing therapeutic benefit and risk, *Thérapie.*, 1999, **54**, 29–34.

293. L. L. Miller, Risk/benefit assessment: the "greased pig" of drug development, *Drug Inf. J.*, 1993, **27**, 1011–1020.

CHAPTER 5

General Anaesthetics

5.1 Introduction

Prior to the mid 1800s the only anaesthetic substances available for surgery in human medicine were alcohol and opiates, despite the fact that Joseph Priestly and Humphrey Davy had commented on the anaesthetic properties of nitrous oxide at the beginning of that century. Some years later, Michael Faraday noted that diethyl ether produced anaesthetic effects similar to those of nitrous oxide. The introduction of diethyl ether and nitrous oxide as anaesthetics was largely due to the efforts of dentists. These agents were followed by chloroform and cyclopropane.[1–2]

These substances are ideal for use as inhalation anaesthetics as they are either gases (nitrous oxide and cyclopropane) or volatile liquids (chloroform and diethyl ether). However, they also have disadvantages. Chloroform is hepatotoxic and induces cardiac depression, while cyclopropane and diethyl ether are flammable and, at certain concentrations, they form explosive mixtures in air. Over time diethyl ether, like some other ethers, forms a peroxide through oxidation and this too is explosive. Nitrous oxide is non-flammable but it supports combustion. At high temperatures, it decomposes to form oxygen and nitrogen and it has been used as a rocket propellant and in high-performance internal combustion engines. These molecules have left a legacy as modern inhalation anaesthetics are either halogenated hydrocarbons (*e.g.* halothane) or halogenated ethers (*e.g.* isoflurane). Nitrous oxide continues to be used as an inhalation anaesthetic, especially in dentistry and in childbirth.[2–5] The major inhalation anaesthetics are shown in Table 5.1.

In veterinary surgery, the major inhalation anaesthetics are halothane, isoflurane and sevoflurane. Nitrous oxide is used, but usually in combination with one of the halogenated compounds.[3]

Issues in Toxicology No. 14
Toxicological Effects of Veterinary Medicinal Products in Humans: Volume 1
By Kevin N. Woodward
© The Royal Society of Chemistry 2013
Published by the Royal Society of Chemistry, www.rsc.org

Table 5.1   Some inhalation anaesthetics.

Common name	Chemical name	Derivative of:	Vapour pressure mmHg (kPa) at 20 °C
Nitrous oxide	Nitrogen oxide; dinitrogen oxide	–	38723 (51550)
Halothane	2-Bromo-2-chloro-1,1,1-trifluroethane	Ethane	243 (32.32)
Isoflurane	1-Chloro-2,2,2-trifluoroethyl difluoromethyl ether	Methyl ethyl ether	238 (3165)
Sevoflurane	1,1,1,2,3,3-Hexafluoro-2-(fluoromethoxy) propane	Methoxy propane; isopropyl methyl ether	1181 (157)
Enflurane	2-Chloro-1,1,2-trifluoroethyl difluoromethyl ether	Methyl ethyl ether	172 (22.8)
Methoxyflurane	2,2-Dichloro-1,1-difluoro-1-methoxy ethane	Methyl ethyl ether	22.5 (2.99)

Injectable anaesthetics are administered to rapidly produce a state of unconsciousness. In most cases they are given prior to an inhalation anaesthetic. Examples include the barbiturates (thiopental and methohexital), ketamine, tiletamine and etomidate. Propofol (2,6-diisopropylphenol) is a rapid acting general anaesthetic used in human and veterinary medicine.[2,3,6,7]

5.2   Human Health Concerns

The general anaesthetics are administered to animals by veterinary professionals trained in their use. They are not used by others involved in the care and welfare of animals such as farmers and the pet-owning public. Although they are potent pharmacologically active agents, these drugs are not generally regarded as toxic except at high concentrations in the case of inhalation anaesthetics or at high doses in the case of injectable anaesthetics. Veterinary personnel may be exposed to the inhalation anaesthetics through faulty administration equipment, through ill-fitting masks and through exhalation from the anaesthetised animal. Occupational exposure to injectable anaesthetics is likely to be due to spillage onto skin or by way of self-injection. However, some of these drugs may also be abused or misused.

5.3   Inhalation Anaesthetics

Several inhalation anaesthetics have been used over the years including diethyl ether and chloroform. These fell out of favour for a number of reasons but notably for the flammability and explosivity of the former and the toxicity of the latter. The inhalation anaesthetics now in veterinary use are discussed below.

5.3.1 Nitrous Oxide

Nitrous oxide (N_2O) is a colourless, odourless gas that is unusual as it is the only inorganic gas suitable for routine anaesthesia.[3–5] It is used either alone or in combination with other volatile anaesthetics where it increases the rate of uptake of the second anaesthetic through the "second gas effect". The main route of elimination is through exhalation.[3]

Nitrous oxide is a dissociative anaesthetic that produces anaesthesia by inhibiting the ascending transmission from the unconscious to the conscious parts of the brain. These agents produce analgesia and anaesthesia without significantly affecting respiratory function.[2,3,8] They also produce delirium, excitement and distorted perception and, in the case of nitrous oxide, euphoria, hence its alternative name "laughing gas". As a result of these effects, nitrous oxide, irrespective of its origins (human or veterinary use), has been the subject of abuse. In addition, nitrous oxide is used as a propellant for whipped cream products and the bulbs containing the gas ("whippet") have been used for abuse purposes.[9,10]

Some of the major effects of nitrous oxide abuse include oxygen deprivation, loss of motor control, hypotension and respiratory depression.[2,11,12] As a result of the extreme cold associated with nitrous oxide liquid, and the cold due to evaporation, physical injury may also result from frostbite.[13–15]

However, the major adverse effect arising from repeated exposure to nitrous oxide, either therapeutically or through abuse, including abuse from nitrous oxide in whipped cream products is a neuropathy or, specifically, a myeloneuropathy similar to that which occurs with vitamin B_{12} deficiency. Indeed, nitrous oxide causes deficiency in this vitamin, probably by lowering its bioavailability, and its toxicity may be even more pronounced in individuals with vitamin B_{12} deficiency. Symptoms include amnesia, limb weakness, numbness and incoordination affecting the extremities, usually as a result of multiple exposures.[9,10,16–27] The condition may mimic Guillain–Barré syndrome.[28]

There is also concern that it may have reproductive toxicity, and there is some evidence to suggest that it induces spontaneous abortion and reduces fertility.[21,29] It may also induce DNA damage in exposed personnel.[30]

No studies of occupational safety or exposure have been conducted with the veterinary use of nitrous oxide. However, medical and dental uses do result in occupational exposure,[31–33] leading others to suggest the need for adequate gas scavenging and ventilation equipment in dental surgeries, operating theatres and recovery rooms.[34,35] Obviously, such sentiments apply equally to veterinary surgeries where nitrous oxide is used.

5.3.2 Halothane

Halothane (Figure 5.1) is an important general anaesthetic in both human and veterinary medicine. However, its use is in decline in human medicine because of concerns over its safety and as alternatives with better efficacy profiles become available. Halothane, along with isoflurane and nitrous oxide, is on the

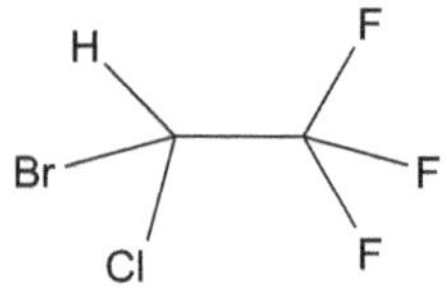

Figure 5.1 Chemical formula of halothane.

World Health Organization's (WHO) Model List of Essential Medicines for human use.[36]

In clinical use in human medicine, halothane causes a dose-dependent reduction of arterial blood pressure. This hypotension arises from direct depression of the myocardium and from depression of the normal baroreceptor mediated tachycardia. Cardiac output may be reduced by 20 to 50% during normal surgical procedures where halothane is used. There is also a depression of ventilation and a degree of muscle relaxation. These effects are unlikely to be experienced in exposed personnel, as they require therapeutic doses of the drug to occur.[2]

One of the major adverse reactions noted with halothane in humans is hepatotoxicity. In an estimated 20–25% of surgical procedures using halothane, there may be mild abnormalities in hepatic enzymes, suggestive of a minor degree of liver toxicity. This quickly resolves following the procedure. However, a more severe form of liver toxicity may develop. Patients develop jaundice around 11 days after a single exposure or 6 days after multiple exposures. The liver injury is severe resulting in fulminant hepatic failure and there is approximately 50% fatality and treatment frequently requires liver transplant. In 1993, deaths due to halothane toxicity were estimated to be around 1 in 35,000, which was much higher than a previous estimate of 1 in 110,000 in 1976. In Sweden, halothane and a number of other drugs including paracetamol and flucloxacillin were the drugs most frequently associated with a fatal outcome and hepatotoxicity. The mechanism underlying this hepatotoxicity is still not fully understood. However, the greater severity and frequency in patients who have previously been given halothane anaesthesia suggests an immunological component.[37–43]

Halothane undergoes biotransformation to trifluoroacetyl chloride and trifluoroacetic acid and the former may acetylate hepatic proteins and other macromolecules to precipitate a toxic response. Antibodies isolated from patients with halothane toxicity or from animal models reacted to specific liver proteins in animals exposed to halothane. Alternatively, the trifluoroacetylated antigenic determinant may be mimicked by an endogenous protein that cross-reacts with antibodies from humans or animals exposed to halothane to initiate liver toxicity.[44–48] Hepatic metabolism of halothane involves the cytochrome P450 superfamily of enzymes, and this may also result in lipid peroxidation while P450 2E1 appears to be an autoantigen associated with halothane hepatitis, possibly through covalent binding of the trifluoroacetyl moiety. A study in mice suggested that interleukin-17 may also be involved in this hepatotoxic response to halothane. Plasma interleukin-17 increased following exposure to halothane, as did hepatic macrophage inflammatory protein 2 expression and neutrophil expression. Neutralisation of interleukin-17 reduced the hepatotoxicity. Neutrophil recruitment in halothane toxicity may be regulated by the actions of natural killer T cells.[49–54]

The toxicity of halothane, combined with its capacity as a gas to pervade and contaminate operating areas and through exhalation by anaesthetised patients in recovery rooms and hospital wards, caused serious concerns over occupational exposure and safety to those involved including surgeons, anaesthetists, dental surgeons and nursing staff and, as a result, efforts have been made to monitor exposure and to reduce it through ventilation and gas scavenging equipment.[55–72] These concerns have been strengthened by reports of neurotoxicity, hepatotoxicity, spontaneous abortions and congenital anomalies among anaesthetists and other exposed medical workers.[44,73–83]

As a consequence, concerns have been expressed over the exposure of veterinary personnel and laboratory animal workers exposed to halothane during surgical procedures and various recommendations have been made for improved ventilation and the use of efficient gas scavenging systems.[84–103] There are no well-documented reports of liver disease associated with halothane exposure in veterinarians although there have been reports of hepatotoxicity in laboratory animal workers potentially exposed.[104,105] However, there are a number of reports that suggest that occupational exposure to halothane by pregnant veterinarians may lead to preterm births, spontaneous abortion and low birth-weights but the data were not entirely convincing due to the retrospective nature of the studies and lack of statistical significance.[105–109] In fact, there is little or no evidence for increases in congenital malformations in children of female veterinarians.[110,111] Despite these comments and the seemingly negative evidence for the induction of birth defects, there is no reason for the relaxation of standards. Normal workplace hygiene considerations demand that employees should not be exposed to undue concentrations of potentially toxic or, for that matter, non-toxic airborne materials. Moreover, in most countries occupational exposure levels have been established for airborne materials in the workplace. In the UK, for example, the long-term exposure limit (8-hour time-weighted average reference period) for halothane is 10 ppm or $82 \, mg/m^3$ in air, and similar limits apply in other European Union countries and elsewhere in the world for halothane and other anaesthetic gases.[112,113] In the USA, the corresponding values established by the American Conference of Governmental Industrial Hygienists (ACGIH) for halothane are 50 ppm or $404 \, mg/m^2$.[114] These, and the occupational exposure limits for some other volatile anaesthetics are shown in Table 5.2.

5.3.3 Isoflurane

Isoflurane (Figure 5.2) is widely used in veterinary anaesthesia.[4] It undergoes very little biotransformation in animals and humans when compared with

Table 5.2   Occupational exposure values for volatile anaesthetics.

Anaesthetic	UK exposure limit (long-term exposure limit, 8-hour time-weighted average reference period)[112]		US American Conference of Governmental Industrial Hygienists (ACGIH) Threshold Limit Values (TLVs) for 8-hour day, 40-hour week[114]	
	ppm	*mg/m³*	*ppm*	*mg/m³*
Nitrous oxide	100	183	50	90
Halothane	10	82	50	404
Isoflurane	50	383	–	–
Sevoflurane	–	–	–	–
Methoxyflurane	–	–	–	–
Enflurane	50	383	75	566

Figure 5.2   Chemical formula of isoflurane.

halothane and only minimal amounts of trifluoroacylated proteins are produced.[4,12,115] Moreover, it is rapidly excreted by the pulmonary route thus reducing the capacity for metabolism.[116]

As with halothane, occupational exposure to isoflurane can occur during human and veterinary surgical procedures.[99,117–121] The hepatotoxicity profile of isoflurane in human patients is far superior to halothane, possibly due to its lack of biotransformation to potentially hepatotoxic metabolites, noted immediately above. Nevertheless, there are concerns over its possible effects on genetic material as a result of occupational exposure to isoflurane, particularly when in combination with nitrous oxide, including the induction of DNA damage and sister chromatid exchanges.[122–124] There are also concerns that isoflurane, along with other general anaesthetics, may affect the development of the brain in neonates and of the embryo *in utero*. Most of these concerns arise from studies in laboratory animals and the major target population is therefore the paediatric surgical one. However, it also raises issues of the safety of pregnant personnel exposed occupationally to isoflurane and to other anaesthetic waste gases.[125–129]

There are also concerns over the drug's ability to deplete T-cells in exposed personnel. The percentages of T-cells were reduced in anaesthetists but the numbers of natural killer cells increased.[130] The biological significance, or more importantly the immunological significance, of these effects, if confirmed, is unclear. Occupational exposure to isoflurane during human surgical procedures has resulted in allergic contact dermatitis and asthma in exposed anaesthetic workers.[131–133]

To date, there have been no reports of ill effects in veterinary or laboratory animal workers despite intensive use of isoflurane as an anaesthetic for animal use. This probably reflects the safer profile of isoflurane when compared to halothane as well as the introduction of better anaesthetic hygiene practices into veterinary medicine.

5.3.4 Sevoflurane

Sevoflurane (Figure 5.3) is a fluorinated isopropyl methyl ether derivative, which, unlike some other halogenated hydrocarbons or ether general anaesthetics, has low irritant potential.[2] It is subject to only limited metabolism *in vivo* but, nevertheless, it is converted to hexafluoroisopropanol and fluoride in mammals, including humans.[134] Studies with human liver microsomes indicate that cytochrome P450 2E1 is the major and specific P450 isoform responsible for this metabolism.[135,136] The hexafluoroisopropanol is rapidly subject to glucuronic acid conjugation and is subsequently excreted in the urine.[136]

Sevoflurane has an excellent safety profile and is not associated with significant hepatotoxicity or nephrotoxicity in human patients.[2,136,137] However, like isoflurane, it produces dose-dependent CNS, cardiovascular and respiratory depressant effects,[138] but these are only expected to occur at therapeutic concentrations and not those that might be encountered under most conditions of occupational exposure. However, and also like isoflurane, there have been reports of genotoxic effects, notably increases in sister chromatid exchanges and DNA damage, in anaesthetists involved in human medicine procedures,[139,140] although the health implications of such findings are not clear. Sevoflurane is known to escape into the operating room area, even to the extent of being detectable in the exhaled air of some operating room personnel.[141–144] Like isoflurane, sevoflurane has been implicated in the development of occupational asthma and contact dermatitis in staff involved in anaesthesia in human medicine.[132] Thus far, there have been no reports of adverse effects in veterinarians potentially exposed to sevoflurane.

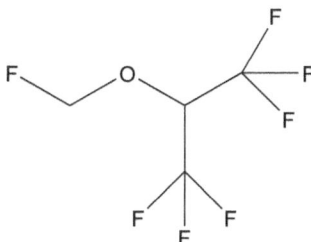

Figure 5.3 Chemical formula of sevoflurane.

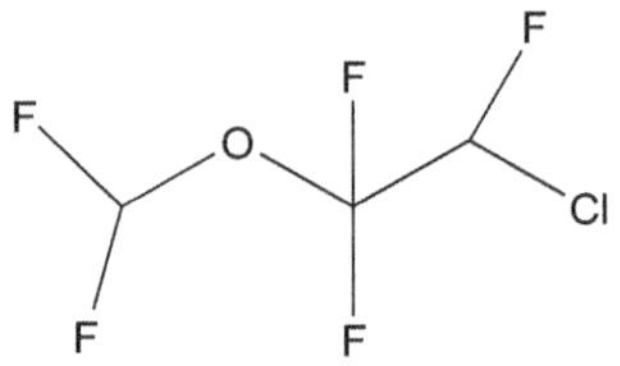

Figure 5.4 Chemical formula of enflurane.

5.3.5 Enflurane

As with halothane, enflurane (Figure 5.4) produces a decrease in arterial blood pressure in human patients as the depth of anaesthesia progresses. It also results in respiratory and CNS depression.[2,145,146] Like other halogenated anaesthetics, enflurane is metabolised to fluoride and trifluoroacyl derivatives *in vivo* in humans[115,147–149] and, as with sevoflurane, possibly involving the intermediacy of cytochrome P450 2E1.[150] In addition, a number of thioether and thiol compounds, which subsequently lead to S-conjugates, are also formed.[151]

Enflurane is hepatotoxic, but not to the same degree as halothane, and it is also nephrotoxic. Moreover, the formation of trifluoroacylated proteins by both halothane and enflurane may lead to cross-reactivity with immune-mediated hepatotoxicity in patients exposed to both compounds.[147,152] Occupational exposure of operating theatre personnel to enflurane is known to occur.[69,153,154] Hence, the biotransformation products of enflurane, including plasma fluoride and urinary thiol compounds, have been detected in operating room personnel exposed to enflurane.[148,155] As with other halogenated anaesthetics, the major adverse effects reported following occupational enflurane exposure (or *in vitro* exposure) are chromosome anomalies, sister chromatid exchanges and DNA damage.[156–159]

5.4 Injectable Anaesthetics

There are a number of agents available for use as injectable veterinary anaesthetic drugs and of these the most important currently in use are propofol, the barbiturates, etomidate and the dissociative drugs ketamine and tiletamine. These drugs have found uses in both small- and large-animal medicine as well as in human medicine.

5.4.1 Propofol

Propofol (2,6-diisopropylphenol; Figure 5.5) is a non-barbiturate sedative and hypnotic agent. It is poorly soluble in water and so is supplied as a lecithin-containing emulsion. This formulation is capable of sustaining microbial growth and unused propofol must be discarded.[3] Propofol is normally

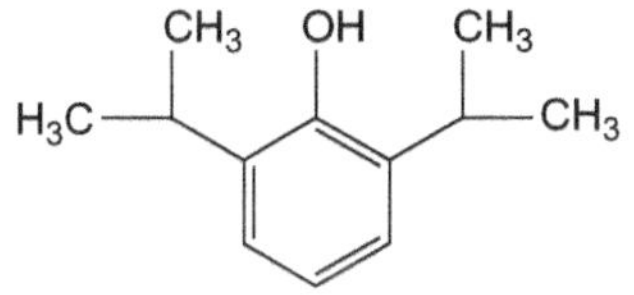

Figure 5.5 Chemical formula of propofol.

administered as a bolus intravenous dose for the induction and maintenance of anaesthesia in human and animal patients. It permits rapid recovery with few side effects. Those that do occur include excitement during induction and recovery, pain on injection and muscle tremors, although respiratory depression and apnoea may occasionally occur.[2,3,160–162] Keratitis has also been reported in humans.[163] However, the most important, albeit rare, reaction with propofol during normal human clinical use is known as propofol infusion syndrome. Common clinical features of this include hyperkalaemia, hepatomegaly, lipaemia, metabolic acidosis, myocardial failure and rhabdomyolysis.[164–166] The mechanism underlying this syndrome is unknown but it appears to be related to a number of factors including impaired tissue oxygenation, sepsis, serious cerebral injury and propofol dosage and duration of anaesthesia. Mitochondrial injury, which may also be related to poor oxygenation, may also be involved.[164–168] A similar syndrome has been observed in rabbits after prolonged administration with relatively high doses of the drug. Here, organ toxicity occurred in the lungs, liver, gallbladder and urinary bladder.[169] Despite this, propofol is recognised as a safe general anaesthetic that has the added benefit of reducing occupational exposure to volatile anaesthetics, although low-level exposure to the drug itself may occur in operating rooms for human surgery.[170–173] None of the adverse effects noted above in human (or animal) patients are likely to be observed following occupational exposure in human or veterinary medicine as these tend to occur at therapeutic doses.

At doses higher than the optimal therapeutic doses, signs of pharmacological or toxicological significance may occur. These cases tend to arise after systematic abuse of the drug, and they occasionally involve individuals who have access to the drug such as health professionals, including anaesthetists. In young children and infants (less than two years), where the induction dose for anaesthesia is higher (2.9 mg/kg bw) than in older children or adults (around 2.2 mg/kg bw), accidental overdoses of up to five times the therapeutic dose may result in mild hypotension, reduced heart rates and abnormal blood oxygenation, while higher doses may result in myocardial dysfunction.[174,175] In one case, a dose of 20 mg/kg bw per hour infused over 15 hours was initially survived by a 3-year-old child who had developed respiratory perturbation and metabolic acidosis. However, on recovery the patient was given further propofol (4 mg/kg bw per hour) and this resulted in intractable bradycardic dysrhythmias that led to fatal cardiac insufficiency.[176] Hence, medication errors may lead to exaggerated pharmacological responses and eventually to frank toxicity. These effects may be exacerbated by faulty medical equipment.[177]

However, medication errors do not pose the greatest risks. Propofol is frequently abused. As noted by one poison control centre, "propofol has alluring and addictive properties that lend itself to potential recreational abuse dependence". This may lead to recreational abuse, tolerance, dependence, withdrawal effects and death.[178] Propofol is also favoured for use in suicide attempts, frequently successful, and in homicides.[179–186]

All of the effects noted with propofol underline the need for proper medical or veterinary supervision of the use of the drug during anaesthesia procedures, something that was emphasised by the death of the singer Michael Jackson following propofol administration for non-medical use. In the hospital environment, human or veterinary, propofol is a very safe and effective anaesthetic agent. However, following self-administration, the drug may have lethal effects that are sometimes the intent of the abuse. On other occasions, it may be used for homicide attempts. As the veterinary and human propofol formulations currently available are identical, then for practical purposes it is immaterial as to the source of the product. Clearly, whether intended for veterinary or human clinical use, propofol should be securely kept when not in use.

5.4.2   Barbiturates

The barbiturates are derivatives of barbituric acid (malonylurea; Figure 5.6), a substance that is only slightly soluble in water. However, conversion of this into water-soluble derivatives has allowed the development of many compounds that have found use as therapeutic agents. Several barbiturates are used in veterinary medicine and the choice of drug is frequently determined by the desired duration of activity (Table 5.3) and the structures of two of these, phenobarbital sodium and pentobarbital, are shown in Figure 5.6. The barbiturates may be used as injectable anaesthetics or as induction agents prior to use of other anaesthetic drugs such as isoflurane.[3,6] They are also used as veterinary euthanasia agents and for the treatment of epileptic seizures, especially in dogs.[186–190]

The major effect of the barbiturates in animals and humans is depression of the central nervous system from increased inhibitory activity, which leads to fatigue, changes in cognitive function, anaesthesia or at higher doses to death and, consequently, barbiturates are frequently used in suicides.[191–199] As physicians have access to drugs, barbiturates are frequently used in suicides by this occupational group, especially anaesthetists.[200] Although veterinarians may be at elevated risk of suicide, there are no substantive data to suggest that the ready availability of barbiturates or indeed other drugs plays a role in this.[201,202] However, barbiturate formulations specifically marketed for veterinary use have featured in suicides including suicides by veterinarians.[203–206]

Barbiturates are known to induce hepatic microsomal enzymes and hence to enhance the metabolism and sometimes the toxicity of other chemicals including other drugs. Indeed, in experimental toxicology and carcinogenesis, phenobarbital has long been used for such purposes.[207]

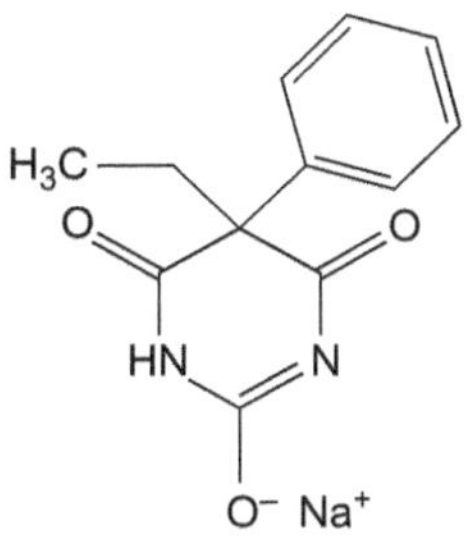

Barbituric acid

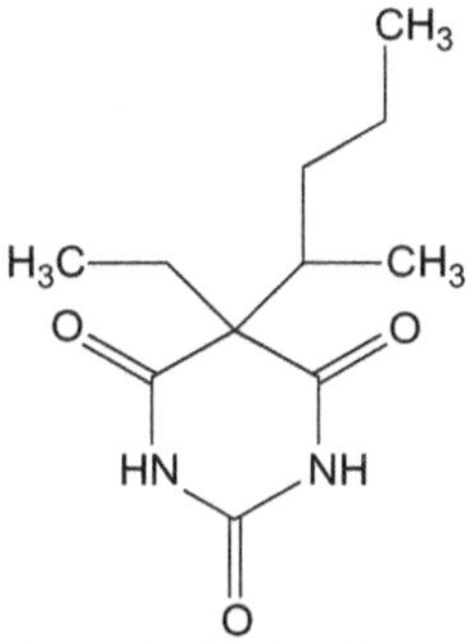

Phenobarbital sodium

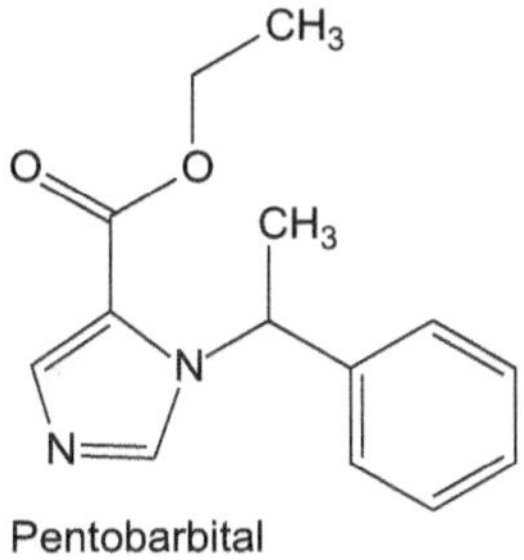

Pentobarbital

Figure 5.6 Chemical formulae of barbituric acid, phenobarbital sodium and pentobarbital.

5.4.3 Etomidate

Etomidate (ethyl 1-(1-phenylethyl)-1H-imidazole-5-carboxylate; Figure 5.7) is a unique drug, being the only anaesthetic in this chemical class in clinical use, although several other candidate compounds were synthesised.[208] In veterinary and human medicine, intravenously administered etomidate is frequently used for short surgical procedures and it is preferred to barbiturates due to its high therapeutic index.[6,208] Etomidate possesses a chiral carbon atom, resulting in a chiral centre and two enantiomers, the R(+) and S(−) compounds. Studies have demonstrated that the R(+) isomer is around 10- to 20-fold more potent as a hypnotic drug than the S(−) isomer.[208–210] Etomidate has been shown to

Table 5.3 Some barbiturates used in veterinary medicine.

Barbiturate	Duration of action
Phenobarbital sodium	Long acting
Barbital sodium	Long acting
Amobarbital sodium	Intermediate acting
Pentobarbital/pentobarbital sodium	Short acting
Secobarbital sodium	Short acting
Thiopental sodium	Ultrashort acting
Thiamylal sodium	Ultrashort acting
Thialbarbital sodium	Ultrashort acting
Methohexital sodium	Ultrashort acting

Figure 5.7 Chemical formula of etomidate.

interact with the $GABA_A$ receptors, the major inhibitory neurotransmitter receptors in the brain.[208–213]

It has been shown to be an exceptionally safe drug when used for general anaesthesia. Side effects include pain on injection, myoclonic movements, post-operative nausea and vomiting.[208] Adrenal toxicity has been reported in human patients after prolonged etomidate infusions.[214–216] It has been shown to suppress adrenocortical activity in humans and in experimental animals.[217–222] Etomidate, or a metabolite of etomidate, may block ascorbic acid metabolism and, subsequent to this, inhibit steroidogenesis.[223]

It may also inhibit mitochondrial function, at least in part through the inhibition of nitric oxide synthase, producing ischaemic injury in the brain.[224] Etomidate (and propofol) may also severely depress neuronal firing of neurons in the cat cortex, thalamus and reticular formation.[225]

Clearly, the side effects and toxicity noted with etomidate are related to clinical use of the drug and are unlikely to be seen following occupational exposure, even accidental self-injection, during normal veterinary use.

5.4.4 Ketamine

Ketamine (2-(chlorophenyl)-2-(methylamino)cyclohexanone; Figure 5.8) is a dissociative anaesthetic structurally related to phencyclidine (1-(1-phenylcyclohexyl)piperidine), a substance previously used as an anaesthetic but which is now solely used as a recreational drug under the names PCP or angel dust. Ketamine is also structurally related to tiletamine (2-(ethylamino)-2-(2-thienyl)cyclohexanone).

Phencyclidine was developed for use in human medicine but its use was abandoned because of hallucinations and psychological problems and it was replaced with ketamine, which has a lower frequency of such effects.[2,226,227] Both ketamine and tiletamine are used as anaesthetic agents in veterinary medicine. Indeed, they have a wide range of uses in companion, farm and exotic animals. Both are frequently used in combination with other drugs, and tiletamine is supplied as a fixed combination with zolazepam (Telazol).[2,6,228–255]

Phencyclidine, ketamine and related drugs are *N*-methyl-D-aspartate (NMDA) antagonists and this activity may be associated with the induction of apoptosis in the rat and primate brain, and notably in young rats during the period of synaptogenesis.[256–263] Anaesthesia for periods of 9 hours or greater was associated with significant nerve cell death in monkeys.[260] Certain agents, including yohimbine, lithium and xenon, exert a protective effect in this neurotoxicity.[264–266] The exact mechanism is not yet understood but it may involve enhanced expression of the NMDA receptor subunit mRNA and interactions with neuronal growth factors.[256–258,260,261] Such findings raise concern over the paediatric use of ketamine, although simple overdose in children, even with 100 times the recommended dose, appears to result mainly in prolonged sedation.[267,268] However, the effects may not be restricted to neonatal animals thus giving rise to concerns for older patients and for drug abusers.[269] Intrathecal and subarachnoid administration of ketamine is also associated with neuronal degeneration in animals.[270–273] Similar effects have been reported in human patients given ketamine intrathecally for the control of cancer pain.[274,275] Ketamine given by continuous subcutaneous infusion appears to be a safer treatment option for the treatment of refractory cancer pain.[276]

Ketamine also may induce hepatotoxicity, adverse effects on the urogenital system and, in mice at least, cardiotoxicity when given with alcohol.[277–279] Ketamine was used to treat American soldiers injured in the Vietnam war and, shortly afterwards, along with phencyclidine, it became a drug of abuse.[227] Its effects include an altered state of consciousness, and a feeling of being "high". However, its abuse can result in memory deficits and behavioural changes.[280,281] In animal models, it produces behavioural changes and effects that are suggestive of a schizophrenia-like state.[282–285] In humans, it produces changes in speech that mimic some aspects of schizophrenia.[286] Chronic abuse may result in cholestasis and biliary dilatation.[287] In animal models, ketamine has been shown to induce hepatic microsomal enzymes and hence it may affect the metabolism and toxicity of other chemical agents.[288–291] Such findings are

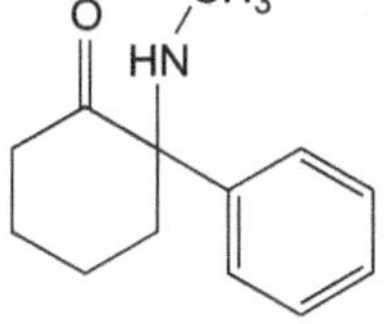

Figure 5.8 Chemical formula of ketamine.

important as ketamine continues to be abused, especially as a "club" drug, along with rohypnol, methamphetamine and gamma-hydroxybutyrate.[227,292–299] Clearly, the origins of the drug, whether intended for use in human or in veterinary medicine, are irrelevant but, whatever use is intended, the evidence suggests that ketamine should be kept securely. Nevertheless, ketamine is frequently abused by health professionals, including anaesthetists.[300] Tiletamine, as the tiletamine-zolazepam formulation, induced a movement disorder after abuse of the product by a veterinarian over a 2-week period.[301] In another case, a zoo worker who injected herself with the veterinary formulation and a diazepam product became obtunded and arousable only to deep painful stimuli but quickly recovered. She was found to be a regular abuser of the veterinary formulation.[302] Fatalities with Telazol have included at least one veterinarian.[303,304]

5.5   Conclusions

Some of the volatile anaesthetics offer significant potential for adverse effects in circumstances that provide prolonged or repeated exposures such as those that pertain with occupational exposure. The associated risks can be mitigated with normal occupational hygiene measures including adequate ventilation and gas scavenging measures as well as ensuring that anaesthetic delivery devices are well maintained and, crucially, are free from leaks.

Injectable anaesthetics also need to be used with normal occupational hygiene measures in mind, including the avoidance of needlestick injuries and self-injection. However, under most circumstances, it is unlikely that pharmacological effects will be evoked due to the very small amounts of substance that are likely to be delivered in such accidents. The major concern with these drugs (and to an extent with nitrous oxide) is substance abuse, especially with ketamine. The drugs need to be kept in a secure environment to prevent them from becoming available for any purpose other than their intended therapeutic uses. Veterinarians and other veterinary staff have free access to these drugs and, clearly, the prevention of abuse under these circumstances may be problematic. Adequate record keeping of the amounts of these drugs being employed in practice may serve to highlight missing quantities that may be being used for illicit purposes.

References

1. S. K. Kennedy and D. E. Longnecker, History and principles of anesthesiology in *Goodman and Gilman's The Pharmacological Basis of Therapeutics*, ed. J. G. Hardman and L. E. Limbird, McGraw-Hill, London, 9th edn, 1996, pp. 295–306.
2. B. E. Marshall and D. E. Longnecker, General anesthetics in *Goodman and Gilman's The Pharmacological Basis of Therapeutics*, ed. J. G. Hardman and L. E. Limbird, McGraw-Hill, London, 9th edn, 1996, pp. 307–330.

3. E. A. Martinez, Anaesthetic agents in *Small Animal Clinical Pharmacology and Therapeutics*, ed. D. M. Boothe , W. B. Saunders Company, London, 2001, pp. 425–430.

4. E. P. Steffey, Inhalation anesthetics in *Veterinary Pharmacology and Therapeutics*, ed. H. R. Adams, Iowa State Press, Ames, 8th edn, 2001, pp. 184–212.

5. L. W. Hall, K. W. Clarke and C. M. Trim, *Veterinary Anaesthesia*, Saunders, London, 10th edn, 2001.

6. K. R. Bransom, Injectable anesthetics in *Veterinary Pharmacology and Therapeutics*, ed. H. R. Adams, Iowa State Press, Ames, 8th edn, 2001, pp. 213–267.

7. L. W. Hall, K. W. Clarke and C. M. Trim, General pharmacology of the injectable agents used in anaesthesia in *Veterinary Anaesthesia*, Saunders, London, 10th edn, 2001, pp. 113–132.

8. H. C. Lin, Dissociative anesthetics in *Lumb and Jones' Veterinary Anesthesia*, ed. J. C. Thurman, W. J. Tranquili and G. J. Benson, Williams & Wilkins, Baltimore, 1996, pp. 241–296.

9. Z. Sahenk, J. R. Mendel, D. Couri and J. Nachtman, Polyneuropathy from inhalation of N_2O through a whipped-cream dispenser, *Neurology*, 1978, **28**, 485–487.

10. A. Brett, Myeloneuropathy from whipped cream bulbs presenting as conversion disorder, *Aust. N. Z. J. Psychiatry*, 1997, **31**, 131–132.

11. R. D. Sanders, J. Weimann and M. Maze, Biologic effects of nitrous oxide: a mechanistic and toxicologic review, *Anesthesiology*, 2008, **109**, 707–722.

12. G. Torri, Inhalation anesthetics: a review, *Minerva Anestesiol.*, 2010, **76**, 215–228.

13. J. C. Hwang, H. N. Himmel and R. F. Edlich, Frostbite of the face after recreational use of nitrous oxide, *Burns*, 1996, **22**, 152–153.

14. N. Svartling, S. Ranta, J. Vuola and O. Takkunen, Life-threatening airway obstruction from nitrous oxide induced frostbite of the oral cavity, *Anaesth. Intensive Care.*, 1996, **24**, 717–720.

15. M. Yamashita, K. Motokawa and S. Watanabe, Do not use the "innovated" cylinder valve handle for cracking the valve, *Anesthesiology*, **64**, 658–659.

16. G. W. Paulson, "Recreational" misuse of nitrous oxide, *J. Am. Dent. Assoc.*, 1979, **98**, 410–411.

17. R. B. Layzer, R. A. Fisher and J. A. Schafer, Neuropathy following abuse of nitrous oxide, *Neurology*, 1978, **28**, 504–506.

18. M. A. Nevins, Neuropathy after nitrous oxide abuse, *J. Am. Med. Assoc.*, 1980, **244**, 2264.

19. H. Manji, Toxic neuropathy, *Curr. Opin. Neurol.*, 2011, **24**, 484–490.

20. A. J. Waclawik, C. C. Luzzio, K. Juhasz-Pocsine and V. Hamilton, Myeloneupathy from nitrous oxide abuse: unusually high methylmalonic acid and homocysteine levels, *Wisc. Med. J.*, 2003, **102**, 43–45.

21. R. T. Louis-Ferdinand, Myelotoxic, neurotoxic and reproductive effects of nitrous oxide, *Adverse Drug React. Toxicol. Rev.*, 1994, **13**, 193–206.

22. H. Butzkueven and J. O. King, Nitrous oxide myelopathy in an abuser of whipped cream bulbs, *J. Clin. Neurosci.*, 2000, **7**, 73–75.
23. K. Iwata, G. B. O'Keefe and A. Karanas, Neurologic problems associated with chronic nitrous oxide abuse in a non-healthcare worker, *Am. J. Med. Sci.*, 2001, **322**, 173–174.
24. J. Weimann, Toxicity of nitrous oxide, *Best Pract. Res. Clin. Anaesthesiol.*, 2003, **17**, 47–61.
25. R. M. Shulman, T. J. Geraghty and M. Tadros, A case of unusual substance abuse causing myeloneuropathy, *Spinal Cord*, 2007, **45**, 314–317.
26. P. J. Pema, H. A. Horak and R. H. Wyatt, Myelopathy caused by nitrous oxide toxicity, *Am. J. Neuroradiol.*, 1998, **19**, 894–896.
27. P. G. Richardson, Peripheral neuropathy following nitrous oxide abuse, *Emerg. Med. Australas.*, 2010, **22**, 88–90.
28. W. O. Tatum, D. D. Bui, E. G. Grant and R. Murtagh, Pseudo-guillain-barré syndrome due to "whippet"-induced myeloneuropathy, *J. Neuroimaging*, 2010, **20**, 400–401.
29. S. M. Olfert, Reproductive outcomes among dental personnel: a review of selected exposures, *J. Can. Dent. Assoc.*, 2006, **72**, 821–825.
30. T. Wrońska-Nofer, J. Paulus, W. Krajewski, J. Jajte, M. Kucharska, J. Stetkiewska, W. Wasowicz and K. Rydzyński, DNA damage induced by nitrous oxide: study in medical personnel of operating rooms, *Mutat. Res.*, 2009, **666**, 39–43.
31. H. Westburg, L. Egelrud, C. C. Ohlson, M. Hygerth and C. Lindholm, Exposure to nitrous oxide in delivery suites at six Swedish hospitals, *Int. Arch. Occup. Environ. Health*, 2008, **81**, 828–836.
32. J. B. Brodsky, E. N. Cohen, B. W. Brown, M. L. Wu and C. E. Whitcher, Exposure to nitrous oxide and neurologic disease among dental professionals, *Anesth. Analg.*, 1981, **60**, 297–301.
33. A. Nayebzadeh, Exposure to exhaled nitrous oxide in hospitals in post-anesthesia care units, *Ind. Health*, 2007, **45**, 334–337.
34. M. G. Irwin, T. Trinh and C. L. Yao, Occupational exposure to anaesthetic gases: a role for TVA, *Expert Opin. Drug Saf.*, 2009, **8**, 473–483.
35. W. Krajewski, M. Kucharska, W. Wesolowski, J. Stetkiewicz and T. Wrońska-Nofer, Occupational exposure to nitrous oxide – the role of scavenging and ventilation systems in reducing the exposure level in operating rooms, *Int. J. Hyg. Environ. Health*, 2007, **210**, 133–138.
36. World Health Organization, *WHO Model List of Essential Medicines*, WHO, Geneva, 17th edn, March 2011. Available at: http://www.who.int/medicines/publications/essentialmedicines/en/.
37. H. M. Mehendale, R. A. Roth, A. J. Gandolfi, J. E. Klaunig, J. J. Lemasters and L. R. Curtis, Novel mechanisms in chemically induced hepatotoxicity, *FASEB J.*, 1994, **8**, 1285–1295.
38. J. Neuberger and R. Williams, Halothane hepatitis, *Digest. Dis.*, 1988, **61**, 52–64.
39. G. L. Bird and R. Williams, Anaesthesia-induced liver disease, *Monogr. Allergy*, 1992, **30**, 174–191.

40. E. D. Kharasch, Adverse drug reactions with halogenated anesthetics, *Clin. Pharmacol. Ther.*, 2008, **84**, 158–162.
41. J. Neuberger, Halothane hepatitis, *Eur. J. Gastroenterol. Hepatol.*, 1998, **10**, 631–633.
42. J. K. Aronson, ed., Inhalational anaesthetics – halogenated in *Meyler's Side Effects of Drugs Used in Anaesthesia*, Elsevier, Oxford, 2009, pp. 15–41.
43. E. Björnsson, P. Jerlstad, A. Bergqvist and R. Olsson, Fulminant drug-induced hepatic failure leading to death or liver transplantation on Sweden, *Scand. J. Gastroenterol.*, 2005, **40**, 1095–1101.
44. J. Neuberger, G. Mieli-Vergani, J. M. Tredger, M. Davis and R. Williams, Oxidative metabolism of halothane in the production of altered hepatocyte membrane antigens in acute halothane-induced hepatic necrosis, *Gut*, 1981, **22**, 669–672.
45. G. L. Bird and R. Williams, Detection of antibodies to a halothane metabolite hapten in sera from patients with halothane-associated hepatitis, *J. Hepatol.*, 1989, **9**, 366–373.
46. P. M. Dansette, E. Bonierbale, C. Minoletti, P. H. Beaune, D. Passsayre and D. Mansuy, Drug-induced immunotoxicity, *Eur. J. Drug Metab. Pharmacokinet.*, 1998, **23**, 443–451.
47. A. K. Hubbard, T. P. Roth, S. Schuman and A. J. Gandolfi, Localisation of halothane-induced antigen in situ by specific anti-halothane metabolite antibodies, *Clin. Exp. Immunol.*, 1989, **76**, 422–427.
48. J. Gut, U. Christen and J. Huwyler, Mechanisms of halothane toxicity: novel insights, *Pharmacol. Ther.*, 1993, **58**, 133–155.
49. Y. Masobuchi and T. Horie, Toxicological significance of mechanism-based inactivation of cytochrome p450 enzymes by drugs, *Crit. Rev. Toxicol.*, 2007, **37**, 389–342.
50. E. D. Kharasch, D. C. Hankins, K. Fenstamaker and K. Cox, Human halothane metabolism, lipid peroxidation, and cytochrome P(450)2A6 and P(450)3A4, *Eur. J. Clin. Pharmacol.*, 2000, **55**, 853–859.
51. M. Bourdi, W. Chen, R. M. Peter, J. L. Martin, J. T. Buters, S. D. Nelson and L. R. Pohl, Human cytochrome P450 2E1 is a major autoantigen associated with halothane hepatitis, *Chem. Res. Toxicol.*, 1996, **9**, 1159–1166.
52. E. Kobayashi, M. Kobayashi, K. Tsuneyama, T. Fukami, M. Nakajima and T. Yokoi, Halothane-induced liver injury is mediated by interleukin-17 in mice, *Toxicol. Sci.*, 2009, **111**, 302–310.
53. L. Cheng, Q. You, H. Yin, M. P. Holt and C. Ju, Involvement of natural killer T cells in halothane-induced liver injury in mice, *Biochem. Pharmacol.*, 2010, **80**, 255–261.
54. C. M. Dugan, A. M. Fullerton, R. A. Roth and P. E. Ganey, Natural killer cells mediate severe liver injury in a murine model of halothane hepatitis, *Toxicol. Sci.*, 2011, **120**, 507–518.
55. S. Koda, S. Kumagaj, M. Toyota, N. Yasuda and H. Chara, A study of waste anaesthetic gases monitoring and working environmental controls in hospital operating rooms, *Sangyo Eiseigaku Zasshi.*, 1997, **39**, 38–45.

56. F. D. Smith, Management of exposure to waste anesthetic gases, *AORN J.*, 2010, **91**, 482–494.
57. K. Homishak, S. Widmer and R. Stauffer, Scavenging anesthetic gas from a membrane oxygenator during cardiopulmonary bypass, *J. Extra Corpor. Technol.*, 1996, **28**, 88–90.
58. S. Merdl, C. Byhahn, U. Abdel-Rahman, G. Mattheis and K. Westphal, Occupational exposure to inhalational anesthetics during cardiac surgery on cardiopulmonary bypass, *Ann. Thorac. Surg.*, 2003, **75**, 1924–1927.
59. H. W. Linde and D. L. Bruce, Occupational exposure of anaesthetists to halothane, nitrous oxide and radiation, *Anaesthesiol.*, 1969, **30**, 363–368.
60. T. H. Cohen, B. W. Brown, D. L. Bruce, H. F. Sascorbi, T. H. Corbett, T. W. Jones and C. E. Whichter, A survey of anesthetic health hazards among dentists, *J. Amer. Dent. Assoc.*, 1975, **90**, 1291–1296.
61. L. Hunter, An occupational health approach to anaesthetic air pollution, *Med. J. Aust.*, 1976, **1**, 465–468.
62. C. Whitcher and R. Piziali, Monitoring occupational exposure to inhalation anesthetics, *Anesth. Analg.*, 1977, **56**, 778–785.
63. K. Korttila, P. Pfaffli, M. Linnoila, E. Blomgren, H. Hanninen and S. Hakkinen, Operating nurses' psychomotor and driving skills after occupational exposure to halothane and nitrous oxide, *Acta Anesthesiol. Scand.*, 1978, **22**, 33–39.
64. H. T. Davenport, M. J. Halsey, B. Wardley-Smith and P. E. Bateman, Occupational exposure to anaesthetics in 20 hospitals, *Anaesthesia*, 1980, **35**, 354–359.
65. R. Harrison, Medical surveillance for workplace hepatotoxins, *Occup. Med.*, 1990, **5**, 515–530.
66. T. E. Kole, Environmental and occupational hazards of the anesthesia workplace, *Am. Assoc. Nurse Anesth. J.*, 1990, **58**, 327–331.
67. K. A. Henderson and I. P. Matthews, Staff exposure to anaesthetic gases in theatre and non theatre areas, *Eur. J. Anaesthesiol.*, 2000, **17**, 149–151.
68. K. Sitarek, W. Wesolowski, M. Kucharska and G. Celichowski, Concentrations of anaesthetic gases in hospital operating theatres, *Int. J. Occup. Med. Environ. Health*, 2000, **13**, 61–66.
69. C. Byhahn, H. J. Wilke and K. Westphal, Occupational exposure to volatile anaesthetics: epidemiology approaches to reducing the problem, *CNS Drugs*, 2001, **15**, 197–215.
70. J. Stachnik, Inhaled anaesthetic agents, *Am. J. Health Syst. Pharm.*, 2006, **63**, 623–634.
71. S. Babich and R. P. Burakoff, Occupational hazards of dentistry. A review of literature from 1990, *N. Y. State Dent. J.*, 1997, **63**, 26–31.
72. D. J. Culley, Z. Xie and G. Crosby, General anaesthetic-induced neurotoxicity: an emerging problem for young and old? *Curr. Opin. Anaesthesiol.*, 2007, **20**, 408–413.
73. K. Teschke, Z. Abaanto, L. Arbour, K. Beking, Y. Chow, B. Chong, N. D. Le, P. A. Ratner, J. J. Spinelli and H. Dimich-Ward, Exposure to

anesthetic gases and congenital anomalies in offspring of female registered nurses, *Am. J. Ind. Med.*, 2011, **54**, 118–127.

74. S. Belfrage, I. Ahlgren and S. Axelson, Halothane hepatitis in an anaesthetist, *Lancet*, 1966, **ii**, 1466–1467.

75. T. H. Corbett, R. G. Cornell, J. L. Endres and K. Lieding, Birth defects among the children of nurse-anesthetists, *Anesthesiol.*, 1974, **41**, 341–345.

76. J. M. Duvaldestin, R. I. Mazze, Y. Nivoche and J. M. Desmonts, Occupational exposure to halothane results in enzyme induction in anesthetists, *Anesthesiol.*, 1981, **54**, 57–61.

77. G. Franco, Occupational exposure to anesthetics: liver injury, microsomal enzyme induction and preventive aspects, *G. Ital. Med. Lav.*, 1989, **11**, 205–208.

78. H. Grimmeisen, Chronic exposure to halothane: liver damage in anaesthetists, *Anaesthetist*, 1973, **22**, 41–46.

79. S. Keiding, M. Dossing and F. Hardt, A nurse with liver injury associated with occupational exposure to halothane in a recovery unit, *Dan. Med. Bull.*, 1984, **31**, 255–256.

80. G. Klatskin and D. V. Kimberg, Recurrent hepatitis attributable to halothane sensitization in an anesthetist, *N. Engl. J. Med.*, 1969, **280**, 515–522.

81. S. Lings, Halothane related liver affection in an anaesthetist, *Br. J. Ind. Med.*, 1988, **45**, 716–717.

82. R. Luchini, D. Placidi, F. Toffoletto and L. Alessio, Neurotoxicity in operating room personnel working with gaseous and nongaseous anesthesia, *Int. Arch. Occup. Environ. Med.*, 1996, **68**, 188–192.

83. S. Popova, A. Krüsteva and P. Traĭkova, Toxic hepatitis and spontaneous abortion in female anesthesiologists, *Khirurgiia*, 1980, **33**, 118–120.

84. J. E. Burkhart and T. J. Stobbe, Real-time measurement and control of waste gases during veterinary surgeries, *Am. Ind. Hyg. Assoc. J.*, 1990, **51**, 640–645.

85. D. W. Dreesen, G. L. Jones, J. Brown and J. L. Rawlings, Monitoring for trace anesthetic gases in a veterinary hospital, *J. Am. Vet, Med. Assoc.*, 1981, **179**, 797–799.

86. R. J. Gardner, J. Hampton and J. S. Causton, Inhalation anaesthetics – exposure and control during veterinary surgery, *Ann. Occup. Hyg.*, 1991, **35**, 377–388.

87. C. J. Green, Anaesthetic gases and health risks to laboratory personnel: a review, *Lab. Anim.*, 1981, **15**, 397–403.

88. R. E. Korczynski, Anaesthetic gas exposure in veterinary clinics, *Appl. Occup. Environ. Hyg.*, 1999, **14**, 384–390.

89. J. E. Milligan, J. L. Sablan and C. E. Short, A survey of waste anesthetic gas concentrations in the U.S. Air Force veterinary surgeries, *J. Am. Vet. Med. Assoc.*, 1980, **177**, 1021–1022.

90. R. M. Moore, Y. M. Davis and R. G. Kaczmarek, An overview of occupational hazards among veterinarians with particular reference to pregnant women, *Am. Ind. Hyg. Assoc. J.*, 1993, **54**, 113–120.

91. D. L. Potts and B. F. Craft, Occupational exposure of veterinarians to waste anesthetic gases, *Appl. Ind. Hyg.*, 1988, **3**, 132–138.

92. S. M. Schuchman, F. L. Frye and R. P. Barrett, Toxicities and hazards for clinicians in small animal practice, *Vet. Clin. North Am.*, 1975, **5**, 727–735.

93. T. M. Stimpfel and E. L. Gershey, Selecting anaesthetic agents for human safety and animal recovery after surgery, *FASEB J.*, 1991, **5**, 2099–2104.

94. G. S. Ward and R. R. Byland, Concentrations of halothane in veterinary operating and treatment rooms, *J. Am. Vet. Med. Assoc.*, 1982, **180**, 174–177.

95. G. S. Ward and R. R. Byland, Concentrations of methoxyfluorane and nitrous oxide in veterinary operating rooms, *Am. J. Vet. Res.*, 1982, **43**, 360–362.

96. W. E. Wingfield, D. L. Ruby, R. M. Buchan and B. J. Gunther, Waste anesthetic gas exposure to veterinarians and animal technicians, *J. Am. Vet. Med. Assoc.*, 1981, **178**, 399–402.

97. C. E. Short, Thoughts on studies linking occupational exposure to anesthetic waste gases, *J. Am. Vet. Med. Assoc.*, 2009, **235**, 660–661.

98. J. A. Smith, Anesthetic pollution and waste anesthetic gas scavenging, *Semin. Vet. Med. Surg.*, 1993, **8**, 90–103.

99. R. E. Meyer, Anesthesia hazards to animal workers, *Occup. Med.*, 1999, **14**, 225–234.

100. C. E. Short and R. C. Harvey, Anesthetic waste gases in veterinary medicine: analysis of the problem and suggested guidelines for reducing personnel exposures, *Cornell Vet.*, 1983, **73**, 363–374.

101. L. Fritschi, A. Shirangi, I. D. Robertson and L. M. Day, Trends in exposure of veterinarians to physical and chemical hazards and use of protection practices, *Int. Arch. Occup. Environ. Med.*, 2008, **81**, 371–378.

102. A. Shirangi, L. Fritschi and C. D. Holman, Prevalence of occupational exposures and protective practices in Australian female veterinarians, *Aust. Vet. J.*, 2007, **85**, 32–38.

103. D. L. Ruby, R. M. Buchan and B. J. Gunter, Waste anesthetic gas and vapour exposures in veterinary hospitals and clinics, *Am. Ind. Hyg. Assoc. J.*, 1980, **41**, 229–231.

104. C. I. Johnson and F. Mendelsohn, Halothane hepatitis in a laboratory technician, *Aust. N. Z. J. Med.*, 1971, **1**, 171–173.

105. D. E. Sutherland and W. A. Smith, Chemical hepatitis associated with occupational exposure to halothane in a research laboratory, *Vet. Hum. Toxicol.*, 1992, **34**, 423–424.

106. S. Shuhaiber and G. Koren, Occupational exposure to inhaled anesthetic, *Can. Fam. Phys.*, 2000, **46**, 2391–2392.

107. A. Shirangi, L. Fritschi and C. D. Holman, Maternal occupational exposures and risk of spontaneous abortion in veterinary practice, *Occup. Environ. Med.*, 2008, **65**, 719–725.

108. J. A. Johnson, R. M. Buchan and J. S. Reif, Effect of waste gas and vapour exposure on reproductive outcome in veterinary personnel, *Am. Ind. Hyg. Assoc. J.*, 1987, **48**, 62–66.

109. A. Shirangi, L. Fritschi and C. D. Holman, Associations of unscavenged anesthetic gases and long working hours with preterm delivery in female veterinarians, *Obstet. Gynecol.*, 2009, **113**, 1008–1017.

110. A. Shirangi, L. Fritschi, C. D. Holman and C. Bower, Birth defects in offspring of female veterinarians, *J. Occup. Environ. Med.*, 2009, **51**, 525–533.

111. S. Shuhaiber, A. Einarson, I. C. Radde, M. Sarkar and G. Koren, A prospective-controlled study of veterinary staff exposed to inhaled anesthetics and x-rays, *Int. J. Occup. Med. Environ. Health*, 2002, **15**, 363–373.

112. Health and Safety Executive, EH40/2005 *Workplace Exposure Limits*, Health and Safety Executive, Bootle, 2nd edn, 2011. Available at: http://www.hse.gov.uk/pubns/priced/EH40.pdf.

113. For occupational exposure limits in various European Union countries, see http://osha.europa.eu/en/topics/ds/oels/members.stm.

114. American Conference of Governmental Industrial Hygienists, http://acgih.org/home.htm.

115. D. Njoku, M. J. Laster, D. H. Gong, E. I. Eger, G. F. Reed and J. L. Martin, Biotransformation of halothane, enflurane, isoflurane and desflurane to trifluoroacetylated liver proteins: association between protein acylation and hepatic injury, *Anesth. Analg.*, 1997, **84**, 173–178.

116. B. A. Hitt and R. I. Mazze, Effect of enzyme induction on nephrotoxicity of halothane-related compounds, *Environ. Health Perspect.*, 1977, **21**, 179–183.

117. J. C. Smith and B. Bolon, Comparison of three commercially available activated charcoal canisters for passive scavenging of waste isoflurane during conventional anesthesia, *Contemp. Top. Lab. Anim. Sci.*, 2003, **42**, 10–15.

118. H. Säre, T. D. Ambrisko and Y. Moens, Occupational exposure to isoflurane during anaesthesia induction with standard and scavenging double masks in dogs, pigs and ponies, *Lab. Anim.*, 2011, **45**, 191–195.

119. J. C. Smith and B. Bolon, Atmospheric waste isoflurane concentrations using conventional equipment and rat anaesthesia protocols, *Contemp. Top. Lab. Anim. Sci.*, 2002, **41**, 10–17.

120. F. E. Bennetts and C. M. Carnegie, Isoflurane sedation and atmospheric pollution, *Intensive Care Med.*, 1994, **20**, 460.

121. S. Mierdl, C. Byhahn, U. Abdel-Rahman, G. Matheis and K. Westphal, Occupational exposure to inhalational anesthetics during cardiac surgery or cardiopulmonary bypass, *Ann. Thorac. Surg.*, 2003, **75**, 1924–1927.

122. Anon, Anesthetic may affect chromosomes, *J. Am. Dent. Assoc.*, 1999, **130**, 1276.

123. K. H. Hoerauf, G. Wiesner, K. F. Schroegendorfer, B. P. Jobst, A. Spacec, M. Harth, S. Sator-Katzenschlager and H. W. Rüdiger, Waste

anaesthetic gases induce sister chromatid exchanges in lymphocytes of operating personnel, *Br. J. Anaesth.*, 1999, **82**, 764–766.

124. K. Hoerauf, M. Lierz, G. Wiesner, K. Schroegendorfer, P. Lierz, A. Spack, L. Brunnberg and M. Nüsse, Genetic damage in operating room personnel exposed to isoflurane and nitrous oxide, *Occup. Environ. Med.*, 1999, **56**, 433–437.

125. T. D. Shear, Is a weekend too long? *Anesthesiology*, 2011, **115**, 899–905.

126. G. K. Istaphanous and A. W. Loepke, General anesthetics and the developing brain, *Curr. Opin. Anaesthesiol.*, 2009, **22**, 368–373.

127. N. Lunardi, C. Ori, A. Erisir and V. Jevtovic-Todorovic, General anesthesia causes long-lasting disturbances in the ultrastructural properties of developing synapses in young rats, *Neurotox. Res.*, 2010, **17**, 179–188.

128. G. Liang, C. Ward, J. Peng, Y. Zhao, B. Huang and H. Wei, Isoflurane causes greater neurodegeneration than an equivalent exposure of Sevoflurane in the developing brain of neonatal mice, *Anesthesiol*, 2010, **112**, 1325–1334.

129. E. I. Eger, Fetal injury and abortion associated with occupational exposure to inhaled anesthetics, *AANA J.*, 1991, **59**, 309–312.

130. A. Bargellini, S. Rovesti, A. Barbieri, R. Vivoli, R. Roncaglia, E. Righi and P. Borella, Effects of chronic exposure to anaesthetic gases on some immune parameters, *Sci. Total Environ.*, 2001, **270**, 149–156.

131. S. Caraffini, F. Ricci, D. Assalve and P. Lisi, Isoflurane: an uncommon cause of occupational airborne contact dermatitis, *Contact Dermatitis*, 1998, **38**, 286.

132. A. D. Vellore, V. J. Drought, D. Sherwood-Jones, V. C. Moore, A. S. Robertson and P. S. Burge, Occupational asthma and allergy to sevoflurane and isoflurane in anaesthetic staff, *Allergy*, 2006, **61**, 1485–1486.

133. T. M. Finch, A. Muncaster, L. Prais and I. S. Foulds, Occupational airborne contact dermatitis from isoflurane vapour, *Contact Dermatitis*, 2000, **42**, 46.

134. E. D. Kharasch, Biotransformation of sevoflurane, *Anesth. Analg.*, 1995, **81**, S27–S38.

135. E. D. Kharasch and K. E. Thummel, Identification of cytochrome P450 2E1 as the predominant enzyme catalysing human liver microsomal defluorination of sevoflurane, isoflurane and methoxyflurane, *Anesthesiology*, 1993, **79**, 795–807.

136. E. D. Kharasch, Metabolism and toxicity of the new anesthetic agents, *Acta Anaesthesiol. Belg.*, 1996, **47**, 7–14.

137. M. Nuscheler, P. Conzen and K. Peter, Sevoflurane: metabolism and toxicity, *Anaesthetist*, 1998, **47**(1), S24–S32.

138. S. S. Patel and K. L. Goa, Sevoflurane. A review of its pharmacodynamic and pharmacokinetic properties and its clinical use in general anaesthesia, *Drugs*, 1996, **51**, 658–700.

139. K. Szyfter, R. Szulc, A. Mikstacki, I. Stachecki, M. Rydzanicz and P. Jaloszyński, Genotoxicity of inhalation anaesthetics: DNA lesions generated by sevoflurane *in vitro* and *in vivo*, *J. Appl. Genet.*, 2004, **45**, 369–374.

140. G. Wiesner, F. Schiewe-Langgartner and M. Gruber, Increased formation of sister-chromatid exchanges, but not of micronuclei, in anaesthetists exposed to low levels of sevoflurane, *Anaesthesia*, 2008, **63**, 861–865.

141. G. Summer, P. Lirk, K. Hoerauf, U. Riccabona, F. Bodrogi, H. Raifer, M. Deibl, J. Rieder and W. Schobersberger, Sevoflurane in exhaled air of operating room personnel, *Anesth. Analg.*, 2003, **97**, 1070–1073.

142. B. Tankó, C. Molnár, T. Budi, C. Peto, L. Novák and B. Fülesdi, The relative exposure of the operating room staff to sevoflurane during intracerebral surgery, *Anesth. Analg.*, 2009, **109**, 1187–1192.

143. M. Laisalmi, A. Soikkeli, H. Markkanen, A. Yli-Hankala, P. Rosenburg and L. Lindgren, Fluoride metabolism in smokers and non-smokers following enflurane anaesthesia, *Br. J. Anaesth.*, 2003, **91**, 800–804.

144. M. W. Anders, Formation and toxicity of anaesthetic degradation products, *Annu. Rev. Pharmacol. Toxicol.*, 2005, **45**, 147–176.

145. A. B. Seifen, E. Seifen, R. H. Kennedy, J. P. Bray, G. A. Bushman and G. E. Loss, Myocardial recovery from the cardiac depressant effects of enflurane and halothane, *J. Cardiothorac. Anesth.*, 1988, **2**, 463–471.

146. O. Dale and B. R. Brown, Clinical pharmacokinetics of the inhalational anaesthetics, *Clin. Pharmacokinet.*, 1987, **12**, 145–167.

147. D. D. Christ, H. Satoh, J. G. Kenna and L. R. Pohl, Potential metabolic basis for enflurane hepatitis and the apparent cross-sensitization between enflurane and halothane, *Drug Metab. Disp.*, 1988, **16**, 135–140.

148. P. Carlsson, J. Ekstrand and B. Hallén, Plasma fluoride and bromide concentrations during occupational exposure to enflurane or halothane, *Acta Anaesthesiol. Scand.*, 1985, **29**, 669–673.

149. M. Morio, O. Yuge and K. Fujii, Biotransformation and toxicity of inhalational anaesthetics, *Can. J. Anaesth.*, 1990, **37**, Scxvi–Scxxiii.

150. J. L. Raucy, J. C. Kraner and J. M. Lasker, Bioactivation of halogenated hydrocarbons by cytochrome P4502E1, *Crit. Rev. Toxicol.*, 1993, **23**, 1–20.

151. H. Orhan, N. P. Vermeulen, G. Sahin and J. N. Commandeur, Characterisation of thioether compounds formed from alkaline degradation products of enflurane, *Anaesthesiology*, 2001, **95**, 165–175.

152. G. L. Bird and R. Williams, Anaesthesia-related liver disease, *Monogr. Allergy*, 1992, **30**, 174–191.

153. A. M. Sass-Kortsak, I. P. Wheeler and J. T. Purdham, Exposure of operating room personnel to anaesthetic agents: an examination of the effectiveness of scavenging systems and the importance of maintenance programs, *Can. Anaesth. Soc. J.*, 1981, **28**, 22–28.

154. K. Hoerauf, T. Mayer and J. Hobbhahn, Occupational exposure to enflurane and laughing gas in operating rooms, *Zentralbl. Hyg. Umweltmed.*, 1996, **198**, 265–274.

155. R. Pasquini, S. Monarca, G Scassellati-Sforzolini, F. A. Baueleo, G. Angeli and F Cerami, Thioethers, mutagens, and D-glucaric acid in urine of operating personnel exposed to anaesthetics, *Teratog. Carcinog. Mutagen.*, 1989, **9**, 359–368.

156. P. Bigatti, L. Lamberti, G. Ardito, F. Armellino and C. Malanetto, Chromosome aberrations and sister chromatid exchanges in occupationally exposed workers, *Med. Lav.*, 1985, **76**, 334–339.

157. L. Lamberti, P. Bigatti, G. Ardito and F. Armellino, Chromosome analysis in operating room personnel, *Mutagenesis*, 1989, **4**, 95–97.

158. M. Reitz, K. DasGupta, G. Löber and P. Kleemann, Variations of DNA damage in human lymphocytes after enflurane exposure *in vitro*, *Arzneimittelforschung*, 1998, **48**, 120–124.

159. R. Pasquini, G. Scassellati-Sforzolini, C. Fatigoni, M. Marcarelli, S. Monarca, F. Donato, S. Concetti and F. M. Cerami, Sister chromatid exchanges and micronuclei in lymphocytes of operating room personnel occupationally exposed to enflurane and nitrous oxide, *J. Environ. Pathol. Toxicol. Oncol.*, 2001, **20**, 119–126.

160. J. A. Smith, J. S. Gaynor, R. M. Bednarski and W. W. Muir, Adverse effects of administration of propofol with various preanesthetic regimens in dogs, *J. Am. Vet. Med. Assoc.*, 1993, **202**, 1111–1115.

161. J. H. Kanto, Propofol, the newest induction agent of anaesthesia, *Int. J. Clin. Pharmacol. Ther. Toxicol.*, 1988, **26**, 41–57.

162. W. W. Muir and J. E. Gadawski, Respiratory depression and apnea induced by propofol in dogs, *Am. J. Vet. Res.*, 1998, **59**, 157–161.

163. M. B. Reddy, Can propofol cause keratitis? *Anaesthesia*, 2002, **57**, 206.

164. T. M. Kang, Propofol infusion syndrome in critically ill patients, *Ann. Pharmacother.*, 2002, **36**, 1453–1456.

165. D. E. Withington, M. K. Decell and T. Al Ayed, A case of propofol toxicity: further evidence for a causal mechanism, *Paediatr. Anaesth.*, 2004, **14**, 505–508.

166. A. Chukwuemeka, R. Ko and A. Ralph-Edwards, Short-term low-dose propofol anaesthesia associated with severe metabolic acidosis, *Anaesth. Intensive Care*, 2006, **34**, 651–655.

167. K. Ahlen, C. J. Buckley, D. B. Goodale and A. H. Pulsford, The 'propofol infusion syndrome': the facts, their interpretation and implications for patient care, *Eur. J. Anaesthesiol.*, 2006, **23**, 990–998.

168. T. G. Short and Y. Young, Toxicity of intravenous anaesthetics, *Best Pract. Res. Clin. Anaesthesiol.*, 2003, **17**, 77–89.

169. P. Ypsilantis, M. Politou, D. Mikroulis, M. Pittiakoudis, M. Lambropoulou, M. Tsigalou, V. Didilis, G. Bourgioukas, N. Papadopoulos, C. Manolas and C. Simopoulos, Organ toxicity and mortality in propofol-sedated rabbits under prolonged mechanical ventilation, *Anesth. Analg.*, 2007, **105**, 155–166.

170. T. Kiringoda, A. E. Thurm, M. E. Hirschtritt, D. Koziol, R. Wesley, S. E. Swedo, N. P. O'Grady and Z. M. Quezado, Risks of propofol sedation/anesthesia in a clinical research center, *Arch. Pediatr. Adolesc. Med.*, 2010, **164**, 554–560.

171. J. W. Devlin, S. Mallow-Corbett and R. R. Riker, Adverse drug events associated with the use of analgesia, sedatives and antipsychotics in the intensive care unit, *Crit. Care Med.*, 2010, **38**(6), S231–S243.

172. M. M. Zestos, D. Bhattacharya, S. Rajan, S. Kemper and M. Haupert, Propofol decreases waste anesthetic gas exposures during pediatric bronchoscopy, *Laryngoscope*, 2004, **114**, 212–215.

173. J. L. Merlo, B. A. Goldberger, D. Kolodner, K. Fitzgerald and M. S. Gold, Fentanyl and propofol exposure in the operating room: sensitization hypotheses and further data, *J. Addict. Dis.*, 2008, **27**, 67–76.

174. B. Patemann, S. Buzello, M. Dück, M. Paul and S. Kampe, Accidental overdose of propofol in a 6-month old infant undergoing elective craniosynostosis repair, *Anaesthesia*, 2004, **59**, 912–914.

175. M. Seyedhejazi, G. Abafattash and R. Taheri, Accidental five fold over-dosage of propofol for induction in a 38-days-old infant undergoing emergency bilateral inguinal hernia repair, *Saudi J. Anaesth.*, 2011, **5**, 417–418.

176. J. Holzki, C. Aring and A. Gillor, Death after re-exposure to propofol in a 3-year-old child, *Paediatr. Anaesth.*, 2004, **14**, 265–270.

177. C. Koch, C. Hollister and P. H. Breen, Infusion pump delivers over-dosage of propofol as a result of missing syringe support, *Anesth. Analg.*, 2006, **102**, 1154–1156.

178. C. Wilson, P. Canning and E. M. Caravati, The abuse potential of propofol, *Clin. Toxicol.*, 2010, **48**, 165–170.

179. R. R. Kirby, J. M. Colaw and M. M. Douglas, Death from propofol: accident, suicide, or murder, *Anesth. Analg.*, 2009, **108**, 1182–1184.

180. E. F. Kranioti, A. Mavroforou, P. Mylonakis and M. Michalodimitrakis, Lethal self administration of propofol (Diprivan). A case report and review of the literature, *Forensic Sci. Int.*, 2007, **167**, 56–58.

181. T. C. Lee, D. S. Lo, P. P. Chui and T. H. Koh, The first fatal dose of 2,6-di-isopropylphenol (propofol) poisoning in Singapore: a case report, *Forensic Sci. Int.*, 1994, **66**, 1–7.

182. S. Iwersen-Bergmann, P. Rösner, H. C. Kühnau, M. Junge and A. Schmoldt, Death after excessive propofol abuse, *Int. J. Legal Med.*, 2001, **114**, 248–251.

183. R. J. Levy, Clinical effects and lethal forensic aspects of propofol, *J. Forensic Sci.*, 2011, **56**(1), S142–147.

184. G. Klausz, K. Róna, I. Kristóf and K. Töro, Evaluation of a fatal pro-pofol intoxication due to self administration, *J. Forensic Leg. Med.*, 2009, **16**, 287–289.

185. O. H. Drummer, A fatality due to propofol poisoning, *J. Forensic Sci.*, 1992, **37**, 1186–1189.

186. E. P. Steffey, Euthanizing agents in *Veterinary Pharmacology and Therapeutics*, ed. H. R. Adams, Iowa State Press, Ames, 8th edn, 2001, pp. 397–402.

187. K. Chandler, Canine epilepsy: what we can learn from human seizure disorders, *Vet. J.*, 2006, **172**, 207–217.

188. M. Podell, Antiepileptic drug therapy, *Clin. Tech. Small Anim. Pract.*, 1998, **13**, 185–192.

189. Y. Chang, D. J. Mellor and T. J. Anderson, Idiopathic epilepsy in dogs: owners' perspectives on management with phenobarbital and/or potassium bromide, *J. Small Anim. Pract.*, 2006, **47**, 574–581.

190. P. M. Dowling, Management of canine epilepsy with phenobarbital and potassium bromide, *Can. Vet. J.*, 1994, **35**, 724–725.

191. M. R. Trimble, Anticonvulsant drugs and cognitive function: a review of the literature, *Epilepsia*, 1987, **28**(3), S37–S45.

192. K. Michel, V. Waeber, L. Valch, G. Arestegui and T. Spuhler, A comparison of the drugs taken in fatal and nonfatal self-poisoning, *Acta Psychiatr. Scand.*, 1994, **90**, 184–189.

193. B. Colac, L. Başer, N. Yayci, N. Etiler and M. A. Inanici, Deaths from drug overdose and toxicity in Turkey: 1997–2001, *Am. J. Forensic Med. Pathol.*, 2006, **27**, 50–54.

194. N. Retterstøl, Norwegian data on death due to overdose of antidepressants, *Acta Psychiatr. Scand.*, 1989, **354**(Suppl.), 61–68.

195. S. M. Coupey, Barbiturates, *Pediatr. Rev.*, 1997, **18**, 260–264.

196. C. Tomaszewski, J. Runge, M. Gibbs, S. Colucciello and M. Price, Evaluation of a rapid bedside screen in patients suspected of drug toxicity, *J. Emerg. Med.*, 2005, **28**, 389–394.

197. D. A. Zlott and M. Byrne, Mechanisms by which pharmacologic agents may contribute to fatigue, *PMR*, 2010, **2**, 451–455.

198. C. Brandt-Casadevall, T. Krompecher, C. Giroud and P. Mangin, A case of suicide disguised as natural death, *Sci. Justice*, 2003, **43**, 41–43.

199. F. L. McGuire, H. Birch, L. A. Gottschalk, J. F. Heiser and E. C. Dinovo, A comparison of suicide and non-suicide deaths involving psychotropic drugs in four major U.S. cities, *Am. J. Public Health*, 1976, **66**, 1058–1061.

200. K. Hawton, S. Clements, S. Simkin and A. Malmberg, Doctors who kill themselves: a study of the methods used for suicide, *Q. J. Med.*, 2000, **93**, 351–357.

201. B. Platt, K. Hawton, S. Simkin and R. J. Mellanby, Systematic review of the prevalence of suicide in veterinary surgeons, *Occup. Med. (Lond.)*, 2010, **60**, 436–446.

202. D. J. Bartram and D. S. Baldwin, Veterinary surgeons and suicide: a structured review of possible influences on increased risk, *Vet. Rec.*, 2010, **166**, 388–397.

203. J. Magdalan and A. Antończyk, Three cases of suicidal intoxication – preparation for euthanasia of small animals, *Pol. Arch. Med. Wewn.*, 2006, **115**, 139–143.

204. A. Poklis and A. Z. Hameli, Two unusual barbiturate deaths, *Arch. Toxicol.*, 1975, **34**, 77–80.

205. N. Romain, C. Giroud, K. Michaud and P. Mangin, Suicide by injection of a veterinarian barbiturate euthanasia agent: report of a case and toxicological analysis, *Forensic Sci. Int.*, 2003, **131**, 103–107.

206. M. A. Clark and J. W. Jones, Suicide by intravenous injection of a veterinary euthanasia agent: report of a case and toxicologic studies, *J. Forensic Sci.*, 1979, **24**, 762–767.

207. A. Parkinson, Biotransformation of xenobiotics in *Casarett and Doull's Toxicology. The Basic Science of Poisons*, ed. C. D. Klaassen, McGraw-Hill, London, 5th edn, 1996, pp. 113–186.
208. S. A. Forman, Clinical and molecular pharmacology of etomidate, *Anesthesiology*, 2011, **114**, 695–707.
209. S. L. Tomlin, A. Jenkins, W. R. Lieb and N. P. Franks, Stereoselective effects of etomidate optical isomers on gamma-aminobutyric acid Type A receptors and animals, *Anesthesiology*, 1998, **88**, 708–717.
210. S. S. Husain, M. R. Ziebell, D. Ruesch, F. Hong, E. Aravalo, J. A. Kosterlitz, R. W. Olsen, S. A. Forman, J. B. Cohen and K. W. Miller, 2-(3-methyl-3H-diaziren-3-yl)ethyl 1-(1-phenylethyl)-1H-imidazole-5-carboxylate: a derivative of the stereoselective general anesthetic etomidate for photolabeling ligand-gated ion channels, *J. Med. Chem.*, 2003, **46**, 1257–1265.
211. C. Vanlersberghe and F. Camu, Etomidate and other non-barbiturates, *Handb. Exp. Pharmacol.*, 2008, **182**, 267–282.
212. K. Solt and S. A. Forman, Correlating the clinical actions and molecular mechanisms of general anesthetics, *Curr. Opin. Anaesthesiol.*, 2007, **20**, 300–306.
213. D. Belelli, A. L. Muntoni, S. D. Merrywest, L. J. Gentet, A. Casula, H. Callachan, P. Madau, D. K. Gemmell, N. M. Hamilton, J. J. Lambert, K. T. Sillar and J. A. Peters, The *in vitro* and *in vivo* enantioselectivity of etomidate implicates the GABAA receptor in general anaesthesia, *Neuropharmacology*, 2003, **45**, 57–71.
214. I. M. Ledingham and I. Watt, Influence of sedation on mortality in crtically ill multiple trauma patients, *Lancet*, 1983, **321**, 1270.
215. I. Watt and I. M. Ledingham, Mortality amongst multiple trauma patients admitted to an intensive care therapy unit, *Anesthesia*, 1984, **39**, 973–981.
216. J. L. McKee and W. E. Finlay, Cortisol replacement in severely stressed patients, *Lancet*, 1983, **321**, 484.
217. P. Preziosi and M. Vacca, Etomidate and corticotrophic axis, *Arch. Int. Pharmacodyn. Ther.*, 1982, **256**, 308–310.
218. R. L. Wagner, P. F. White, P. B. Rosenthal and D. Felfman, Inhibition of adrenal steroidogenesis by the anesthetic etomidate, *N. Engl. J. Med.*, 1984, **310**, 1415–1421.
219. R. L. Wagner and P. F. White, Etomidate inhibits adrenocortical function in surgical patients, *Anesthesiology*, 1984, **61**, 647–651.
220. R. J. Fragen, C. A. Franks, A. Molteni and M. J. Avram, Effects of etomidate on hormonal responses to surgical stress, *Anesthesiology*, 1984, **61**, 652–656.
221. M. Wanscher, F. Tonnesen, M. Huttel and K. Larsen, Etomidate infusion and adrenocortical function: A study in elective surgery, *Acta Anaesthesiol. Scand.*, 1985, **29**, 483–485.
222. P. Igaz, Z. Tömböl, P. M. Szabó, I. Likó and K. Rácz, Steroid biosynthesis inhibitors in the therapy of hypercortisolism: theory and practice, *Curr. Med. Chem.*, 2008, **15**, 2734–2747.

223. M. P. Boidin, W. E. Erdmann and N. S. Faithful, The role of ascorbic acid in etomidate toxicity, *Eur. J. Anesthesiol.*, 1986, **3**, 417–422.

224. J. C. Drummond, L. D. McKay, D. J. Cole and P. M. Patel, The role of nitric oxide synthase inhibition in the adverse effects of etomidate in the setting of focal cerebral ischemia in rats, *Anesth. Analg.*, 2005, **100**, 841–846.

225. J. Andrada, P. Livingston, B. J. Lee and J. Antognini, Propofol and etomidate depress cortical, thalamic and reticular formation neurons during anesthetic-induced unconsciousness, *Anesth. Analg.*, 2012, **144**, 661–669.

226. E. F. Domino, P. Chodoff and G. Corssen, Pharmacologic effects of CI-581, a new dissociative anesthetic, in man, *Clin. Pharmacol. Ther.*, 1965, **6**, 279–291.

227. E. F. Domino, Taming the ketamine tiger, *Anesthesiology*, 2010, **113**, 678–686.

228. T. Bouts, N. Harrison, K. Berry, P. Taylor, A. Routh and F. Gasthuys, Comparison of three anaesthetic protocols in Bennett's wallabies (*Macropus rufogriseus*), *Vet. Anaesth. Analg.*, 2010, **37**, 207–214.

229. T. G. Raske, S. Pelkey, A. E. Wagner and A. S. Turner, Effect of intra-venous ketamine and lidocaine on isoflurane requirement in sheep undergoing orthopaedic surgery, *Lab. Anim (NY)*, 2010, **39**, 76–79.

230. R. Borkowski, S. Citino, M. Bush, P. Wollenman and B. Irvine, Surgical castration of subadult giraffe (*Giraffa camelopardalis*), *J. Zoo Wildl. Med.*, 2009, **40**, 786–790.

231. R. S. Larsen, M. L. Sauther and F. P. Cuozzo, Evaluation of modified techniques for immobilization of wild ring-tailed lemurs (*Lemur catta*), *J. Zoo Wildl. Med.*, 2011, **42**, 623–633.

232. T. Bouts, D. Karunaratna, K. Berry, J. Dodds, F. Gasthuys, A. Routh and P. Taylor, Evaluation of medetomidine-alfaxalone and medetomi-dine-ketamine in semi-free ranging Bennett's wallabies (*Macropus rufo-griseus*), *J. Zoo Wildl. Med.*, 2011, **42**, 617–622.

233. R. Bednarski, K. Grimm, R. Harvey, V. M. Lukasik, W. S. Penn, B. Sargent and K. Spelts, AAHA anesthesia guidelines for dogs and cats, *J. Am. Anim. Hosp. Assoc.*, 2011, **47**, 377–385.

234. K. A. Harrison, S. A. Robertson, J. K. Levy and N. M. Isaza, Evaluation of medetomidine, ketamine and buprenorphine for neutering feral cats, *J. Feline Med. Surg.*, 2011, **13**, 896–902.

235. F. A. Al-Sobayil and O. H. Omer, Serum biochemical values of adult ostriches (*Struthio camelus*) anesthetized with xylazine, ketamine, and isoflurane, *J. Avian Med. Surg.*, 2011, **25**, 97–101.

236. J. R. Elfenbein, S. A. Robertson, A. A. Corser, R. J. Urion and L. C. Sanchez, Systemic effects of prolonged continuous infusion of ketamine in healthy horses, *J. Vet. Intern. Med.*, 2011, **25**, 1134–1137.

237. C. M. Brim and C. Braun, Anesthetic agents and complications in Vietnamese potbellied pigs: 27 cases (1999–2006), *J. Am. Vet. Med. Assoc.*, 2011, **239**, 114–121.

238. C. Walzer, F. Goritz, R. Hermes, S. Nathan, P. Kretzschmar and T. Hildebrandt, Immobilization and intravenous anesthesia in a Sumatran rhinoceros (*Dicerorhinus sumatrensis*), *J. Zoo Wildl. Med.*, 2010, **41**, 115–120.

239. A. Valverde, G. J. Crawshaw, N. Cribb, G. Gianotti, L. Arroyo, J. Koenig, M. Kummrow and M. C. Costa, Anesthetic management of a white rhinoceros (*Ceratotherium simum*) undergoing an emergency exploratory celiotomy for colic, *Vet. Anaesth. Analg.*, 2010, **37**, 280–285.

240. A. S. Chohan, Anesthetic considerations in orthopaedic patients with or without trauma, *Top. Companion Anim. Med.*, 2010, **25**, 107–119.

241. A. R. Ajadi, T. A. Olussa, O. F. Smith, E. S. Ajibola, O. E. Adeleye, O. T. Adenubi and F. A. Makinde, Tramadol improved the efficacy of ketamine-xylazine anaesthesia in young pigs, *Vet. Anaesth. Analg.*, 2009, **36**, 562–566.

242. R. Gehring, J. F. Coetzee, J. Tarus-Sang and M. D. Apley, Pharmacokinetics of ketamine and its metabolite norketamine administered at a sub-anesthetic dose together with xylazine to calves prior to castration, *J. Vet. Pharmacol. Ther.*, 2009, **32**, 124–128.

243. A. R. Sohayati, C. M. Zaini, L. Hassan, J. Epstein, A. Siti Suri, P. Daszak and S. H. Sharifah, Ketamine and xylazine combinations for short-term immobilization of wild variable flying foxes (*Pteropus hypomelanus*), *J. Zoo Wildl. Med.*, 2008, **39**, 674–676.

244. L. A. Lamont, Adjunctive analgesic therapy in veterinary medicine, *Vet. Clin. North Am. Small Anim. Pract.*, 2008, **38**, 1187–1203.

245. S. Hazra, D. Da, B. Roy, S. Nandi and A. Konar, Use of ketamine, xylazine, and diazepam anesthesia with retrobulbar block for phacoemulsification in dogs, *Vet. Ophthalmol.*, 2008, **11**, 255–259.

246. F. F. Barros, J. P. Queiroz, A. C. Filho, E. A. Santos, V. V. Paula, C. I. Freitas and A. R. Silva, Use of two anesthetic combinations for semen collection by electroejaculation from captive coatis (*Nasua nasua*), *Theriogenology*, 2009, **71**, 1261–1266.

247. T. M. Prado, T. J. Doherty, E. B. Boggan, H. M. Airasmaa, T. Martin-Jiminez and B. W. Rohrbach, Effects of acepromazine and butorphanol on tiletamine-zolazepam anesthesia in llamas, *Am. J. Vet. Res.*, 2008, **69**, 182–188.

248. J. L. Belant, Tiletamine-zolazepam-xylazine immobilization of fishers (*Martes pennanti*), *J. Wildl. Dis.*, 2007, **43**, 279–285.

249. M. Jacquier, P. Aarhaug, J. M. Arnemo, H. Bauer and B. Enriquez, Reversible immobilization of free-ranging African lions (*Panthera leo*) with medetomidine-tiletamine-zolazepam and atipamezole, *J. Wildl. Dis.*, 2006, **42**, 432–436.

250. J. C. Ko and A. G. Berman, Anesthesia in shelter medicine, *Top. Companion Anim. Med.*, 2010, **25**, 92–97.

251. M. Re, F. J. Blanco-Murcia and I. A. Gómez de Segura, Chemical restraint and anaesthetic effects of tiletamine-zolazepam/ketamine/detomidine combination in cattle, *Vet. J.*, 2011, **190**, 66–70.

252. U. Auer, S. Wenger, C. Beigelböck, W. Zenker and M. Mosing, Total intravenous anesthesia with midazolam, ketamine, and xylazine or detomidine following induction with tiletamine, zolazepam, and xylazine in red deer (*Cervus elaphus hippelaphus*) undergoing surgery, *J. Wildl. Dis.*, 2010, **46**, 1196–1203.

253. S. D. Langton, S. E. Moss, P. P. Pomeroy and K. E. Borer, Effect of induction dose, lactation stage and body condition on tiletamine-zolazepam anaesthesia in adult female grey seals (*Halichoerus grypus*) under field conditions, *Vet. Rec.*, 2011, **168**, 457.

254. J. Y. Lee and M. C. Kim, Anesthesia of growing pigs with tiletamine-zolazepam and reversal with flumazenil, *J. Vet. Med. Sci.*, 2012, **74**, 335–339.

255. H. C. Lin, J. C. Thurmon, G. J. Bensom and W. J. Tranquilli, Telazol – a review of its pharmacology and use in veterinary medicine, *J. Vet. Pharmacol. Ther.*, 1993, **16**, 383–418.

256. C. Wang, N. Sadovova, X. Fu, L. Schmued, A. Scallett, J. Hanig and W. Slikker, The role of N-methyl-D-aspartate receptor in ketamine-induced apoptosis in rat forebrain, *Neuroscience*, 2005, **132**, 967–977.

257. W. Slikker, X. Zou, C. E. Hotchkiss, R. L. Divine, N. Sadovova, N. C. Twaddle, D. R. Doerge, A. C. Scallet, T. A. Patterson, J. P. Hanig, M. G. Paule and C. Wang, Ketamine-induced neuronal cell death in the perinatal rhesus monkey, *Toxicol. Sci.*, 2007, **98**, 145–158.

258. H. Viberg, E. Pontén, P. Eriksson, T. Gordh and A. Fredriksson, Neonatal ketamine exposure results in changes in biochemical substrates of neuronal growth and synaptogenesis and alters adult behavior irreversibly, *Toxicology*, 2008, **249**, 153–159.

259. J. C. Ibla, H. Hayashi, D. Bajic and S. G. Soriano, Prolonged exposure to ketamine increases brain derived neurotrophic factor levels in developing rat brains, *Curr. Drug Saf.*, 2009, **4**, 11–16.

260. X. Zou, T. A. Patterson, R. L. Divine, N. Sadovova, X. Zhang, J. P. Hanig, M. G. Paule, W. Slikker and C. Wang, Prolonged exposure to ketamine increases neurodegeneration in the developing monkey brain, *Int. J. Dev. Neurosci.*, 2009, **27**, 727–731.

261. X. Zou, T. A. Patterson, N. Sadovova, N. C. Twaddle, D. R. Doerge, X. Zhang, X. Fu, J. P. Hanig, M. G. Paule, W. Slikke and C. Wang, Potential neurotoxicity of ketamine in the developing rat brain, *Toxicol. Sci.*, 2009, **108**, 149–158.

262. T. M. Beyers, J. A. Richardson and M. D. Prince, Axonal degeneration and self-mutilation as a complication of the intramuscular use of ketamine and xylazine in rabbits, *Lab. Anim. Sci.*, 1991, **41**, 519–520.

263. N. B. Farber and J. W. Olney, Drugs of abuse that cause developing neurons to commit suicide, *Brain Res. Dev. Brain Res.*, 2003, **147**, 37–45.

264. M. M. Straiko, C. Young, D. Cattano, C. E. Creeley, H. Wang, D. J. Smith, S. A. Johnson, E. S. Li and J. W. Olney, Lithium protects against anesthesia-induced developmental neuroapoptosis, *Anesthesiology*, 2009, **110**, 862–868.

265. D. Ma, S. Wilhelm, M. Maze and N. P. Franks, Neuroprotective and neurotoxic properties of the 'inert' gas, xenon, *Br. J. Anaesth.*, 2002, **89**, 739–746.
266. K. Kilander and H. Williams, Yohimbine reduces neuropathology induced by ketamine/xylazine anesthesia, *Physiol. Behav.*, 1992, **51**, 657–659.
267. J. Persson, Wherefore ketamine? *Curr. Opin. Anesthesiol.*, 2010, **23**, 455–460.
268. S. M. Green, R. Clark, M. A. Hostetler, M. Cohen, D. Carlson and S. G. Rothrock, Inadvertent ketamine overdose in children: clinical manifestations and outcome, *Ann. Emerg. Med.*, 1999, **34**(4 Part 1), 492–497.
269. J. K. Beals, L. B. Carter and V. Jevtovic-Todorovic, Neurotoxicity of nitrous oxide and ketamine is more severe in aged than in young rat brain, *Ann. N. Y. Acad. Sci.*, 2003, **993**, 115.
270. S. M. Walker, B. D. Westin, R. Deumens, R. Grafe and T. L. Yaksh, Effects of intrathecal ketamine in the neonatal rat: evaluation of apoptosis and long-term functional outcome, *Anesthesiology*, 2010, **113**, 147–159.
271. L. M. Gomes, J. B. Garcia, J. S. Ribamar and A. G. Nascimento, Neurotoxicity of subarachnoid preservative-free S(+)-ketamine in dogs, *Pain Physician*, 2011, **14**, 83–90.
272. J. M. Malinovsky, J. Y. Lepage, A. Cozian, J. M. Mussini, M. Pinaudt and R. Souron, Is ketamine or its preservative responsible for neurotoxicity in the rabbit? *Anesthesiology*, 1993, **78**, 109–115.
273. J. H. Vranken, D. Troost, P. de Haan, F. A. Pennings, M. H. van der Vegt, M. G. Dijkgraaf and M. W. Hollmann, Severe toxic damage to the rabbit spinal cord after intrathecal administration of preservative-free S(+)-ketamine, *Anesthesiology*, 2006, **105**, 813–818.
274. N. Karpinski, J. Dunn, L. Hansen and E. Masliah, Subpial vacuolar myelopathy after intrathecal ketamine: a case report, *Pain*, 1997, **73**, 103–105.
275. J. H. Vranken, D. Troost, J. T. Wegener, M. R. Kruis and M. H. van der Vegt, Neuropathological findings after continuous intrathecal administration of S(+)-ketamine for the management of neuropathic cancer pain, *Pain*, 2005, **117**, 231–235.
276. K. Jackson, M. Ashby, D. Howell, J. Petersen, D. Brumley, P. Good, M. Pisasale, S. Wein and R. Woodruff, The effectiveness and adverse effects profile of "burst" ketamine in refractory cancer pain: The VCOG PM 1-00 study, *J. Palliat. Care*, 2010, **26**, 178–183.
277. I. M. Noopers, M. Niesters, L. P. Aarts, M. C. Bauer, A. M. Drewes, A. Dahan and E. Y. Sarton, Drug-induced liver injury following a repeated course of ketamine treatment for chronic pain in CRPS type 1 patients: a report of 3 cases, *Pain*, 2011, **152**, 2173–2178.
278. S. Tan, W. M. Chan, M. S. Chai, L. K. Hui, A. E. James, L. Y. Yeung and D. T. Yew, Ketamine effects on the urogenital system – changes in the urinary bladder and sperm motility, *Microsc. Res. Tech.*, 2011, **74**, 1192–1198.

279. W. M. Chan, Y. Liang, M. S. Mai, A. S. Hung and D. T. Yew, Cardio-toxicity induced in mice by long-term ketamine and ketamine plus alcohol treatment, *Toxicol. Lett.*, 2011, **207**, 191–196.
280. R. A. Hiney, D. C. Turner, G. D. Honey, S. R. Sharar, D. Kumaran, E. Pomarol-Clotet, P. McKenna, B. J. Sahakian, T. W. Robbins and P. C. Fletcher, Subdissociative dose ketamine produces a deficit in manipulation but not maintenance of the contents of working memory, *Neuropsychopharmacology*, 2003, **28**, 2037–2044.
281. J. J. Chrobak, J. R. Hinman and H. R. Sabolek, Revealing past memories: proactive interference and ketamine-induced memory deficits, *J. Neurosci.*, 2008, **28**, 4512–4520.
282. A. Becker and G. Grecksch, Ketamine-induced changes in rat behaviour: a possible animal model of schizophrenia. Test of predictive validity, *Prog. Neuropsychopharmacol. Biol. Psychiatry*, 2004, **28**, 1267–1277.
283. G. Keilhof, H. G. Bernstein, A. Becker, G. Grecksch and G. Wolf, Increased neurogenesis in a rat ketamine model of schizophrenia, *Biol. Psychiatry*, 2004, **56**, 317–322.
284. H. R. Hsu, Y. Y. Mei, C. Y. Wu, P. H. Chiu and H. H. Chen, Behavioural and toxic interaction profile of ketamine in combination with caffeine, *Basic Clin. Pharmacol. Toxicol.*, 2009, **104**, 379–383.
285. T. Hayase, Y. Yamamoto and K. Yamamoto, Behavioural effects of ketamine and toxic interactions with psychostimulants, *BMC Neurosci.*, 2006, **7**, 25.
286. M. A. Covington, W. J. Riedel, C. Brown, C. He, E. Morris, S. Weinstein, J. Semple and J. Brown, Does ketamine mimic aspects of schizophrenic speech? *J. Psychopharmacol.*, 2007, **21**, 338–346.
287. R. S. C. Lo, R. Krishnamoorthy, J. G. Freeman and A. S. Austin, Cholestasis and biliary dilatation associated with chronic ketamine abuse: a case series, *Singapore Med. J.*, 2011, **52**, e52–e55.
288. C. M. Contreras, M. L. Marvan, G. Mexicano, A. Puente and A. Morfin, Ketamine antagonises toxic action of anticholinesterases, *Bol. Estud. Med. Biol.*, 1990, **38**, 10–15.
289. W. H. Chan, W. Z. Sun and T. H. Ueng, Induction of rat hepatic cyto-chrome P-450 by ketamine and its toxicological implications, *J. Toxicol. Environ. Health*, 2005, **68**, 1581–1597.
290. M. R. Mever and H. H. Maurer, Absorption, distribution, metabolism and excretion pharmacogenomics of drugs of abuse, *Pharmacogenomics*, 2011, **12**, 215–233.
291. M. S. Abdel-Rahman and E. E. Ismail, Teratogenic effect of ketamine and cocaine in CF-1 mice, *Teratology*, 2000, **61**, 291–296.
292. K. A. Graeme, New drugs of abuse, *Emerg. Med. Clin. North Am.*, 2000, **18**, 625–636.
293. K. A. Parks and C. L. Kennedy, Club drugs: reasons for and con-sequences of use, *J. Psychoactive Drugs*, 2004, **36**, 295–302.

294. G. C. Britt and E. F. McCance-Katz, A brief overview of the clinical pharmacology of "club drugs", *Subst. Use Misuse*, 2005, **40**, 1189–1201.

295. T. E. Freese, K. Miotto and C. J. Freeback, The effects and consequences of selected club drugs, *J. Subst. Abuse Treat.*, 2002, **23**, 151–156.

296. P. M. Gahlinger, Club drugs: MDMA, gamma-hydroxybutyrate (GHB), rohypnol, and ketamine, *Am. Fam. Physician*, 2004, **69**, 2619–2626.

297. R. S. Gable, Acute toxic effects of club drugs, *J. Psychoactive Drugs*, 2004, **36**, 303–313.

298. D. M. Wood, M. Nicholau and P. I. Dargan, Epidemiology of recreational drug toxicity in a nightclub environment, *Subst. Use Misuse.*, 2009, **44**, 1495–1502.

299. D. M. Wood, S. Davies, M. Puchnarewicz, A. Johnson and P. I. Dargan, Acute toxicity associated with the recreational use of the ketamine derivative methoxetamine, *Eur. J. Clin. Pharmacol.*, 2012, **68**, 853–856.

300. N. N. Moore and J. M. Bostwick, Ketamine dependence in anaesthesia providers, *Psychosomatics*, 1999, **40**, 356–359.

301. C. C. Lee, Y. Y. Lin, C. W. Hsu, S. J. Chu and S. H. Tsai, Movement disorder caused by abuse of veterinary anesthesia containing tiletamine, *Am. J. Emerg. Med.*, 2009, **28**, e5–e6.

302. M. Y. Quail, P. Weimersheimer, A. D. Woolf and B. Magnani, Abuse of telazol: an animal tranquilizer, *J. Toxicol. Clin Toxicol.*, 2001, **39**, 399–402.

303. C. J. Cording, R. DeLuca, T. Camporese and E. Spratt, A fatality related to the veterinary anesthetic telazol, *J. Anal. Toxicol.*, 1999, **23**, 552–555.

304. H. Chung, H. Choi, E. Kim, W. Jin, H. Lee and Y. Yoo, A fatality due to the injection of tiletamine and zolazepam, *J. Anal. Toxicol.*, 2000, **24**, 305–308.

CHAPTER 6

Veterinary Products Containing Pesticide Active Ingredients

6.1 Introduction

Veterinary medicinal products containing active ingredients also used as pesticides, usually insecticides, are used to treat a number of conditions in animals, usually ectoparasites. In most countries, including the European Union, ectoparasiticides applied topically to animals are regulated as veterinary medicinal products as they are used to treat diseases of animals. Hence the regulatory authorities that deal with pharmaceuticals and biological products such as vaccines usually control them. The notable exception is the United States where the Environmental Protection Agency (EPA) regulates pesticides, including those used as ectoparasiticides, whereas pharmaceuticals are controlled by the Food and Drug Administration's Center for Veterinary Medicine (CVM) and vaccines and other biologicals by the United States Department of Agriculture. In contrast, products given orally or parenterally are controlled by drug regulatory authorities.[1-4]

Cat and dog fleas and other external parasites are conveniently susceptible to external treatments such as insecticides, including the synthetic pyrethroids (excluding cats, as these are susceptible to the toxic effects of this group) and selamectin.[5-8] Nuisance and other flies and ticks of sheep and cattle can be controlled with a variety of agents including pour-on formulations and insecticidal ear tags.[9-17] Sheep, cattle and other animals are prone to attack from blow-fly strike and myiasis, a condition where the larvae of various flies infest living or necrotic tissues.[18-21] In addition, sheep suffer from sheep scab caused by the sheep scab mite *Psoroptes ovis*.[22,23] These diseases can be treated, and frequently prevented, by a variety of chemotherapeutic agents including those

Issues in Toxicology No. 14
Toxicological Effects of Veterinary Medicinal Products in Humans: Volume 1
By Kevin N. Woodward
© The Royal Society of Chemistry 2013
Published by the Royal Society of Chemistry, www.rsc.org

containing organophosphorus compounds, synthetic pyrethroids, dicyclanil and cyromazine. They are applied by spraying, plunge dipping or topical applications.[22,24–32] Newer agents have been introduced in recent years including imidacloprid, spinosad, lufenuron and fipronil for the treatment of fleas on cats and dogs.[33–40]

In aquaculture (fish farming), several agents are used for the treatment and control of sea lice infestations caused by *Lepeophtheirus salmonis* and *Caligus* spp. on Atlantic salmon. Azamethiphos, cypermethrin, deltamethrin, hydrogen peroxide, emamectin benzoate, diflubenzuron and teflubenzuron are currently used or have been used as chemotherapeutic agents, while in the past dichlorvos and trichlorfon have been widely used.[41–46]

6.2 Toxicity of Individual Substances

6.2.1 Pyrethroids

Pyrethroids that do not contain an α-cyano group such as permethrin and allethrin give rise to pronounced repetitive activity in sense organs and sensory nerve fibres resulting in the so-called T-syndrome. This is characterised by fine or coarse tremor, hypersensitivity to stimuli and aggressive sparring. Pyrethroids in this group are classified as Type I pyrethroids. The data available suggest that these compounds act directly on the axon through interference with sodium channel gating mechanisms.[47–50]

Pyrethroids that possess an α-cyano group such as deltamethrin, cyhalothrin, cyfluthrin and cypermethrin produce the so-called CS-syndrome. This is characterised by marked choreoathetosis (sinuous writhing), salivation (hence, CS), coarse tremor, and convulsions. Pyrethroids in this group are classified as Type II pyrethroids. The data demonstrate that α-cyano pyrethroids act on sodium channels in the nerve membrane and cause persistent prolongation of the transient increase in sodium permeability of the membrane during excitation. Type II pyrethroids tend to be more toxic than Type I compounds, and more potent than the naturally occurring pyrethrins obtained from *Chrysanthemum cinerariaefolium*.[47,51–53] It has been postulated that Type II pyrethroids exert some of their effects through binding to the GABA receptor although they are only moderately inhibitory to this.[54]

Type I pyrethroids act on peripheral nerves whereas Type II act primarily on the CNS. The results of studies indicate, for example, that deltamethrin concentrations in the brains of mice correlate with the severity of the Type II response and Type II agents injected intracerebrally are more potent than when given by the intraperitoneal route, and when compared with those causing Type I responses.[55–57]

The main mode of action is thought to involve alteration of the sodium channels in the excitable membrane of nerve cells resulting in prolonged sodium permeability of the neuronal membrane.[49,50] Cyhalothrin (and permethrin) has been shown to be a potent inhibitor of the mitochondrial complex I *in vitro*. Using rat liver isolated mitochondria, there was a concentration-dependent inhibition of glutamate and succinate stage 3 respiration suggesting that an effect on cellular respiration may be a contributory factor to the effects of pyrethroids.[58]

6.2.1.1 Type II Pyrethroids

The toxicity of cyhalothrin typifies the effects of the Type II pyrethroids. Cyhalothrin is the ISO name for (RS)-α-cyano-3-phenoxybenzyl (Z)-$(1RS,3RS)$-2(chloro-3,3,3-trifluoropropenyl)-2,2-dimethylcyclopropanecarboxylate and it consists of 4 of a possible 16 isomers. These isomers comprise two pairs of enantiomers, A and B, in a ratio of 60 : 40, as shown in Figure 6.1. The related compound, lambda-cyhalothrin, contains only the B isomers but this substance is no longer used for veterinary purposes.

A pair of enantiomers $Z(1R)$ *cis* (R)α-CN   **and** $Z(1S)$ *cis* (S)α-CN

B pair of enantiomers $Z(1R)$*cis* (S)α-CN   **and** $Z(1S)$*cis* (R)α-CN

Hence, commercial products contain the following combinations of cyhalothrin isomers:

~30% $Z(1R)$ *cis* (R)α-CN

~30% $Z(1S)$ *cis* (S)α-CN } **A pair of enantiomers**

~20% $Z(1R)$ *cis* (S)α-CN

~20% $Z(1S)$ *cis* (R)α-CN } **B pair of enantiomers**

Cyhalothrin is well absorbed after oral administration in corn oil to rats with around 40% being recovered in urine and the remainder in faeces. Around 4 to

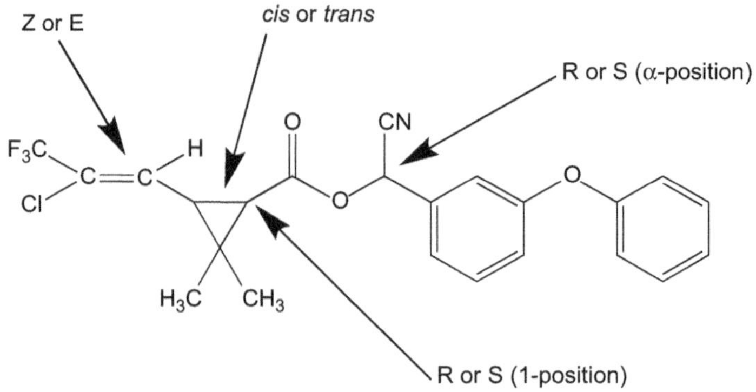

Figure 6.1 Chemical formula of cyhalothrin.

10% was excreted in bile. In dogs and rats, metabolism is similar and yields the 3-phenoxybenzoic acid and the triflurochloropropenylcyclopropyl carboxylic acid moieties, through hydrolysis of the ester bond, a common pathway in pyrethroid metabolism.[59] The former is hydroxylated to 3-(4'hydroxyphenoxy) benzoic acid in the rat and dog and this is converted to the sulfate conjugate, and in the dog to the glycine and glucuronide conjugates. The latter is conjugated to yield the glucuronide in both species. Similar biotransformation pathways have been reported in cattle and goats. The majority of absorbed cyhalothrin is found in the liver and adipose tissues.[60] In humans exposed to lambda-cyhalothrin during pesticide applications, the three main metabolites found in the dog, namely the triflurochloropropenylcyclopropyl carboxylic acid, 3-phenoxybenzoic acid and 3-(4'-hydroxyphenoxy) benzoic acid were the major urinary metabolites.[61]

Cyhalothrin was moderately acutely toxic after oral administration in corn oil to rats, with LD_{50} values being in the range 114 to 240 mg/kg bw, although higher toxicity has been noted in some studies. It was more toxic to mice after oral administration in corn oil with LD_{50} values of 37 and 62 mg/kg bw being calculated. It was much less acutely toxic after dermal application with LD_{50} values being in excess of 3500 mg/kg bw. Signs of toxicity were indicative of neurotoxicity with salivation, incontinence, ataxia, piloerection and abnormalities of gait being reported.[60]

In repeat dose studies, signs of neurotoxicity, occasionally severe, were noted in mice and rats in oral studies ranging from 5 days to 4 weeks for mice and 10 days to 3 months for rats. Like the acute toxicity studies, these signs included ataxia, piloerection and abnormal gait. Muscle trembling, collapse, convulsions and gait abnormalities have been reported in dogs given cyhalothrin for periods of 4 to 26 weeks.

Cyhalothrin has been tested in a range of studies for genotoxic potential, including the reverse mutation test for point mutations, an *in vivo* cytogenetics test in the rat and a mouse lymphoma assay but only negative results were obtained and, where tested, similar effects were seen with lambda-cyhalothrin.[60,62] However, some studies with lambda-cyhalothrin have yielded anomalous results.[63,64] It produced no evidence of a carcinogenic effect in mice or rats.[60]

The substance provided no evidence of reproductive toxicity in a three-generation study in mice and only a small decrease in litter size in a three-generation study in rats.[60,65] In a teratology study in rats given cyhalothrin orally in corn oil, there was no evidence of foetal abnormalities even at doses that produced maternal toxicity.[60] In other studies, it produced delays in development.[66]

As might be expected, cyhalothrin did not induce delayed neurotoxicity in the hen.[60] In a study of neurobehavioral effects cyhalothrin was tested in the inclined plane test in the rat. However, at the lowest dose used, 50 mg/kg bw/day, signs of neurotoxicity occurred including lethargy, writhing, ataxia, splayed gait, salivation, increased activity and vocalisation. These effects possibly masked any subtle signs of neurobehavioral toxicity. To further investigate any possible effects, cyhalothrin was tested in the acute startle response test with auditory habituation after dosing. In the main part of this study, rats were given oral doses of between 5 and 75 mg/kg bw cyhalothrin. Clinical signs of toxicity, including ataxia, hypersensitivity to touch and a high-stepping gait, occurred in high-dose animals but not in those given 5 or 15 mg/kg bw/day. There was, however, no effect on time to maximum amplitude in the acute startle reflex test itself performed 1 or 8 days after dosing.[60] Six functional domains have been suggested for the investigation of neurobehavioral effects of chemicals – sensorimotor, autonomic, neuromuscular, physiological, activity and excitability.[67–69] It can be argued that cyhalothrin has been subjected to standard toxicity tests, described above, where these end-points have been addressed. Most effects were only seen at relatively high doses and, even in the acute startle test, signs of toxicity were only seen at the highest dose employed and a clear NOEL of 15 mg/kg bw/day was identified. Moreover, in a functional observational battery in rats with supermethrin (a congener of cyhalothrin), lambda-cyhalothrin was used as a "model compound".[70] Some but not all of the proposed functional domains mentioned above were affected by lambda-cyhalothrin, a substance that is generally more toxic than cyhalothrin, at a dose of 18 mg/kg bw. Taken together, these data confirm that the standard toxicity studies are sufficient in the case of cyhalothrin to investigate its neurobehavioral effects.

Deltamethrin (ISO, (*S*)-α-cyano-3-phenoxybenzyl (1*R*3*R*)-3-(2,2-dibromovinyl)-2,2-dimethylcyclopropanecarboxylate) is very similar structurally to cyhalothrin, the only difference being that two bromine atoms replace a chlorine atom and a trifluoromethyl group on the terminal vinyl group. As a result, there are eight possible stereoisomers for deltamethrin as the two bromine atoms remove the possibility for *cis : trans* isomerisation about the vinyl group. Its toxicology has been reviewed by the International Programme on Chemical Safety and by the Joint FAO/WHO Meeting on Pesticide Residues (JMPR).[71,72]

Absorption of deltamethrin after oral administration is vehicle-dependent. It is well absorbed when given in polyethylene glycol 400 or glycerol formal, but less well absorbed when given in vegetable oil. Following oral administration to rats in sesame oil, deltamethrin was rapidly but incompletely absorbed. Soon after an oral dose of 26 mg/kg bw, plasma levels reached almost 1 μg/ml, as did concentrations of the major metabolite, 4′-hydroxydeltamethrin.[73] When given to rats in an aqueous vehicle, it was virtually non-toxic, suggesting poor absorption. Around 70% of an orally administered dose was excreted in the urine. In rats and mice, deltamethrin and its metabolites are widely distributed to all parts of the body but concentrations were higher in lipid rich tissue including the fat and myelin.[74,75]

The biotransformation of deltamethrin is complex. In rats, the first metabolite is probably 4′-hydroxydeltamethrin followed by further hydroxylation and cleavage of the ester linkage. Many of the metabolites formed are converted to glucuronic acid, sulfate and glycine conjugates. Metabolism in other species has many similarities, but some notable differences.[72,73,76–82]

The acute oral toxicity of deltamethrin varies widely depending on the vehicle used and on the species. In rodents, the compound was very toxic to rats and mice when given in PEG 200 but marginally less so when given in sesame oil. Oral LD_{50} values were in the range 18 to 40 mg/kg bw. These correspond to values cited in published articles where oral LD_{50} values in the range of 25–140 mg/kg bw in rodents with arachis oil as vehicle have been reported,[83–85] and 25–63 mg/kg bw in rats administered the substance in glycerol formal.[55] The compound appears to be less toxic after oral administration to dogs with the LD_{50} value in excess of 300 mg/kg bw despite the use of PEG 200, which appeared to exacerbate the acute toxicity in rodents. When given to mice in aqueous methylcellulose, the acute toxicity was very low with the LD_{50} value being 6800 mg/kg bw.[86] The studies also showed that deltamethrin was highly toxic to rodents and dogs after intraperitoneal and intravenous administration.[83,85,87] Topical administration of deltamethrin resulted in low toxicity in rats and rabbits despite the use of occlusive dressing techniques. LD_{50} values were in the range 2–3 g/kg bw.[86] Inhalation toxicity using acute exposures was investigated in rats, mice and guinea pigs. However, these studies were conducted using a complex exposure media including isophorone, BHT and oil. The studies were poorly reported and, overall, little interpretative value can be placed on the results although the studies suggested a low order of toxicity. A more conventional acute inhalation study in the rat using deltamethrin dust suggested a higher order of toxicity with a 6-hour LC_{50} value of 600 mg/m^3. This is in keeping with published values of 940 and 785 mg/m^3 in male and female Sprague-Dawley rats using approximately 2-hour exposures.[85]

Signs of toxicity noted in these studies included muscular stiffening, clonic-tonic convulsions, ataxia, weakness, salivation and cyanosis in rodents with hyperexcitability, hind limb stiffness and vomiting in dogs. These signs are typical of those noted with Type II pyrethroids and have been reported in published studies.[85,88,89]

When mice were administered deltamethrin orally at 5 or 25 mg/kg bw/day for 28 days, no major signs of overt toxicity were noted, in keeping with the majority of findings in the studies described above.[90] However, these co-workers also examined hepatic, haematopoietic and other effects in some detail and found that even the lower of the two doses caused liver, kidney and splenic degenerative changes, while deltamethrin at both doses caused stimulation of erythropoiesis, increased haematocrit and increased numbers of leucocytes in males but not in females. Oral studies in rabbits using a 1-week dosing period failed to produce any major adverse effects although it was not clear what doses were used.[91] Others have reviewed 21-day dermal toxicity studies in the rat with doses of up to 1000 mg/kg bw/day and PEG 400 as vehicle.[89] There were no signs of systemic toxicity, probably reflecting poor absorption by this route. Rats exposed to 6 or 12 mg/m^3 deltamethrin as an aerosol, 30 minutes each day for 45 days, showed a variety of pulmonary effects including pneumonia, focal haemorrhage, foamy macrophage accumulation, emphysema and damage to alveolar lining cells.[92] However, it was unclear as to how the aerosol was generated or even what its components were. Moreover, the nature of the controls (no exposure or exposure to aerosol components only) was not stated. Consequently, it is difficult to derive any useful information from this study. Intraperitoneal administration to rats of deltamethrin at 7.2 mg/kg bw/day for 28 days produced no evidence of pyrethroid toxicity, although minor hepatic effects did occur (increase in mitochondria, change in their morphology).[93]

Although there are no standard reproductive studies available in the open literature with deltamethrin, other reports suggest that it may induce testicular degeneration, at least in the rat.

Administration of doses of 1 or 2 mg/kg bw/day to male rats for 65 consecutive days in order to cover a complete spermatogenic cycle resulted in decreases in weights of the testes, seminal vesicles and prostates. There were also reductions in sperm counts and plasma testosterone concentrations. These findings were accompanied by a reduction in male fertility following mating with untreated female rats.[94] In a study where rats were given daily intraperitoneal injections of 1 mg/kg bw deltamethrin for 21 days, arrest of spermatogenesis occurred, accompanied by degenerative changes in the testes and increases in the rate of apoptosis in basal germ cells and primary and secondary spermatocytes. Plasma levels of nitric oxide were increased over control values.[95] Deltamethrin produced slight changes in ejaculate volume and declines in sperm numbers in treated rabbits, although it was not entirely clear what doses had been used (cited as fractions of the LD_{50} value).[96]

When rats were exposed *in utero* to deltamethrin and its metabolites by treating pregnant female rats with the substance using oral gavage doses of 0, 1, 2 or 4 mg/kg bw/day from day 1 of gestation to day 21 of lactation, there were reductions in testicular weights of male offspring at the highest dose. The time to reach sexual maturity was not affected and there were no effects on sperm morphology or plasma testosterone levels.[97]

In vitro studies suggested that several pyrethroids had estrogenic effects, whereas a number of organophosphorus compounds were devoid of such activity.[98] However, studies in immature female rats and castrated males treated with up to 4 mg/kg bw/day deltamethrin for 3 days by oral gavage showed no estrogenic or androgenic effects.[99] Similar negative results were obtained when rats were treated with a combination of deltamethrin and endosulfan.[100] Administration of deltamethrin resulted in testicular degenerative changes accompanied by reductions in testosterone and the arrest of spermatogenesis.[101]

The results of these studies suggest that deltamethrin may adversely affect the male reproductive system causing degenerative changes and reductions in sperm count, possibly involving an increase in apoptosis. It does not appear to have significant estrogenic activity *in vivo*. Two multigeneration studies have been reviewed elsewhere. In one of these studies where there were three generations and two litters per generation, deltamethrin was given at 0, 20 or 50 ppm in the diet. The only effects seen were at the highest dietary concentration where there was reduced body weight in F_0 females and reduced food consumption in F_1 males. There were no effects on reproductive performance.[89] The NOEL was 20 ppm or 2 mg/kg bw/day using the WHO conversion factor.[102] In a second multigeneration study, rats were given dietary deltamethrin at 0, 5, 20, 80 or 320 ppm deltamethrin. The animals were dosed for 12 weeks before a 3-week mating period, and then throughout gestation and lactation. Deltamethrin-related deaths occurred in the F_1 generation accompanied by ataxia, impaired righting reflex, urine-stained fur and dark material in the stomachs of animals given the highest dietary concentration. Surviving animals also showed signs of pyrethroid induced toxicity at this dietary level. The body weights of rats were also significantly reduced at 320 ppm. However, in this study there were no effects on reproductive performance. The NOEL for toxicity was 80 ppm or approximately 4.3 mg/kg bw/day as the calculated dose while the NOEL for reproductive effects was the highest concentration tested, 320 ppm or 18 mg/kg bw as the calculated dose.[103]

Deltamethrin has been tested in adequate developmental studies in the mouse, rat and rabbit at sensitive periods of gestation, where it produced evidence of maternal toxicity in the rabbit for which the NOEL was 4 mg/kg bw/day. There were few signs of toxicity in mice and rats and no evidence for any teratogenic effects in any species tested.[103] Similar findings have been reported in published studies where mice were given up to 38 mg/kg bw/day or rats up to 5 mg/kg bw/day during gestation. Although maternal signs of pyrethroid toxicity were noted, there was no evidence of teratogenic effects.[85,104,105] There is thus no evidence for teratogenic potential for deltamethrin.

There have been several publications dealing with the genotoxicity of deltamethrin. In these studies, negative results were obtained in *Salmonella* reversion assays, in the V79 Chinese hamster mutation test, in a dominant lethal assay in mice and in *in vivo* studies for clastogenicity in mice and the substance did not induce excision repair.[106–109]

Some studies, largely for clastogenic activity, have reported positive or equivocal results with deltamethrin and other substances including other synthetic pyrethroids. Thus, positive results were seen in mouse micronucleus tests and clastogenicity studies using human lymphocytes. In the micronucleus test, positive results were generally only seen at high doses, while in the human lymphocyte studies, the results appeared to depend on the donor rather than on the substance being tested.[110–117] For some substances, including deltamethrin, some of these effects may be due to contaminants and impurities.[118] Overall, the available data suggest that deltamethrin is not a genotoxic material in accordance with the findings of others and of regulatory bodies.[81,89,103,119]

Carcinogenicity studies (mouse and rat) were commenced with deltamethrin. These were reported at 12 months as interim reports and they are discussed here under repeat dose toxicity. However, the final reports covering the entire 2-year period are not available, probably because agreement between the sponsor and the supplier of deltamethrin (and owner of the studies) was terminated. It seems that the carcinogenicity studies were finalised and discussed at JMPR, EMEA and European Commission.[81,103,119] In the mouse study, mice were fed diets containing 0, 1, 5, 25 and 100 ppm deltamethrin for 2 years. As described here, there were no significant findings at the 12-month interim report. Proliferative lesions were noted in some organs at 24 months but these were of similar incidence in treated and control animals and were considered to be spontaneous. There was no increased incidence of neoplasms in treated mice when compared to control values.[103]

In the rat study, animals were given diets containing 0, 5, 20 or 50 ppm deltamethrin for 2 years. Again, as described here, there were no untoward findings at the 12-month interim time point. There were no major signs of toxicity noted during the 2-year study and at termination there was no increased incidence of tumours in treated animals when compared with controls.[103]

Other carcinogenicity studies in rats and mice have been conducted but the results are not available. Thus, deltamethrin was given in the diets of mice at levels of up to 2000 ppm for 2 years. There was no increased incidence of tumours in treated animals. Similarly, rats were given diets containing up to 800 ppm deltamethrin for 2 years. Evidence of toxicity was noted in some animals but at termination there was no increased incidence of any tumour type.[103]

In studies conducted by the International Agency for Research on Cancer (IARC), mice were given gavage doses of deltamethrin in arachis oil at doses of 0, 1, 4 or 8 mg/kg bw/day for 2 years. There was no compound-related increased incidence of any tumour type. Similarly, rats were given doses of 0, 3 or 6 mg/kg bw/day deltamethrin for 2 years. Again, there was no evidence of compound-related carcinogenic effects and the authors concluded that deltamethrin does not appear to be carcinogenic in rats or mice.[120]

In mechanistic studies using topical application, deltamethrin was not carcinogenic in a mouse model. There was some evidence to suggest that it had some initiating activity when applied to mouse skin and the area treated with phorbol esters but there were no data to suggest that it was a complete carcinogen.[121] It gave negative results in a rat model of hepatocarcinogenesis where animals were treated with diethylnitrosamine, followed by deltamethrin and then subjected to partial hepatectomy.[122]

As discussed earlier, Type II pyrethroids are neurotoxic and many of their toxic effects can be attributed to this. All the pyrethroids affect motor function, but Type II pyrethroids, including deltamethrin, are the most potent in this respect.[123] Deltamethrin has been shown to produce prolonged increases of excitability following nerve impulses in rats[124] and in the giant axons of the annelid worm *Myxicola infundibulum*[125] while the substance reduced the amplitude of the action potential in isolated frog sciatic nerve.[126] When injected directly into the CNS, deltamethrin is extremely toxic with fatalities at doses of approximately 11 µg/kg bw in rats after intraventricular administration.[127,128] Intraperitoneal doses of 12.5 mg/kg bw to rats induce degenerative changes in the brain including apoptosis. Apoptosis also occurs in cultured cerebral cortex neurons *in vitro*.[129,130]

Deltamethrin has been tested in a range of neurobehavioral toxicity studies. The compound was found to increase spontaneous activity in both rats (7 mg/kg bw in corn as a commercial pesticide emulsion, orally) and mice (0.7 mg/kg bw in arachis oil-egg lecithin aqueous emulsion, orally). In the rat study, aggressive behaviour and the relearning index were also increased whereas there was no effect on learning and memory.[131,132] Oral doses of up to 8 mg/kg bw in corn oil resulted in decreases in maze behaviour in rats; the NOEL was 2 mg/kg bw/day. In this same work, deltamethrin resulted in a dose-dependent decrease in amplitude and an increase in latency of the acute startle reflex again with an NOEL of 2 mg/kg bw.[133] When rats were studied in the acute startle reflex test with oral doses of up to 6 mg/kg bw deltamethrin in corn oil, the acute startle reflex was attenuated at the highest dose. The NOEL was 4 mg/kg bw.[134]

In a study of the scheduled-controlled response in mice given 0.3 to 3 mg/kg bw deltamethrin by the intraperitoneal route, responses were reduced by doses greater than 0.1 mg/kg bw (the NOEL). The ED_{50} was approximately 1 mg/kg bw.[135] A similar study in rats used intraperitoneal doses of 2 mg/kg bw, which reduced the operant response by 80%.[136] Unfortunately, no other doses were used and so an NOEL could not be identified.

Deltamethrin (15 and 150 mg/kg bw orally) was subjected to a number of tests in a study of neuropharmacological studies. These comprised a test for motor coordination using a rotarod and the effects on pentobarbitone sleeping time and pentylenetetrazole-induced convulsions. Deltamethrin treatment significantly decreased sleeping time while it increased the duration of convulsions. In the rotarod test, significant ataxia occurred.[137] The latter findings are perhaps not surprising in view of the induction of ataxia and convulsions in standard toxicity studies.

Deltamethrin at 0.08 mg/kg bw led to alterations in swimming behaviour, motor activity and striatal dopamine concentrations when exposed prenatally.[138] The data suggested a higher level of dopaminergic activity but the implications of these observations are unknown.

Rats treated with inducers of cytochrome P450 showed increases in some neurobehavioral parameters while those treated with cobalt chloride to deplete cytochrome P450 showed decreases, indicating that a metabolite of deltamethrin may be responsible for some of the effects seen in rodents.[139]

As noted in the discussion on cyhalothrin, it has been suggested that the neurobehavioral effects of substances should be assessed by reference to six functional domains – sensorimotor, autonomic, neuromuscular, physiological, activity and excitability.[67,69] These effects have not been investigated systematically in the studies described here nor have dose-response relationships been established. However, in GLP-compliant 2 studies reviewed by JMPR, deltamethrin was administered to rats at oral doses of 0, 5, 15 or 50 mg/kg bw in corn oil. This battery included posture, convulsions, tremors, biting, eyelid closure, faecal consistency, ease of handling, lachrymation, salivation, respiration rate, muscular tone, motility, rearing, convulsions, tremors, bizarre or stereotypical behaviour, gait, startle, touch, tail pinch, grip strength, rotarod performance, body temperature and locomotor activity. At the highest dose, tremors, clonic and tonic convulsions and numerous behavioural changes occurred and all six domains described previously were affected.[69] At 15 mg/kg bw, slight salivation, slightly stained fur and impaired ability were noted in individual animals. The

NOEL was 5 mg/kg bw. In a further study by the same authors, rats were given diets containing 0, 50, 200 or 800 ppm deltamethrin for 91 days, and subjected to the same battery of tests and observations as described immediately previously. Signs of toxicity and notably neurotoxicity were seen in animals given the highest dietary concentration and the lowest dietary concentration without adverse effect was 200 ppm equivalent to 54 mg/kg bw/day.[103]

In conclusion therefore, deltamethrin induces neurotoxicity characterised by tremors, clonic and tonic convulsions and ataxia in rodents. It also produces more subtle neuropharmacological/toxicological effects. The oral NOELs for these effects is in the range of 2 to 5 mg/kg bw although this was higher at 54 mg/kg bw in a 90-day neurobehavioral study.

Deltamethrin has been tested in a study in the hen. This test has been developed to demonstrate organophosphorus-induced delayed neuropathy (OPIDN), which occurs following an initial cholinergic crisis, and involves a selective degeneration of long and large fibres of the spinal cord and peripheral nervous system.[140] The domestic chicken has been shown to be a model, albeit with some limitations for this effect of organophosphorus compounds, and it is widely used to investigate or predict this specific toxicity.

Synthetic pyrethroids have not been shown to cause this effect and their mode of action would not suggest that it is likely and neuropathy target esterase (NTE) is almost exclusively a target for organophosphorus compounds.[141] Hence, this study can be considered to be superfluous. Unsurprisingly, the study was negative and there was no indication of the induction of a delayed neuropathy.

Cypermethrin (ISO; (*RS*)-α-cyano-3-phenoxybenzyl (1*RS*,3*RS*;1*RS*,3*SR*)-3-(2,2-dichlorovinyl)-2,2-dimethylcyclopropanecarboxylate) is a Type II pyrethroid similar in structure to deltamethrin but here two chlorine atoms replace the two bromine atoms on the vinyl structure. Like deltamethrin, cypermethrin is a mixture of eight isomers. α-Cypermethrin (ISO) is a racemate composed of the 1*R*, *cis* and 1*S*, *cis* isomers.[142,143] Cypermethrin is well absorbed after oral administration and rapidly excreted in urine and faeces. As with other pyrethroids, the ester bond is cleaved to yield the 3-phenoxybenzoyl moiety, which is further oxidised and subject to sulfate conjugation, and the corresponding cyclopropane carboxylic acid. Minor metabolites include the glycine conjugate of 3-phenoxybenzoic acid and 3-(4-hydroxyphenoxy)benzoic acid.[144] Cypermethrin residues are found in most tissues in several animal species, but concentrations are significantly higher in adipose tissues.[142–144]

Like other pyrethroids, cypermethrin and α-cypermethrin are more toxic orally when administered in oil than when given in predominantly aqueous solvents. For example, the oral LD_{50} value for cypermethrin in rats was 251 mg/kg bw in corn oil but 4000 mg/kg bw when given in 40% aqueous dimethyl sulfoxide and 3423 mg/kg bw when given as a 50% aqueous suspension. Similar results were seen with α-cypermethrin but this was more acutely toxic than cypermethrin with LD_{50} values in the rat of 64 mg/kg bw when given in corn oil. However, as with cypermethrin, toxicity was reduced when given in aqueous dimethyl sulfoxide (LD_{50} 4000 mg/kg bw) or as an aqueous suspension

(LD$_{50}$ >5000 mg/kg bw). Signs of toxicity included ataxia, splayed gait, tip-toe walking, tremors and clonic convulsions.[142–144]

In repeat-dose studies where mice were given a variety of dietary concentrations of α-cypermethrin for 29 days, animals developed signs of neurotoxicity at doses 1200 or 800 mg per kg feed and above. Signs included ataxia, abnormal gait, over activity and hunched posture. The no-observed effect level was approximately 57 mg/kg bw/day. When groups of mice were given the substance at up to 1000 mg per kg feed for 13 weeks, the major adverse sign noted was hair loss at all dose levels. Other signs included ungroomed fur, and encrustations of the dorsal body surfaces. There were a number of variations in organ weights but no frank evidence of neurotoxicity.[144] Effects on the bactericidal activity of neutrophils, and increase in the numbers of monocytes and lymphocytes seen in one study with α-cypermethrin in mice, are difficult to interpret in the absence of data from other pyrethroids and in other species.[145]

Cypermethrin and α-cypermethrin have been tested in a range of repeat-dose studies in rats ranging from 35 to 90 or 95 days. With cypermethrin, the main effects were decreases in haemoglobin, mean corpuscular volume and eosinophil counts and increases in relative liver weights. The NOEL from these studies was 5 mg/kg bw/day. α-Cypermethrin caused decreases in mean corpuscular volume and haemoglobin. Animals given 800 and 1200 mg/kg feed showed signs of neurotoxicity including high stepping, splayed gait, abasia and hypersensitivity, with cachexia in severe cases. Similar effects were seen in a separate study with doses of 540 mg/kg feed. The NOEL from these studies was equivalent to 3 mg/kg bw/day. Signs of neurotoxicity have also been reported in dogs given cypermethrin or α-cypermethrin in repeat-dose studies. These included tremors, ataxia, incoordination and hyperaesthesia. At 1500 mg/kg feed, 50% of animals in a dose group had to be sacrificed due to the toxic effects of cypermethrin. The NOEL from this particular study was 12.5 mg/kg bw/day. Similar signs were reported with α-cypermethrin, although this substance appeared to be more toxic than cypermethrin. The lowest NOEL with α-cypermethrin was 1.5 mg/kg bw/day.[144]

Cypermethrin had no adverse effects on reproductive performance in a three-generation study in rats. Both substances produced signs of maternal toxicity in teratogenicity studies in rats while α-cypermethrin produced fetotoxicity at higher doses. Neither compound produced any evidence of teratogenicity. Similarly, both substances have been tested in teratogenicity studies in rabbits. Neither produced evidence of embryotoxicity or teratogenicity. The NOELs from these studies were 70 mg/kg bw/day for cypermethrin and 9 mg/kg bw/day for α-cypermethrin in rats and 120 mg/kg bw/day for cypermethrin and 30 mg/kg bw/day for α-cypermethrin in rabbits.[144]

Both substances have been investigated in a number of *in vitro* and *in vivo* studies of genotoxicity covering a variety of end-points including the induction of mutations and clastogenicity. All of these studies yielded negative results. There was no evidence of carcinogenicity with cypermethrin in long-term studies in mice and rats,[144] and in view of this result, and the results from genotoxicity studies, there is no reason to believe that α-cypermethrin would be carcinogenic.

Cypermethrin produced a significant but transient functional impairment in the inclined plane test in rats that was maximal after 7 days of administration. However, there were no adverse effects in the acute startle reflex test.[146,147] α-Cypermethrin was investigated in a functional observational battery of tests for measurements of fore and hind limb grip strength, hind limb landing foot splay and motor activity. Signs of toxicity included abnormal and splayed gaits, prostration, vocalisation, piloerection and hunched posture while gait abnormalities were observed during the functional observational battery phase of the study. At higher doses, slight degeneration of the fibres of the sciatic nerve occurred at higher doses. The NOEL for this study was 4 mg/kg bw.

6.2.1.2   Type I Pyrethroids

As mentioned earlier, permethrin (ISO; 3-phenoxybenzyl(1*RS*,3*RS*;1*RS*,3*SR*)-3-(2,2-dichlorovinyl)-2,2-dimethylcyclopropanecarboxylate) is a pyrethroid which lacks the cyano group that characterises cyhalothrin, deltamethrin, cypermethrin and other similar synthetic pyrethroids (Figure 6.2). Unlike these substances, permethrin, like allethrin and resmethrin, is a Type I pyrethroid, whose actions are thought to be due to its effects on ion channels in axons.[148,149] The metabolism of permethrin, like that of many other pyrethroids, is complex. In the rat, the major metabolites arise from cleavage of the ester bonds to yield the hydroxyphenoxybenzoic acid derivatives, which are conjugated with sulfate. Phenoxybenzoic acid, probably *via* phenoxybenzyl alcohol, is also formed and this is converted to the glucuronide and glycine conjugates.[148,149]

In the absence of an oily vehicle, the acute oral toxicity of permethrin is low with LD_{50} values in excess of 2000 mg/kg bw, or even 8000 mg/kg bw in rats. However, when administered in corn oil the toxicity increases markedly. LD_{50} values in the range 230 to 1700 mg/kg bw have been reported in mice, and 220 to 1600 mg/kg bw in rats. The toxicity also depends on the isomeric composition of the material used with permethrin with a *cis*: *trans* ratio of 80–100:20–0 being up to 24 times more toxic than that with a *cis*: *trans* ratio of 10–25:90–75. In rabbits, the oral LD_{50} value was >2000 mg/kg bw for *cis*: *trans* 55:45 and 40:60 permethrin.[149]

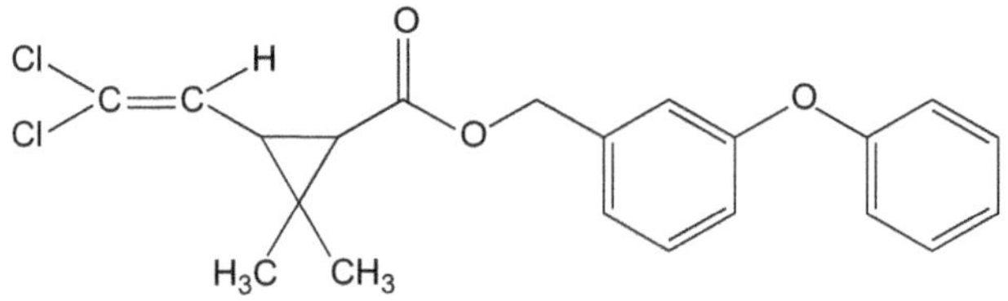

Figure 6.2   Chemical formula of permethrin.

In repeat dose studies in mice, no significant clinical findings occurred when animals were given permethrin (*cis*: *trans* 39 : 56) in the diet at concentrations equivalent to up to 560 mg/kg bw/day for 28 days. There were no major gross or microscopic findings except for increased liver weights at the two highest concentrations with some eosinophilia in centrilobular hepatocytes. The NOEL was equivalent to 140 mg/kg bw/day. In rats given a similar isomeric composition of permethrin in the diet for 28 days, 63% of those given the equivalent of 500 mg/kg bw/day and 100% of those given the equivalent of 1000 mg/kg bw/day died. Animals showed whole-body tremors, hyperactivity and piloerection. In a similar study where the highest dietary level was equivalent to 630–660 mg/kg bw/day for 30 days, all the high-dose animals died within 24 hours to one week of the start of the study. There was very high mortality at the next dietary level equivalent to around 250 mg/kg bw/day. The main clinical signs included slight to moderate tremors and staining of fur. The NOEL values from these two studies were 50 and 250 mg/kg bw/day, respectively.[149]

When rats were given dietary permethrin at concentrations of 0, 20, 50, 100, 250, 500 and 1000 mg/kg bw/day for 28 days, all animals given the highest dietary intake died within three days of the start of the study. There was also high mortality at the 500 mg/kg bw/day dose. Prior to death, animals displayed whole body tremors, hyperactivity and piloerection while surviving animals given 500 mg/kg bw/day showed urinary incontinence. At the end of the study, animals given ≥ 250 mg/kg bw/day had increased absolute and relative liver weights. The NOEL in this study was equal to 50 mg/kg bw/day. Similar qualitative findings were made in other repeat dose studies of similar durations and in other studies extending to 90 days or six months. Hypersensitivity was also seen in these studies.[140]

In dogs given repeat oral doses of permethrin of up to 500 mg/kg bw/day for 90 days, a range of clinical signs of toxicity have been reported including tremors, emesis, transient narcosis, nystagmus, ataxia and aggressive behaviour at the highest dose employed. However, when given at 250 mg/kg bw/day for 180 days, no major signs except emesis were observed. At 1000 mg/kg bw/day in a 52-week study, convulsions, muscle tremor and lack of coordination occurred. Lower doses produced reductions in body weight. The lowest NOEL from studies in dogs was 5 mg/kg bw/day.[140]

Permethrin was not a skin irritant in studies in rabbits and produced only signs of mild eye irritation in this species. It was tested in a number of maximisation tests in the guinea pig but produced no evidence of dermal sensitisation.[140]

In a battery of tests for various end-points of genotoxicity, permethrin gave negative results. These tests included those for gene mutations, the induction of unscheduled DNA synthesis and DNA repair. It has not been tested for clastogenic activity *in vivo* but there was evidence of clastogenicity, or at least equivocal results, in mammalian cells *in vitro*.[149–162]

In CD-1 mice, a slightly elevated incidence of alveolar adenoma and alveolar carcinoma were seen in an oral carcinogenicity study with permethrin. However, the incidence of the former was lower in test animals than in controls, while the incidence of the latter was only slightly increased in females (0% in all males and in female controls and in 1 each in 59 or 60 mice given the low, intermediate and high doses). A second study was conducted and here much higher incidences of both alveolar adenomas and carcinomas were noted than in the previous study. There was no apparent dose relationship in males, but the incidence of both tumour types was increased in females (13, 24, 35 and 49% for adenomas and 8, 9, 15 and 20% for carcinomas in controls, low (3 mg/kg bw/day), intermediate (15 mg/kg bw/day) and high (75 mg/kg bw/day), respectively). There were also slight increases in hepatocellular adenoma as is often seen in long-term mouse studies, but the incidence of hepatocellular carcinoma was not increased. In a separate study using Alderley Park mice, and dietary concentrations equivalent to 0, 38, 150 or 380 mg/kg bw/day, there was no increased incidence of tumours of any type in these animals. Hence, there is conflicting evidence for the ability of permethrin to induce tumours in mice. However, in two long-term studies in rats (Alderley Park and Long Evans) there was no evidence of a carcinogenic effect. In the CD-1 mice studies where lung tumours were seen, there was a high background (controls) of alveolar adenomas in mice of both sexes in one study and of adenomas and carcinomas in the other, whereas a third study gave negative results. In view of this, the overwhelming number of negative results in tests for genotoxicity, and negative results in two rat carcinogenicity studies, permethrin can be considered not to be a genotoxic carcinogen in animal models.[149,163]

Permethrin has been tested in a number of studies of neurotoxicity. After intravenous administration to mice, permethrin induced hyperactivity, increased sensitivity to external stimuli and whole body tremor. This eventually led to prostration and death with the ED_{50} being 20 mg/kg bw for the *cis* isomer, 36 mg/kg bw for the technical mixture and 93 mg/kg bw for the *trans* isomer. The ED_{50} was much lower after intracerebroventricular administration (0.09, 0.15 and 1.1 mg/kg bw, respectively). The neurotoxicology of permethrin has been investigated in functional observational studies in rats. In one study where animals were given permethrin orally in corn oil, those given the highest dose had whole body tremors, exaggeration of flexion of the hind limbs, staggered gait, splayed hind limbs and abnormal posture with convulsions on the first day of the observational tests. The NOEL for this study was 150 mg/kg bw. In another observational battery study, rats were given diets containing permethrin for 13 weeks. Signs of toxicity appeared at dietary concentrations of ≥ 1500 ppm and included staggered gait, splayed hind limbs and tremors. The NOEL was equivalent to 15 mg/kg bw day.[149,164,165]

6.2.2 Overview of the Toxic Effects of the Pyrethroids in Animals

The synthetic pyrethroids are characterised by their neurotoxicity. They are not reproductive toxicants or teratogens and in general they yield negative results in genotoxicity and carcinogenicity studies. However, regardless of the type of study, if high enough doses are given, then neurotoxicity will occur. As mentioned at the beginning of this section on synthetic pyrethroids, this toxicity is dependent on the presence or absence of the α-cyano group and is perhaps more advantageously characterised after intracerebroventricular administration.[48,57] Despite the advances made in research in recent years, the biochemical and molecular mechanisms of pyrethroid toxicity are still not fully understood and new information continues to become available. For example, although it is known that the pyrethroids cause decreases in the voltage-gated sodium channel inactivation rates, it is not known how these effects result in the characteristic toxicities of different synthetic pyrethroids and why the Type I and II compounds differ so markedly in their activities. However, this could be related to differential effects on glutamergic and other neuronal networks.[166] Moreover, some sodium channels may be more sensitive to the effects of those pyrethroids containing the α-cyano group.[167] Deltamethrin may also affect the dopaminergic system, specifically in the hippocampus and striatum, and may even result in nerve cell damage through induction of mitochondrial-mediated apoptosis.[168–171] Deltamethrin is a potent inducer of brain-derived neurotropic factors in neurons, suggesting its capacity to act as an inducer of neuronal hyperexcitation.[172] However, none of these findings, or those discussed elsewhere in this chapter, fully explain the range of signs of toxicity elicited in mammals by the synthetic pyrethroids.

Permethrin and other synthetic pyrethroids are widely used as ectoparasiticides for the treatment of dogs. These are usually applied as spot-on formulations and are used largely to control fleas or, in combination with other active substances, to control other parasitic organisms. Problems occur when these pyrethroid products are used in cats. Their use in cats can, and often does, result in severe toxicity and frequently in death. In fact, a recent survey of 286 cases found that 96.9% of cats exposed to permethrin developed clinical effects and over 10% died or were euthanized. Warnings have been issued, and continue to be issued, by regulatory authorities to try to minimise this problem. This extreme toxicity in cats is probably related to a number of factors including the animal's grooming habits and the inabilities of felines (large as well as small) to conjugate xenobiotics, thus ensuring that they are not adequately detoxified and excreted.[173–180]

6.2.3 Toxicity to Humans

Neurotoxicity occurs in animals exposed to relatively high doses of synthetic pyrethroids. Such doses are higher than human beings are likely to encounter during the normal use of veterinary medicinal products or indeed during the normal use of pyrethroid-containing pesticides. In fact, the major form of adverse effect associated with exposure to synthetic pyrethroids in humans is cutaneous paraesthesia.[181–184] This develops some time, usually hours, after exposure, and produces a burning or stinging sensation on the skin. It is associated with Type II pyrethroids. However, when exposure to higher doses occurs, dizziness, burning and tingling sensations, epigastric pain, vomiting, anorexia, chest tightness, blurred vision, palpitations, muscular fasciculations, and disturbances of consciousness may occur. In severe poisoning cases, convulsions and loss of consciousness ensue. All of these effects are reversible except when death occurs.[184–193]

6.3 Imidacloprid

Imidacloprid (ISO; 1-(6-chloro-3-pyridinylmethyl)-*N*-nitroimidazolidin-2-ylideneamine; Figure 6.3) is a relatively new insecticide that is used as a pest control agent on crops and as a veterinary medicinal product. It is the main neonicotinoid used in veterinary products. These are chemically related to naturally occurring nicotine and in addition to imidacloprid the class includes nitenpyram, thiacloprid and acetamiprid. Imidacloprid, like many neonicotinoids, is water soluble (0.6 g/l) and most of an oral dose is excreted unchanged in the urine although a significant quantity may be excreted in the bile in rats. The substance is widely distributed in the body. It is extensively metabolised to yield *inter alia* 6-hydroxynicotinic acid, 6-methylmercaptonicotinic acid and its glycine conjugate and various metabolites derived from the nitro-2-imidazolidinimine moiety.[194,195]

The neonicotinoid agents act as agonists for the nicotinic acetylcholine receptors (nAChR) in insects and mammals, and particularly for the α4β2 subtype.[192]

Imidacloprid is moderately acutely toxic in rodents with oral LD_{50} values in the range 380–650 mg/kg bw in rats and 130–170 mg/kg bw in mice. It was practically non-toxic ($LD_{50} > 5000$ mg/kg bw) following dermal application to rats. Where toxicity occurred, signs included transient trembling and spasms, motility abnormalities, respiratory signs, and behavioural effects.[194,195] In repeat dose studies in rodents, the main signs of toxicity were frequently limited to elevated enzymes and depressed protein, albumin, cholesterol and triglycerides. In rats, there was decreased activity of acetylcholine in serum and in the brain.[195,196] In dogs, ataxia, vomiting and tremor occurred.[193]

There was no evidence of carcinogenic effects in long-term studies in mice and rats, although there was evidence of mineralisation of the thalamus in mice and an increased incidence of mineralisation of the thyroid in rats.[193] Imidacloprid has been tested in a number of studies for genotoxic potential covering a wide range of end-points including those for mutations, DNA damage, sister chromatid exchange and the induction of micronuclei. In the vast majority of those studies where imidacloprid was tested alone, negative results were

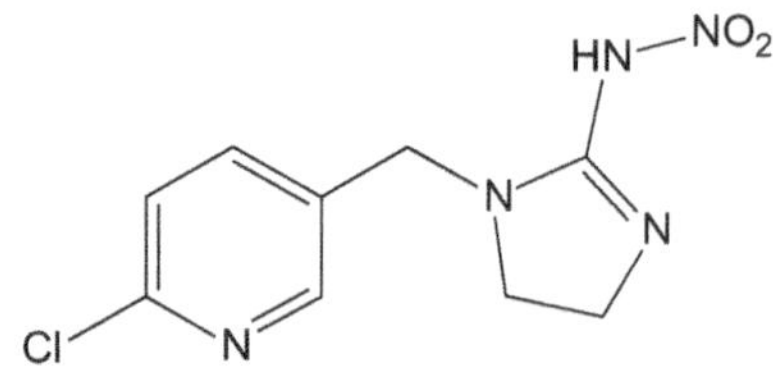

Figure 6.3 Chemical formula of imidacloprid.

obtained, except in one test for sister chromatid exchange where a positive result was noted.[195] When tested in combination with the organophosphorus insecticide methamidophos, positive results were noted in a *Salmonella* reversion assay, in a rat bone marrow chromosome aberration assay and in a mouse micronucleus test; similar results were noted when the compounds were tested individually.[197] The significance of these results remains unclear in the light of the results of the numerous (16) studies mentioned above, and overall the data strongly suggest that imidacloprid is not genotoxic.

In a multigeneration study in rats, the major effects were reduced body weights in parental and F_1 and F_2 animals. There was no evidence of teratological effects in rats or rabbits but fetotoxicity was seen (wavy ribs, delayed ossification) in offspring from animals that showed signs of maternotoxicity.[195]

In studies of neurotoxicity, tremors, gait abnormalities, decreased activity and coolness to touch have been reported. The lowest NOEL from these studies was 9.3 mg/kg bw/day.[195]

6.3.1 Effects in Humans

The major adverse effects in humans exposed to imidacloprid appear to be occasional mild cases of dermatitis in pet owners who had treated their animals with a commercial formulation of the product. However, these effects were probably due to other constituents of the formulation rather than to the active substance itself.[195] In a double-blind crossover study of tree planters who had handled trees treated with imidacloprid and cypermethrin, no adverse effects were found.[198] No signs of toxicity were seen in a 4-year-old child who ingested approximately 200 mg of imidacloprid, equivalent to about 10 mg/kg bw.[195] Ingestion of relatively large quantities of imidacloprid formulations that resulted in measurable plasma concentrations (mean 10.58 ng/l; range 0.02–51.25 ng/l) resulted in mild symptoms such as nausea, vomiting, headache and diarrhoea. One patient had respiratory failure and another prolonged sedation, but no deaths occurred.[199]

6.4 Organophosphorus Compounds

The toxicity of the organophosphorus compounds in mammals, including humans, is well documented.[200,201] Their acute toxicity is characterised by inhibition of acetylcholine esterase resulting in the accumulation of acetylcholine and overstimulation of nicotinic and muscarinic receptors.[201–203] However, there is also an intermediate phase characterised by weakness and paralysis of proximal limb and other muscles and delayed peripheral neuropathy, and these occur after the initial cholinergic phase, although the latter, rarely, may occur in its absence.[201–204] Organophosphorus-induced delayed neuropathy (OPIDN), which only occurs with certain compounds, ensues around 5 weeks after acute poisoning and the molecular target is thought to be neuropathy target esterase.[201–204] Organophosphorus compounds may cause a variety of other effects on a number of organ systems and many of them possess genotoxic properties.

In the past, a number of these substances have been used in veterinary medicine including phosmet, propetamphos, chlorfenvinphos and dichlorvos. However, the major uses are now restricted to diazinon and azamethiphos. The organophosphorus compounds are discussed in more detail in Chapter 10.

6.4.1 Diazinon

Diazinon (ISO; formerly dimpylate, *O,O*-diethyl *O*-[4-methyl-6-(propan-2-yl)pyrimidin-2yl] phosphorothioate; Figure 6.4) is an organophosphorus compound that is widely used in agriculture but whose use in veterinary medicine is now largely restricted to sheep-dipping for the treatment and control of ectoparasites. Its toxicity has been reviewed by JMPR.[205] Diazinon is well absorbed in rats after oral administration with up to 80% of the administered dose being excreted in urine. Similarly, after oral administration to mice, guinea pigs and dogs, absorption was extensive. Following topical application to rats, up to 80% of the applied dose was recovered in urine, demonstrating facile dermal absorption.

The biotransformation of diazinon is complex with both minor and major pathways being identified.[205] The major metabolites are the oxon (diazoxon), diethylphosphate and diethylthiophosphate along with 2-isopropyl-4-methyl-6-hydroxypyrimidine. The activation to the oxon has been shown to be due to the action of cytochrome P450 and in human liver *in vitro*, through CYP2C19.[205–209] Although diazinon itself is considered to be a weak inhibitor of acetylcholinesterase, the oxons are known to be potent inhibitors.

Diazinon is acutely toxic with oral LD_{50} values in rats being in the range 200–1250 mg/kg bw. Following topical exposure, LD_{50} values were >2150 mg/kg bw in the rat and >2020 mg/kg bw in the rabbit.[205] Signs of toxicity were typical of organophosphorus compounds and those expected from acetylcholinesterase inhibitors, namely decreases in activity, sedation, dyspnoea, ataxia, tremors, convulsions, lacrimation and diarrhoea. These signs resolved in animals that survived. In repeat dose toxicity studies, the major signs were again those associated with acetylcholinesterase inhibition, and, where

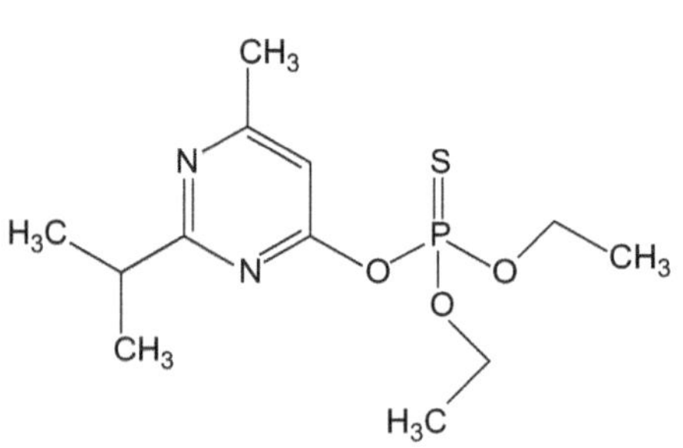

Figure 6.4   Chemical formula of diazinon.

measured, there were significant reductions in erythrocyte, and more importantly in brain acetylcholinesterase activities.[205] Diazinon has been tested for the induction of delayed neuropathy in the hen. There was no evidence of this effect and no adverse histopathological findings.[205]

Diazinon gave negative results in the majority of the studies for genotoxic activity, with the exception of the mouse lymphoma assay for forward mutations and an *in vitro* test for chromosome aberrations.[205] These results are perhaps not surprising because, as mentioned earlier, it is recognised that some organophosphorus compounds are genotoxic, although diazinon fell into the category of "mainly negative results".[206] Nevertheless, in some studies diazinon has given positive results including those for chromosomal aberrations and DNA damage.[210–218] This too is not surprising given that many organophosphorus compounds are alkylating agents.[217] However, although diazinon has been evaluated in carcinogenicity studies in mice and rats, there was no evidence for the induction of tumours.[205]

Diazinon has been tested in reproductive and in developmental studies. In reproduction studies, the main findings were reduced viability of pups and reduced weight gain of dams. The substance did not induce birth defects in the offspring of rats or rabbits treated during sensitive periods of gestation.[205] However, diazinon and other organophosphorus compounds may adversely affect the testes, sperm quality and motility, effects for which melatonin may be protective.

Many of the organophosphorus compounds are immunotoxic and immunosuppressive. The mechanisms by which diazinon and other organophosphorus compounds cause immunotoxicity are not fully understood but diazinon is cytotoxic and results in necrotic areas of the spleen and thymus in mice. It also leads to hyperplasia of the medulla of the thymus and lymph nodes, and hyperplasia of the white and red pulp in the spleen. Some of these changes may result in decreases in cytokines such as interleukins and interferons.[219–223]

6.4.1.1 Toxicity to Humans

There have been several incidents involving toxicity with diazinon. Some of these were deliberate and some accidental.[224–227] Of the accidental cases, these usually involved ingestion of stored liquid formulations.[228–230] Some cases involved topical exposure during applications for lice treatment while others involved children.[228–234] The majority of cases resulted in acute toxicity and signs were typical of acetylcholinesterase inhibition. Most cases responded well to atropine and oxime inhibition. In severe cases, death has resulted.[227]

There have been several cases of intermediate toxicity with diazinon. These resulted in paralysis of the proximal limb muscles, the neck flexor muscles and respiratory muscles. These signs are not responsive to atropine therapy.[225,235,236]

There have also been reports of occupational exposure to diazinon, resulting in toxicity. Occasionally this was due to contamination with TEPP or monothio-TEPP and other impurities. In some of these cases deaths have occurred and, in addition, several cattle died in one incident, almost certainly as a result of exposure to monothio-TEPP present as a contaminant in the formulation.[237–239] In the period 1945 to 1989 pesticides were responsible for 1012 of the 87,385 deaths due to poisoning in the UK. Of these deaths, only one was due to diazinon.[240]

In the United Kingdom, reports began to appear of adverse reactions in farm workers and shepherds following exposure to sheep dips, particularly those containing organophosphorus compounds, and notably diazinon (see Chapters 10 and 15). These reactions included a transient influenza-like illness widely referred to as "dipper's 'flu" and longer term clinical signs and symptoms that were frequently vague in nature but included loss of memory, depression, pyrexia and headaches.[241–243] A considerable amount of research was commissioned to try to obtain data that might cast some light on this phenomenon but none of the efforts provided conclusive evidence to associate it with exposure to diazinon during sheep dipping and, although dipping of sheep continues, the numbers of reports of adverse reactions has fallen markedly.[241,244,245]

In addition to the anticholinergic effects of organophosphorus compounds, there are other, more subtle effects on the nervous system, some of which may contribute to the long-term effects. Indeed, some of these effects occur at concentrations that are unlikely to inhibit acetylcholinesterase. These include effects on other enzymes and transcriptional changes in genes involved in neuronal cell differentiation and in cell signalling and enhancement of the toxicity of other xenobiotics. There may also be developmental effects arising from exposure to diazinon.[246–262] As an example, increases in sister chromatid exchange in peripheral lymphocytes have been reported in sheep dip workers after dipping at exposures that did not result in an increase in diazinon urinary metabolites.[263] Moreover, there may be genetic components in the activity of certain enzymes as there appears to be with paraoxonase, an enzyme that can hydrolyse several oxons, including diazoxon.[264] Sheep farmers with lower paraoxonase activity had a greater risk of being affected by ill health allegedly associated with sheep dipping.[265]

6.4.2   Azamethiphos

Azamethiphos (ISO; *S*-6-chloro-2,3-dihydro-2-oxo-1,3-oxazolo[4,5-*b*]pyridine-3-ylmethyl *O,O*-dimethyl phosphorothioate; Figure 6.5) is an organophosphorus compound that has been used to control flies and other insects in animal houses, and to control mosquitoes, tsetse flies, cockroaches and other insects that pose a public hygiene problem. In veterinary medicine it is used for the treatment of sea lice on farmed Atlantic salmon and other fish.[45,266–268]

Compared with many other pesticides, the metabolism and toxicity of azamethiphos are poorly documented. In fact there are more publications available on its environmental and ecotoxicological effects than there are on its toxicological effects. The only readily available document describing the toxicity of

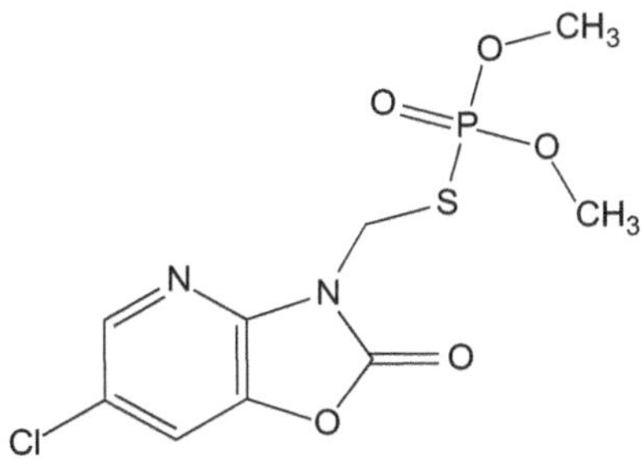

Figure 6.5 Chemical formula of azamethiphos.

azamethiphos is that published by the European Medicines Agency as a summary of the data that supported its application for a European maximum residues limit (MRL).[275] This documents that azamethiphos is well absorbed after oral administration to rats, with the majority of the administered dose being found in urine. The substance was poorly absorbed after topical administration.[269] A number of metabolites are formed in rats and goats including the sulfate and glucuronic acid conjugates of the chloro amino pyridine moiety, suggesting cleavage of the dimethyl phosphorothioate group and of the five-membered heterocyclic ring.[270]

Azamethiphos is of moderate toxicity to rodents with the acute oral LD_{50} value of 1180 mg/kg bw and the acute dermal LD_{50} value of >2150 mg/kg bw. The major signs of toxicity are those associated with cholinesterase inhibition. In a 13-week repeat dose study in rats, the major sign of toxicity was a reduction in blood cholinesterase activity, which persisted for the duration of a 28-day recovery period. Unfortunately, brain cholinesterase was not monitored. In one study, azamethiphos decreased serum cholinesterase in rats while cholinesterase isozyme fractions gave conflicting results with some decreasing and some increasing.[271] In a three-generation study in rats, the major effects were on parental body weights. In developmental studies in rats and mice fetotoxicity was noticed at the highest doses employed but there was no evidence of teratogenic effects.[269]

Like diazinon and other organophosphorus compounds azamethiphos gave equivocal results in genotoxicity tests. For example, it gave positive results in the *Salmonella* reverse mutation test, in a test for DNA damage in mammalian cells *in vitro*, in the *Saccharomyces cerevisiae* D7 mutation assay and in the *Drosophila* wing spot test,[216,269] and it has been shown to be a proficient alkylating agent.[272] However, it gave negative results in a dominant lethal assay and in a test for unscheduled DNA repair. Despite the occurrence of positive results in these tests, azamethiphos gave negative results in two carcinogenicity studies in rats and in a study, unfortunately not conducted in accordance with Good Laboratory Practice. In mice it did not induce delayed neuropathy.[269]

There are no data on the toxicity of azamethiphos to humans.

6.4.2.1 Adverse Effects of Diazinon and Azamethiphos in Animals

In view of the large number of sheep dipped in the UK each year, and the large numbers of sheep and cattle dipped or sprayed in other countries, it is perhaps surprising that there are virtually no reports of organophosphorus-related toxicity in treated animals. This may be related to the dilutions involved, to the poor absorption through skin and because, in sheep at least, lanolin forms a protective barrier to absorption of the aqueous formulation. In one of the few cases reported, several sheep died after a 15-year-old sheep dip was used and this was found to have a high concentration of monothio-TEPP. In a separate incident in the same report, four yearling bulls were affected by cholinergic symptoms soon after treatment. One animal died but the others recovered.[273] As a formulated product, azamethiphos has been shown to be safe under normal circumstances of use in the Atlantic salmon, European eel, sea bass and trout. Unlike the comparable medication containing dichlorvos, there have been no reports of organophosphorus toxicity in fish treated with azamethiphos-containing formulations.[274–278]

6.5 Metaflumizone

Metaflumizone (ISO; (*EZ*)-2′-[2-(4-cyanophenyl)-1-(α,α,α-trifluoro-*m*-tolyl)-ethylidene]-4-(trifluoromethoxy)carbanilhydrazide; Figure 6.6) is a new semicarbazone insecticide. Its mode of action involves state-dependent blockage of sodium channels in insects leading to paralysis. This probably involves selective binding to the slow-inactivated state of the sodium channel, which is characteristic of the mode of action of the pyrazoline sodium channel insecticides developed during the 1970s and from which metaflumizone was derived.[279,280]

After oral administration to rats, the majority of the administered dose is excreted in faeces ($\sim$90%), with only small amounts in bile and urine. Maximum plasma concentrations were achieved after 10 to 48 hours. Once

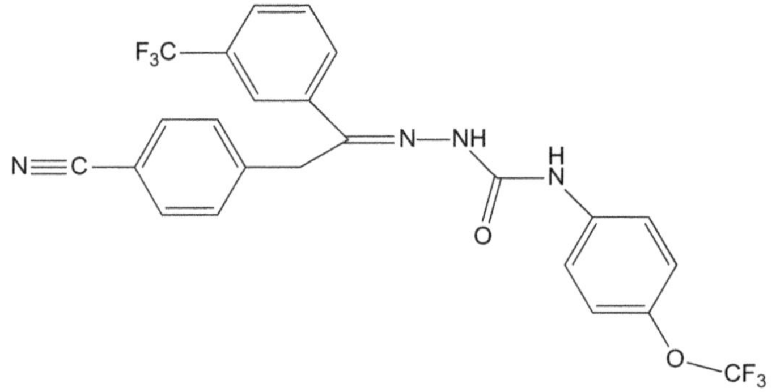

Figure 6.6   Chemical formula of metaflumizone.

absorbed, metaflumizone is metabolised by hydroxylation and hydrolysis and the metabolites formed are subject to sulfate and glucuronic acid conjugation. After dermal administration to rats for 6 hours, absorption was only 0.08 to 0.13%. Following topical application to cats and dogs, plasma levels were virtually undetectable soon after administration. Metaflumizone was well distributed throughout the hair of cats and dogs. These results suggest that metaflumizone acts locally and not systemically, at least in cats and dogs.[281,282]

As metaflumizone is a new insecticide in veterinary medicine, there are no reports of significant health effects either in treated animals or in exposed humans. The substance is of very low acute toxicity in the rat and the mouse with the acute oral LD_{50} values being > 5000 mg/kg bw in both species. It had low toxicity after inhalation exposure (4 hour, nose only) in the rat (LC_{50} > 5.2 mg/l). It was only a slight eye irritant in the rabbit and was not a skin irritant. There was no evidence of skin sensitising potential in the guinea pig maximisation test.[283]

Metaflumizone has been tested in a range of repeat-dose studies including 28-day and 13-week oral gavage studies in the rat and 90-day and 1-year studies in the dog. There were no notable effects in the rat except for a slight liver lesion at the highest dose and the NOEL was established at 60 mg/kg bw/day. Toxicity was more marked in the dog where it was given in gelatine capsules. At doses of 30 mg/kg bw/day and above, reduced food intake was seen and animals had reduced body weight gain and body weight loss. The NOEL in the dogs was 12 mg/kg bw/day. Repeat-dose studies using the inhalation route showed metaflumizone to be of low toxicity in rats. Similarly, it was of low toxicity in a 90-day dermal toxicity study, again in the rat.[283]

The substance was tested in a range of genotoxicity studies, both *in vitro* and *in vivo*, covering a range of end-points. These included studies for gene mutation, for clastogenicity and for the induction of DNA damage. Negative results were obtained for the majority of these studies but a positive result occurred in an *in vitro* assay for chromosome aberrations. However, this only occurred in the absence of metabolic activation. Moreover, negative results were obtained in an *in vivo* study for clastogenic activity, and in the mouse micronucleus test, and the compound did not induce unscheduled DNA synthesis in an assay in rats. Overall, there are no data to suggest that metaflumizone is genotoxic. In combined chronic toxicity and carcinogenicity studies in the mouse and rat, there was no increased incidence of any tumour type. In these studies, the only adverse effects were microscopic liver lesions at the two highest doses used (60 and 300 mg/kg bw/day) in rats, and brown pigment deposition in the spleen of mice at the highest dose (1000 mg/kg bw/day). The NOELs in these studies were 30 mg/kg bw/day and 250 mg/kg bw/day in rats and mice, respectively.[283]

In a two-generation study in the rat, the highest dose (75 mg/kg bw/day) resulted in maternotoxicity characterised by poor general health and reduced body weights. This resulted in high pup mortality. The NOEL for maternotoxicity was determined to be 20 mg/kg bw/day. For successive generations, the maximum dose used was 50 mg/kg bw/day, which had no effects on reproductive performance. There were no indications of teratogenic potential in the rat and rabbit although maternal toxicity occurred in both species and this was accompanied by fetotoxicity.[289]

In specific studies for neurotoxicity in the rat, one an acute study and the other a 90-day oral study, the only signs seen were of general toxicity largely in the form of poor condition. However, there were no signs indicative of neurotoxicity.[283]

There are no reports of adverse effects in humans.

6.6   Indoxacarb

Indoxacarb (Figure 6.7), like metaflumizone, is a sodium channel-blocking insecticide that has been used against lepidopteran pests. However, it has recently been given a positive opinion in the European Union by the Committee for Medicinal Products for Veterinary Use (CVMP) for use against fleas in dogs and cats by topical application. Indoxacarb is the ISO name for methyl (*S*)-*N*-[7-chloro-2,3,4a,5-tetrahydro-4a-(methoxycarbonyl)-indeno[1,2*e*][1,3,4]oxadiazin-2-ylcarbonyl]-4′-(trifluoromethoxy)carbanilate.[284–286] Indoxacarb exists as two enantiomers (*S* : *R*), also known as DPX-KN128 and DPX-KN127, respectively, but only the *S* enantiomer has insecticidal activity. There are no widely available data on indoxacarb, but it has been reviewed by the JMPR.[287]

After oral administration in aqueous vehicles, absorption in rats was saturable and was estimated to be 70 to 80% following a dose of 5 mg/kg bw but only 8 to 14% following 150 mg/kg bw. When the substance was radiolabelled in the indanone group, the half-life in rats was 45–59 hours. When radiolabelled in the trifluoromethoxy phenyl moiety, the half-life was 92 and 114 hours for males and females, respectively, suggesting some degree of biotransformation. Only low levels of indoxacarb-associated material were found in tissues. Indoxacarb is metabolised both in insects and in rats to the more toxic IN-JT333 (methyl 7-chloro-2,5-dihydro-2-[[[4-(trifluoromethoxy)phenyl]amino]carbonyl]indeno-[1,2*e*][1,3,4]oxadiazine-4a(3H) carboxylate) that was found in relatively high concentrations in fat.[287]

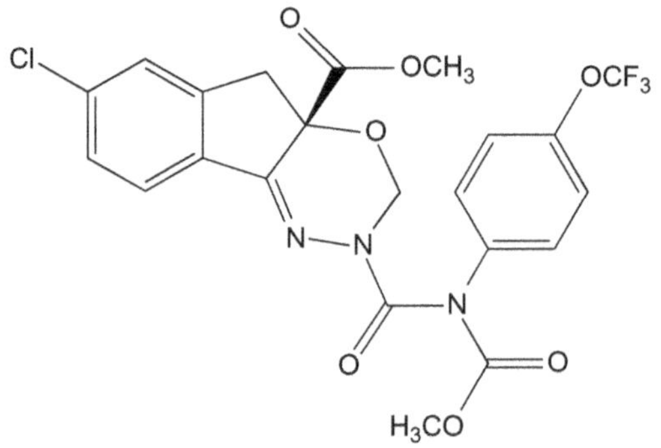

Figure 6.7   Chemical formula of indoxacarb.

Metabolism of indoxacarb is complex and, as well as IN-JT333, a range of other metabolites is formed in rats and these are further converted into sulfate and other conjugates.[287]

In acute oral toxicity studies in rats with DPX-MP062, an isomer blend containing 75% *S* and 25% *R* enantiomers and administered in corn oil, higher toxicity was noted in females where the LD_{50} value was 268 mg/kg bw compared with 1730 mg/kg bw in males. In this study, all rats given the two highest doses (3000 and 5000 mg/kg bw) died with deaths occurring up to 20 days after dosing. Clinical signs included ataxia, hunched posture and ruffled fur. After day 5, signs included general spasms, immobility, lethargy, piloerection and tremors. After dermal administration of the same isomeric mix as an aqueous paste, the LD_{50} was > 5000 mg/kg bw in both sexes. An acute inhalation study was conducted with the racemic mixture of isomers, DPX-JW062. Toxicity was low with the 4-hour LC_{50} values being 5400 mg/m^3 and 4200 mg/m^3 in males and females, respectively. Signs of toxicity included lethargy, abnormal gait and hunched posture.[287]

In mice given DPX-JW062 in the diet for 28 days, signs of toxicity included abnormal gait, head tilt and tremors. The NOEL based on reduced body weights in females was equivalent to 35.3 mg/kg bw/day. In a 90-day study in mice, similar clinical signs occurred. There were also haematological findings characterised by Heinz bodies within erythrocytes, increases in neutrophil and lymphocytes counts and an increased incidence of haemosiderosis in the spleen and liver. These effects are typical of mild haemolysis. The NOEL in this study was 5.5 mg/kg bw based on haematological effects.[287]

When rats were given DPX-JW062 in the diets for 28 days, there were no major signs of toxicity in males at dietary levels of up to 235 ppm except for reductions in body weight when compared with control values. However, three out of five females given 400 ppm and two out of five females given 235 ppm died and signs of toxicity included abnormal gait, dehydration and ruffled fur. The NOELs based on effects on body weights were 8.9 and 2.6 mg/kg bw/day for male and female rats, respectively. When administered in the diets of rats at dietary levels of up to 250 ppm for 90 days, there were no signs of toxicity except for decreased body weights and reduced food consumption in animals given the highest dietary concentrations. Evidence of haemolysis occurred in treated animals with haemosiderosis in spleens, increased reticulocyte counts and erythrocytic hyperplasia. The NOELs based on haematological effects were 2.3 mg/kg bw/day for females and 3.9 mg/kg bw/day for males. In another 90-day dietary study with rats but using DPX-MP062, evidence of haemolysis was again the main finding. Haematological findings included reductions in erythrocyte numbers and haemoglobin and increases in mean corpuscular volume accompanied by haemosiderosis, increased splenic haematopoiesis and bone marrow hyperplasia. The overall NOEL in this study was 2.1 mg/kg bw/day in females based on haemolysis.[287] Similar haemolytic effects were seen in dogs fed diets containing DPX-JW062 for periods of up to 1 year. In the 1-year dog study, the NOEL was 1.1 mg/kg bw/day based on haemolytic effects.[287]

These haemolytic effects are similar to the methaemoglobinaemia noted with aniline and its derivatives such as *p*-chloroaniline, the urea herbicides and other compounds that result in haemolysis and methaemoglobinaemia.[300–306] Some of the metabolites of indoxacarb are aniline derivatives or compounds closely related to these.

Indoxacarb gave negative results in a battery of short-term tests for genotoxicity and was not carcinogenic in animal bioassays in rats and mice. In multigeneration studies in rats, the only notable effects were parental toxicity and in developmental studies in rats and rabbits there was no evidence of teratogenic effects. However, maternal toxicity was noted in these studies and this was accompanied by decreased foetal weights.[287]

As with metaflumizone, the veterinary use of indoxacarb is new and there are no reports of adverse effects in occupationally exposed humans. Humans who have ingested indoxacarb formulations have developed methaemoglobinemia requiring methylene blue treatment and supportive care.[295–300] These effects are predictable from the animal studies (see above).

6.7   Fipronil

Fipronil (ISO; (±)-5-amino-1-(2,6-dichloro-α, α, α-trifluoro)-4-trifluoromethylsulfinylpyrazole-3-carbonitrile; Figure 6.8), a phenylpyrazole, has been used as an insecticide in agriculture for many years but has recently been introduced as an ectoparasiticide for use in companion animals. It acts by blocking chloride channels at the $GABA_A$ receptor and it is believed that it is more selective at this receptor through the β3 subunit in insects than it is in mammals, although this selectivity may be less pronounced with the sulfone metabolite and with the desulfinyl photodegradation product.[301–303]

In rats, fipronil was well absorbed after oral administration with maximum blood concentrations being achieved after approximately 6 hours. The elimination half-lives were 183 and 245 hours in male and female rats, respectively. After dermal application to rats, absorption was poor with less than 1% of the applied dose being recovered in blood, carcasses, urine, faeces and cage washings.[304]

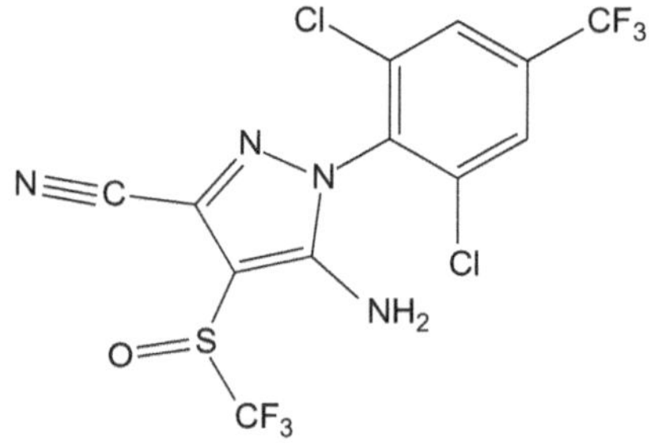

Figure 6.8   Chemical formula of fipronil.

In mammals, fipronil is metabolised through reduction, oxidation and hydrolysis. The major product of reductive metabolism is the sulfinyl compound, which is found in rat faeces and, as a conjugate, in rat urine. The sulfoxide is formed through oxidative metabolism and this is also found in the faeces of rats and, again as a conjugate, in rat urine as well as in tissues and milk of goats. The product formed from the hydrolysis of the carbonitrile group is found in the faeces and urine of rats and in goat tissues. The sulfoxide may undergo further metabolism through cleavage of the pyrazole ring or by loss of the sulfoxide moiety.[304]

Fipronil has high acute toxicity in rats and mice with oral LD_{50} values being in the range 91 to 103 mg/kg bw. The major signs seen were attributable to neurotoxicity and included convulsions, tremors, abnormal gait and hunched posture. The substance was also toxic following inhalation exposure with 4-hour nose-only LC_{50} values of 0.36 to 0.68 mg/l in rats. However, it was much less toxic after dermal application with LD_{50} values of greater than 2000 mg/kg bw in the rat when given using an aqueous vehicle. It was more toxic in the rabbit by this route when given moistened with corn oil and the LD_{50} values were 445 and 354 mg/kg bw in males and females, respectively, probably reflecting greater absorption with this lipid material.[304]

When mice were given fipronil in the diet for 13 weeks at concentrations of up to 25 ppm (equal to 3.2 and 4.5 mg/kg bw/day) there were no major sings of toxicity and the only notable effects were reduced body weight gains at the dietary level. Histopathological examination revealed the main effect to be a periacinar hypertrophy of the liver. Focal necrosis was observed in one male given the highest dietary level. As the hepatic effects were seen in mice given even the lowest dietary concentration, an NOEL could not be identified.[304]

In rats given diets containing up to 400 ppm fipronil for four weeks, there were no clinical signs of toxicity. At termination, males given 20 and 400 ppm fipronil, and females given all dietary concentrations showed increased liver weights. There was thyroid follicular cell hypertrophy in almost all treated animals and, because of this and the hepatic effects, an NOEL could not be identified. In a separate study, rats were given diets containing up to 300 ppm fipronil for 13 weeks. There was a clonic convulsion in one male given the highest dietary level of fipronil but there were no other signs attributable to compound intake. At necropsy, changes were again seen in the liver and thyroid. There were increases in relative liver weights in animals given the two highest dietary levels of 30 and 300 ppm. There was an increased incidence of thyroid follicular cell hyperplasia in animals given the highest dietary level. Based on these and other minor effects, some of which were probably related to effects on thyroid function, the NOEL was 5 ppm equal to 0.333 mg/kg bw/day.[304]

In dogs given up to 10 mg/kg bw/day fipronil orally in gelatin capsules, significant signs of toxicity were seen in high-dose animals. These included emaciation, lack of activity and hunched posture. Two dogs had to be euthanized. Other signs at the high dose included those suggestive of neurotoxicity including hypothermia, excessive salivation, convulsions, head nodding, tremors, limb jerk, ataxia and muscle twitching. Some animals also had an irregular heart rate. There were no histopathological findings that were considered to be compound related. The NOEL was 0.5 mg/kg bw/day. In a 1-year study in dogs given up to 5 mg/kg bw/day as gelatin capsules, signs of toxicity, some related to neurotoxicity, were seen at the high and intermediate (2 mg/kg bw/day) doses. These included convulsions, tremors, twitches, ataxia, abnormal gait and aggression. One male given the intermediate dose and two males given the highest dose had to be euthanized. There were no consistent histopathological findings and the NOEL in this study was 0.2 mg/kg bw/day. In a further study in dogs, fipronil was given in the diet at doses equivalent to 0, 0.075, 0.3, 1 or 3 mg/kg bw/day. As well as routine observations, neurological examinations were also carried out and blood samples were taken and analysed for triiodothyronine (T3) and thyroxine (T4). One animal given the highest dietary level was euthanized on day 32 because of poor health and evidence of neurotoxicity. Neurological examination showed an absence of visual placing reactions, depressed menace and startle reactions and abnormal gait. Other signs of toxicity included convulsions, head nodding and twitching or tremors of muscles. There were no effects on T3 or T4.[304]

Fipronil has been tested in a battery of genotoxicity tests and, generally, negative results were obtained. However, in one study, a test for the induction of chromosome aberrations in a Chinese hamster lung cell line, a positive result was obtained. This only occurred under conditions of a 6-hour pulse treatment and in the absence of metabolic activation and fipronil can be considered to be non-genotoxic.[304]

In a carcinogenicity study in mice, animals were given fipronil in the diet at concentrations of up to 60 ppm for 18 months. The only notable effects were an increased incidence of hepatocellular carcinoma in animals given the highest dietary level. This incidence was similar to that in historical controls for the testing facility concerned and was not considered to be compound related. In a study in rats, animals were given fipronil in the diet at concentrations of up to 300 ppm for one year to assess chronic toxicity while other groups were given the substance in the diet for two years. In this study evaluations were made of thyroid function by measuring T3 and T4 as well as thyroid stimulating hormone (TSH). At the highest dietary level, convulsions, sometimes fatal, were observed as well as other signs of neurotoxicity. Signs of neurotoxicity also occurred at the next dietary level, 30 ppm. T3 concentrations were not affected during treatment but were increased in females given 30 and 300 ppm from 4 weeks after treatment while T4 concentrations were depressed in male and female rats. TSH concentrations were increased in animals given 300 ppm and in males given 30 ppm fipronil in the diet. At necropsy, there was an increased incidence of thyroid follicular cell adenomas and carcinomas in animals given dietary fipronil.[304]

This increase in thyroid follicular tumours is not restricted to fipronil. Similar effects have been noted with a range of substances including several pesticides such as amitrole and fenbuconazole and with a number of pharmaceuticals including sulfadimidine (sulfamethazine), a sulfonamide antimicrobial agent. These agents are goitrogenic in rats resulting in constant stimulation of the thyroid by TSH and the eventual induction of thyroid tumours. Humans are insensitive to this mechanism of carcinogenesis and hence the results have no significance for human health.[305–316]

In a two-generation study with fipronil in rats, the main signs of toxicity were thyroid and liver hypertrophy in parental animals along with signs of neurotoxicity such as convulsions. It also resulted in decreased litter size and body weights and reduced the fertility index of parental animals. There were also reductions in post-implantation and post-natal survival. The NOEL for reproductive toxicity was 2.5 mg/kg bw/day.

Fipronil may lengthen the oestrous cycle in rats and alter concentrations of progesterone and oestradiol. In this study, where fipronil was applied topically to rats, the fertility index was also reduced.[315]

Fipronil was not teratogenic in rats and rabbits but there were indications of some degree of maternal toxicity.[304]

6.7.1 Toxicity to Humans

Ingestion of or dermal contact with small quantities of fipronil are either asymptomatic or result in short-lived, non-specific effects.[317–318] In seven cases of fipronil ingestion in Sri Lanka, generalised tonic-clonic convulsions occurred in two patients who had peak fipronil plasma concentrations of 1600 and 3744 μg/l. These patients were managed with diazepam. Another patient with a peak plasma concentration of 1040 μg/l was asymptomatic. In another case where fipronil ingestion had occurred, the patient required intubation and ventilation, and he developed seizures and pneumonia and died.[318] However, this patient may have either ingested a large dose of the agent or another substance such as endosulfan.[319,320] Surveillance data from 11 states in the USA for the period 2001 to 2007 for individuals exposed to fipronil identified 103 cases where exposure had occurred.[321] The majority of these (86%) experienced exposure in a private dwelling and of these 37% had exposure to companion animal products and 26% had occupational exposures. Most of these individuals had mild and temporary effects including headaches, dizziness and paraesthesia. Other effects included ocular, gastrointestinal, respiratory and dermal signs.[331]

6.8 Amitraz

Amitraz (ISO; *N*-methylbis(2,4-xylyliminomethyl)amine; Figure 6.9) is a formamidine insecticide that has been in widespread use in agriculture since the early 1970s.[322] It is an α_2-adrenergic receptor agonist with some partial structural similarities with the therapeutic drugs clonidine, guanfacine and guanabenz,[323] and with the acaricide chlordimeform (*N'*-(4-chloro-2-methyl-phenyl)-*N*,*N*-dimethylimidoformamide).[322,324]

The substance prolongs gastric transit time and induces bradycardia in dogs and, through its actions on central and peripheral adrenoreceptors, it may induce CNS depression and neurotoxicity, and some of its actions may be

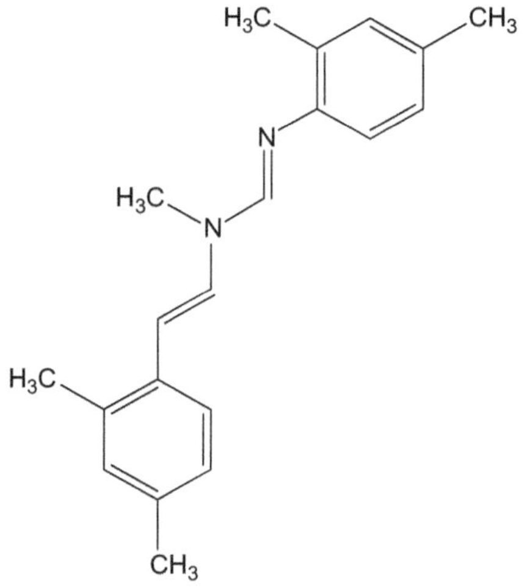

Figure 6.9   Chemical formula of amitraz.

antagonised by the action of yohimbine.[325–330] Amitraz induces glucose intolerance in rats, possibly by the inhibition of insulin release through its action on
α_2-adrenoceptors.[331] Like other α_2-adrenoceptor agonists, amitraz can
adversely affect the mammalian reproductive system by binding to presynaptic
α_2-adrenoceptors in the hypothalamus, thus inhibiting noradrenalin release and
decreasing the secretion of gonadotropin-releasing hormone. This can result in
a number of effects in mammals including decreased ovulation, decreases in
litter size and, in males, reduced sperm production.[332–334] In human luteinised
granulosa cells *in vitro*, amitraz inhibited basal and human chorionic gona-
dotropin-stimulated oestrogen production but had no effect on oestrogen.[335]
Hence, amitraz might be expected to have adverse effects on reproduction in
animal toxicology studies.

   In mice given dietary amitraz, the majority of a radiolabelled dose was
excreted in the urine. Similarly, in rats given amitraz orally, up to 85% was
excreted in urine with the remainder in the faeces. In dogs, around 80% of an
oral dose was excreted in urine, while in pigs and baboons the major part of the
oral dose was subject to urinary excretion. Following topical administration to
animals, the majority of the dose ($\sim 99\%$) was found at the application site and
systemic absorption was very low. In mammals, amitraz is cleaved to yield the
formamide and formamidine derivatives of 2,4-xylidine that may then be
subject to conjugation. In addition, the former is metabolised to 4-*N*-methyl-
formidoyl amino-*m*-toluic acid while the latter may be subject to further
biotransformation ultimately to give 4-acetamido-*m*-toluic acid and 4-amino-
m-toluic acid.[336,337]

   The major signs of acute toxicity of amitraz in mice and rats were hyperexcitability, ataxia, tremor and ptosis. Rabbits developed CNS depression,
decreased rectal temperatures and decreased pulse rates while dogs had CNS

depression, ataxia, muscular weakness and spasms, micturition and decreased rectal temperatures and pulse rates. The oral LD_{50} values in the mouse and rat were $> 1600 \, mg/kg \, bw$ and $600 \, mg/kg \, bw$, respectively, while in the dog the value was $100 \, mg/kg \, bw$.[336]

In repeat-dose studies in mice and rats, the main findings were increased aggression or irritability. Rats also had ataxia, increased nasal secretion, polyuria and body weight loss. In rabbits, decreased heart rates and rectal temperatures with a transient sedative effect were the main findings. Reduced rectal temperatures, decreased heart rates, vomiting, ataxia and CNS depression were the major findings in dogs. The lowest NOEL from these repeat dose studies was $0.25 \, mg/kg \, bw/day$ in the dog.[336]

Amitraz gave uniformly negative results in a battery of genotoxicity tests. In a mouse carcinogenicity study, there was an increased incidence of hepatocellular carcinomas in animals given in excess of the maximum tolerated dose, but in rats there was no increased incidence of any tumour type. The main findings in these studies were increases in aggressive behaviour of male mice and rats.[356]

In a rat multigeneration study, the most notable finding was a reduction in fertility and viability of offspring from the F_0 generation. The dose that produced this effect ($16 \, mg/kg \, bw$) was removed for the next generation but, nevertheless, the numbers of young alive at day 21 was reduced in all generations and the NOEL was $4.4 \, mg/kg \, bw$.[336]

There were no major effects reported in teratology studies in rats and rabbits at doses of up to $30 \, mg/kg \, bw/day$ in rats and up to $25 \, mg/kg \, bw/day$ in rabbits, administered at sensitive periods of gestation.[357] However, in a separate teratology study in rats using doses of up to $30 \, mg/kg \, bw/day$ from days 1 to 19 of pregnancy, there were increases in foetal death rates, decreases in litter size and a reduction in foetal body weight gain. There were also increases in the incidences of foetal external, visceral and skeletal anomalies at the maternotoxic dose ($30 \, mg/kg \, bw/day$) and the NOEL was $3 \, mg/kg \, bw/day$.[338] In a cross-fostering study, control pups were nursed by control dams, control pups were nursed by treated dams, treated pups were nursed by treated dams and treated pups were nursed by control dams. Pups with pre-natal exposure to amitraz showed decreases in the age for vaginal opening. Those from the group comprising treated pups and treated dams had higher locomotor activity and rearing frequency. There were no effects on the acute startle reflex or on open field behaviour.[339] Amitraz prolonged pro-oestrous in mice and resulted in lower concentrations of progesterone. Rats treated with amitraz had longer oestrous cycles resulting from prolonged oestrous or dioestrous.[336] Amitraz given orally to rats for 28 days resulted in increased relative adrenal weights; there were also decreases in mean corpuscular volume, in splenic plaque-forming cells and in the delayed hypersensitivity reactions.[340]

6.8.1 Toxicity to Humans

The major signs of acute amitraz poisoning in humans are somnolence, coma, miosis, mydriasis, bradycardia, respiratory failure, hypo- and hyperthermia and increased blood glucose concentrations. The respiratory failure may require mechanical ventilation in severe cases.[341–345] A dose of around 10 g of amitraz, accompanied by around 35 g of xylene (a commercial amitraz formulation), proved almost fatal in a 72-year-old man who drank the product by mistake. He developed dizziness, coma, miosis, respiratory failure and hyperglycaemia. However, instead of bradycardia, atrial fibrillation developed, which was successfully treated with digoxin. The individual gradually recovered over a 3-day period.[346] From double-blind cross-over trials in humans and from volunteer studies, the NOEL for effects in humans is around 0.13 to 0.3 mg/kg bw/day.[336]

In children, the main sign of toxicity is altered consciousness along with nausea and vomiting. The other major signs were coma, convulsions, respiratory depression, hyperglycaemia, miosis, mydriasis, bradycardia, hypotension, hypothermia and polyuria.[347,348]

6.9   Dicyclanil

Dicyclanil (ISO; 4,6-diamino-2-(cyclopropylamino)pyrimidine-5-carbonitrile) is an insect growth regulator used primarily to prevent blowfly strike on sheep, although it can be used against other ectoparasites (Figure 6.10).[32,349–355] It exerts its actions through the inhibition of chitin synthesis.[356–358]

Absorption from the gastrointestinal tract of rats is extensive with around 85% of the administered dose being excreted in urine. The highest concentrations of test compound were found in liver, kidneys and carcase. In the rat, a number of metabolites are formed but the major fraction ($\sim$50% of the dose) was N-4,6-diamino-5-cyanopyrimidin-2-yl)proprionamide. Other metabolites identified included 2,4,6-triaminopyrimidin-5-carbonitrile, 3-(4,6-diamino-5-cyanopyrimidin-2-ylamino)propionic acid and 2-(diamino-5-cyano-pyrimidin-2-ylamino)-3-hydroxypropionic acid as well as unchanged parent compound.[359]

In rats, the acute oral LD_{50} values were 560 mg/kg bw in males and 500 mg/kg bw in females. Signs of toxicity included piloerection, hunched posture and dyspnoea. There was reduced locomotor activity and ataxia in some males. After dermal application the LD_{50} value was $>$2000 mg/kg bw. In a 4-hour

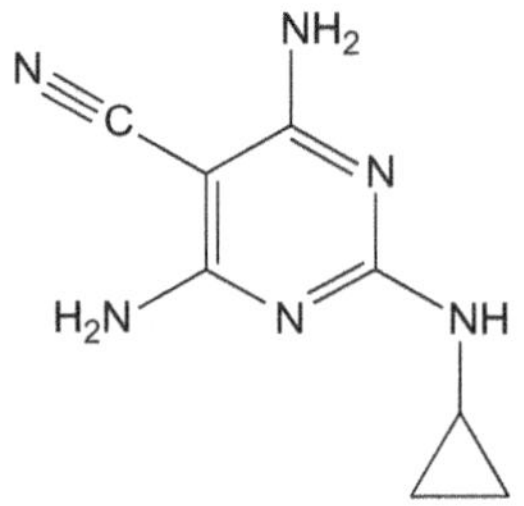

Figure 6.10   Chemical formula of dicyclanil.

nose-only acute inhalation toxicity test, the LC_{50} value was 3400 and 3000 mg/ m^3, respectively, and signs of toxicity included piloerection, hunched posture, dyspnoea and reduced locomotor activity.[359]

When groups of rats were given diets containing dicyclanil at concentrations of up to 2000 mg/kg of diet for 28 days in a range-finding study, the main sign of toxicity was piloerection. Dose-related reductions in food consumption, body weight gain and final body weights occurred in all treatment groups. Reduced spermatogenesis was noted in males given the high and intermediate (500 mg/kg of feed) dietary levels. In the corresponding females, polyovular ovaries occurred. In a 3-month dietary study in rats with dietary concentrations of up to 500 mg/kg of diet, there were no treatment-related deaths and no signs of toxicity except for reductions in body weight at dietary concentrations of 125 or 500 mg/ kg of feed. The NOEL in this study was 1.6 mg/kg bw/day. No significant signs of toxicity occurred in a 4-week study in rats where dicyclanil was applied topically at doses of up to 1000 mg/kg bw/day. Microscopic examination showed hepatic hypertrophy at 300 and 1000 mg/kg bw/day in females and at 1000 mg/kg bw/ day in males. The NOEL in this study was 30 mg/kg bw/day.[359]

Dietary concentrations of up to 2500 mg/kg of diet given to beagle dogs for four weeks resulted in those given the highest dietary concentration developing tremors, vomiting and dyspnoea. There was some evidence of testicular atrophy and focal hepatic necrosis in this group. When groups of beagles were given diets containing dicyclanil at concentrations of up to 1500 mg/kg of feed for 3 months, one high-dose male was found dead at the end of week 11 of the study. Animals in this group began to show signs of toxicity from week 11 and these included slight ataxia, raised tails and frequent shaking. At necropsy, microscopic examination revealed focal or multifocal subcapsular inflammation of the liver with fibrosis in some male and female dogs given the highest dietary concentration. High-dose males had a degree of tubular atrophy of the testes with a marked reduction in spermatogenesis. There was also an increase in inflammatory changes of the urinary bladder associated with epithelial hyperplasia in females given the 100, 500 and 1500 mg/kg of diet concentrations. The NOEL in this dog study was 0.6 mg/kg bw/day based on a number of findings including the bladder changes, increased plasma cholesterol and changes in the prostate. In a 1-year beagle dog study, animals were given diets containing up to 750 mg/kg of food. One high-dose female was found dead on day 13 of the study and one high-dose male was euthanized *in extremis* on day 32. Females given the highest dietary concentration vomited and food consumption was reduced in this group. Throughout the study, plasma cholesterol levels were increased in animals given the highest dietary level and in males given the next lower level of 150 mg/kg food. This persisted during the 4-week recovery period. Microscopic findings were limited to the two animals that died or were euthanized before the end of the study and these were considered to be incidental findings and not related to compound treatment. The NOEL in this study was 0.7 mg/kg bw/day based on increased cholesterol concentrations in plasma.[359]

Dicyclanil gave only negative results in a battery of genotoxicity tests.[359,360] In a mouse carcinogenicity study conducted over 18 months, animals were given diets containing up to 1500 mg/kg of feed. Males and females given the highest dietary concentration showed injuries obtained through excessive scratching and this group was terminated during weeks 58 to 59. At termination, the major findings were in the liver where Kupffer cell pigmentation and hepatocellular necrosis occurred in males given ≥ 100 mg/kg of dicyclanil in feed. Increases in the numbers of hepatocytes with mitotic figures and multinucleated hepatocytes occurred in high-dose males. There was an increased incidence of hepatocellular adenomas in females given the two highest doses and of hepatocellular carcinomas in females given the highest dose. The increased incidence of liver tumours occurred in animals where the maximum tolerated dose was given.[359]

Despite liver tumours in mice being common in mouse carcinogenicity studies, some workers have investigated the association between the occurrence of these neoplasms and exposure to dicyclanil. It has been suggested that they may arise from DNA damage caused by oxidative stress in the absence of direct genotoxicity and initiation activity, in combination with inhibition of apoptosis and failure to repair oxidative DNA damage.[360–364] Thus, dicyclanil-induced oxidative damage may mediate liver tumour promotion in mice.[365,390]

Dicyclanil had no notable effects in a two-generation study in rats at doses of up to 500 mg/kg bw/day and it was not teratogenic in rats or rabbits.[356]

There are no reports of significant effects in exposed humans.

6.10   Cyromazine

Cyromazine (ISO; *N*2-cyclopropyl-1,3,5-triazine-2,4,6-triamine) is a triazine derivative that, nonetheless, is similar in structure to dicyclanil (Figure 6.11) and has the same mode of action.[27,30,351,353,354,357,366,367]

After oral administration to rats, the major route of excretion is urinary with approximately 94% of the administered dose being recovered. Only small amounts (3.8%) were recovered in faeces. In a separate experiment where rats were given single oral or intravenous doses of cyromazine, similar results were obtained irrespective of the route of administration, which suggested that around 70 to 80% of the administered dose was excreted in the urine with up to 7.5% in

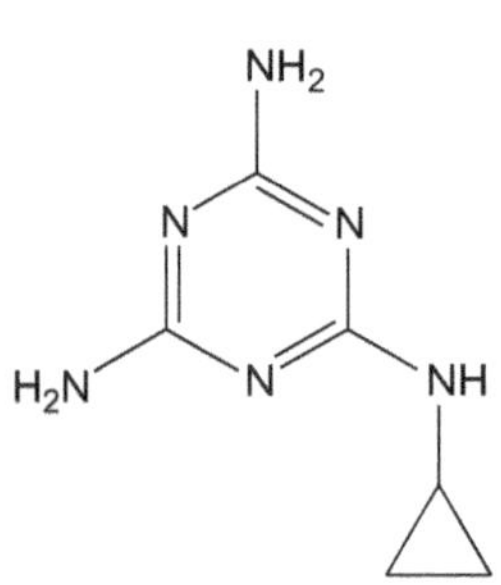

Figure 6.11   Chemical formula of cyromazine.

faeces. Plasma concentrations reached a maximum approximately 30 minutes after oral administration and rapidly declined over the next 24 hours. Extremely low concentrations were found in the tissues and carcases of treated animals. Similar findings were made in monkeys (*Macaca fascicularis*) given single oral doses of cyromazine with up to 83% of the administered dose being recovered in urine and less than 2% in faeces. After dermal application to rats, only around 5% of the applied dose was found in urine and faeces with the remainder being recovered from the application site suggesting poor absorption.[368]

The major component in rat urine was unchanged parent compound. However, there were small quantities of melamine (1,3,5-triazine-2,4,6-triamine) present along with methylcyromazine and hydroxycyromazine. In monkeys, there was a slightly higher quantity of melamine produced than in rats.[368]

The acute toxicity of cyromazine in rats is low with the acute and dermal LD_{50} values being 3387 and >3170 mg/kg bw, respectively. Similarly, acute toxicity following inhalation exposure is also low (4 hour LC_{50} 3.6 mg/l). The major signs of toxicity seen in the acute toxicity studies were sedation, dyspnoea and a curved body posture and animals recovered within 9 to 12 days. After inhalation exposure the main signs were decreased activity, piloerection and nasal discharge and animals recovered by the second day following exposure.[368]

Cyromazine was of low toxicity in repeat-dose toxicity studies where rats were given the substance for up to 90 days in the diet and rabbits were given topical administrations for 6 hours each day for 3 weeks. The NOEL values were 232 mg/kg bw/day and 2000 mg/kg bw/day, respectively. In dogs given diets containing up to 3000 ppm cyromazine for 90 days, the main findings were reductions in body weight gain at the highest dietary level. Treated animals also had increased incidences of slightly relaxed nictitating membranes when compared with controls. There were no macroscopic or microscopic findings associated with compound intake. The lowest NOEL was 300 ppm equal to 12 mg/kg bw/day based on reductions in body weight gain.[368]

In a 1-year dog study, animals were given diets containing up to 3500 ppm cyromazine. One female in the high-dose group was found dead during week 3 and one male in a group given 200 ppm cyromazine in the diet had to be euthanized during week 29 due to aggressiveness. There were no other signs of toxicity in treated animals but females given the highest dietary level had reduced body weights in the first weeks of treatment. Haematological changes included a slight hypochromic and microcytic anaemia with lower haemoglobin concentrations, erythrocyte volume fraction, mean corpuscular volume and mean corpuscular haemoglobin in high-dose males and females. The absolute and relative weights of the heart and liver were increased in high-dose males and females and in females given 800 ppm dietary cyromazine. Relative kidney weights were also increased in high-dose females. The main macroscopic and microscopic findings were in high-dose animals with a hard myocardium and severe chronic myocarditis in the right atria. There was also chronic epithelial regeneration of the kidney tubules and hypercellularity of bone marrow. The NOEL in this study was 5.7 mg/kg bw/day based on haematological findings.[368]

Cyromazine was tested in an extensive battery of tests for genotoxicity but gave uniformly negative results except in the mouse spot test where the result was inconclusive.[368]

In a carcinogenicity study in mice, animals were given diets containing up to 3000 ppm cyromazine for 2 years. There were no effects on survival. Males, but not females, showed reductions in body weight at 1000 and 3000 ppm. At termination, there was no significant increase in the incidence of tumours when compared with controls, except for a slight increase in the incidences of hepatocellular adenoma and carcinomas, notably in male mice. These were not considered to be treatment related as there was no evident dose response and the effect was limited to males. In a carcinogenicity study in rats, animals were given diets containing up to 3000 ppm cyromazine for 2 years. There were no effects on condition, behaviour or survival but there were decreases in body weights in rats given the highest dietary level. There was a higher incidence of mammary tumours in females given the highest dietary level but the values were within those of historical controls.[368]

The metabolite melamine is of low acute oral toxicity. In repeat-dose toxicity studies in mice and rats, the main findings were urinary tract calculi, with bladder ulceration associated with inflammation. Calculi were occasionally found in the kidneys.[369–371] In a mouse carcinogenicity study the major findings were in the urinary tract and consisted of acute and chronic inflammation and epithelial hyperplasia and urinary bladder calculi. In rats, chronic inflammation of the kidney was observed in some females given diets contacting melamine, and calculi were also found. Examination of the calculi showed them to be composed of melamine.[369] In a separate study in rats, administration of melamine was associated with an increased incidence of papillomas and carcinomas of the urinary bladder and ureters.[371] Similar findings were made in a further study with melamine in rats but at low doses of melamine with sodium chloride, the incidence of urinary tract lesions diminished suggesting that the associated increased urinary outputs decreased the incidence of inflammation and associated pathology.[371]

Melamine has been shown to be non-genotoxic.[368] Other chemicals that induce calculi in the urinary tract, such as saccharin, *o*-phenylphenol and uracil, have also been shown to induce tumours in the bladder and associated organs. These calculi induce inflammation, which may in turn lead to carcinogenesis.[372–380] Most of these substances probably cause calculi because of their poor solubility in water or, more specifically, in urine. It seems likely that the small quantities of melamine formed from the biotransformation of cyromazine are sufficient to result in concentrated solutions in urine and therefore in the deposition of calculi.

In a multigeneration study, dietary concentrations of 1000 and 3000 ppm cyromazine resulted in reduced parental body weights. Male fertility was reduced at 3000 ppm but reproductive performance was not affected. The lowest NOEL for parental toxicity and minor effects on offspring was 51 mg/kg bw/day.[368]

Cyromazine was not teratogenic in rats and rabbits, but maternotoxicity was observed in both species. In rabbits, this resulted in maternal deaths, abortions and decreases in body weight with embryotoxicity. The lowest NOEL from these studies was 10 mg/kg bw/day based on maternotoxicity.[368]

6.10.1 Effects in Humans

Despite extensive use of cyromazine in veterinary medicine and in crop protection, there are no reports of adverse effects in humans. There have been reports of suicide attempts with substances of the triazine class but these were generally asymptomatic, suggesting low toxicity to humans as might be expected from their low acute toxicity to animals.[381]

6.11 Benzoylureas – Diflubenzuron/Lufenuron/ Teflubenzuron

The benzoylureas, or at least those referred to here, are derivatives of 2,6-difluorobenzoylurea and they differ only in the substitution pattern of the phenyl ring attached to the terminal nitrogen of the urea group (Figure 6.12). They are insect growth regulators that act through the inhibition of chitin synthesis.[382–386] Lufenuron is used to control fleas and ticks on companion animals and, unlike many agents used to control external parasites, it is effective after oral administration; diflubenzuron and teflubenzuron are used for the control of sea lice, largely on Atlantic salmon.[42,44–46,387–391]

There are few data available on lufenuron and teflubenzuron but diflubenzuron has been reviewed by both the JMPR and by the International Programme on Chemical Safety.[392,393]

Diflubenzuron (ISO; 1-(4-chloropheny)-3-(2,6-difluorobenzoyl)urea) is well absorbed in rats and mice after oral administration with up to ∼30% of the

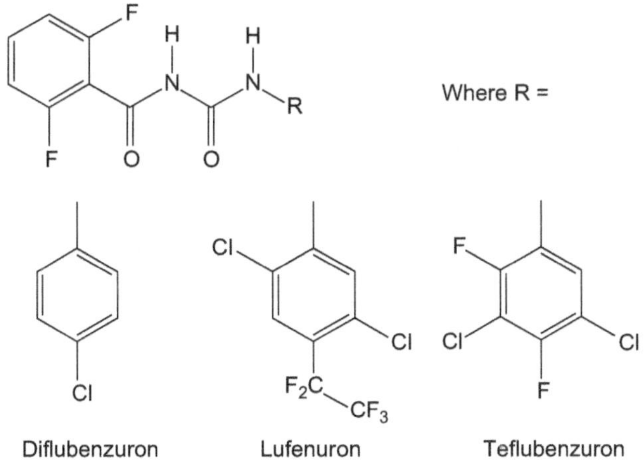

Figure 6.12 Chemical formulae of diflubenzuron, lufenuron and teflubenzuron.

administered dose being recovered from urine. The remainder was voided in faeces and only a small amount is accounted for by biliary excretion. The degree of absorption decreases with increasing dose. Thus, at 4 mg/kg bw in rats, around 42% of the dose was excreted in urine but at 1000 mg/kg bw this was reduced to only 1%. When applied topically to rats, <0.5% of the applied dose was absorbed. Similar results were obtained when diflubenzuron, as an aqueous suspension, was applied topically to rabbits.[393]

A number of metabolites are produced in rats but the major metabolic pathways give rise to 2,5-diflurobenzoic acid and 3-chloro-5-hydroxyaniline. The aniline moiety of diflubenzuron itself is hydroxylated and this and the 3-chloro-5-hydroxyaniline are subject to conjugation with sulfate and glutamate. The main metabolites formed in rats are 2-hydroxydiflubenzuron (7–10%), 4-chlorophenylurea (5–6%) and 2,6-difluorobenzamide (2–4%).[393]

Diflubenzuron has low acute toxicity with oral LD_{50} values in the mouse and rat being >4600 mg/kg bw. In rats, the dermal LD_{50} was >10,000 mg/kg bw while with whole body exposure, the LC_{50} with an unspecified exposure time was >2.9 mg/l air. No clinical signs were noted in these studies.[393]

In a 13-week feeding study in rats with dietary concentrations of up to 50,000 ppm, the main findings were chronic hepatitis, haemosiderosis, congestion of the spleen and erythroid hyperplasia of the bone marrow. These lesions increased in severity with increasing dose. There was also a degree of methaemoglobinemia. As adverse effects, notably methaemoglobinemia, occurred at all dose levels, including the lowest dose employed (160 ppm equal to 8 mg/kg bw/day), an NOEL could not be identified.[393]

In a study using dermal application, rats were given diflubenzuron in 0.25% aqueous gum tragacanth using 6-hour semi-occlusive dressings and doses of up to 1000 mg/kg bw/day. The only death in this study was incidental and there were no signs of toxicity including effects on body weights and food consumption. There were reductions in erythrocyte parameters in females given 500 mg/kg bw/day and in animals of both sexes given 1000 mg/kg bw/day. Those given 500 mg/kg bw/day also showed polychromasia, hyperchromasia and anisocytosis. The NOEL in this study was 20 mg/kg bw/day.[393]

Reductions in haemoglobin and in erythrocyte volume occurred in rats exposed to diflubenzuron by inhalation for 4 weeks. This only occurred at the highest exposure concentration (110 mg/m^3) and the NOEL was 34 mg/m^3 of air.[393]

In dogs given up to 160 ppm in food for 13 weeks, there were no mortalities and no signs of toxicity. The main findings in this study were haematological and consisted of reductions in erythrocytes and increases in haemoglobin and methaemoglobin. The NOEL was 40 ppm equal to 1.6 mg/kg bw/day. When diflubenzuron was given to beagle dogs at doses of up to 250 mg/kg bw/day for 52 weeks, there were two deaths thought not to be related to compound treatment but no other consistent differences between controls and treated animals. As with the 13-week study, the major findings in this study were haematological with increases in sulfhaemoglobin and methaemoglobin at weeks 4, 13, 26 and 52. In addition, there were decreases in haemoglobin and increases in Heinz bodies and pigmented Kupffer cells. These were seen at all dose levels (10, 50 and 250 mg/kg bw/day) but were marginal at the lowest dose of 2 mg/kg bw/day. The NOEL in this study was 2 mg/kg bw/day.[393]

Diflubenzuron has been tested in an extensive battery of tests for genotoxicity and uniformly negative results were obtained.[393,394]

In a mouse carcinogenicity study where animals were given diets containing up to 10,000 ppm diflubenzuron for 91 weeks, the major findings were again haematological and included methaemoglobinemia. However, there was no evidence of any carcinogenic effects. Rats were given diflubenzuron in the diet at concentrations of up to 160 ppm for 2 years. Once again, the major findings were haematological and included methaemoglobinemia. There was no increased incidence of any tumour type.[418]

It can be concluded that diflubenzuron is not a genotoxic carcinogen.

There were no major effects in a multigeneration study in rats, except for a reduction in pup body weight gain during lactation, with significant decreases in F_1 pup weights at days 4, 8 and 21 of lactation. The NOEL for effects on offspring was equal to 430 mg/kg bw/day. There was no evidence that diflubenzuron was teratogenic in rats or rabbits and the NOEL in both studies was the highest dose tested, 1000 mg/kg bw/day.

In summary, therefore, diflubenzuron has low mammalian toxicity and is not genotoxic or carcinogenic. However, it does cause haematotoxicity largely through the induction of methaemoglobinemia. As with indoxacarb (see earlier) some of the metabolites of diflubenzuron are aniline derivatives, compounds that are known to cause methaemoglobinaemia.[288–294]

The toxicities of lufenuron (ISO; (*RS*)-1-[2,5-dichloro-4-(1,1,2,3,3,3-hexafluoropropoxy)phenyl]-3-(2,6-difluorobenzoyl)urea and teflubenzuron (ISO; 1-(3,5-dichloro-2,4-difluorophenyl)-3-(2,6-difluorobenzoyl)urea) might be expected to be at least qualitatively similar to that of diflubenzuron. There are no toxicity data publicly available on lufenuron. However, there is a brief summary report available for teflubenzuron published by the European Medicines Agency as part of the consideration for an MRL.[395]

This shows that teflubenzuron is metabolised in rats to give similar products to those noted with diflubenzuron but in extremely low quantities and most of the orally administered dose was excreted unchanged. Like diflubenzuron, the acute toxicity was low after oral administration to mice and rats with the LD_{50} value in excess of 5000 mg/kg bw. However, in repeat dose toxicity studies in rats, mice and dogs, there was no apparent haematotoxicity, including methaemoglobinemia, perhaps reflecting the small quantities of aniline-related metabolites formed. Like diflubenzuron, teflubenzuron was not genotoxic and gave negative results in carcinogenicity studies in mice and rats. It had no appreciable effects in a two-generation study in rats and was not teratogenic in rats or rabbits.

It seems likely, therefore, that for the benzoylureas to produce haematotoxicity, and specifically to produce methaemoglobinemia, significant oral absorption is required accompanied by conversion to appreciable quantities of aniline-related metabolites. In a study of haematological effects of five benzoylphenyl urea compounds, only diflubenzuron and triflumuron resulted in haematological effects in rats.[396]

The only report of exposure in humans concerns a lactating and breast-feeding woman who accidentally ingested lufenuron. The infant was exposed to an average lufenuron dose of 0.032 mg/kg/day but no adverse effects were noted during a 7-month follow-up period.[397]

6.12 Spinosad

Spinosad (ISO; 50–95% (2*R*,3a*S*,5a*R*,5b*S*,9*S*,13*S*,14*R*,16a*S*,16b*R*)-2-(6-deoxy-2,3,4-tri-*O*-methyl-α-L-mannopyranosyloxy)-13-(4-dimethylamino-2,3,4,6-tetra-deoxy-β-D-erythropyranosyloxy)-9-ethyl-2,3,3a,5a,5b,6,7,9,10,11,12,13,14,15,16a,-16b-hexadecahydro-14-methyl1*H*-*as*-indaceno[3,2-*d*]oxacyclododecine-7,15-dione [spinosyn A] and 50–5% (2*S*,3a*R*,5a*S*,5b*S*,9*S*,13*S*,14*R*,16a*S*,16b*R*)-2-(6-deoxy-2,3,4-tri-*O*-methyl-α-L-mannopyranosyloxy)-13-(4-dimethylamino-2,3,4,6-tetra-deoxy-β-D-erythropyranosyloxy)-9-ethyl-2,3,3a,5a,5b,6,7,9,10,11,12,13,14,15,16a,-16b-hexadecahydro-4,14-dimethyl1*H*-*as*-indaceno[3,2-*d*]oxacyclododecine-7,15-dione [spinosyn D]) is a novel insecticide (Figure 6.13).[398–400] It is a biological product derived from the soil actinomycete *Saccharopolyspora spinosa* and it is active against a number of insect pests.[398]

Spinosad appears to act on the CNS causing involuntary muscle contractions and excitation of the nervous system.[401,402] However, it seems to act at a receptor site that as yet remains unidentified.[403] It is extremely effective against fleas on dogs,[404] and against head-lice in humans.[405]

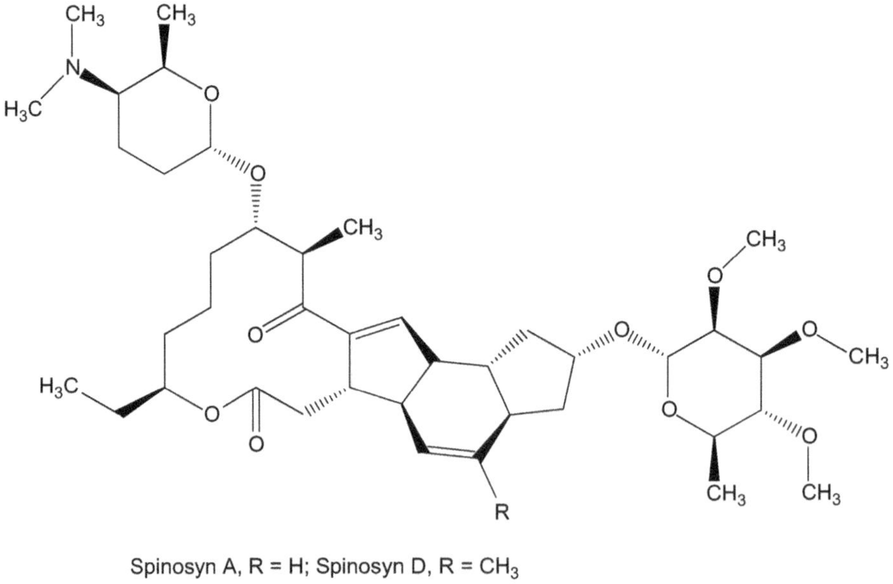

Spinosyn A, R = H; Spinosyn D, R = CH$_3$

Figure 6.13 Chemical formula of spinosad.

After oral administration to rats, the main route of excretion was faecal with up to 88% of the administered dose being voided by this route with 6 to 10% being excreted in the urine. Faecal elimination was biphasic, suggesting biliary excretion and in a study with bile duct cannulated rats 28 to 40% of the orally administered dose was excreted in the bile. The highest concentrations of substance were found in the kidneys, lymph nodes, fat and thyroid and, in males, in the liver.[393]

The major routes of biotransformation in rats were *N*-demethylation and *O*-demethylation of spinosyns A and D. The demethylation products and parent compounds were subject to conjugation with glutathione.[393]

Spinosad had low acute toxicity in the rat after oral administration in aqueous vehicles with LD_{50} values being in excess of 5000 mg/kg bw. Similar findings were made for spinosyns A and D. There were no signs of toxicity. After dermal application to rabbits the LD_{50} was in excess of 5000 mg/kg.[393]

In repeat-dose studies in mice where animals were given diets containing spinosad for 13 weeks, the main findings were intracellular vacuolation of histiocytic and epithelial cells in numerous tissues and organs including the kidneys, liver, spleen, thymus, pancreas, ovaries, cervix, vagina and epididymis, probably as a result of phospholipidosis. The NOEL for these effects was 6 mg/kg bw/day.[393,406] Similar effects were seen in repeat-dose studies in rats with dosing periods of up to 1 year and the lowest NOEL was 7.7 mg/kg bw/day.[393,407]

In a range-finding study with one animal of each sex per dose level, dogs were given diets containing up to 4000 ppm spinosad for 4 weeks. The two dogs given 4000 ppm (equal to 120 mg/kg bw/day for the male and 92 mg/kg bw/day for the female) were euthanized on day 23 because of extremely poor condition. These animals had loose or watery faeces with blood and mucous, and vomiting. There was occult blood in the urine of these animals. At 2000 ppm, there was vacuolation of several organs and tissues similar in appearance to those noted in rodent studies, while at 200 ppm microgranulomas of the liver and spleen with focal haemorrhage of the caecum occurred. A further study used dietary concentrations of up to 900 ppm for females and 1350 ppm for males, and this was given to dogs for 13 weeks. The 1350 ppm dietary level for males had to be reduced to 900 ppm at day 38 as one animal was euthanized *in extremis*. Loose and black faeces occurred in high-dose females and at week 13 the body weights of animals of both sexes given the highest concentrations were markedly reduced compared to control values. Dogs given spinosad had numerous haematological and blood biochemical abnormalities including reductions in erythrocytes, haemoglobin, lymphocytes and platelets. The haematological findings, along with bone marrow necrosis and hypercellularity seen on microscopic examination, are suggestive of the early phases of aplastic anaemia. At termination, there was vacuolation of several tissue and organ systems and the NOEL from this study was 150 ppm equal to 4.9 mg/kg bw/day. In a 12-month study in dogs where animals were given diets containing up to 300 ppm spinosad, only slight effects were noted. There were some abnormalities in clinical chemistry and the vacuolation of various tissues but only at the 300 ppm level. The NOEL in this study was 100 ppm equal to 2.7 mg/kg bw/day.[393]

Spinosad has been tested in a battery of tests for genotoxicity and only negative results were observed. It was tested in carcinogenicity studies in rats and mice with dietary concentrations of up to 360 ppm for 18 months in mice and up to 1000 ppm for up to 2 years in rats. There was no evidence of any carcinogenic effects in these studies but the vacuolation effects noted in repeat dose studies were seen in both the mouse and the rat. An NOEL of 80 ppm equal to 11 mg/kg bw/day was identified in mice and 50 ppm equal to 2.4 mg/kg bw/day in rats.[393,406,407]

The main finding in a two-generation study with rats and dietary doses equal to 0, 3, 10 or 100 mg/kg bw/day was parental toxicity with effects on the offspring. There were increases in relative and absolute liver, kidney, heart, spleen and kidney weights and vacuolation of various tissues and organs at the highest dietary concentration used. Litter sizes were reduced at this concentration and survival of pups was reduced. The NOEL for this study was 10 mg/kg bw/day.[393,408]

Spinosad was not teratogenic in developmental toxicity studies in rats and rabbits at doses of up to 200 mg/kg bw/day and 50 mg/kg bw/day, respectively. However, significant maternal toxicity was noted in both species, with some embryo- and fetotoxicity. The NOEL values for maternal toxicity were 50 and 10 mg/kg bw/day and for embryo- and fetotoxicity 200 and 50 mg/kg bw/day, in rats and rabbits, respectively.[393,409]

Hence, spinosad is of low acute toxicity but is more toxic in repeated dose studies where the major effects are vacuolation of various organs and tissues due to phospholipidosis. Phospholipidosis usually arises from inhibition of phospholipase activity and is caused by cationic amphiphilic drugs and chemicals including amiodarone, tamoxifen, gentamicin, chlorphentermine and chloroquine.[410–413]

Treatment of human patients suffering from head lice with a 0.9% spinosad topical medication resulted in only occasional and mild ocular hyperaemia and application site erythema and irritation.[405] There are no other data concerning its effects in humans.

6.13 Macrocyclic Lactones

Drugs such as abamectin and ivermectin were first introduced as anthelmintic agents and are active against a wide range of nematodes including *Ostertagia* spp. and *Strongyloides papillosus*. However, they are also active against a number of arthropod parasites of cattle and sheep including cattlegrubs and warbles (*e.g. Hypoderma bovis*), screwworm fly larvae (*e.g. Chrysoma bezziana*), mange mites including the organism responsible for sheep scab, *Psoroptes ovis*, and various ticks.[414–419] They are used in veterinary medicine to treat and control internal and external parasites and may be given orally, by subcutaneous injection or as pour-on formulations for topical application. As they are active against internal and external parasites, they are usually referred to as endectocides.

Ivermectin, a member of the avermectin group, was the first member of that group to be used in veterinary medicine and was introduced in many countries in the early 1980s.[420] Since then, a number of related compounds have been registered. These include abamectin, eprinomectin, doramectin, selamectin and emamectin benzoate. They are 16-membered macrocyclic lactones with a spiroketal component and are derivatives of naturally occurring avermectins formed as fermentation products of *Streptomyces avermitilis*.[421,422] Ivermectin itself is 22, 23-dihydroavermectin (Figure 6.14), while abamectin is a mixture of avermectin B_{1a} and avermectin B_{1b} while emamectin and eprinomectin are substituted derivatives.

Doramectin is closely related to abamectin and ivermectin but it has a cyclohexyl substituent at the 25 position, while selamectin is a derivative of doramectin. Moxidectin is a member of the milbemycin group. These are closely related structurally to the avermectins but lack the bisoleandrosyl substituent at the C-13 position (Figure 6.15).

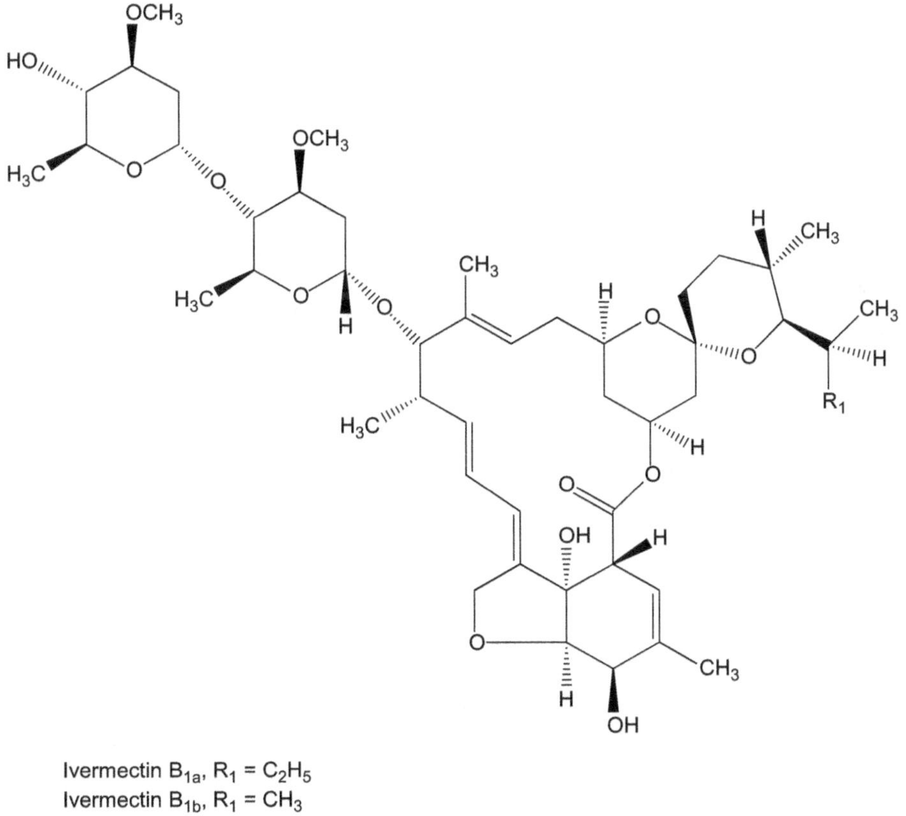

Ivermectin B_{1a}, $R_1 = C_2H_5$
Ivermectin B_{1b}, $R_1 = CH_3$

Figure 6.14 Chemical formula of ivermectin.

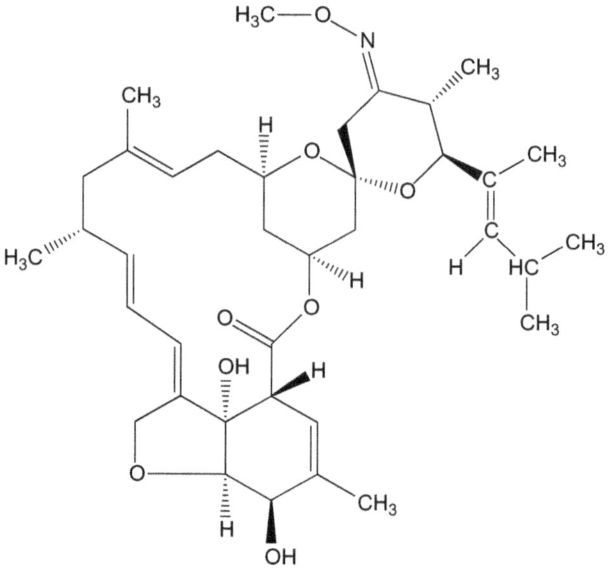

Figure 6.15   Chemical formula of moxidectin.

Eprinomectin has been developed as a broad spectrum endectocide for use topically in cattle.[423,424] As a result of its residues depletion profile, it is the only avermectin with an EU maximum residue limit (MRL) for lactating cattle or, specifically, for milk. However, the milbemycin compound, moxidectin, has MRLs for bovine and ovine milk. Selamectin is used topically for the treatment of external parasites of cats and dogs such as fleas and ear mites, and for the treatment of internal parasites including heartworm and *Toxocara* species.[425–427]

Emamectin has been widely used as an insecticide on crops and trees.[15] The major ectoparasites of farmed and wild salmon are the copepods *Caligus* spp. and *Lepeophtheirus salmonis* and emamectin benzoate and ivermectin are active against these organisms.[43,44,428–435] The use of emamectin benzoate has successfully supplemented the few other available treatments (*e.g.* hydrogen peroxide, organophosphorus compounds and cypermethrin) and replaced the off-label or illegal use of other chemotherapeutics, notably that of ivermectin.[42,436]

6.13.1   Metabolism

Virtually all of the metabolism and toxicology data on the avermectins and milbemycins have been generated to support marketing authorisation or approval dossiers in the EU, the USA or elsewhere, or dossiers for European Union maximum residue limit (MRL) applications.[2,307,436–438] As a consequence, these data are not publically available. However, the metabolism and toxicological studies for several avermectins and for moxidectin have been reviewed by the Joint FAO/WHO Expert Committee on Food Additives (JECFA), which proposes MRL values for veterinary drugs for use in the Codex Alimentarius process, while abamectin has been reviewed by the Joint Meeting on Pesticide Residues (JMPR), which conducts a similar function for pesticides.[306] Hence, there are adequate data on the safety of these substances in the public domain. Emamectin benzoate has not been formally reviewed by JECFA but it is discussed in the eprinomectin monograph. There is also a summary of the MRL evaluation prepared by the European Medicines Agency and this will be referred to here.[439–449]

After oral administration of ivermectin to rats in sesame oil, the majority of the administered dose (up to 90%) was excreted in the faeces, suggesting poor absorption from the gastrointestinal tract but absorbed ivermectin is subject to intestinal secretion.[450] Ivermectin is extremely lipophilic, and the highest concentrations were found in fat, followed by kidney, liver and muscle. Absorption is slow and peak plasma levels were reached ten days after administration.

However, after subcutaneous administration, bioavailability is much higher, at least in cattle, with 40 to 55% of the administered dose being absorbed, depending on the formulation. In pigs, plasma ivermectin concentrations were significantly higher after subcutaneous administration when compared with oral dosing.

The major compound found *in vivo* is unchanged ivermectin but there is a degree of hepatic metabolism. The major liver metabolite is 24-hydroxymethyl-H_2B_{1a} in cattle, sheep and rats. In pigs, the $3''$-O-desmethyl-H_2B_{1a} and $3''$-O-desmethyl-H_2B_{1b} compounds are the major metabolites. Similar patterns of desmethylation and hydroxylation occur with doramectin, while eprinomectin is subject to N-deacetylation. Moxidectin is excreted largely unchanged, although some minor metabolites are formed in the liver.

6.13.2 Toxicology

These compounds have been tested in a range of toxicology studies. As already mentioned, many of these data are available only as JECFA or JMPR reports, or from regulatory sources.

6.13.2.1 Acute Toxicity

Abamectin was moderately toxic to mice, rats, dogs and monkeys when given orally with LD_{50} values in the range of 11 to 41 mg/kg body weight (bw) in mice, 8.7 to 12.8 mg/kg bw in rats, approximately 8 mg/kg bw in dogs and >24 mg/kg bw in monkeys. In all cases, the major clinical signs were ataxia and tremors. The substance was less toxic when applied dermally with LD_{50} values of >330 mg/kg bw in the rat and >1600 mg/kg in the rabbit.[439,440]

When beagles were given oral doses of ivermectin in sesame oil of up to 10 mg/kg bw, signs of toxicity including emesis and salivation were noted at the two highest doses employed (5 and 10 mg/kg bw). Tremors also occurred and one dog given the highest dose became ataxic and comatose but it later recovered. In another study in beagles, mortalities occurred with doses of 40 and 80 mg/kg bw and clinical signs included emesis and salivation. It was more toxic after subcutaneous administration. No deaths occurred at doses of 20 mg/kg bw. Mydriasis and negative pupillary responses were seen in all treated animals along with tremors, ataxia, salivation and decreased activity.[441]

Reports from in-use treatment of collie dogs had already suggested that ivermectin was more toxic in some animals in this breed than in other breeds. In a study with collies, groups of four dogs were given oral doses of 50, 200 or 600 µg/kg bw ivermectin in fractionated coconut oil with 2% benzyl alcohol. One dog given 200 and one given 600 µg/kg bw ivermectin developed severe signs of toxicity including ataxia, depression, tremors, recumbency and mydriasis. The affected dog given 600 µg/kg bw was euthanized while the animal from the 200 µg/kg bw group died approximately 50 hours after administration. The affected dogs had higher concentrations of ivermectin in the central nervous system than did unaffected animals.[442]

With ivermectin, LD_{50} values were in the range 43 to 53 mg/kg bw in the rat. However, in the specific strain of mouse used in the studies, the CF-1 mouse, the LD_{50} values were in the range 12 to 57 mg/kg bw. Again, the major signs noted were tremor and ataxia with paresis, paralysis and death. Neonatal rats were more susceptible to the acute toxicity of ivermectin than adult animals with an oral LD_{50} value of 2.3 mg/kg bw. In the dog, oral LD_{50} values varied from >10 to around 80 mg/kg bw. After subcutaneous administration to this species the LD_{50} values were in the 8 to 10.5 mg/kg bw range.[441] Signs of systemic toxicity including tremor, bradypnoea and anorexia were seen in rabbits treated topically with 165, 330 or 660 mg/kg bw ivermectin and the percutaneous LD_{50} value was estimated to be 406 mg/kg bw.

Signs of neurotoxicity including depression and ataxia have been noted in cattle given 4 mg/kg bw ivermectin – four times the therapeutic dose. When given 8 mg/kg bw ivermectin, increased respiratory rate, muscular tremors, rigidity of the extremities and deaths occurred. Sheep given 4 mg/kg bw ivermectin showed signs of depression including recumbency and lack of co-ordination. Animals given 8 mg/kg bw ivermectin became ataxic and depressed. All animals were mildly depressed and lacked co-ordination 24 hours after dosing. Similar signs have been seen in horses and pigs.[441,442]

Eprinomectin appeared to be less orally toxic than either abamectin or ivermectin. Oral LD_{50} values were in the range of 70 and 55 mg/kg bw in the mouse and rat, respectively.[37] Similarly, emamectin benzoate as the solvate and as the hydrate was less toxic orally than ivermectin and abamectin, and the oral LD_{50} values in CD-1 mice were 120 and 107 mg/kg bw, respectively. However, the substance was more toxic to CF-1 mice with LD_{50} values for the hydrochloride salt of 22 and 31 mg/kg bw for male and female animals, respectively. In rats, the acute oral LD_{50} values were 88 and 76 mg/kg bw, respectively. Signs of toxicity included tremors, ataxia, ptosis, bradypnoea and loss of righting reflex.[444,445] Doramectin appeared to be slightly less toxic to mice and rats than some of the other compounds.[446]

When given orally in sesame oil to groups of mice, doses of 30, 100 and 300 mg/kg bw selamectin produced no mortalities. The major signs of toxicity were ptosis and mild piloerection at 100 and 300 mg/kg bw and increased respiration rates and moderate muscle weakness. No adverse effects occurred at 30 mg/kg bw.[425]

Moxidectin was moderately toxic to mice after oral administration with LD_{50} values of 84 (male and female) and 42–50 (female) mg/kg bw. In male and female rats, the oral LD_{50} value was 106 mg/kg bw. In mice, the main signs of toxicity were decreased activity, while in rats decreased activity, tremors, prostration, decreased respiration, hypersensitivity to touch and sound and epistaxis occurred.[447]

The acute toxicity studies with these compounds demonstrate a number of points:

- The main signs of toxicity are those of neurotoxicity
- The avermectins and moxidectin are moderately toxic after oral administration
- The CF-1 mouse, where used in these studies, appears to be more sensitive to the acute toxicity of these compounds
- Ivermectin is highly toxic to some collies and certainly more toxic in some individuals of this breed than it is to laboratory beagles
- On the limited data available, the toxicity is affected by vehicle effects with higher toxicity being seen with edible oils and less with aqueous vehicles. This is undoubtedly due to the greater solubility of these substances in lipid solvents.

6.13.2.2 Repeat-dose Toxicity

A number of repeat-dose toxicity studies have been performed with these compounds although there are no data in the public domain for selamectin. The data generated emphasise the findings from acute toxicity studies, mainly that these substances are relatively toxic and that neurotoxicity is the major form of toxicity noted.

In these studies, typical signs of neurotoxicity included decreased activity, lethargy, tremors, mydriasis, ataxia and salivation. When tested in the CF-1 mouse, emamectin, but not moxidectin, was more toxic than in the CD-1 strain. Beagles were the only breed tested in these repeat dose studies so no comparisons can be made with sensitive individuals within the collie population.[306,439–446]

Further evidence for the neurotoxic effects of these drugs was provided by histopathological examination in some studies. Dogs given 2 mg/kg bw eprinomectin for a year in an aqueous vehicle showed degeneration of some neurons in the pons area or in the cerebellar nuclei.[441] Neuronal vacuolation or degeneration in the spinal cord and sciatic nerve occurred in rats given emamectin hydrochloride in the diet for 14 weeks or longer, while emamectin hydrochloride and emamectin benzoate produced neuronal degeneration in dogs in both the peripheral and central nervous systems.[38,445]

6.13.2.3   Carcinogenicity Studies

Abamectin, emamectin and moxidectin have been tested in rodent carcinogenicity bioassays. They were not carcinogenic in these studies. There are no
publicly available data for selamectin and carcinogenicity studies are not
available for ivermectin, eprinomectin or doramectin. However, ivermectin is
similar in structure to abamectin, while eprinomectin is similar to emamectin.
Doramectin shares close similarities with the other avermectins. Moreover, all
of these substances have been tested in batteries of tests for genotoxic potential,
including tests for point mutations in bacterial systems, tests for forward
mutations in mammalian cells *in vitro* and in *in vivo* studies *e.g.* cytogenetic
assay in rat bone marrow, tests for unscheduled DNA synthesis and in the
mouse bone marrow micronucleus test.[439–441,443–447,451–459] These tests overall
gave convincingly negative results. Hence, taken together, the data strongly
suggest that these compounds are not genotoxic and are not mammalian
carcinogens.

In these long-term studies the main effects reported were neurotoxicity with
tremors, vocalisation, decreased activity and hypersensitivity to external
stimuli.

6.13.2.4   Studies of Reproductive Performance

A number of studies of reproductive performance and teratogenicity have been
conducted with these compounds with dosing usually occurring prior to conception, throughout gestation, at sensitive periods of organogenesis and into
lactation.[439–441,443–447] The doses used in these studies were limited by neonatal
or maternal toxicity and notably by neurotoxicity in some studies.[447–449,451–455]

Neurotoxicity was frequently the limiting factor in teratology studies where
the compounds were administered to experimental animals in gestation,
including through periods of critical organogenesis.[439–441,443–447] There was no
evidence for frank teratogenic effects in these studies. As with acute and repeat
dose studies, the CF-1 mouse, where used in the studies, appeared to be
uniquely susceptible to the toxic effects of these compounds.

6.13.3   Summary of Laboratory Animal Toxicity Studies

The compounds discussed here together display one main feature, that of
neurotoxicity. This is typified by mydriasis, tremors and convulsions, ataxia
and abnormalities of locomotion and, where examined, neuronal degeneration
at higher doses. Moreover, there is evidence that ivermectin may induce
behavioural effects in rats, including following perinatal exposure,[452,453] while
histopathological examination revealed degenerative lesions in the central and
peripheral nervous systems in some animals in longer term studies. From the
studies available, the CF-1 mouse and the collie dog appear to be more susceptible than other species or breeds to these effects. Of course it could well be
that the neurotoxicity is so dose limiting that other toxic effects and signs of

toxicity, which might appear at higher doses, are thus being prevented or being masked.

6.13.4 Factors Affecting Toxicity

The avermectins and milbemycins are highly lipophilic drugs. In target organisms, there is a high-affinity binding site and the physiological response to binding is an increase in permeability to chloride ions through γ-aminobutyric acid- (GABA) gated chloride ion channels.[454,455] GABA is a major neurotransmitter in target parasites and in mammals and it is likely that the avermectins and milbemycins are agonists resulting in interference with the transmission of nerve impulses.[456–464] Ivermectin and other analogues bind to GABA receptors in rat brain.[457] In mammals, GABA receptors are found largely in the central nervous system and any disruption of nerve impulses could plausibly explain the toxicity noted in both laboratory animal studies and, as will soon become apparent, in target animal adverse reactions. It is likely that many of these adverse reactions are due to overdosing. The toxicity in the CF-1 mouse provides some interesting insights.

In fact, subsequent studies have shown that a subpopulation of CF-1 mice is deficient in P-glycoprotein in the intestinal epithelium and brain endothelium and concentrations of radiolabelled ivermectin were found to be higher in brains of sensitive mice when compared to non-sensitive animals.[465] This deficiency allows greater intestinal absorption of orally administered avermectins, and higher brain penetration.[466] This sensitive population of CF-1 mice is also more susceptible to the reproductive effects of the avermectins. In a susceptible population of CF-1 mice, 100% of animals were affected by cleft palate while in the non-sensitive population there was almost a zero incidence at the same doses.[467] P-glycoprotein is a protein pump encoded for by a gene known as *MDR1* or *ABCB1*. It is one of a number of proteins belonging to an ATP-binding class and where present can lead to drug resistance (or lowered susceptibility to toxicity).[468] It was so named because of the over-expression noted in multidrug resistant human tumour cells.[469] Deficiency or disruption of this gene or inhibition of P-glycoprotein leads to enhanced absorption or organ exposure, including enhanced brain penetration, to a number of drugs including ivermectin.[470–476] P-glycoprotein deficiency also leads to higher foetal exposure to some drugs.[477] Similar effects can be achieved by pharmacological blocking of P-glycoprotein.[416,478]

In the CF-1 mouse, this sensitive population constitutes around 25% of the animals. These mice have been shown to have low or absent P-glycoprotein in brain endothelial cells and they are those with the higher sensitivity to the effects of the macrocyclic lactones.[465–467]

There may be significant differences in the disposition of these macrocyclic lactones. For example, in P-glycoprotein-deficient mice, ivermectin and eprinomectin, but to a much lesser extent moxidectin, were excreted by the intestine through a P-glycoprotein-dependent pathway, whereas moxidectin excretion was P-glycoprotein independent. All three drugs accumulated in the brains of these mice but eprinomectin concentrations were lower, possibly because eprinomectin disposition is controlled by P-glycoprotein efflux.[479]

6.14   Adverse Effects in Target Species

Data on adverse effects in target animals are often difficult to access. Much of this information is reported to regulatory authorities by veterinarians, by manufacturers and by the public, under regulatory pharmacovigilance schemes, and it largely remains confidential.[1,480,481] However, some data can be accessed from the website of the US Food and Drug Administration's CVM, where there are cumulative summaries from 1987 to 2009.[482] Some caution must be applied to these data because, although there is a numerator in these lists in the form of the numbers of animals with adverse events, there is no indication of the total numbers of animals treated. Hence no measure of incidence can be applied to the numbers. Similarly, for all drugs cited in the list there is no way of relating the number of animals affected with each clinical sign. There are also no data on doses given and so it is not possible to relate adverse drug reactions and clinical toxicity to (for example) overdosing.

In cats, the adverse drug reactions signs include those typical of neurotoxicity including ataxia, depression, mydriasis, staggering, collapse and facial trembling.[482] These have similarities with case reports where recumbency, lethargy, weakness, blindness, ataxia, tachycardia and coma have been noted.[483–486] Many of the findings are typical of toxicity resulting from overdose.[487,488] Doses of 200 to 1330 µg/kg bw are said to be generally tolerated in cats,[487] but the oral therapeutic dose is between 24 and 48 µg/kg bw/day,[489] and higher doses may be toxic in individual animals.

Selamectin has been developed specifically for use in cats and dogs and has been shown to be effective against internal parasites and fleas in both species.[425–427,490] Its safety has been studied extensively in cats at the therapeutic topical dose range of 6 to 12 mg/kg bw and no adverse effects were seen.[491]

In dogs, the therapeutic oral dose of ivermectin is between 6 and 12 µg/kg bw[489] and doses of 50 to 500 µg/kg bw may be tolerated.[487,492] Adverse reactions in 1165 dogs given ivermectin orally included the familiar signs of neurotoxicity.[116] Similar signs have been reported in the literature.[493]

Moxidectin is authorised in some countries for the treatment of heartworm in dogs with oral therapeutic doses of 3 µg/kg bw.[489,492] The well recognised signs of neurotoxicity with moxidectin in dogs are similar to those noted with the avermectins.[488] These effects were among those observed and reported among 369 dogs exposed orally to moxidectin and in 6 dogs exposed topically and reported to the CVM.[482]

As already alluded to, one of the major concerns with the use of ivermectin or other macrocyclic lactones in dogs is the increased sensitivity to these compounds shown by some animals in the collie dog population as a result of the homozygous occurrence of the nt230 (del 4) deletion in the *MDR1* gene and defective P-glycoprotein allowing greater intestinal and brain permeability.

Ivermectin and the related compounds are more toxic to susceptible individuals in this breed,[442,487] and this has been noted with ivermectin, doramectin and moxidectin,[494–502] although moxidectin appears to be less toxic than ivermectin,[500–506] while ivermectin was less toxic when administered in a beef formulation.[505] The young of other breeds may be more sensitive.[100] Some breeds including the White Swiss shepherd dog, Australian shepherds and long-haired whippets also have this mutation and may be susceptible not only to the macrocyclic lactones but also to other drugs dependent on P-glycoprotein.[480,507–516] It should be noted that as with the CF-1 mouse and collie dog, not all animals are susceptible and only a proportion of animals in these breeds are likely to be exquisitely sensitive to the effects of these drugs.[487,496] For example, in a small population (40) of collie dogs, 22% were homozygous for the normal gene, 42% were heterozygous and 35% were homozygous for the mutant.[514]

Reactions including anorexia, lethargy, pyrexia and emesis and a shock-like syndrome have been seen following ivermectin treatment of dogs infected with microfilariae.[517–520] These reactions may be attributable to toxicity but they may also be due to the effects of dying parasites and thus may be analogous to the Mazzotti reaction noted in humans (see the next section). They have been noted with other drugs used in dogs for this condition including moxidectin.[173,521–525] Consumption of moxidectin-containing equine products has resulted in toxicity in dogs, which in turn has given rise to regulatory concerns.[526–528]

Selamectin, as already described, has been developed as an endectocide specifically for use in cats and dogs.[425,426,488,529] It has been extensively studied for safety in the dog at its topical target dose range of 6 to 12 mg/kg bw.[530] Examination of the CVM cumulative list reveals 98 dogs orally exposed to selamectin displaying a range of clinical signs including depression and lethargy, hypersalivation, convulsions, trembling, weakness, ataxia and collapse.[482] For topical application there are a total of 11,427 animals that have been evaluated with a spectrum of clinical signs including lack of expected efficacy and signs that are unrelated to neurotoxicity. However, reactions suggestive of neurotoxicity have been noted.

Signs of neurotoxicity with ivermectin and eprinomectin have also been reported in horses and cattle.[482] In equines, these signs may include blindness and convulsions.[531–538] Similarly, in cattle, oral exposure to ivermectin has produced anorexia, depression, lethargy and collapse.[524] Neurotoxicity has been observed in cattle after treatment with doramectin and eprinomectin.[539–541] Neurological signs have been reported in Murray Grey cattle given therapeutic doses of abamectin.[541] Protruding tongues resulting from lingual paralysis were noted in some animals and there were a number of deaths. In a clinical investigation under controlled conditions, 208 Murray Grey cattle were given the drug strictly in accordance with label requirements and one animal developed neurological signs. These findings suggest that this breed may be more sensitive to the effects of avermectins than others. The authors suggested that the drug may be able to reach the CNS in this breed more easily than in other breeds. This is reminiscent of the P-glycoprotein phenomenon discussed in relationship to other animal strains and breeds. However, there is no firm evidence to support this in Murray Grey cattle, although, not surprisingly, P-glycoprotein plays a role in ivermectin transport in bovine blood vessels.[542] However, this breed also has other mutations that result in neurological signs, including those that lead to spinal myelinopathy and mannosidosis,[543–545] and such conditions might confound the effects of drugs.

Adverse reactions, including signs of neurotoxicity with ivermectin, doramectin, selamectin and moxidectin, have been reported in several species including goats, sheep, pigs, ferrets and rabbits, as well as in some exotic species.[546]

6.15 Human Toxicity

Other species or breeds known to be susceptible to the toxicity of the avermectins and other drugs, such as the collie mentioned earlier and the White Swiss Shepherd dog, have been shown to have individuals with mutations of the *MDR1* gene[547–549] and there are concerns that P-glycoprotein polymorphisms in humans could result in increased susceptibility to the toxicity of ivermectin.[550–554] Ivermectin, as *Mectizan*, has been widely used in humans for the treatment and prophylaxis of filariasis due to *Wucheria bancrofti*, onchocerciasis caused by *Onchocerca volvulus*, loiasis, scabies and strongyloidiasis.[2,555–568] Treatments usually consist of 150 μg/kg body weight (or approximately 10 mg for a 70 kg adult) and adverse reactions are rare and mild.[563–569] A high oral dose of avermectin (414 mg/kg bw) resulted in coma, myoclonus and polyneuropathy.[570] The most common adverse reaction seen with ivermectin in humans is also a marker of its success. This is the Mazzotti reaction, which is an immune response to dying parasites characterised by urticaria, fever, swollen lymph nodes, arthralgias, hypotension, tachycardia, oedema and abdominal pain.[571–574] Under some circumstances, particularly when the initial parasite burden is high, this may be severe[571–576] and has been observed with other drugs including diethylcarbamazine and praziquantel.[577–579] This may be due to neutrophil granule activation,[546,580] possibly induced by a myosin-like antigen released from the muscle of the parasite.[581] An encephalopathy associated with ivermectin treatment of onchocerciasis-infected patients in *Loa loa* endemic areas remains of uncertain origin although this too is probably associated with parasite burden.[582,583] However, treatment with ivermectin or with ivermectin plus diethylcarbamazine is generally safe.[584] When toxicity does occur in humans it is usually as a result of doses higher than those for therapeutic purposes. Patients are likely to experience hypotension, respiratory failure, coma and, in extreme circumstances, death.[585]

Oral ingestion of small amounts of abamectin was generally asymptomatic. However, oral doses of around 23 mg/kg bw produced minor symptoms. More severe effects were produced by doses of around 15 mg/kg bw ivermectin and 115 mg/kg bw abamectin, including coma, aspiration with respiratory failure and hypotension. Of seven affected patients, six recovered after intensive supportive care but one later died with multiple organ failure.[586]

6.16 Conclusions

There are a number of agents, indeed classes of agents, available to treat animals suffering from ectoparasitic disease, or indeed to prevent such disease. Their pharmacologic effects are exerted through a number of mechanisms, although the majority are neurotoxic. They can exert a variety of toxic effects and, quite frequently, these effects are related to the pharmacodynamic activity of the agent. However, these compounds are important components of the armoury against parasitic disease in animals (and occasionally, in humans), and when used properly and, in accordance with label recommendations, are effective and safe for users and for others potentially exposed.

The macrocyclic endectocides are exceptionally effective veterinary drugs that have revolutionised the treatment of several diseases including those caused by internal and external parasites. Prior to their introduction there were only two classes of drug available for the treatment of internal parasites, levamisole/tetramisole and the benzimidazoles. The introduction of the macrocyclic lactones not only provided a third class of drugs but also offered greater scope for the rotation of drug class as an aid in avoiding the build-up of parasite resistance. Over the years since their individual introductions, countless millions of doses have been administered safely and effectively to animals and, in the case of ivermectin, to humans. These are very important pieces of information that cannot be overemphasised – these drugs are highly effective, offer alternatives to existing drug classes and when used according to label recommendations are extremely safe.

However, these compounds do exert toxic effects and neurotoxicity is the predominant finding. This is particularly true in subpopulations of laboratory and other animals with mutations in the *MDR1* gene, which predisposes to nervous system exposure.

In clinical veterinary use, adverse drug reactions to these drugs do occur. Neurological effects, typical of those noted in preclinical toxicity, studies are frequently observed. Although the data do not allow for further analysis it is likely that the majority of these arise from overdosing, from miscalculation of doses during off-label use and in animals with sensitivity to the toxic effects of this group of drugs.[456,587] In fact there are several reports of ivermectin toxicity in animals following off-label use, including mice, rhesus macaque, fruit bats, a chameleon, chelonians and chickens.[588–593] Off-label use of ivermectin in farmed salmon may result in toxicity with listlessness, inappetance and death.[594–596] Younger animals with more permeable blood-brain barriers may be more susceptible to the toxic effects of these substances than adults.

There have been no major reports of toxicity in humans potentially exposed to the macrocyclic lactones and the data available suggest that ivermectin is safe, at least at therapeutic doses.[587,597]

References

1. K. N. Woodward, Veterinary pharmacovigilance in the European Union in *Veterinary Pharmacovigilance: Adverse Reactions to Veterinary Medicinal Products*, ed. K. N. Woodward, Wiley-Blackwell, Chichester, 2009, pp. 19–46.

2. K. N. Woodward, Regulation of veterinary drugs in *General and Applied Toxicology*, ed. B. Ballantyne, T. Marrs and T. Syversen, MacMillan Reference, Basingstoke, 2nd edn, 2000, pp. 1633–1652.
3. K. N. Woodward, Veterinary Pharmacovigilance. Part 1. The legal basis in the European Union, *Vet. Pharmacol. Ther.*, 2005, **28**, 131–147.
4. P. Frank and J. H. Schafer, Animal health products in *Regulatory Toxicology*, ed. S. C. Gad, Taylor and Francis, London, 2nd edn, 2001, pp. 70–84.
5. R. G. Endris, V. E. Reuter, J. D. Nelson and J. O. Nelson, Efficacy of 65% permethrin applied as a topical spot-on against walking dandruff caused by the mite, *Cheyletiella yasguri*, in dogs, *Vet. Ther.*, 2000, **1**, 273–279.
6. R. G. Endris, R. Everett, J. Cunningham, T. L. Katz and K. Thompson, Efficacy of two 65% permethrin spot-on formulations against canine infestations of *Ctenocephalides felis* and *Rhipicephalus sanguineus*, *Vet. Ther.*, 2002, **3**, 326–332.
7. R. G. Endris, D. Cooke, D. Amodie, D. L. Sweeney and T. l. Katz, Repellency and efficacy of 65% permethrin and selamectin spot-on formulations against *Ixodes ricinus* ticks on dogs, *Vet. Ther.*, 2002, **3**, 64–71.
8. R. Molina, J.-M. Lohse and J. Nico, Evaluation of a topical solution containing 65% permethrin against the Sandfly (*Phlebotomus perniciosus*) in dogs, *Vet. Ther.*, 2001, **2**, 261–267.
9. J. E. Hillerton, A. M. Bramley and N. H. Yarrow, Control of flies (Diptera: *muscidae*) on dairy heifers by Flectron ear-tags, *Br. Vet. J.*, 1985, **141**, 160–167.
10. N. French, A. J. Wright, W. R. Wilson and D. B. R. Nichols, Control of headfly on sheep, *Vet. Rec.*, 1977, **100**, 40–43.
11. H. D. Bailie and D. W. T. Morgan, Field trials to assess the efficacy of permethrin for the control of flies on cattle, *Vet. Rec.*, 1980, **106**, 124–127.
12. J. A. Harris, J. E. Hillerton and S. V. Morant, Effect on milk production of controlling muscid flies, and reducing fly-avoidance behaviour, by the use of fenvalerate ear tags during the dry period, *J. Dairy Res.*, 1987, **54**, 165–171.
13. J. E. Hillerton, S. V. Morant and J. A. Harris, Control of Muscidae on cattle by flucythrinate ear-tags, the behaviour of these flies on cattle and the effects on fly-dislodging behaviour, *Entomol. Exp. Appl.*, 1986, **41**, 213–218.
14. R. N. Titchener, Insecticidal ear tags control cattle ectoparasiticides, *Parasitol. Today*, 1986, **2**, 26–27.
15. J. A. Shemanechuk, Repellent action of permethrin, cypermethrin and resmethrin against black flies (*Simulium* spp.) attacking cattle, *Pestic. Sci.*, 1981, **12**, 412–416.
16. M. H. Muma, B. E. Hill, E. Hixon and L. Harries, Control of sheep-ticks on feeder lambs, *J. Econ. Entomol.*, 1952, **45**, 833–838.
17. D. W. Tarry, The sheep head fly and the problem of pasture flies, *ADAS Q. Rev.*, 1976, **23**, 283–293.

18. M. J. Hall, Traumatic myiasis of sheep in Europe: a review, *Parassitologia*, 1997, **39**, 409–413.
19. J. M. Brougham and R. Wall, Fly abundance and climate as determinants of sheep blowfly strike incidence in southwest England, *Med. Vet. Entomol.*, 2007, **21**, 231–238.
20. B. Bisdorf and R. Wall, Sheep blowfly strike risk and management in Great Britain: a survey of current practice, *Med. Vet. Entomol.*, 2008, **22**, 303–308.
21. S. E. Aiello and A. Mays (ed.), Flies in *The Merck Veterinary Manuel*, Merck & Co. Inc., New Jersey, 8th edn, 1998, pp. 637–658.
22. P. Bates, Sheep scab (*Psoroptes ovis*) in *Diseases of Sheep*, ed. I. D. Aitken, Blackwell Publishing, Oxford, 2007, pp. 321–325.
23. A. H. van den Broek and J. F. Huntley, Sheep scab: the disease, pathogenesis and control, *J. Comp. Pathol.*, 2003, **128**, 79–81.
24. P. Bates, M. Rankin, D. Clifford and L. Stubbings, Shower dipping in diazinon or cypermethrin dipwash to control ovine psoroptic mange (sheep scab), *Vet. Rec.*, 2005, **156**, 655.
25. R. Wall and P. Bates, Sheep scab control using trans-cinnamic acid, *Vet. Parasitol.*, 2011, **175**, 129–134.
26. B. Harvey, M. Bakewell, T. Felton, K. Stafford, G. C. Coles and R. Wall, Comparison of traps for the control of sheep blowfly in the U.K., *Med. Vet. Entomol.*, 2010, **24**(2), 210–213.
27. B. Lonsdale, D. W. Tarry, F. L. Bowen and D. G. Stansfield, Cyromazine pour-on for the prevention of cutaneous myiasis of sheep, *Vet. Rec.*, 1990, **126**, 207–210.
28. W. N. Beesley, Sheep dipping, with special reference to the UK, *Pest. Outlook*, 1994, **5**, 16–21.
29. R. Wall, N. P. French and A. Fenton, Sheep blowfly strike: a model approach, *Res. Vet. Sci.*, 2000, **69**, 1–9.
30. D. J. O'Brien and G. Fahey, Control of blowfly strike in sheep by means of a pour-on formulation of cyromazine, *Vet. Rec.*, 1991, **129**, 351–353.
31. F. L. Bowen, P. Fisara, P. Junquera, D. T. Keevers, R. H. Mahoney and H. R. Schmid, Long-lasting prevention against blowfly strike using the insect growth regulator dicyclanil, *Aust. Vet. J.*, 1999, **77**, 454–460.
32. B. Lonsdale, H. R. Schmid and P. Junquera, Prevention of blowfly strike on lambs with the insect growth regulator dicyclanil, *Vet. Rec.*, 2000, **147**, 540–544.
33. B. L. Blagburn, D. R. Young, J. A. Meyer, A. Leigh-Effron, T. Paarlberg, A. G. Zimmermann, D. Mowrey, S. Wiseman and D. E. Snyder, Effects of orally administered spinosad (Comfortis) in dogs on adult and immature stages of the cat flea (*Ctenocephalides felis*), *Vet. Parasitol.*, 2010, **168**, 312–327.
34. D. E. Snyder, A. G. Zimmermann, M. Qiao, S. J. Gissendanner, L. R. Cruthers, R. L. Slone and D. R. Young, Preliminary studies on the effectiveness of the novel pulicide, spinosad, for the treatment and control of fleas on dogs, *Vet. Parasitol.*, 2007, **150**, 345–351.

35. M. K. Rust, Advances in the control of *Ctenophalides felis* (cat flea) on cats and dogs, *Trends Parasitol.*, 2005, **21**, 232–236.
36. R. Marsella, Advances in flea control, *Vet. Clin. North Am. Small Anim. Pract.*, 1999, **29**, 1407–1424.
37. M. W. Dryden, Flea and tick control in the 21st century: challenges and opportunities, *Vet. Dermatol.*, 2009, **20**, 435–440.
38. T. Schneider, S. Wolken and N. Mencke, Comparative efficacy of imidacloprid, selamectin, fipronil-(S)methoprene, and metaflumizone against cats experimentally infested with *Ctenocephalides felis*, *Vet. Ther.*, 2008, **9**, 176–183.
39. M. Franc and E. Bouhsira, Efficacy of a combination of fipronil-(S)-methoprene spot-on formulation and a deltamethrin-impregnated collar in controlling fleas and sandflies on dogs, *Vet. Ther.*, 2009, **10**, 71–77.
40. B. L. Blagburn and M. W. Dryden, Biology, treatment and control of flea and tick infestations, *Vet. Clin. North Am. Small Anim. Pract.*, 2009, **39**, 1173–1200.
41. K. N. Woodward, Veterinary pesticides in *Mammalian Toxicology of Insecticides. Issues in Toxicology No. 12*, ed. T. C. Marrs, Royal Society of Chemistry, Cambridge, 2012, pp. 348–426.
42. M. Roth, R. H. Richards and C. Sommerville, Current practices in the chemotherapeutic control of sea lice infestations in aquaculture: a review, *J. Fish Dis.*, 1993, **16**, 1–26.
43. J. Stone, I. H. Sutherland, C. S. Sommerville, R. H. Richards and K. J. Varma, The efficacy of emamectin benzoate as an oral treatment of sea lice, *Lepeophtheirus salmonis* (Krøyer) infestations in Atlantic salmon, *Salmo salar* L, *J. Fish Dis.*, 1999, **22**, 261–270.
44. B. M. MacKinnon, Sea lice: a review, *World Aquac.*, 1997, **28**, 5–10.
45. M. Roth, The availability and use of chemotherapeutant sea lice control products, *Contrib. Zool.*, 2000, **69**, http:dpc.uva.nl/ctz/vol69/nr01/art12.
46. M. J. Costello, Review of methods to control sea lice (Caligidae: Crustacea) infestations on salmon (*Salmo salar*) farms in *Pathogens of Wild and Farmed Fish: Sea Lice*, ed. G. A. Boxall and D. Defaye, Ellis Horwood, London, 1993, pp. 219–252.
47. W. N. Aldridge, An assessment of the toxicological properties of pyrethroids and their neurotoxicity, *Crit. Rev. Toxicol.*, 1990, **21**, 89–103.
48. D. W. Gammon, M. A. Brown and J. E. Casida, Two classes of pyrethroid action in the cockroach, *Pest. Biochem. Physiol.*, 1981, **15**, 181–191.
49. H. P. M. Vijverberg and J. van den Bercken, Neurotoxicological effects and the mode of action of pyrethroid insecticides, *Crit. Rev. Toxicol.*, 1990, **21**, 105–126.
50. H. P. M. Vijverberg, J. M. van den Zalm and J. van den Bercken, Similar mode of action of pyrethroids and DDT on sodium channel gating in myelinated nerves, *Nature*, 1982, **295**, 601–603.
51. J. R. Coats, Mechanisms of toxic action and structure relationships for organochlorine and synthetic pyrethroid insecticides, *Environ. Health Persp.*, 1990, **87**, 255–262.

52. T. Narahashi, Nerve membrane ionic channels as the primary target of pyrethroids, *Neurotoxicology*, 1985, **2**, 3–22.
53. L. Pap, D. Bajomi and I. Székely, The pyrethroids. An overview, *Int. Pest Control*, 1996, **38**, 15–19.
54. J. R. Bloomquist, P. M. Adams and D. M. Soderlund, Inhibition of gamma-amino butyric acid-stimulated chloride flux in mouse brain vesicles by polychlorocycloalkane and pyrethroid insecticides, *Neurotoxicology*, 1986, **7**, 11–20.
55. J. M. Barnes and R. D. Verschoyle, Toxicity of new pyrethroid insecticides, *Nature*, 1974, **248**, 711.
56. L. O. Ruzo, J. L. Engel and J. E. Casida, Decamethrin metabolites from oxidative, hydrolytic and conjugative reactions in mice, *J. Agric. Food Chem.*, 1979, **27**, 725–731.
57. L. J. Lawrence and J. E. Casida, Pyrethroid toxicology: mouse intracerebral structure-toxicity relationships, *Pest. Biochem. Physiol.*, 1982, **18**, 9–14.
58. B. Gassner, A. Wüthrich, A, G. Scholtysik and M. Solioz, The pyrethroids permethrin and cyhalothrin are potent inhibitors of the mitochondrial complex I, *J. Pharmacol. Exp. Ther.*, 1997, **281**, 855–860.
59. J. Miyamoto, Degradation, metabolism and toxicity of synthetic pyrethroids, *Environ. Health Perspect.*, 1976, **14**, 15–28.
60. Joint FAO/WHO Expert Committee on Food Additives, *Toxicological Evaluation of Certain Veterinary Drug Residues in Food*, WHO Food Additive Series 45, The Fifty-fourth Meeting of the Joint FAO/WHO Expert Committee on Food Additives International Programme on Chemical Safety, World Health Organization, Geneva, 2000, pp. 41–74.
61. G. Chester, N. N. Sabathy and B. H. Woollon, Exposure and health assessment during application of lambda-cyhalothrin for malaria vector control in Pakistan, *Bull. World Health Organ.*, 1992, **70**, 615–619.
62. International Programme on Chemical Safety, Environmental Health Criteria 99, *Cyhalothrin*, World Health Organization, Geneva, 1990.
63. M. A. Campana, A. M. Panzeri, V. J. Moreno and F. N. Dulout, Genotoxic evaluation of the pyrethroid lambda-cyhalothrin using the micronucleus test in erythrocytes of the fish *Cheirodon interruptus interruptus*, *Mutat. Res.*, 1999, **438**, 155–161.
64. A. Çelik, B. Mazmanci, Y. Çamlica, A. Aşkin and U. Çömelekoğlu, Induction of micronuclei by lambda-cyhalothrin in Wistar rat bone marrow and gut epithelial cells, *Mutagenesis*, 2005, **20**, 125–129.
65. P. B. Desmukh, Three-generation study of a synthetic pyrethroid – cyhalothrin, *Toxicol. Letters*, 1992, **64/65**, 770–781.
66. M. de Silva Gomes, M. M. Bernardi and H. de Souza Spinosa, Effects of prenatal pyrethroid insecticide exposure on the sexual development of rats, *Vet. Hum. Toxicol.*, 1991, **33**, 427–428.
67. V. C. Moser, Screening approaches to neurotoxicity: A functional observational battery, *J. Am. Coll. Toxicol.*, 1989, **8**, 85–93.

68. V. C. Moser, J. P. McCormick, J. P. Creason and R. C. MacPhail, Comparison of chlordimeform and carbaryl using a functional observational battery, *Fund. Appl. Toxicol.*, 1988, **11**, 189–206.
69. V. C. Moser and R. C. MacPhail, Comparative sensitivity of neurobehavioral tests for chemical screening, *Neurotoxicol.*, 1990, **11**, 335–354.
70. M. Hornychová, E. Frantik, J. Kubát and J. Formánek, Neurotoxicity profile of supermethrin, a new pyrethroid insecticide, *Centr. Eur. J. Publ. Health*, 1995, **3**, 210–218.
71. International Programme on Chemical Safety, Environmental Health Criteria 97, *Deltamethrin*, World Health Organization, Geneva, 1990.
72. Joint FAO/WHO Meeting on Pesticide Residues. Pesticide Residues in Food – 2000, Evaluations 2000. Part II – Toxicological, World Health Organization, Geneva, 2001.
73. A. Anadón, M. R. Larrañaga, M. Fernandez-Cruz, M. J. Diaz, M. C. Fernandez and M. A. Martinez, Toxicokinetics of deltamethrin and its 4′-hydroxy metabolite in rat, *Toxicol. Appl. Pharmacol.*, 1996, **141**, 8–16.
74. L. M. Cole, L. O. Ruzo, E. J. Wood and J. E. Casida, Decamethrin metabolites from oxidative, hydrolytic, and conjugative reactions in mice, *J. Agric. Food Chem.*, 1979, **27**, 725–731.
75. L. O. Ruzo, T. Unai and J. E. Casida, Pyrethroid metabolism. Comparative fates in rats of tralomethrin, tralocythrin, deltamethrin and (1R, alpha S)-cis-cypermethrin, *J. Agric. Food Chem.*, 1982, **30**, 631–636.
76. K. E. Appel and S. Gericke, Neurotoxicity and toxicokinetics of pyrethroids, *Bundesgesundheitblatt.*, 1993, **6**, 219–228.
77. S. S. Anand, K.-B. Kim, J. W. Fisher and J. V. Bruckner, Ontogeny of hepatic and plasma metabolism of deltamethrin *in vitro*. Role in age-dependent acute neurotoxicity, *Drug. Metab. Rev.*, 2006, **34**, 389–397.
78. M. H. Akhtar, Metabolism of deltamethrin by cow and chicken liver enzyme preparations, *J. Agric. Food Chem.*, 1984, **32**, 258–262.
79. M. H. Akhtar, R. M. G. Hamilton and H. L. Trenholm, Metabolism, distribution and excretion of deltamethrin by leghorn hens, *J. Agric. Food Chem.*, 1985, **33**, 753–756.
80. M. H. Akhtar, K. E. Hartin and H. L. Trenholm, Fate of [^{14}C] deltamethrin in the lactating dairy cow, *J. Agric. Food Chem.*, 1986, **34**, 753–756.
81. European Medicines Agency/Committee for Veterinary Medicinal Products. Deltamethrin. MRL Summary Report (3), EMEA/MRL/779/01-FINAL, 2001. Available at: www.ema.europa.eu/, accessed January 2011.
82. M. A. Saleh, N. A. Ibrahim, N. Z. Soliman and M. K. El Sheimy, Persistence and distribution of cypermethrin, deltamethrin and fenvalerate in laying chickens, *J. Agric. Food Chem.*, 1986, **34**, 895–898.
83. P. H. Chanh, C. Navarro-Delmasure, A. Chanh, P. Clavel, G. Van Haverbeke and S. L. Cheav, Toxicological studies of deltamethrin, *Int. J. Tiss. Reac.*, 1984, **VI**, 127–133.
84. T. B. Gaines and R. E. Linder, Acute toxicity of pesticides in adult and weanling rats, *Fundam. Appl. Toxicol.*, 1986, **7**, 299–308.

85. R. Kavlock, N. Chernoff, R. Baron, R. Linder, E. Rogers, B. Carver, J. Dilley and V. Simmon, Toxicity studies with decamethrin, a synthetic pyrethroid insecticide, *J. Environ. Pathol. Toxicol.*, 1979, **2**, 751–765.

86. S. H. Kowalczyk-Bronisz, J. Gieldanowski and B. Bubak, Immunological profile of animals exposed to pesticide – deltamethrin, *Arch. Immunol. Ther. Exp.*, 1990, **38**, 229–238.

87. M. Bleys, J. Cotonat and P. Foulhoux, Letter to the editor, *J. Toxicol. Clin. Exper.*, 1986, **6**, 211–212.

88. P. H. Chanh, C. Navarro-Delmasure, A. Chanh, S. L. Cheav, F. Ziade and F. Samaha, Pharmacological studies of deltamethrin on the central nervous system, *Arzneim. Forsch.*, 1984, **34**, 175–181.

89. S. M. Barlow, F. M. Sullivan and J. Lines, Risk assessment of the use of deltamethrin on bednets for the prevention of malaria, *Food. Chem. Toxicol.*, 2001, **39**, 407–422.

90. S. Tós-Luty, A. Haratym-Maj, J. Latuszyńska, D. Obuchowska-Przebirowska and M. Tokarska-Rodak, Oral toxicity of deltamethrin and fenvalerate in Swiss mice, *Ann. Agric. Environ. Med.*, 2001, **8**, 245–254.

91. N. Shaker, G. A. Hassan, F. D. El-Nouty, Z. Abo-Elezz and G. A. Abd-Allah, *In vivo* chronic effect of dimethoate and deltamethrin on rabbits, *J. Environ. Sci. Health*, 1988, **B23**, 387–399.

92. S. Erdogan, E. H. Zeren, M. Emre, O. Aydin and D. Gumurdulu, Pulmonary effects of deltamethrin inhalation: an experimental study in rats, *Ecotoxicol. Environ. Safety*, 2006, **63**, 318–323.

93. J. Cotonat, M. Bleys and P. Foulhoux, Antagonistic effect of phenprobamate and mephenesin carbamate on deltamethrin toxicity, *J. Toxicol. Clin. Exper.*, 1987, **7**, 5–19.

94. M. I. Abd-El-Aziz, A. M. Sahlab and M. Adb El-Khalik, Influence of diazinon and deltamethrin on reproductive organs and fertility of male rats, *Dtsch. Tierärztl. Wschr.*, 1994, **101**, 213–248.

95. M. El-Gohary, W. M. Awara, S. Nassar and S. Hawas, Deltamethrin-induced testicular apoptosis in rats: the protective effect of nitric oxide synthase inhibitor, *Toxicology*, 1999, **132**, 1–8.

96. M. H. Salem, Z. Abo-Elezz, G. A. Abd-Allah, G. A. Hassan and N. Shaker, Effects of organophosphorus (dimethoate) and pyrethroid (deltamethrin) pesticides on semen characteristics in rabbits, *J. Environ. Sci. Health*, 1988, **B23**, 279–290.

97. A. J. M. Andrade, S. Araújo, G. M. Santana, M. Ohi and P. R. Dalsenter, Screening for *in vivo* (anti)estrogenic and (anti)androgenic activities of technical and formulated deltamethrin, *Regul. Toxicol. Pharmacol.*, 2002, **35**, 379–382.

98. H. Chen, J. Xiao, G. Hu, J. Zhou, H. Xiao and X. Wang, Estrogenicity of organophosphorus and pyrethroid pesticides, *J. Toxicol. Environ. Health*, 2002, **65**, 1419–1435.

99. A. J. M. Andrade, S. Araújo, G. M. Santana, M. Ohi and P. R. Dalsenter, Reproductive effects of deltamethrin on male offspring of rats exposed during pregnancy and lactation, *Regul. Toxicol. Pharmacol.*, 2002, **36**, 310–317.

100. K. M. Presibella, D. H. Kita, C. B. Carneiro, A. J. M. Andrade and P. R. Dalsenter, Reproductive evaluation of two pesticides combined (deltamethrin and endosulfan) in female rats, *Reprod. Toxicol.*, 2005, **20**, 95–101.
101. C. Issam, H. Samir, H. Zohra, Z. Monia and B. Cheikh Hassen, Toxic responses to deltamethrin on gonads, sex hormones and lipoperoxidation in male rats following subcutaneous implants, *J. Toxicol. Sci.*, 2009, **34**, 663–670.
102. World Health Organization, Principles for the Safety Assessment of Food Additives and Contaminants in Food, Environmental Health Criteria 70, WHO, Geneva, 1987.
103. Joint FAO/WHO Meeting on Pesticide Residues. Evaluations 2000, Part II. Toxicological. Deltamethrin. International Programme on Chemical Safety, Geneva, 200, pp. 79–110.
104. M. M. Abdel-Khalik, M. S. M. Hanafy and M. I. Abdel Aziz, Studies on the teratogenic effects of deltamethrin in rats, *Dtsch. Tierärztl. Wschr.*, 1993, **100**, 142–143.
105. R. J. Kavlock, N. Chernoff and E. H. Rogers, The effect of acute maternal toxicity on fetal development in the mouse, *Teratog. Carcinog. Mutagen.*, 1985, **5**, 3–13.
106. H. Poláková and M. Vargová, Evaluation of the mutagenic effects of decamethrin: cytogenetic analysis of bone marrow, *Mutat. Res.*, 1983, **120**, 167–171.
107. M. Pluijmen, M. Drevon, R. Montesano, A. Malaveille, A. Hautefeuille and H. Bartsch, Lack of mutagenicity of synthetic pyrethroids in *Salmonella typhimurium* strains and in V79 hamster cells, *Mutat. Res.*, 1984, **137**, 7–15.
108. Y. Shukla and P. Taneja, Mutagenic evaluation of deltamethrin using rodent dominant lethal assay, *Mutat. Res.*, 2000, **467**, 119–127.
109. J. Surrallés, N. Xamena, A. Creus and R. Marcos, The suitability of the micronucleus assay in human lymphocytes as a new biomarker of excision repair, *Mutat. Res.*, 1995, **342**, 43–59.
110. D. K. Agarwal, L. K. S. Chauhan, S. K. Gupta and V. Sundararaman, Cytogenetic effects of deltamethrin on rat bone marrow, *Mutat. Res.*, 1994, **311**, 133–139.
111. S. P. Bhunya and P. C. Pati, Effect of deltamethrin, a synthetic pyrethroid, on the induction of chromosome aberrations, micronuclei and sperm abnormalities in mice, *Mutagenesis*, 1990, **5**, 229–232.
112. L. K. S. Chauhan, D. K. Agarwal and V. Sundararaman, In vivo induction of sister chromatid exchange in mouse bone marrow following oral exposure to commercial formulations of alpha-cyano pyrethroids, *Toxicol. Letters*, 1997, **93**, 153–157.
113. P. Dolara, M. Salvadori, T. Capobianco and F. Torricelli, Sister-chromatid exchanges in human lymphocytes induced by dimethoate, omethoate, deltamethrin, benomyl and their mixture, *Mutat. Res.*, 1992, **283**, 113–118.

114. G. Gandhi, J. B. Chowdhury, P. K. Sareen and V. P. S. Dhillon, Genotoxic effects of deltamethrin in the mouse bone marrow micronucleus assay, *Mutat. Res.*, 1995, **346**, 203–206.
115. C. K. Grisolia, A comparison between mouse and fish micronucleus test using cyclophosphamide, mitomycin C and various pesticides, *Mutat. Res.*, 2002, **518**, 145–150.
116. J. Surrallés, N. Xamena, A. Creus, J. Catalán, H. Norppa and R. Marcos, Induction of micronuclei by five pyrethroid insecticides in whole-blood and isolated human lymphocytes cultures, *Mutat. Res.*, 1995, **341**, 169–184.
117. M. Villarini, M. Moretti, P. Pasquini, G. Scassellati-Sforzolini, C. Fatigoni, M. Marcarelli, S. Monarca and A. V. Rodríguez, In vitro genotoxic effects of the insecticide deltamethrin in human peripheral blood leukocytes: DNA damage ('comet' assay) in relation to the induction of sister-chromatid exchanges and micronuclei, *Toxicology*, 1998, **130**, 129–139.
118. W. Hadnagy, N. H. Seemayer, K.-H. Kühn, G. Leng and H. Idel, Induction of mitotic cell division disturbances and mitotic arrest by pyrethroids in V79 cell cultures, *Toxicol. Letters*, 1999, **107**, 81–87.
119. European Commission, Review report for the active substance deltamethrin, 2002, 6504/VI/99-Final.
120. J. R. P. Cabral, D. Galendo, M. Laval and N. Lyandrat, Carcinogenicity studies with deltamethrin in mice and rats, *Cancer Lett.*, 1990, **49**, 147–152.
121. Y. Shukla, A. Arora and A. Singh, Tumourigenic studies on deltamethrin in Swiss albino mice, *Toxicology*, 2001, **163**, 1–9.
122. K. Hakoi, R. Cabral, T. Hoshiya, R. Hasegawa, T. Shirai and N. Ito, Analysis of carcinogenic activity of some pesticides in a medium-term liver bioassay in the rat, *Teratog. Carcinog. Mutagen.*, 1992, **12**, 269–276.
123. M. J. Wolansky, C. Gennings and K. M. Crofton, Relative potencies for acute effects of pyrethroids on motor function in rats, *Toxicol. Sci.*, 2006, **89**, 271–277.
124. M. Takahashi and P. M. Le Quesne, The effects of the pyrethroids deltamethrin and cismethrin on nerve excitability in rats, *J. Neurol. Neurosurg. Psychiatr.*, 1982, **45**, 1005–1011.
125. H. Duclohier and D. Georgescauld, The effects of the insecticide decamethrin on action potential and voltage-clamp currents of *Myxicola* giant axon, *Comp. Biochem. Physiol.*, 1979, **62C**, 217–223.
126. G. Theophilidis, M. Benaki and E. Papadopoulou-Mourkidou, Neurotoxic action of six pyrethroid insecticides on the isolated sciatic nerve of a frog (*Rana ridibunda*), *Comp. Biochem. Physiol.*, 1997, **118C**, 97–103.
127. M. E. Brodie, Deltamethrin infusion into different sites in the neuraxis of freely-moving rats, *Neurobehav. Toxicol. Teratol.*, 1985, **7**, 51–55.

128. A. J. Gray and J. Rickard, Toxicity of pyrethroids to rats after direct injection into the central nervous system, *NeuroTox.*, 1982, **3**, 25–35.

129. A. Wu and Y. Liu, Apoptotic death in rat brain following deltamethrin treatment, *Neurosci. Letters*, 2000, **279**, 85–88.

130. A. Wu, L. Li and Y. Liu, Deltamethrin induces apoptotic cell death in cultured cerebral cortical neurons, *Toxicol. Appl. Pharmacol.*, 2003, **187**, 50–57.

131. P. Eriksson and A. Fredriksson, Neurotoxic effects of two different pyrethroids, bioallethrin and deltamethrin, on immature and adult mice: changes in behavioural and muscarinic receptor variables, *Toxicol. Appl. Pharmacol.*, 1991, **108**, 78–85.

132. R. Husain, R. Husain, V. M. Adhami and P. K. Seth, Neurobehavioral, neurochemical, and neuromorphological effects of deltamethrin in adult rats, *J. Toxicol. Environ. Health*, 1996, **48**, 515–526.

133. K. M. Crofton and L. W. Reiter, Effects of two pyrethroid insecticides on motor activity and the acoustic startle response in the rat, *Toxicol. Appl. Pharmacol.*, 1984, **75**, 318–328.

134. T. H. Hijzen and J. L. Slanger, Effects of Type I and Type II pyrethroids on the startle response in rats, *Toxicol. Lett.*, 1988, **40**, 141–152.

135. J. R. Glowa, Acute and sub-acute effects of deltamethrin and chlordimeform on schedule-controlled responding in the mouse, *Neurobehav. Toxicol. Teratol.*, 1986, **8**, 97–102.

136. A. S. Bloom, G. Staatz and T. Dieringer, Pyrethroid effects on operant responding and feeding, *Neurobehav. Toxicol. Teratol.*, 1983, **5**, 321–324.

137. S. Manna, D. Bhattacharyya, T. K. Mandal and S. Dey, Neuropharmacological effects of deltamethrin in rats, *J. Vet. Sci.*, 2006, **7**, 133–136.

138. C. A. Lazarini, J. C. Florio, I. P. Lemonica and M. M. Bernardi, Effects of prenatal exposure to deltamethrin on forced swimming behaviour, motor activity, and striatal dopamine levels in male and female rats, *Neurotoxicol. Teratol.*, 2006, **23**, 665–673.

139. M. Dayal, D. Parmar, A. Dhawan, M. Ali, U. N. Dwivedi and S. K. Seth, Effect of pre-treatment of cytochrome P450 (P450) modifiers on neurobehavioral toxicity induced by deltamethrin, *Food Chem. Toxicol.*, 2003, **41**, 431–437.

140. B. Veronesi Validation of a rodent model of organophosphorus-induced delayed neuropathy in *Clinical and Experimental Toxicology of Organophosphates and Carbamates*, ed. B. Ballantyne and T. C. Marrs, Butterworth-Heinemann, Oxford, 1992, pp. 114–125.

141. M. J. Wolansky and J. A. Harrill, Neurobehavioral toxicology of pyrethroid insecticides in adult animals: a critical review, *Neurotoxicol. Teratol.*, 2008, **30**, 55–78.

142. International Programme on Chemical Safety, Environmental Health Criteria 82, *Cypermethrin*, WHO, Geneva, 1989.

143. International Programme on Chemical Safety, Environmental Health Criteria 142, *Alpha-cypermethrin*, WHO, Geneva, 1992.

144. Joint FAO/WHO Expert Committee on Food Additives, Toxicological Evaluation of Certain Veterinary Drug Residues in Food, WHO Food Additive Series 38, The Forty-seventh Meeting of the Joint FAO/WHO Expert Committee on Food Additives International Programme on Chemical Safety, World Health Organization, Geneva, 1996, pp. 133–170.

145. S. Luty, J. Latuszyńska, D Obuchowska-Przebirowska, M. Tokarska and A. Haratym-Maj, Subacute toxicity of orally applied alpha-cypermethrin in Swiss mice, *Ann. Agric. Environ. Med.*, 2000, **7**, 33–41.

146. G. P. Rose and A. J. Dewar, Intoxication with four synthetic pyrethroids fails to show any correlation between neuromuscular dysfunction and neurobiochemical abnormalities in rats, *Arch. Toxicol.*, 1983, **53**, 297–316.

147. T. H. Hijzen, R. de Beun and J. L. Slanger, Effects of pyrethroids on acoustic startle reflex in the rat, *Toxicology*, 1988, **49**, 271–276.

148. International Programme on Chemical Safety, Environmental Health Criteria 94, *Permethrin*, WHO, Geneva, 1990.

149. Joint FAO/WHO Meeting on Pesticide Residues, Evaluations 1999, Part II – Toxicological, WHO, Geneva, 2000.

150. H. Bartsch, C. Malaveille, A. M. Camus, G. Martel-Planche, G. Brun, A. Huatefeuille, N. Sabadie, A. Barbin, T. Kuroki, C. Drevon, C. Piccoli and R. Montesano, Validation and comparative studies on 180 chemicals with *S. typhimurium* strains and V79 hamster cells in the presence of various metabolizing systems, *Mutat. Res.*, 1980, **76**, 1–50.

151. M. Moriya, T. Ohta, K. Watanabe, T. Miyazawa, K. Kato and Y. Shirasu, Further mutagenicity studies on pesticides in bacterial reversion assay systems, *Mutat. Res.*, 1983, **116**, 185–216.

152. N. Kornuta, E. Bagley and N. Nedopitanskaya, Genotoxic effects of pesticides, *J. Environ. Pathol. Toxicol. Oncol.*, 1996, **15**, 75–78.

153. M. D. Pednekar, S. R. Gandhi and M. S. Netrawali, Evaluation of mutagenic activities of endosulfan, phosalone, malathion and permethrin, before and after metabolic activation, in the Ames *Salmonella* test, *Bull. Environ. Contam. Toxicol.*, 1987, **38**, 925–933.

154. A. Herrera and E. Laborda, Mutagenic activity in synthetic pyrethroids in *Salmonella typhimurium*, *Mutagenesis*, 1988, **3**, 509–514.

155. A. Herrera, C. Barrueco, C. Caballo and E. de la Peña, Effect of permethrin on the induction of sister chromatid exchanges and micronuclei in cultured human lymphocytes, *Environ. Mol. Mutagen.*, 1992, **20**, 218–222.

156. R. C. Woodruff, J. P. Phillips and D. Irwin, Pesticide-induced complete and partial chromosome loss in screens with repair-defective females of *Drosophila melanogaster*, *Environ. Mutagen.*, 1983, **5**, 835–846.

157. R. K. Gupta, Z. A. Mehr, D. W. Korte and L. C. Routledge, Mutagenic potential of permethrin in *Drosophila melanogaster* (Diptera: Drosophilidae) sex-linked recessive lethal test, *J. Econ. Entomol.*, 1990, **83**, 721–724.

158. C. Barrueco, A. Herrera, C. Caballo and E. de la Peña, Cytogenetic effects of permethrin in cultured human lymphocytes, *Mutagenesis*, 1992, **7**, 433–437.

159. C. Barrueco, A. Herrera, C. Caballo and E. de la Peña, Induction of structural chromosome aberrations in human lymphocyte cultures and CHO cells by permethrin, *Teratog. Carcinog. Mutagen.*, 1994, **14**, 31–38.

160. J. Surrallès, N. Xamena, A. Creus, J. Catalan, H. Norppa and R. Marcos, Induction of micronuclei by five pyrethroid insecticides in whole-blood and isolated human lymphocyte cultures, *Mutat. Res.*, 1995, **341**, 169–164.

161. J. Surrallès, N. Xamena, A. Creus and R. Marcos, The suitability of the micronucleus assay in human lymphocytes as a new biomarker of excision repair, *Mutat. Res.*, 1995, **342**, 43–59.

162. J. Flodström, L. Warngard, S. Lundquist and U. G. Ahlborg, Inhibition of metabolic cooperation *in vitro* and enhancement of enzyme foci incidence in rat liver by the pyrethroid insecticide fenvalerate, *Arch. Toxicol.*, 1988, **61**, 218–223.

163. J. Ishmael and M. H. Litchfield, Chronic toxicity and carcinogenic evaluation of permethrin in rats and mice, *Fundam. Appl. Toxicol.*, 1988, **11**, 308–322.

164. C. G. Staatz, A. S. Bloom and J. J. Lech, A pharmacological study of pyrethroid toxicity in mice, *Pest. Biochem. Physiol.*, 1982, **17**, 287–292.

165. D. W. Gammon, L. J. Lawrence and J. E. Casida, Pyrethroid toxicology: protective effects of diazepam and phenobarbital in the mouse and cockroach, *Toxicol. Appl. Pharmacol.*, 1982, **66**, 290–296.

166. T. J. Shafer, S. O. Rijal and G. W. Gross, Complete inhibition of spontaneous activity in neuronal networks in vitro by deltamethrin and permethrin, *NeuroToxicol.*, 2008, **29**, 203–212.

167. C. A. Meacham, P. D. Brodfuehrer, J. A. Watkins and T. Shafer, Developmentally-regulated sodium channel subunits are differentially sensitive to α-cyano containing pyrethroids, *Toxicol. Appl. Pharmacol.*, 2008, **231**, 273–281.

168. S. K. Tayebati, M. A. Di Tullio, A. Ricci and F. Amenta, Influence of dermal exposure to the pyrethroid insecticide deltamethrin on rat brain microanatomy and cholinergic/dopaminergic neurochemistry, *Brain Res.*, 2009, **1301**, 180–188.

169. D. Chen, X. Huang, L. Lin and N. Shi, Deltamethrin induces mitochondrial membrane permeability an altered expression of cytochrome c in rat brain, *J. Appl. Toxicol.*, 2007, **27**, 368–372.

170. T. Morikawa and K. Furuhama, Effects of NMDA receptor antagonists on deltamethrin-induced striatal dopamine release in conscious unrestrained rats, *J. Vet. Med. Sci.*, 2009, **71**, 1129–1132.

171. D. E. Ray, S. A. Burr and T. Lister, The effects of combined exposure to the pyrethroids deltamethrin and *S*-bioallethrin on hippocampal inhibition and skeletal muscle hyperexcitability in rats, *Toxicol. Appl. Pharmacol.*, 2006, **216**, 354–362.

172. L. Isamura, M. Yasuda, K. Kuramitsu, D. Hara, A. Tabuchi and M. Tsuda, Deltamethrin, a pyrethroid insecticide, is a potent inducer for the activity-dependent gene expression of brain-derived neurotrophic factor in neurons, *J. Pharmacol. Exp. Ther.*, 2006, **316**, 136–143.

173. K. N. Woodward, Adverse effects of veterinary pharmaceutical products in animals in *Veterinary Pharmacovigilance: Adverse Reactions to Veterinary Medicinal Products*, ed. K. N. Woodward, Wiley-Blackwell, Chichester, 2009, pp. 393–421.

174. W. M. Valentine, Pyrethrin and pyrethroids insecticides, *Vet. Clin. North Am. Small Anim. Pract.*, 1990, **20**, 375–382.

175. P. A. Volmer, S. A. Kahn, M. W. Knight and S. R. Hansen, Warning against use of some permethrin products in cats, *J. Am. Vet. Med. Assoc.*, 1998, **213**, 800.

176. E. K. Meyer, Toxicosis in cats erroneously treated with 45 to 65% permethrin products, *J. Am. Vet. Med. Assoc.*, 1999, **215**, 198–203.

177. N. Sutton, N. Bates and A. Campbell, Seasonal rise in permethrin 'spot-on' poisoning in cats, *Vet. Rec.*, 2007, **161**, 244.

178. N. M. Sutton, N. Bates and A. Campbell, Clinical effects and outcome of feline permethrin spot-on poisonings reported to the Veterinary Poisons Information Service (VPIS), London, *J. Feline Med. Surg.*, 2007, **9**, 335–339.

179. P. J. Linnett, Permethrin toxicosis in cats, *Austral. Vet. J.*, 2008, **86**, 32–35.

180. R. Malik, M. P. Ward, A. Seavers, A. Fawcett, E. Bell, M. Govendir and S. Page, Permethrin spot-on intoxication of cats. Literature review and survey of veterinary practitioners in Australia, *J. Feline Med. Surg.*, 2010, **12**, 5–14.

181. S. A. Box and M. R. Lee, A systemic reaction following exposure to a pyrethroid insecticide, *Hum. Exp. Toxicol.*, 1996, **15**, 389–390.

182. P. M. LeQuesne, I. C. Maxwell and S. T. Butterworth, Transient facial sensory symptoms following exposure to synthetic pyrethroids: a clinical and electrophysiological assessment, *Neurotoxicol.*, 1980, **2**, 1–11.

183. S. B. Tucker and S. A. Flannigan, Cutaneous effects from occupational exposure to fenvalerate, *Arch. Toxicol.*, 1983, **54**, 195–202.

184. F. He, L. Liu, S. Chen, Z. Zhang and J. Sun, Clinical manifestations and diagnosis of acute pyrethroid poisoning, *Arch. Toxicol.*, 1989, **63**, 54–58.

185. A. T. Proudfoot, Poisoning due to pyrethrins, *Toxicol. Rev.*, 2005, **24**, 107–113.

186. D. E. Ray and J. R. Fry, A reassessment of the neurotoxicity of pyrethroid insecticides, *Pharmacol. Ther.*, 2006, **111**, 174–193.

187. L. G. Costa, G. Giordano, M. Guizetti and A. Vitalone, Neurotoxicity of pesticides: a brief review, *Front. Biosci.*, 2008, **13**, 1240–1249.

188. K. Hammond and J. B. Leikin, Topical pyrethrin toxicity leading to acute-onset stuttering in a toddler, *Am. J. Ther.*, 2008, **15**, 323–324.

189. J. Magdalan, M. Zawadzki and A. Merwid-Lad, Fatal intoxication with hydrocarbons in deltamethrin preparation, *Hum. Exp. Toxicol.*, 2009, **28**, 791–793.

190. N. Gunay, Z. Kekec, Y. Cete, C. Eken and A. T. Demiryurek, Oral deltamethrin ingestion due in a suicide attempt, *Bratisl. Lek. Listy.*, 2010, **111**, 303–305.

191. R. Ahdab, S. S. Ayache, F. Maltoni, P. Brugières and J. P. Lefaucheur, Motor neuron disorder with tongue spasms due to pyrethroid insecticide toxicity, *Neurology*, 2011, **76**, 196–197.

192. S. M. Bradberry, S. A. Cage, A. T. Proudfoot and J. A. Vale, Poisoning due to pyrethroids, *Toxicol. Rev.*, 2005, **24**, 93–106.

193. S. A. Flannigan, S. B. Tucker, M. M. Key, C. E. Ross, E. J. Fairchild, B. A. Grimes and R. B. Harrist, Synthetic pyrethroid insecticides: a dermatological evaluation, *Br. J. Ind. Med.*, 1985, **42**, 363–372.

194. M. Tomizawa and J. E. Casida, Neonicotinoid insecticide toxicology: mechanisms of selective action, *Annu. Rev. Pharmacol.*, 2005, **45**, 247–268.

195. Joint FAO/WHO Meeting on Pesticide Residues, Pesticide Residues in Food – 2001, Evaluations 2001, Part II – Toxicological, World Health Organization, Geneva, 2002.

196. S. Bhardwaj, M. K. Srivastava, U. Kapoor and L. P. Srivastava, A 90 days oral toxicity of imidacloprid in female rats: morphological, biochemical and histopathological examination, *Food Chem. Toxicol.*, 2010, **48**, 1185–1190.

197. N. U. Karabay and M. G. Oguz, Cytogenetic and genotoxic effects of the insecticides, imidacloprid and methamidophos, *Genet. Mol. Res.*, 2005, **4**, 653–662.

198. L. Elfman, C. Hogstedt, K. Engvall, E. Lampa and C. H. Lindh, Acute health effects on planters of conifer seedlings treated with insecticides, *Ann. Occup. Hyg.*, 2009, **53**, 383–390.

199. F. Mohamed, I. Gawarammana, T. A. Robertson, M. S. Roberts, C. Palangasinghe, S. Zawahir, S. Jayamanne, J. Kandasamy, M. Eddleston, N. A. Buckley, A. H. Dawson and D. M. Roberts, Acute human self-poisoning with imidacloprid compound: a neonicotinoid insecticide, *PLoS One*, 2009, **4**, e5127.

200. B. Ballantyne and T. C. Marrs, Overview of the biological and clinical aspects of organophosphates and carbamates in *Clinical and Experimental Toxicology of Organophosphates and Carbamates*, ed. B. Ballantyne and T. C. Marrs, Butterworth Heinemann, London, 1992, pp. 3–14.

201. M. Lotti, Central neurotoxicity and behavioural effects of anticholinesterases in *Clinical and Experimental Toxicology of Organophosphates and Carbamates*, ed. B. Ballantyne and T. C. Marrs, Butterworth Heinemann, London, 1992, pp. 75–83.

202. M. K. Johnson and P. Glynn, Neuropathy target esterase (NTE) and organophosphorus-induced delayed polyneuropathy (OPIDP): recent advances, *Toxicol. Lett.*, 1995, **82/83**, 459–463.

203. M. B. Abou-Donia, Organophosphorus ester-induced chronic neurotoxicity, *Arch. Environ. Health*, 2003, **58**, 484–497.

204. A. Moretto, Experimental and clinical toxicology of anticholinesterase agents, *Toxicol. Lett.*, 1998, **102–103**, 509–513.
205. Joint FAO/WHO Meeting on Pesticide Residues. Pesticide Residues in Food – 1993, Evaluations 1993, Part II – Toxicological, World Health Organization, Geneva, 1994.
206. E. Mutch and F. Williams, Diazinon, chlorpyrifos and parathion are metabolised by multiple cytochromes P450 in human liver, *Toxicology*, 2006, **224**, 22–32.
207. T. S. Poet, H. Wu, A. A. Kousba and C. Timchalk, *In vitro* rat hepatic and intestinal metabolism of the organophosphate pesticides chlorpyrifos and diazinon, *Toxicol. Sci.*, 2003, **72**, 193–200.
208. W. A. Kappers, R. J. Edwards, S. Murray and A. R. Boobis, Diazinon is activated by CYP2C19 in human liver, *Toxicol. Appl. Pharmacol.*, 2001, **177**, 68–76.
209. M. Jokanović, Biotransformation of organophosphorus compounds, *Toxicology*, 2001, **166**, 139–160.
210. K. M. Atherton, F. M. Williams, S. Jameson and E. Mutch, DNA damage by single doses of five organophosphate pesticides, *Toxicology*, 2008, **253**, 8–9.
211. E. Salazar-Arredondo, M. de Jesús Solis-Heredia, E. Rojas-García, I. Hernández-Ochoa and B. Quintanilla-Vega, Sperm chromatin alteration and DNA damage by methyl-parathion, chlorpyrifos and diazinon and their oxon metabolites in human spermatozoa, *Reprod. Toxicol.*, 2008, **25**, 455–460.
212. M. Tisch, P. Schmezer, M. Faulde, A. Groh and H. Maier, Genotoxicity studies on permethrin, DEET and diazinon in primary human nasal mucosal cells, *Eur. Arch. Otorhinolaryngol.*, 2002, **259**, 150–153.
213. K. Kuroda, Y. Yamaguchi and G. Endo, Mitotic activity, sister chromatid exchange, and rec assay of pesticides, *Arch. Environ. Contam. Toxicol.*, 1992, **23**, 13–18.
214. D. Lopez, C. Aleixandre, M. Merchan and E. Carrascal, *In vitro* induction of alterations in peripheral blood lymphocytes by different doses of diazinon, *Bull. Environ. Contam. Toxicol.*, 1986, **37**, 517–522.
215. D. Lopez and E. Carrascal, Sensitivity of human lymphocyte chromosome to diazinon at different times during cell culture, *Bull. Environ. Contam. Toxicol.*, 1987, **38**, 125–130.
216. Ş. Çakir and R. Sarikaya, Genotoxicity testing of some organophosphate insecticides in the *Drosophila* wing spot test, *Food Chem. Toxicol.*, 2005, **43**, 443–450.
217. N. E. Garrett, H. F. Stack, M. A. Jackson and M. D. Waters, Genotoxic and carcinogenic potential of anticholinesterases in *Clinical and Experimental Toxicology of Organophosphates and Carbamates*, ed. B. Ballantyne and T. C. Marrs, Butterworth Heinemann, London, 1992, pp. 223–240.
218. D. B. MacGregor, A. Brown, P. Cattenach, I. Edwards, D. McBride, C. Riach and W. J. Caspary, Responses of the L5178 TK$^+$/TK$^-$ mouse lymphoma cell forward mutation assay: III. 72 coded chemicals, *Environ. Mol. Mutagen.*, 1988, **12**, 85–154.

219. E. Zabihi Neishabouri, Z. M. Hassa, E. Azizi and S. N. Ostad, Evaluation of immunotoxicity induced by diazinon in C57bl/6 mice, *Toxicology*, 2004, **196**, 173–179.

220. G. J. Oostingh, G. Wichmann, M. Schmittner, I. Lehmann and A. Duschl, The cytotoxic effects of the organophosphates chlorpyriphos and diazinon differ from their immunomodulating effects, *J. Immunotoxicol.*, 2009, **6**, 136–145.

221. R. D. Handy, H. A. Abd-El Samei, M. F. F. Bayomy, A. M. Mahran, A. M. Abdeen and E. A. El-Elaimy, Chronic diazinon exposure: pathologies of spleen, thymus, blood cells and lymph nodes are modulated by dietary protein or lipid in the mouse, *Toxicology*, 2002, **172**, 13–34.

222. T. Galloway and R. Handy, Immunotoxicity of organophosphorus pesticides, *Ecotoxicol.*, 2003, **12**, 345–363.

223. A. M. Alluwaimi and Y. Hussein, Diazinon immunotoxicity in mice: modulation of cytokines level and their gene expression, *Toxicology*, 2007, **236**, 123–131.

224. V. N. Kabrawala, R. M. Shah and G. G. Oza, Diazinon poisoning (a study of 25 cases, *Indian Pract.*, 1965, **18**, 711–717.

225. R. S. Wadia, C. Sadagopan, R. B. Amin and H. V. Sardesai, Neurological manifestations of organophosphorus poisoning, *J. Neurol. Neurosurg. Psychiatry*, 1974, **37**, 841–847.

226. H. W. Klemmer, E. R. Reichert and W. L. Yauger, Five cases of intentional ingestion of 25 per cent diazinon with treatment and recovery, *Clin. Toxicol.*, 1978, **12**, 435–444.

227. A. Poklis, F. W. Kutz, J. F. Sperling and D. P. Morgan, A fatal diazinon poisoning, *Forensic Sci. Int.*, 1980, **15**, 135–140.

228. R. J. Zwiener and C. M. Ginsberg, Organophosphate and carbamate poisoning in infants and children, *Pediatrics*, 1988, **81**, 121–126.

229. Z. Weizman and S. Sofer, Acute pancreatitis in children with anticholinesterase insecticide intoxication, *Pediatrics*, 1992, **90**, 204–206.

230. International Programme on Chemical Safety, Environmental Health Criteria 198, *Diazinon*, World Health Organization, Geneva, 1998.

231. F. Muratore, H. Faiolo and G. Ponzetta, On four cases of poisoning by organophosphorus acid esters (antiparasitic) with recovery, with special reference to hepatic involvement, *Minerva Med.*, 1960, **51**, 3342–3345.

232. A. Halle and D. D. Sloas, Percutaneous organophosphate poisoning, *South. Med. J.*, 1987, **80**, 1179–1181.

233. A. M. Mizra, N. Schaub, L. Samler and T. E. Reuchelderfer, Organophosphate insecticide diazinon poisoning in children, *Med. Ann. DC.*, 1972, **41**, 559–560.

234. S. L. Wagner and D. L. Orwick, Chronic organophosphate exposure associated with transient hypertonia in an infant, *Pediatrics*, 1994, **94**, 94–97.

235. S. W. Hall and B. B. Baker, Intermediate syndrome from organophosphate poisoning, *Vet. Hum. Toxicol.*, 1989, **31**, 355.

236. K. K. Samal and C. S. Sahu, Organophosphorus poisoning and inter-mediate neurotoxic syndrome., *J. Assoc. Phys. India*, 1990, **38**, 181–182.
237. S. A. Soliman, G. W. Sovocol, A. Curley, N. S. Ahmed and A. K. El-Fiki El-Sabae, Two acute human poisoning cases resulting from exposure to diazinon transformation products in Egypt, *Arch. Environ. Health*, 1982, **37**, 207–212.
238. D. Mello, F. Rodrigues Puga and R. Benintendi, Intoxications produced by degradation products of diazinon in its use as a tick killer, *Biologico*, 1972, **38**, 136–139.
239. L. Wecker, R. E. Mrak and W. D. Dettbran, Evidence of necrosis in human intercostal muscle following inhalation of an organophosphorus insecticide, *J. Environ. Pathol. Toxicol. Oncol.*, 1985, **6**, 171–175.
240. P. Casey and J. A. Vale, Deaths from pesticide poisoning in England and Wales: 1945–1989, *Hum. Exp. Toxicol.*, 1994, **13**, 95–101.
241. T. C. Marrs and P. Edwards, Medicines used to control and treat external parasites of sheep – toxicology and the phenomenon of reported adverse human responses to organophosphorus sheep dips in *Veterinary Pharmacovigilance: Adverse Reactions to Veterinary Medicinal Products*, ed. K. N. Woodward, Wiley-Blackwell, Chichester, 2009, pp. 517–527.
242. D. Swanston and I. Shaw, Organophosphorus compounds, *Sheep Farmer*, 1990, **10**, 31–33.
243. G. A. Jamal, Long term neurotoxic effects of organophosphate compounds, *Adverse Drug React. Toxicol. Rev.*, 1995, **14**, 85–99.
244. K. N. Woodward, Adverse reactions in humans following exposure to veterinary drugs in *Veterinary Pharmacovigilance: Adverse Reactions to Veterinary Medicinal Products*, ed. K. N. Woodward, Wiley-Blackwell, Chichester, 2009, pp. 475–515.
245. K. N. Woodward, Veterinary Pharmacovigilance. Part 4. Adverse reactions in humans to veterinary medicinal products, *J. Vet. Pharmacol. Ther.*, 2005, **28**, 185–201.
246. J. C. Axelrad, C. V. Howard and W. G. McLean, The effects of acute pesticide exposure on neuroblastoma cells chronically exposed to diazinon, *Toxicology*, 2003, **185**, 67–78.
247. W. G. Carter, M. Tarhoni, A. J. Rathbone and D. E. Ray, Differential protein adduction by seven organophosphorus pesticides in both brain and liver, *Hum. Exp. Toxicol.*, 2007, **26**, 347–353.
248. L. Sarabia, I. Maurer and E. Bustos-Obregón, Melatonin prevents damage by the organophosphorus pesticide diazinon on the mouse testis, *Ecotoxicol. Environ. Safety*, 2009, **72**, 938–942.
249. S. H. Swan, R. L. Kruse, F. Liu, D. B. Barr, E. Z. Drobnis, J. B. Redmon, C. Wang, C. Brazil and J. W. Overstreet, Study for Future Families Research Group, *Environ. Health Perspect.*, 2003, **111**, 1478–1484.
250. A. Okamura, M. Kamijima, K. Ohtani, O. Yamanoshita, D. Nakamura, Y. Ito, J. Ueyama, T. Suzuki, R. Imai, K. Takagi and T. Nakajima, Broken sperm, cytoplasmic droplets and reduced sperm motility are

principal markers of decreased sperm quality due to organophosphorus pesticides in rats, *J. Occup. Health*, 2009, **51**, 478–487.

251. T. Rush, X. Q. Liu, J. Hjelmhaug and D. Lobner, Mechanisms of chlorpyrifos and diazinon induced neurotoxicity in cortical culture, *Neuroscience*, 2010, **166**, 899–906.

252. T. A. Slotkin, I. T. Ryde, E. D. Levin and F. J. Seidler, Developmental neurotoxicity of low-dose diazinon exposure of neonatal rats: effects of serotonin systems in adolescence and adulthood, *Brain Res. Bull.*, 2008, **75**, 640–647.

253. E. Sidiropoulou, M. Sachana, J. Flaskos, W. Harris, A. J. Hargreaves and Z. Woldehiwet, Diazinon oxon interferes with differentiation of rat C6 glioma cells, *Toxicol. In Vitro*, 2009, **23**, 1548–1552.

254. C. S. Roegge, O. Timofeeva, F. J. Seidler, T. A. Slotkin and E. D. Levin, Developmental neurotoxicity in rats: later effects on emotional response, *Brain Res. Bull.*, 2008, **75**, 166–172.

255. T. A. Slotkin, B. E. Bodwell, E. D. Levin and F. J. Seidler, Neonatal exposure to low doses of diazinon: long-term effects on neural cell development and acetylcholine systems, *Environ. Health Perspect.*, 2008, **116**, 340–348.

256. T. A. Slotkin and F. J. Seidler, Comparative developmental neurotoxicity of organophosphates in vivo: transcriptional responses of pathways for brain cell development, cell signalling, cytotoxicity and neurotransmitter systems, *Brain Res. Bull.*, 2007, **72**, 232–274.

257. T. A. Slotkin, F. J. Seidler and F. Fumagalli, Exposure to organophosphates reduces the expression of neurotrophic factors in neonatal rat brain regions: similarities and differences in the effects of chlorpyriphos and diazinon on the fibroblast growth factor superfamily, *Environ. Health Perspect.*, 2007, **115**, 909–916.

258. T. A. Slotkin, E. D. Levin and F. J. Seidler, Comparative developmental neurotoxicity of organophosphate insecticides: effects on brain development are separable from systemic toxicity, *Environ. Health Perspect.*, 2006, **114**, 746–751.

259. T. A. Slotkin, C. A. Tate, I. T. Ryde, E. D. Levin and F. J. Seidler, Organophosphate insecticides target the serotonergic system in developing rat brain regions: disparate effects of diazinon and parathion at doses spanning the threshold for cholinesterase inhibition, *Environ. Health Perspect.*, 2006, **114**, 1542–1546.

260. O. A. Timofeeva, C. S. Roegge, F. J. Seidler, T. A. Slotkin and E. D. Levin, Persistent cognitive alterations in rats after early postnatal exposure to low doses of the organophosphate pesticide, diazinon, *Neurotoxicol. Teratol.*, 2008, **30**, 38–45.

261. M. Guizzetti, S. Pathak, G. Gennaro and L. G. Costa, Effect of organophosphorus insecticides and their metabolites on astroglial cell proliferation, *Toxicology*, 2005, **215**, 182–190.

262. D. E. Ray and P. G. Richards, The potential for toxic effects of chronic, low-dose exposure to organophosphates, *Toxicol. Lett.*, 2001, **120**, 343–351.

263. K. O'Leary, R. J. Edwards, M. M. Town and A. R. Boobis, Genetic and other sources of variation in the activity of serum paraoxonase/diazoxonase in humans: consequences for risk from exposure to diazinon, *Pharmacogenet. Genomics*, 2005, **15**, 51–60.

264. B. A. Hatjian, E. Mutch, F. M. Williams, P. G. Blain and J. W. Edwards, Cytogenetic response without changes in peripheral cholinesterase enzymes following exposure to a sheep dip containing diazinon in vivo and in vitro, *Mutat. Res.*, 2000, **472**, 85–92.

265. B. Mackness, P. Durrington, A. Povey, S. Thompson, M. Dippnall, M. Mackness, T. Smith and N. Cherry, Paraoxonase and susceptibility to organophosphorus poisoning in farmers dipping sheep, *Pharmacogenetics*, 2003, **13**, 81–88.

266. J. O'Halloran and W. E. Hogans, First use in North America of azamethiphos to treat Atlantic salmon for sea lice infestations: procedures and efficacy, *Can. Vet. J.*, 1996, **37**, 610–611.

267. A. N. Grant, Medicines for sea lice, *Pest. Manag. Sci.*, 2002, **58**, 521–527.

268. L. Burridge, J. S. Weis, F. Cabello, J. Pizarro and K. Bostock, Chemical use in salmon aquaculture: A review of current practices and possible environmental effects, *Aquaculture*, 2010, **306**, 7–23.

269. Committee for Veterinary Medicinal Products, Azamethiphos, Summary Report (1). EMEA/MRL/001/95-FINAL.

270. T. Roberts and D. Hutson (ed.), in *Metabolic Pathways of Agrochemicals. Part two. Insecticides and Fungicides*, Royal Society of Chemistry, Cambridge, 1999, pp. 205–206.

271. K. Kohzaki, T. Masaoka, M. Nagayama, F. Akahori, K. Kakaguchi and R. Kohzaki, Effects of azamethiphos, an organophosphorus insecticide, on serum cholinesterase activity and isoenzymes in the rats, *Vet. Hum. Toxicol.*, 1991, **33**, 575–578.

272. V. Zitco, Alkylating potency of azamethiphos, *Bull. Environ. Contam. Toxicol.*, 2001, **66**, 283–286.

273. R. T. Sharpe, C. T. Livesey, I. H. Davies, J. R. Jones and A. Jones, Diazinon toxicity in sheep and cattle arising from misuse of unlicensed and out-of-date products, *Vet. Rec.*, 2006, **159**, 16–19.

274. C. Pretti, G. Soldani, A. M. Cognetti-Varriale, G. Monni, V. Meucci and L. Intorre, Efficacy and safety of azamethiphos for the treatment of pseudodactylogyrosis in the European eel, *J. Vet. Pharmacol. Ther.*, 2002, **25**, 155–157.

275. L. Intorre, G. Soldani, A. M. Cognetti-Varriale, G. Monni, V. Meucci and C. Pretti, Safety of azamethiphos in eel, sea bass and trout, *Pharmacol. Res.*, 2004, **49**, 171–176.

276. T. E. Horsberg, T. Høy and I. Nafstad, Organophosphate poisoning of Atlantic salmon in connection with treatment against sea lice, *Acta. Vet. Scand.*, 1989, **30**, 385–390.

277. J. F. Burka, K. L. Hammell, T. E. Horsberg, G. R. Johnson, D. J. Rainnie and D. J. Speare, Drugs in salmonid aquaculture – A review, *J. Vet. Pharmacol. Ther.*, 1997, **20**, 333–349.

278. J. E. Bron, C. Sommerville, R. Wooten and G. H. Rae, Influence of treatment with dichlorvos on the epidemiology of *Lepeophtheirus salmonis* (Krøyer, 1837) and *Caligus elongatus* Nordmann, 1832 on Scottish salmon farms in *Pathogens of Wild and Farmed Fish: Sea Lice*, ed. G. A. Boxall and D. Defaye, Ellis Horwood, London, 1993, pp. 263–274.

279. V. L. Salgado and J. H. Hayashi, Metaflumizone is a novel sodium channel blocker insecticide, *Vet. Parasitol.*, 2007, **150**, 182–189.

280. K. S. Silver, Y. Nomura, V. L. Salgado and K. Dong, Role of the sixth transmembrane segment of domain IV of the cockroach sodium channel in the action of sodium channel-blocker insecticides, *Neurotoxicol.*, 2009, **30**, 613–621.

281. R. L. DeLay, E. Lacoste, S. Delprat and F. Blond-Riou, Pharmacokinetics of metaflumizone in the plasma and hair of cats following topical application, *Vet. Parasitol.*, 2007, **150**, 258–262.

282. R. L. DeLay, E. Lacoste, T. Mezzasalma and F. Blond-Riou, Pharmacokinetics of metaflumizone and amitraz in the plasma and hair of dogs following topical application, *Vet. Parasitol.*, 2007, **150**, 251–257.

283. K. Hempel, F. G. Hess, C. Bögi, E. Fabian, J. Hellwig and I. Fegert, Toxicological properties of metaflumizone, *Vet. Parasitol.*, 2007, **150**, 190–195.

284. B. Lapied, F. Grolleau and D. B. Battelle, Indoxacarb, an oxadiazine insecticide, blocks neuronal sodium channels, *Br. J. Pharmacol.*, 2001, **132**, 587–595.

285. T. Narahashi, Nerve membrane ion channels as the target site for insecticides, *Mini Rev. Med. Chem.*, 2002, **2**, 419–432.

286. European Medicines Agency, European Public Assessment Report, Activyl, EMA/529995/2010, February 2011.

287. Joint FAO/WHO Meeting on Pesticide Residues, Pesticide Residues in Food – 1993, Evaluations 2005. Part II – Toxicological, World Health Organization, Geneva, 2006.

288. H. Singh, E. Purnell and C. Smith, Mechanistic study on aniline-induced erythrocyte toxicity, *Arh. Hig. Rada Toksikol.*, 2007, **58**, 275–285.

289. R. S. Chhabra, M. Thompson, M. R. Elwell and D. K. Gerken, Toxicity of *p*-chloroaniline in rats and mice, *Food Chem. Toxicol.*, 1990, **28**, 717–722.

290. B. E. Watt, A. T. Proudfoot, S. M. Bradberry and J. A. Vale, Poisoning due to urea herbicides, *Toxicol. Rev.*, 2005, **24**, 161–166.

291. J. Umbreit, Methaemoglobin – it's not just blue: a concise review, *Am. J. Haematol.*, 2007, **82**, 134–144.

292. S. M. Bradberry, Occupational methaemoglobinemia. Mechanisms of production, features, diagnosis and management including the use of methylene blue, *Toxicol. Rev.*, 2003, **22**, 13–27.

293. G. Wang, X. Zhang, C. Yao and M. Tian, Four-week oral toxicity of three metabolites of nitrobenzene in rats, *Drug Chem. Toxicol.*, 2010, **33**, 238–243.

294. H. Singh and E. T. Purnell, Aniline derivative-induced methemoglobin in rats, *J. Environ. Pathol. Toxicol. Oncol.*, 2005, **24**, 57–65.
295. Y. J. Wu, Y. L. Lin, H. Y. Huang and B. G. Hsu, Methemoglobinemia induced by indoxacarb intoxication, *Clin. Toxicol.*, 2010, **48**, 766–767.
296. R. Chhabra, I. Singh, M. Tandon and R. Babu, Indoxacarb poisoning: a rare presentation as methaemoglobinemia, *Indian J. Anaesth.*, 2010, **54**, 239–241.
297. L. Prasan, M. S. Rao, V. Singh and R. Kujur, Gowrishankar, Indoxacarb poisoning: a rare presentation as methemoglobinemia, *Ind. J. Crit. Care*, 2008, **12**, 198–200.
298. D. Hainzl, L. M. Cole and J. E. Casida, Mechanisms for selective toxicity of fipronil insecticide and its sulphone metabolite and desulfinyl photo-product, *Chem. Res. Toxicol.*, 1998, **11**, 1529–1535.
299. T. Narahashi, X. Zhao, T. Ikeda, K. Nagata and J. Z. Yeh, Differential actions of insecticides on target sites: basis for selective toxicity, *Hum. Exp. Toxicol.*, 2007, **26**, 361–366.
300. P. Varro, J. Győri and I. Világi, *In vitro* effects of fipronil on neuronal excitability in mammalian and molluscan nervous systems, *Ann. Agric. Environ. Med.*, 2009, **16**, 71–77.
301. G. S. Ratra, G. Kamitra and J. E. Casida, Role of human GABA$_A$ receptor β3 subunit in insecticide toxicity, *Toxicol. Appl. Pharmacol.*, 2001, **172**, 233–240.
302. D. Hainzl and J. E. Casida, Fipronil insecticide: Novel photochemical desulfinylation with retention of neurotoxicity, *Proc. Natl Acad. Sci. USA*, 1996, **93**, 12764–12767.
303. M. Eddleston, Phenylpyrazole insecticides, *Clin Toxicol.*, 2008, **46**, 405.
304. Joint FAO/WHO Meeting on Pesticide Residues, Pesticide Residues in Food – 1997, Evaluations 2005, Part II – Toxicological, World Health Organization, Geneva, 1998.
305. P. M. Hurley, R. N. Hill and R. J. Whiting, Mode of carcinogenic action of pesticides inducing thyroid follicular cell tumors in rodents, *Environ. Health Perspect.*, 1998, **106**, 437–445.
306. K. N. Woodward, The toxicity of particular veterinary drug residues in *Pesticide, Veterinary and Other Residues in Food*, ed. D. H. Watson, CRC Press/Woodhead Publishing Limited, Boca Raton/Cambridge, 2000, pp. 175–223.
307. K. N. Woodward, Veterinary pharmacovigilance. Part 6. Predictability of adverse reactions in animals from laboratory toxicology studies, *J. Vet. Pharmacol. Ther.*, 2005, **28**, 213–231.
308. K. N. Woodward, Carcinogenicity of sulphadimidine, *Hum. Exp. Toxicol.*, 1992, **11**, 60–61.
309. J. E. Heath and N. A. Littlefield, Effects of subchronic oral sulfamethazine administration on Fischer 344 rats and B6C3F1 mice, *J. Environ. Pathol. Toxicol. Oncol.*, 1984, **5**, 201–214.

310. J. E. Heath and N. A. Littlefield, Morphological effects of subchronic oral sulfamethazine on Fischer 344 rats and B6C3F1 mice, *Toxicol. Pathol.*, 1984, **12**, 3–9.

311. N. A. Littlefield, W. G. Sheldon, R. Allen and D. W. Gaylor, Chronic toxicity/carcinogenicity studies of sulfamethazine in Fischer 344/N rats: two-generation exposure, *Food Chem. Toxicol.*, 1990, **28**, 156–167.

312. F. R. Fullerton, R. J. Kushmaul, R. L. Suber and N. A. Littlefield, Influence of oral administration of sulfamethazine on thyroid hormone levels in Fischer F344 rats, *J. Toxicol. Environ. Health*, 1987, **22** 175–185.

313. R. N. Hill, T. M. Crisp, P. M. Hurley, S. L. Rosenthal and D. V. Singh, Risk assessment of thyroid follicular cell tumors, *Environ. Health Perspect.*, 1998, **106**, 447–457.

314. R. M. McClain, Mechanistic considerations for the relevance of animal data on thyroid neoplasia to human risk assessment, *Mutat. Res.*, 1995, **333**, 131–142.

315. L. A. Poirier, D. R. Doerge, D. W. Gaylor, M. A. Miller, R. J. Lorentzen, D. A. Casciano, F. F. Kadlubar and B. A. Schwetz, An FDA review of sulfamethazine toxicity, *Regul. Toxicol. Pharmacol.*, 1999, **30**, 217–222.

316. M. Ohi, R. R. Dalsenter, A. J. M. Andrade and A. J. Nascimento, Reproductive adverse effects of fipronil in Wistar rats, *Toxicol. Lett.*, 2004, **146**, 121–127.

317. H. T. Fung, K. K. Chang, W. M. Ching and C. W. Kam, A case of ingestion of ant bait containing fipronil, *J. Toxicol. Clin. Toxicol.*, 2003, **41**, 245–248.

318. Z. Chodorowski and J. S. Anand, Accidental dermal and inhalation exposure with fipronil – a case report, *J. Toxicol. Clin. Toxicol.*, 2004, **42**, 189–190.

319. F. Mohamed, L. Senarathna, A. Percy, M. Abeyewardene, G. Eaglesham, R. Cheng, S. Azher, A. Hittarage, W. Dissanayake, M. H. Rezvi Sheriff, W. Davies, N. Buckley and M. Eddleston, Acute human self-poisoning with the *N*-phenylpyrazole insecticide fipronil – a GABA$_A$-gated chloride channel blocker, *J. Toxicol. Clin. Toxicol.*, 2004, **42**, 955–963.

320. M. Eddleston, M. H. Rezvi Sheriff and K. Hawton, Deliberate self harm in Sri Lanka: an overlooked tragedy in the developing world, *BMJ*, 1998, **317**, 133–135.

321. S. J. Lee, P. Mulay, B. Diebolt-Brown, M. J. Lackovic, L. N. Mehler, J. Beckman, J. Waltz, J. B. Prado, Y. A. Mitchell, S. A. Higgins, A. Schwartz and G. M. Calvert, Acute illnesses associated with exposure to fipronil – surveillance data from 11 states in the United States, 2001–2007, *Clin. Toxicol.*, 2010, **48**, 737–734.

322. R. M. Hollingworth, Chemistry, biological activity, and uses of formamidine pesticides, *Environ. Health Perspect.*, 1976, **14**, 57–69.

323. B. B. Hoffman and R. J. Lefkowitz, Catecholamines, sympathomimetic drugs, and adrenergic receptor antagonists in *Goodman & Gilman's The*

Pharmacological Basis of Therapeutics, ed. J. G. Hardman and L. E. Limbird, McGraw-Hill, London, 9th edn, 1996, pp. 199–248.

324. F. Matsumura and R. W. Beeman, Biochemical and physiological effects of chlordimeform, *Environ. Health Perspect.*, 1976, **14**, 71–82.

325. L. G. Costa, D. S. Wu, G. Olibet and S. D. Murphy, Formamidine pesticides and alpha 2-adrenoceptors: studies with amitraz and chlordimeform in rats and development of a radioceptor binding assay, *Neurotoxicol. Teratol.*, 1989, **11**, 405–411.

326. W. H. Hsu and D. L. Hopper, Effect of yohimbine on amitraz-induced CNS depression and bradycardia in dogs, *J. Toxicol. Environ. Health*, 1986, **18**, 423–429.

327. L. K. Curren and J. A. Reynolson, Central and peripheral-adrenoceptor actions of amitraz in the dog, *J. Vet. Pharmacol. Ther.*, 1990, **13**, 86–92.

328. L. G. Costa, G. Olibet and S. D. Murphy, Alpha 2-adrenoceptors as a target for formamidine pesticides: *in vitro* and *in vivo* studies in mice, *Toxicol. Appl. Pharmacol.*, 1988, **93**, 319–328.

329. W. H. Hsu, R. N. Shaw, D. D. Schaffer, M. H. Crump and M. H. Greer, Further evidence to support the alpha 2-adrenergic nature of amitraz-induced decrease in intestinal motility, *Arch. Int. Pharmacodym. Ther.*, 1987, **286**, 145–151.

330. W. H. Hsu and S. V. McNeel, Amitraz-induced prolongation of gastrointestinal transit and bradycardia in dogs and their antagonism by yohimbine: preliminary study, *Drug Chem. Toxicol.*, 1985, **8**, 239–253.

331. B. E. Smith, W. H. Hsu and P. C. Yang, Amitraz-induced glucose intolerance in rats: antagonism by yohimbine but not by prazosin, *Arch. Toxicol.*, 1990, **64**, 680–683.

332. D. Altobelli, M. Matire, S. Maurizi and P. Preziosi, Interaction of formamidine pesticides with the presynaptic (alpha(2)-adrenoceptor regulating [^{3}H] noradrenaline release from rat hypothalamic synaptosomes, *Toxicol. Appl. Pharmacol.*, 2001, **172**, 179–185.

333. J. M. Goldman and R. L. Cooper, Assessment of toxicant-induced alterations in the luteinising hormone control of ovulation in the rat in *Female Reproductive Toxicology*, ed. H. Chapin, Academic Press, San Diego, 1993, pp. 79–91.

334. A. S. Al-Thani, A. Al-Thani, A. Elbetieha and H. Darmani, Assessment of reproductive and fertility effects of amitraz pesticides in male mice, *Toxicol. Lett.*, 2003, **138**, 235–260.

335. F. M. Young, M. F. Menadue and T. C. Lavranos, Effects of the insecticide amitraz, an α_2-adrenergic receptor agonist, on human luteinized granulosa cells, *Hum. Reprod.*, 2005, **20**, 3018–3025.

336. Joint FAO/WHO Meeting on Pesticide Residues, Pesticide Residues in Food – 1993, Evaluations 1998, Part II – Toxicological, World Health Organization, Geneva, 1999.

337. T. Roberts and D. Hutson (ed.), Amitraz in *Metabolic Pathways of Agrochemicals. Part Two. Insecticides and Fungicides*, Royal Society of Chemistry, Cambridge, 1999, pp. 729–733.

338. J. C. Kim, J. Y. Shin, Y. S. Yang, D. H. Shin, C. J. Moon, S. H. Kim, S. C. Park, Y. B. Kim, H. C. Kim and M. K. Chung, Evaluation of developmental toxicity of amitraz in Sprague-Dawley rats, *Arch. Environ. Contam. Toxicol.*, 2007, **52**, 137–144.

339. J. Palermo-Neto, J. C. Flório and M. Sakate, Developmental and behavioural effects of prenatal amitraz exposure in rats, *Neurotoxicol. Teratol.*, 1994, **16**, 65–70.

340. L. Institoris, H. Banfi, Z. Lengyel, A. Papp and L. Nagymajtenyi, A study on the immunotoxicological effects of subacute amitraz exposure in rats, *Hum. Exp. Toxicol.*, 2007, **26**, 441–445.

341. S. Ulukaya, K. Demirağ and A. R. Moral, Acute amitraz intoxication in human, *Intensive Care Med.*, 2001, **27**, 930–933.

342. P. G. Jorens, E. Zandijk, L. Belmans, P. J. C. Schepens and L. L. Bossaert, An unusual poisoning case with the unusual pesticide amitraz, *Hum. Exp. Toxicol.*, 1997, **16**, 600–601.

343. J. J. W. Ros and J. van Aken, A case of poisoning with amitraz, an agricultural pesticide, *Ned. Tidschr. Geneeskd.*, 1994, **138**, 776–778.

344. R. Garnier, D. Chataigner and D. Djebbar, Six human cases of amitraz poisoning, *Hum. Exp. Toxicol.*, 1998, **17**, 294.

345. O. Kennel, C. Prince and R. Garnier, Four cases of amitraz poisoning in humans, *Vet. Hum. Toxicol.*, 1996, **38**, 28–30.

346. S. Vucinic, D. Jovanovic, Z. Vucinic, D. Joksovic, Z. Segrt, M. Zlatovic and M. Jovanovic, A near-fatal case of acute poisoning by amitraz/xylene showing atrial fibrillation, *Forensic Toxicol.*, 2007, **25**, 41–44.

347. K. Aydin, S. Kurtoglu, M. H. Poyrazoglu, K. Üzüm, H. B. Üstünbas and I. K. Hallaç, Amitraz poisoning in children: clinical and laboratory findings of eight cases, *Hum. Exp. Toxicol.*, 1997, **16**, 680–682.

348. K. Aydin, H. Per, S. Kurtoglu, M. H. Poyrazoglu, N. Narin and D. Aslan, Amitraz poisoning in children, *Eur. J. Pediatr.*, 2002, **161**, 349–350.

349. H. R. Schmid, G. van Tulder and P. Junquera, Field efficacy of the insect growth regulator dicyclanil for flystrike prevention on lambs, *Vet. Parasitol.*, 1999, **86**, 147–151.

350. R. M. Nottingham, B. C. Hosking, H. R. Schmid, G. Strehlau and P. Junquera, Prevention of blowfly strike on coarse and fine woolled sheep with the insect growth regulator dicyclanil, *Aust. Vet. J.*, 2001, **79**, 51–57.

351. S. Jess, C. Kearns and D. I. Matthews, A survey of annual pesticide usage during the control of sheep ectoparasites in Northern Ireland, 2005, *J. Agric. Sci.*, 2007, **145**, 517–528.

352. P. J. James, A. P. Cramp, J. Winkleman, R. Mophie and G. W. Brown, Strategic use of crutching and dicyclanil to protect unmulesed sheep against breech strike, *Aust. Vet. J.*, 2009, **87**, 138–141.

353. P. Bates, Therapies for ectoparasiticism in sheep, *In Practice*, 2004, **26**, 538–547.

354. M. A. Taylor, Recent developments in ectoparasiticides, *Vet. J.*, 2001, **161**, 253–268.

355. S. Sotiraki, A. Stefanakis, M. J. Hall, R. Frakas and J. F. Graf, Wohlfartiosis in sheep and the role of dicyclanil in its prevention, *Vet. Parasitol.*, 2005, **131**, 107–117.

356. H. Tunaz and N. Uygun, Insect growth regulators for insect pest control, *Turk. J. Agric. For.*, 2004, **28**, 377–387.

357. E. Cohen, Chitin synthesis and inhibition: a revisit, *Pest. Manag. Sci.*, 2001, **57**, 946–950.

358. H. Oberlander and D. L. Silhacek, Mode of action of insect growth regulators in lepidopteran tissue culture, *Pest. Sci.*, 1998, **54**, 300–302.

359. Joint FAO/WHO Expert Committee on Food Additives, Toxicological Evaluation of Certain Veterinary Drug Residues in Food, WHO Food Additive Series 45, The Fifty-fourth Meeting of the Joint FAO/WHO Expert Committee on Food Additives International Programme on Chemical Safety, World Health Organization, Geneva, 2000, pp. 173–179.

360. M. Moto, Y. F. Sasaki, M. Okamura, M. Fujita, Y. Kashida, N. Machida and K. Mitsumori, Absence of *in vivo* genotoxicity and liver initiation activity of dicyclanil, *J. Toxicol. Sci.*, 2003, **28**, 173–179.

361. M. Moto, M. Okamura, M. Mugumura, T. Ito, M. Jin, Y. Kashida and K. Mitsumori, Gene expression analysis of dicyclanil-induced hepatocellular tumors in mice, *Toxicol. Pathol.*, 2006, **34**, 744–751.

362. M. Moto, M. Okamura, T. Muto, Y. Kashida, N. Machida and K. Mitsumori, Molecular pathological analysis on the mechanism of liver carcinogenesis in dicyclanil-treated mice, *Toxicology*, 2005, **207**, 419–436.

363. T. Umemura, Y. Kurolwa, M. Tasaki, T. Okamura, Y. Ishii, Y. Kodama, T. Nohmi, K. Mitumori, A. Nishikawa and M. Hirose, Detection of oxidative DNA damage, cell proliferation and *in vivo* mutagenicity induced by dicyclanil, a non-genotoxic carcinogen, using *gpt* delta mice, *Mutat. Res.*, 2007, **633**, 46–54.

364. M. Moto, T. Umemura, M. Okamura, M. Muguruma, T. Ito, Y. Kashida and M. Mitsumori, Possible involvement of oxidative stress in dicyclanil-induced hepatocarcinogenesis in mice, *Arch. Toxicol.*, 2006, **80**, 694–702.

365. M. Jin, Y. Dewa, M. Kawai, J. Nishimura, Y. Saegusa, S. Kemmochi, T. Harada, M. Shibutani and K. Mitsumori, The threshold dose for liver tumor promoting effects of dicyclanil in ICR mice, *J. Toxicol. Sci.*, 2010, **35**, 69–78.

366. E. E. Grafton-Cardwell, L. D. Godfrey, W. E. Chaney and W. J. Bentley, Various novel pesticides are less toxic to humans, more specific to key pests, *Calif. Agric.*, 2005, **59**, 29–34.

367. G. W. Levot, Resistance and the control of sheep ectoparasites, *Int. J. Parasitol.*, 1995, **25**, 1355–1362.

368. Joint FAO/WHO Meeting on Pesticide Residues, Pesticide Residues in Food – 2000, Evaluations 2006, Part II – Toxicological, World Health Organization, Geneva, 2008.

369. National Toxicology Program, Carcinogenesis bioassay of melamine (CAS No. 108-78-1) in F344/N rats and B6C3F$_1$ mice, National Toxicology Program Technical Report Series No. 245, 1983.

370. M. Okumura, R. Hasegawa, T. Shirai, M. Ito, S. Yamada and S. Fukushima, Relationship between calculus formation and carcinogenesis in the urinary bladder of rats administered non-genotoxic agents thymine or melamine, *Carcinogenesis*, 1992, **13**, 1043–1045.

371. M. Ogasawara, K. Imaida, H. Ishiwata, K. Toyoda, T. Kawanishi, C. Uneyama, S. Hayashi, M. Takahashi and Y. Hayashi, Urinary bladder carcinogenesis induced by melamine in F344 male rats: correlation between carcinogenicity and urolith formation, *Carcinogenesis*, 1995, **16**, 2773–2777.

372. S. Fukushima and T. Mirai, Calculi, precipitates and microcrystalluria associated with irritation and cell proliferation as a mechanism of urinary bladder carcinogenesis in rats and mice, *IARC Sci. Publ.*, 1999, **147**, 159–174.

373. K. Otori, Y. Yano, N. Takad, C. C. Lee, S. Hayashi, S. Otani and S. Fukushima, Reversibility and apoptosis in rat urinary bladder papillomatosis induced by uracil, *Carcinogenesis*, 1997, **18**, 1485–1489.

374. S. M. Cohen, Urinary bladder carcinogenesis, *Toxicol. Pathol.*, 1988, **26**, 121–127.

375. T. Sakata, T. Masui, M. John and S. M. Cohen, Uracil-induced calculi and proliferative lesions of the mouse urinary bladder, *Carcinogenesis*, 1988, **9**, 1271–1276.

376. T. Fujii, K. Nakamura and K. Hiraga, Effects of pH on the carcinogenicity of *o*-phenylphenol and sodium *o*-phenylphenate in the rat urinary bladder, *Food Chem. Toxicol.*, 1987, **25**, 359–362.

377. N. Niho, M. Shibutani, K. Toyoda, H. Sato, A Hirose, K. Imaida, M. Takahashi, Y. Hayashi and M. Hirose, Dose- and time-response studies of sodium *o*-phenylphenate urinary bladder carcinogenicity in rats, *Food Chem. Toxicol.*, 2002, **40**, 715–722.

378. K. N. Woodward, Origins of injection-site sarcomas in cats: The possible role of chronic inflammation – A review, *ISRN Vet. Sci.*, 2011, **2011**, Art. ID: 210982, 16 pp.

379. P. A. Oliveira, A. Colaco, P. L. F. De la Cruz and C. Lopes, Experimental bladder carcinogenesis in rats, *Exp. Oncol.*, 2006, **28**, 2–11.

380. H. A. Milman, Possible contribution of indomethacin to the carcinogenicity of nongenotoxic bladder carcinogens that cause bladder calculi, *Drug Chem. Toxicol.*, 2007, **30**, 161–166.

381. R. Loosli, Triazines, *Toxicology*, 1994, **91**, 59–62.

382. R. Tilak, A. K. Verma and U. B. Wankhade, Effectiveness of diflubenzuron in the control of houseflies, *J. Vector Borne Dis.*, 2010, **47**, 97–102.

383. N. P. Hajjar and J. E. Casida, Insecticidal benzoylphenyl ureas: structure activity relationships as chitin synthesis inhibitors, *Science*, 1978, **30**, 1499–1500.

384. F. Matsumura, Studies on the action mechanism of benzoylurea insecticides to inhibit the process of chitin synthesis in insects: a review on the status of research activities in the past, the present and future prospects, *Pest. Biochem. Physiol.*, 2010, **97**, 133–139.

385. B. D. Hammock and G. B. Quistad, Metabolism and mode of action of juvenile hormone, juvenoids, and other insect growth regulators in *Progress in Pesticide Biochemistry*, ed. D. H. Hutson and T. R. Roberts, John Wiley & Sons, Ltd, Chichester, 1981, vol. 1, pp. 1–83.

386. P. Cabras, Pesticides: toxicology and residues in food in *Food Safety. Contaminants and Toxins*, ed. J. P. F. D'Mello, CABI International, Oxford, 2003, pp. 91–124.

387. G. Ritchie, S. S. Rønsberg, K. A. Hoff and E. J. Bransom, Clinical efficacy of teflubenzuron (Calicide) for the treatment of *Lepeophtheirus salmonis* infestations of farmed Atlantic salmon *Salmo salar* at low water temperature, *Dis. Aquat. Organ.*, 2002, **51**, 101–106.

388. M. Franc and M. C. Cadiergues, Use of injectable Lufenuron for treatment of infestations of *Ctenocephalides felis* in cats, *Am. J. Vet. Res.*, 1997, **58**, 140–142.

389. R. D. Smith, A. J. Paul, U. D. Kitron, J. R. Philip, S. Barnett, M. J. Piel, R. W. Ness and M. Evilsizer, Impact of orally administered insect growth regulator (Lufenuron) on flea infestations of dogs in a controlled simulated home environment, *Am. J. Vet. Res.*, 1996, **57**, 502–504.

390. Y. Nishida, C. Haga, K. Oda and T. Hayama, Disinfestation of experimentally infested cat fleas, *Ctenocephalides felis*, on cats and dogs by oral Lufenuron, *J. Vet. Med. Sci.*, 1995, **57**, 655–658.

391. S. R. Dean, R. W. Meola, S. M. Meola, H. Sittertz-Bhatkhar and R. Schenker, Mode of action of Lufenuron in adult *Ctenocephalides felis* (Siphonaptera: Pulicidae), *J. Med. Entomol.*, 1999, **36**, 486–492.

392. International Programme on Chemical Safety, Environmental Health Criteria 194, *Diflubenzuron*, World Health Organization, Geneva, 1996.

393. Joint FAO/WHO Meeting on Pesticide Residues, Pesticide Residues in Food – 2001, Evaluations, Part II – Toxicological, World Health Organization, Geneva, 2002.

394. J. T. MacGregor, D. H. Gould, A. D. Mitchell and G. P. Sterling, Mutagenicity tests of diflubenzuron in the micronucleus test in E4 mice, the L5178Y mouse lymphoma forward mutation assay and the Ames Salmonella reverse mutation assay, *Mutat. Res.*, 1979, **66**, 45–53.

395. European Medicines Agency/Committee for Veterinary Medicinal Products, Teflubenzuron, MRL Summary Report (3), EMEA/MRL/221/97-FINAL, 1997. Available at: www.ema.europa.eu/.

396. M. Tasheva and V. Hristeva, Comparative study of five benzoylphenylurea insecticides on haematological parameters in rats, *J. Appl. Toxicol.*, 1993, **13**, 67–68.

397. B. Bar-Oz, S. Ito, V. Parks, M. P. Maurer and G. Koren, Estimation of neonatal exposure after accidental ingestion of lufenuron in a breast-feeding mother, *J. Hum. Lact.*, 2000, **16**, 229–230.

398. G. D. Thompson and R. Dutton, Spinosad – a case study: an example from a natural product discovery, *Pest. Manag. Sci.*, 2000, **56**, 696–702.

399. G. Thompson and S. Hutchins, Spinosad, *Pesticide Outlook*, 1999, **10**, 78–81.
400. M. Sarfraz, L. M. Dodsall and B. A. Keddie, Spinosad: A promising new tool for integrated pest management, *Outlook Pest Manag.*, 2005, **16**, 78–84.
401. V. L. Salgado, Studies on the mode of action of spinosad: insect symptoms and physiological correlates, *Pest. Biochem. Physiol.*, 1998, **60**, 91–102.
402. V. L. Salgado, J. J. Sheets, G. B. Watson and A. L. Schmidt, Studies on the mode of action of spinosad. The internal effective concentration and the concentration dependence of neural excitation, *Pest. Biochem. Physiol.*, 1998, **60**, 103–110.
403. N. Orr, A. J. Shaffner, K. Richey and G. D. Crousse, Novel mode of action of spinosad: Receptor binding studies demonstrating lack of interaction with known insecticidal target sites, *Pest. Biochem. Physiol.*, 2009, **95**, 1–5.
404. J. Cisneros, D. Goulson, L. C. Derwent, D. I. Penagos, O. Hernández and T. Williams, Toxic effects of spinosad on predatory insects, *Biol. Control*, 2002, **23**, 156–163.
405. D. Stough, S. Shellabarger, J. Quiring and A. Gabrielsen, Efficacy and safety of spinosad and permethrin crème rinses for pediculosis capitis (head lice), *Pediatrics*, 2009, **124**, e389–e395.
406. K. E. Stebbins, D. M. Bond, M. N. Novilla and M. J. Reasor, Spinosad insecticide: subchronic and chronic toxicity and lack of carcinogenicity in CD-1 mice, *Toxicol. Sci.*, 2002, **65**, 276–287.
407. B. L. Yano, D. M. Bond, M. N. Novilla, L. G. McFadden and M. J. Reasor, Spinosad insecticide: subchronic and chronic toxicity and lack of carcinogenicity in Fischer 344 rats, *Toxicol. Sci.*, 2002, **65**, 288–298.
408. T. R. Hanley, W. J. Breslin, J. F. Quast and E. W. Carney, Evaluation of spinosad in a two-generation dietary reproductive study using Sprague-Dawley rats, *Toxicol. Sci.*, 2002, **67**, 144–152.
409. W. J. Breslin, M. S. Marty, U. Vedula, A. B. Liberacki and B. L. Yano, Developmental toxicity of spinosad administered by gavage to CD rats and New Zealand white rabbits, *Food Chem. Toxicol.*, 2000, **38**, 1103–1112.
410. W. H. Halliwell, Cationic amphiphilic drug-induced phospholipidosis, *Toxicol. Pathol.*, 1997, **25**, 53–60.
411. M. J. Reasor and S. Kacew, Drug-induced phospholipidosis: are there functional consequences? *Exp. Biol. Med.*, 2001, **226**, 825–830.
412. L. A. Chatman, D. Morton, T. O. Johnson and S. D. Anway, A strategy for risk management of drug-induced phospholipidosis, *Toxicol. Pathol.*, 2009, **37**, 997–1005.
413. N. Anderson and J. Borlak, Drug-induced phospholipidosis, *FEBS Lett.*, 2009, **580**, 5533–5540.
414. I. H. Sutherland and W. C. Campbell, Development, pharmacokinetics and mode of action of ivermectin, *Acta Leiden.*, 1990, **59**, 161–168.

415. Q. A. McKellar, Ecotoxicology and residues of anthelmintic agents, *Vet. Parasitol.*, 1997, **72**(3–4), 413–435.
416. Q. A. McKellar and H. A. Benchaoui, Avermectins and milbemycins, *J. Vet. Pharmacol. Ther.*, 1996, **19**, 331–351.
417. J. C. Williams, Anthelmintic treatment strategies: current status and future, *Vet. Parasitol.*, 1997, **72**, 461–470.
418. S. Omura, Ivermectin: 25 years and still going strong, *Int. J. Antimicrob. Agents*, 2008, **31**, 91–98.
419. W. L. Shoop, H. Mrozik and M. H. Fisher, Structure and activity of avermectins and milbemycins in animal health, *Vet. Parasitol.*, 1995, **59**, 139–156.
420. J. Di Netta, List of registrations in *Ivermectin and Abamectin*, ed. W. C. Campbell, Springer-Verlag, New York, 1989, pp. 344–346.
421. M. H. Fisher and H. Mrozik, Chemistry in *Ivermectin and Abamectin*, ed. W. C. Campbell, Springer-Verlag, New York, 1989, pp. 1–23.
422. R. W. Burg and E. O. Stapley, Isolation and characterization of the producing organism in *Ivermectin and Abamectin*, ed. W. C. Campbell, Springer-Verlag, New York, 1989, pp. 24–32.
423. W. L. Shoop, P. Dermontigny, D. W. Fink, J. B. Williams, J. R. Egerton, H. Mrozik, M. H. Fisher, B. J. Skelly and M. J. Turner, Efficacy in sheep and pharmacokinetics in cattle that led to the selection of eprinomectin as a topical endectocide for cattle, *Int. J. Parasitol.*, 1996, **26**, 1227–1235.
424. W. L. Shoop, J. R. Egerton, C. H. Eary, H. W. Haines, B. F. Michael, H. Mrozik, P. Eskola, M. H. Fisher, L. Slayton, D. A. Ostlind, B. J. Skelly, R. K. Fulton, D. Barth, S. Costa, L. M. Gregory, W. C. Campbell, R. L. Seward and M. J. Turner, Eprinomectin: A novel avermectin for use as a topical endectocide for cattle, *Int. J. Parasitol.*, 1996, **26**, 1237–1242.
425. B. F. Bishop, C. I. Bruce, N. A. Evans, A. C. Goudie, K. A. F. Gration, S. P. Gibson, M. S. Pacey, D. A. Perry, N. D. A. Walshe and M. J. Witty, Selamectin: a novel broad spectrum endectocide for dogs and cats, *Vet. Parasitol.*, 2000, **91**, 163–176.
426. M. G. Boy, R. H. Six, C. A. Thomas, M. J. Novotny, C. D. Smothers, T. G. Rowan and A. D. Jernigan, Efficacy and safety of selamectin against fleas and heartworms in dogs and cats presented as veterinary patients in North America, *Vet. Parasitol.*, 2000, **91**, 233–250.
427. R. H. Six, G. H. Sture, C. A. Thomas, R. G. Clemence, H. A. Benchaoui, M. G. Boy, P. Watson, D. G. Smith, A. D. Jernigan and T. G. Rowan, Efficacy and safety of selamectin against gastrointestinal nematodes in cats presented as veterinary patients in North America, *Vet. Parasitol.*, 2000, **91**, 321–331.
428. I. Ishaaya, S. Kontsedalov and A. R. Horowitz, Emamectin, a novel insecticide for controlling field crop pests, *Pest. Manag. Sci.*, 2002, **58**, 1091–1095.
429. J. Brocklebank, Assessing fish health during sea lice infestations, *North. Aquac.*, 1995, **1**, 8–9.

430. R. Armstrong, D. MacPhee, T. Katz and R. Endris, A field efficacy evaluation of emamectin benzoate for the control of sea lice on Atlantic salmon, *Can. Vet. J.*, 2000, **41**, 607–612.

431. L. E. Burridge, N. Hamilton, S. E. Waddy, K. Haya, S. M. Mercer, R. Greenhalgh, R. Tauber, S. V. Radecki, L. S. Crouch, P. G. Wislocki and R. G. Endris, Acute toxicity of emamectin benzoate (SLICE™) in fish feed to American lobster, *Homarus americanus*, *Aquac. Res.*, 2004, **35**, 713–722.

432. K. Willis and N. Ling, The toxicity of emamectin benzoate, an aquaculture pesticide, to planktonic marine copepods, *Aquaculture*, 2003, **221**, 289–297.

433. K. J. Willis, P. A. Gillibrand, C. J. Cromey and K. D. Black, Sea lice treatments on salmon farms have no adverse effects on zooplankton communities: a case study, *Mar. Pollut. Bull.*, 2005, **50**, 806–816.

434. T. C. Telfer, D. J. Baird, J. G. McHenery, J. Stone, I. Sutherland and P. Wislocki, Environmental effects of the anti-sea lice (Copepoda: Caligidae) therapeutant emamectin benzoate under commercial use conditions in the marine environment, *Aquaculture*, 2006, **260**, 163–180.

435. P. R. Smith, M. Maloney, A. McElligott, R. Palmer, J. O'Kelly and F. O'Brien, The efficiency of oral ivermectin in the control of sea lice infestations of farmed Atlantic salmon in *Pathogens of Wild and Farmed Fish: Sea Lice*, ed. G. A. Boxall and D. Defaye, Ellis Horwood Series in Aquaculture and Fisheries Support, London, 1993, pp. 296–307.

436. K. N. Woodward, Maximum residue limits in *Veterinary Pharmacovigilance. Adverse Reactions to Veterinary Medicinal Products*, ed. K. N. Woodward, Wiley-Blackwell, Chichester, 2009, pp. 547–567.

437. K. N. Woodward, The assessment of user safety exposure and risk to veterinary medicinal products in the European Union, *Regul. Pharmacol. Toxicol.*, 2008, **50**, 114–128.

438. K. N. Woodward, The evolution of safety assessments for veterinary medicinal products in the European Union, *Vet. Hum. Toxicol.*, 2004, **46**, 199–205.

439. Joint FAO/WHO Meeting on Pesticide Residues, Pesticide Residues in Food – 1992, Joint FAO/WHO Meeting on Pesticide Residues. Evaluations 1992, Part II – Toxicology, World Health Organization, Geneva, 1993, pp. 3–31.

440. Joint FAO/WHO Meeting on Pesticide Residues, Pesticide Residues in Food – 1994, Joint FAO/WHO Meeting on Pesticide Residues, Evaluations 1994, Part II – Toxicology, World Health Organization, Geneva, 1995, pp. 3–13.

441. Joint FAO/WHO Expert Committee on Food Additives, Toxicological evaluation of Certain veterinary drug residues in food, WHO Food Additive Series 27, The Thirty-sixth Meeting of the Joint FAO/WHO Expert Committee on Food Additives, International Programme on Chemical Safety, World Health Organization, Geneva, 1991, pp. 27–73.

442. J. D. Pulliam, R. L. Seward, R. T. Henry and S. A. Steinberg, Investigating ivermectin toxicity in collies, *Vet. Med.*, 1985, **80**, 33–40.
443. Joint FAO/WHO Expert Committee on Food Additives, Toxicological Evaluation of Certain Veterinary Drug Residues in Food, WHO Food Additive Series 31, The Fortieth Meeting of the Joint FAO/WHO Expert Committee on Food Additives, International Programme on Chemical Safety, World Health Organization, Geneva, 1993, pp. 23–36.
444. Joint FAO/WHO Expert Committee on Food Additives, Toxicological Evaluation of Certain Veterinary Drug Residues in Food, WHO Food Additive Series 41, The Fiftieth Meeting of the Joint FAO/WHO Expert Committee on Food Additives, International Programme on Chemical Safety, World Health Organization, Geneva, 1998, pp. 3–22.
445. Committee for Veterinary Medicinal Products, Emamectin, Summary Report (1), European Medicines Agency, EMEA/MRL/546/99-FINAL, 1999 http://www.ema.europa.eu/ (accessed May 24, 2010).
446. Joint FAO/WHO Expert Committee on Food Additives, Toxicological Evaluation of Certain Veterinary Drug Residues in Food, WHO Food Additive Series 36, The Forty-Fifth Meeting of the Joint FAO/WHO Expert Committee on Food Additives, International Programme on Chemical Safety, World Health Organization, Geneva, 1996, pp. 3–25.
447. Joint FAO/WHO Expert Committee on Food Additives, Toxicological Evaluation of Certain Veterinary Drug Residues in Food, WHO Food Additive Series 36, The Forty-Fifth Meeting of the Joint FAO/WHO Expert Committee on Food Additives, International Programme on Chemical Safety, World Health Organization, Geneva, 1996, pp. 27–50.
448. D. W. Fink and A. G. Porras, Pharmacokinetics of ivermectin in animals and humans in *Ivermectin and Abamectin*, ed. W. C. Campbell, Springer-Verlag, New York, 1989, pp. 113–130.
449. S.-H. L. Chiu and A. Y. H. Lu, Metabolism and tissue residues in *Ivermectin and Abamectin*, ed. W. C. Campbell, Springer-Verlag, New York, 1989, pp. 131–143.
450. C. M. Laffont, P.-L. Toutain, M. Alvinerie and A. Bousquet-Mélou, Intestinal secretion is a major route for parent ivermectin elimination in the rat, *Drug Metab. Dispos.*, 2002, **30**, 626–630.
451. G. R. Lankas, D. H. Minsker and R. T. Robertson, Effects of ivermectin on reproduction and neonatal toxicity in rats, *Food Chem. Toxicol.*, 1989, **27**, 523–529.
452. J. M. Poul, Effects of perinatal ivermectin exposure on behavioural development in rats, *Neurotoxicol. Teratol.*, 1988, **10**, 267–272.
453. I. Nafstad, E. Sannes, A. Hem, P. A. Engen and T. Sagvolden, Behavioural method to detect marginal neurotoxic effects of ivermectin in DA/ Orl rats, *J. Exp. Anim. Sci.*, 1991, **34**, 81–86.
454. G. N. Burkhart, Ivermectin: an assessment of its pharmacology, microbiology and safety, *Vet. Human Toxicol.*, 2000, **42**, 30–35.

455. M. J. Turner and J. M. Schaeffer, Mode of action of ivermectin in *Ivermectin and Abamectin*, ed. W. C. Campbell, Springer-Verlag, New York, 1989, pp. 73–88.

456. J. D. Roder and E. L. Stair, An overview of ivermectin toxicosis, *Vet. Hum. Toxicol.*, 1998, **40**, 369–370.

457. G. R. Dawson, K. A. Wafford, A. Smith, G. R. Marshall, P. J. Bayley, J. M. Schaeffer, P. T. Meinke and R. M. McKernan, Anticonvulsant and adverse effects of avermectins are mediated through the γ-aminobutyric acid$_A$ receptor, *J. Pharmacol. Exp. Ther.*, 2000, **295**, 1051–1060.

458. R. J. Martin, An electrophysiological preparation of *Ascaris suum* pharyngeal muscle reveals a glutamate-gated chloride channel sensitive to the avermectin analogue, Milbemycin D, *Parasitology*, 1996, **112**, 247–252.

459. J. M. Schaeffer and H. W. Haines, Avermectin binding to *Caenorhabditis elegans*. A two-state model for ivermectin binding site, *Biochem. Pharmacol.*, 1989, **38**, 2329–2338.

460. J. Yamazaki, K. Matsumoto, H. Ono and H. Fukuda, Macrolide compounds ivermectin and milbemycin D stimulate chloride channels through GABAergic drugs in cultured chick spinal neurons, *Comp. Biochem. Physiol. C*, 1989, **93**, 97–104.

461. K. L. Mealey, Ivermectin: macrolide parasitic agents in *Small Animal Toxicology*, ed. M. E. Peterson and P. A. Talbot, Elsevier, St. Louis, 2nd edn, 2006, pp. 785–794.

462. D. F. Cully, P. S. Paress, K. K. Liu, J. M. Schaeffer and J. F. Arena, Identification of a *Drosophila melanogaster* glutamate-gated chloride channel sensitive to the antiparasitic agent avermectin, *J. Biol. Chem.*, 1996, **271**, 20187–20191.

463. B. Robertson, Actions of anaesthetics and avermectin on GABA$_A$ chloride channels in mammalian dorsal root ganglion neurones, *Br. J. Pharmacol.*, 1989, **98**, 167–176.

464. A. T. Eldefrawi and M. E. Eldefrawi, Receptors for gamma-aminobutyric acid and voltage-dependent chloride channels as targets for drugs and toxicants, *FASEB J.*, 1987, **1**, 262–271.

465. G. R. Lankas, M. E. Cartwright and D. Umbenhauer, P-glycoprotein deficiency in a subpopulation of CF-1 mice enhances avermectin-induced neurotoxicity, *Toxicol. Appl. Pharmacol.*, 1997, **143**, 357–365.

466. D. R. Umbenhauer, G. R. Lankas, T. R. Pippert, D. Wise, M. E. Cartwright, S. J. Hall and C. M. Beare, Identification of a P-glycoprotein-deficient subpopulation of the CF-1 mouse strain using a restriction fragment length polymorphism, *Toxicol. Appl. Pharmacol.*, 1997, **146**, 88–94.

467. G. R. Lankas, D. Wise, M. E. Cartwright, T. Pippert and D. Umbenhauer, Placental P-glycoprotein deficiency enhances susceptibility to chemically induced birth defects in mice, *Reprod. Toxicol.*, 1998, **12**, 457–463.

468. J. M. Geyer and C. Junko, Treatment of *MDR1* mutant dogs with macrocyclic lactones, *Curr. Pharm. Biotechnol.*, 2012, **13**, 969–986.

469. K. Ueda, C. Cardarelli, M. M. Gottesman and I. Pastan, Expression of a full-length cDNA for the human 'MDR-1' gene confers resistance to colchicine, doxorubicin and vinblastine, *Proc. Natl Acad. Sci. USA*, 1987, **84**, 3004–3008.

470. M. Uhr, T. Steikler, A. Yassouridis and F. Holsboer, Penetration of amitriptyline, but not fluoxetine, into brain is enhanced in mice with blood-brain barrier deficiency due to mdr1a P-glycoprotein gene disruption, *Neuropsychopharmacology*, 2000, **22**, 380–387.

471. M. Uhr, F. Holsboer and M. B. Muller, Penetration of endogenous steroid hormones cortisone, cortisol, aldosterone and progesterone into the brain in mice deficient for both mdr1a and mdr1b P-glycoprotein, *J. Neuroendocrinol.*, 2002, **14**, 753–759.

472. A. H. Schinkel, J. J. Smit, O. van Tellingen, J. H. Beijnen, E. Wagenaar, L. van Deemter, C. A. A. M. Mol, M. A. van der Valk, E. C. Robanus-Maandag, H. P. J. te Riele, A. J. M. Berns and P. Borst, Disruption of the mouse mdr1a P-glycoprotein gene leads to a deficiency in blood-brain barrier and to increased sensitivity to drugs, *Cell*, 1994, **77**, 491–502.

473. A. H. Schinkel, E. Wagenaar, C. A. A. M. Mol and L. van Deempter, P-glycoprotein in the blood-brain barrier of mice influences the brain penetration and pharmacological activity of many drugs, *J. Clin. Invest.*, 1996, **97**, 2517–2524.

474. G. Y. Kwei, R. F. Alvaro, Q. Chen, C. Jenkins, E. A. C. Hop, C. A. Keohane, V. T. Ly, J. R. Straus, R. W. Wang, Z. Wang, T. R. Pippert and D. R. Umbenhauer, Disposition of ivermectin and cyclosporin A in CF-1 mice deficient in mdr1a P-glycoprotein, *Drug Metab. Dispos.*, 1999, **27**, 581–587.

475. J. F. Pouliot, F. L'Hereux, Z. Liu, R. K. Prichard and E. Georges, Reversal of p-glycoprotein-associated multidrug resistance by ivermectin, *Biochem. Pharmacol.*, 1997, **53**, 17–25.

476. L. F. Marques-Santos, R. R. Bernardo, E. F. de Paula and V. M. Rumjanek, Cyclosporin A and trifluoperazine, two resistance-modulating agents, increase ivermectin neurotoxicity in mice, *Pharmacol. Toxicol.*, 1999, **84**, 125–129.

477. J. W. Smit, M. T. Huisman, O. van Tellingen, H. R. Wiltshire and A. H. Schinkel, Absence or pharmacological blocking of placental P-glycoprotein profoundly increases fetal drug exposure, *J. Clin. Invest.*, 1999, **104**, 1441–1447.

478. A. D. Didier and F. Loor, Decreased biotolerability for ivermectin and cyclosporine A in mice exposed to potent p-glycoprotein inhibitors, *Int. J. Cancer*, 1995, **63**, 263–267.

479. S. Kiki-Mvouaka, C. Ménez, C. Borin, F. Lyazrhi, M. Foucaud-Vignault, J. Dupuy, X. Collet, M. Alvinerie and A. Lespine, Role of p-glycoprotein in the disposition of macrocyclic lactones: A comparison between

ivermectin, eprinomectin and moxidectin in mice, *Drug Metab. Dispos.*, 2010, **38**, 73–80.

480. K. N. Woodward, Veterinary pharmacovigilance. Part 2. Veterinary pharmacovigilance in practice – the operation of a spontaneous reporting scheme in a European Union country – the UK, and schemes in other countries, *J. Vet. Pharmacol. Ther.*, 2005, **28**, 149–170.

481. T. M. Hodge, Pharmacovigilance in the US – an industry perspective in *Veterinary Pharmacovigilance. Adverse Reactions to Veterinary Medicinal Products*, ed. K. N. Woodward, Wiley-Blackwell, Chichester, 2009, pp. 231–285.

482. Food and Drug Administration, Center for Veterinary Medicine, http:// www.fda.gov/AnimalVeterinary/SafetyHealth/ProductSafetyInformation/ (accessed January 5, 2011).

483. D. T. Lewis, S. R. Merchant and T. M. Neer, Ivermectin toxicosis in a kitten, *J. Am. Vet. Med. Assoc.*, 1994, **205**, 584–585.

484. H. Frische and L. Hunt, Suspected ivermectin toxicity in kittens, *Can. Vet. J.*, 1991, **32**, 245.

485. J. Pritchard, Treating ivermectin toxicity in cats, *Vet. Rec.*, 2010, **166**, 766.

486. G. Muhammad, A. Jabbar, M. Z. Khan and M. Saqib, Use of neo-stigmine in massive ivermectin toxicity in cats, *Vet. Hum. Toxicol.*, 2004, **46**, 28–29.

487. R. A. Lovell, Ivermectin and piperazine toxicoses in dogs and cats, *Vet. Clin. North Am. Small Anim. Pract.*, 1990, **20**, 453–468.

488. J. D. Roder, Antiparasiticals in *Clinical Veterinary Toxicology*, ed. K. H. Plumlee, Mosby, St. Louis, 2004, pp. 302–305.

489. C. R. Reinemeyer and C. H. Courtney, Chemotherapy of parasitic diseases in *Veterinary Pharmacology and Therapeutics*, ed. H. R. Adams, Iowa State Press, Ames, 2001, pp. 947–991.

490. H. A. Benchaoui, R. G. Clemence, P. J. M. Clements, R. L. Jones, P. Watson, D. J. Shanks, D. G. Smith, G. H. Sture, A. D. Jernigan and T. G. Rowan, Efficacy and safety of selamectin against fleas on dogs and cats presented as veterinary patients in Europe, *Vet. Parasitol.*, 2000, **91**, 223–232.

491. M. J. Krautmann, M. J. Novotny, K. Keulenaer, C. S. Godin, E. I. Evans, J. W. McCall, C. Wang, T. G. Rowan and A. D. Jernigan, Safety of selamectin in cats, *Vet. Parasitol.*, 2000, **91**, 393–403.

492. A. Campbell and M. Chapman, *Handbook of Poisoning in Dogs and Cats*, Blackwell Science, Oxford, 2000, pp. 167–173.

493. P. J. Kenny, K. M. Vernau, B. Puscher and D. J. Maggs, Retinopathy associated with ivermectin toxicosis in two dogs, *J. Am. Vet. Med. Assoc.*, 2008, **233**, 279–284.

494. R. C. Lynn, Drugs for the treatment of heartworm infections in *Small Animal Clinical Pharmacology and Therapeutics*, ed. D. M. Boothe, W. B. Saunders Company, London, 2001, pp. 267–279.

495. K. Hopper, J. Aldrich and S. C. Haskins, Ivermectin toxicity in 17 collies, *J. Vet. Intern. Med.*, 2002, **16**, 89–94.

496. A. J. Paul, W. J. Tranquilli, R. L. Seward, K. S. Todd and J. A. DiPietro, Clinical observations in collies given ivermectin orally, *Am. J. Vet. Res.*, 1987, **48**, 684–685.
497. M. W. Beal, R. H. Poppenga, W. J. Birdsall and D. Hughes, Respiratory failure attributable to moxidectin intoxication in a dog, *J. Am. Vet. Med. Assoc.*, 1999, **215**, 1813–1817.
498. W. J. Tranquilli, A. J. Paul, R. L. Seward, K. S. Todd and J. A. DiPietro, Response to physostigmine administration on collie dogs exhibiting ivermectin toxicosis, *J. Vet. Pharmacol. Ther.*, 1987, **10**, 96–100.
499. E. Yas-Natan, M. Shamir, S. Kleinbart and I. Aroch, Doramectin toxicity in a collie, *Vet. Rec.*, 2003, **153**, 718–720.
500. A. J. Paul, W. J. Tranquilli and D. E. Hutchens, Safety of moxidectin in avermectin-sensitive collies, *Am. J. Vet Res.*, 2000, **61**, 482–483.
501. J. G. Sherman, A. J. Paul and L. D. Firkins, Evaluation of the safety of spinosad and milbemycin 5-oxime orally to collies with the MDR 1 gene mutation, *Am. J. Vet. Res.*, 2010, **71**, 115–119.
502. A. J. Paul, D. E. Hutchens, L. D. Firkins and M. Borgstrom, Dermal safety study with imidacloprid/moxidectin topical solution in the ivermectin-sensitive collie, *Vet. Parasitol.*, 2004, **121**, 285–291.
503. W. J. Tranquilli, A. J. Paul and K. S. Todd, Assessment of toxicosis induced by high-dose administration of milbemycin oxime in collies, *Am. J. Vet. Res.*, 1991, **52**, 1170–1172.
504. N. J. Snowden, C. V. Helyar, S. R. Platt and J. Penderis, Clinical presentation and management of moxidectin toxicity in two dogs, *J. Small Anim. Pract.*, 2006, **47**, 620–624.
505. P. E. Fassler, W. J. Tranquilli, A. J. Paul, M. D. Soll, J. A. DiPietro and K. S. Todd, Evaluation of the safety of ivermectin administered in a beef-based formulation to ivermectin-sensitive collies, *J. Am. Vet. Med. Assoc.*, 1991, **199**, 457–460.
506. D. E. Crandell and G. L. Weinberg, Moxidectin toxicosis in a puppy successfully treated with intravenous lipids, *J. Vet. Emerg. Crit. Care*, 2009, **19**, 181–186.
507. L. L. Sartor, S. A. Bentjen, L. Trepanier and K. L. Mealey, Loperamide toxicity in a collie with the MDR1 mutation associated with ivermectin sensitivity, *J. Vet. Intern. Med.*, 2004, **18**, 117–118.
508. J. Geyer, O. Gavrilova and E. Petzinger, Brain penetration of ivermectin and selamectin in *mdr 1 a, b* P-glycoprotein- and *bcrp*-deficient knockout mice, *J. Vet. Pharmacol. Ther.*, 2008, **32**, 87–96.
509. V. A. Merola, S. Khan and S. Gwaltney-Brant, Ivermectin toxicosis in dogs: a retrospective study, *J. Am. Anim. Hosp. Assoc.*, 2009, **45**, 106–111.
510. P. Dowling, Pharmacogenetics: it's not just about ivermectin in collies, *Can. Vet. J.*, 2006, **47**, 1165–1168.
511. D. M. Houston, J. Parent and K. J. Matushek, Ivermectin toxicosis in a dog, *J. Am. Vet. Med. Assoc.*, 1987, **191**, 78–79.

512. M. K. Hadrick, S. E. Bunch and J. N. Kornegay, Ivermectin toxicosis in two Australian shepherds, *J. Am. Vet. Med. Assoc.*, 1995, **206**, 1147–1150.
513. M. Cotman and J. Zabavnik, Mutation of *MDR 1* gene associated with multidrug sensitivity in Australian shepherds in Slovenia, *Slov. Vet. Res.*, 2007, **44**, 19–24.
514. K. L. Mealey, S. A. Bentjen and D. K. Waiting, Frequency of the mutant MDR1 allele associated with ivermectin sensitivity in a sample population of collies from northwestern United States, *Am. J. Vet. Res.*, 2002, **63**, 479–481.
515. I. Gramer, R. Leidolf, B. Döring, S. Klintzsch, E. M. Krämer, E. Yalcin, E. Petzinger and J. Geyer, Breed distribution of the nt230(del 4) MDR1 mutation in dogs, *Vet. J.*, 2011, **189**, 67–71.
516. J. Geyer and C. Janko, Treatment of MDR1 mutant dogs with macrocyclic lactones, *Curr. Pharm. Biotechnol.*, 2012, **13**, 969–986.
517. L. S. Blair, P. F. Malatesta and D. W. Ewanciw, Dose-response study of ivermectin against *Dirofilaria immitis* in dogs with naturally acquired infections, *Am. J. Vet. Res.*, 1983, **44**, 475–477.
518. E. C. McManus and J. D. Pulliam, Histopathologic features of canine heartworm microfilarial infection after treatment with ivermectin, *Am. J. Vet. Res.*, 1984, **45**, 91–97.
519. M. T. Suderman and T. M. Craig, Efficacy of ivermectin against *Dirofilaria immitis* microfilariae in naturally infected dogs, *Am. J. Vet. Res.*, 1984, **45**, 1031–1032.
520. P. F. Boreham and R. B. Atwell, Absence of shock-like reactions to ivermectin in dogs infected with *Dirofilaria immitis*, *J. Helminthol.*, 1983, **57**, 279–281.
521. P. F. Boreham, R. B. Atwell and J. M. Euclid, Studies on the mechanism of the DEC reaction in dogs infected with *Dirofilaria immitis*, *Int. J. Parasitol.*, 1985, **15**, 543–549.
522. C. H. Carlisle, C. W. Prescott, P. J. McCosker and A. A. Seawright, The toxic effects of thiacetarsemide sodium in normal dogs and in dogs infested with *Dirofilaria immitis*, *Aust. Vet. J.*, 1974, **50**, 204–208.
523. Y. Sasaki, H. Kitagawa and K. Ishihara, Clinical application of milbemycin D as a prophylactic agent against *Dirofilaria immitis* infection in dogs: clinical findings in dogs with shock-like reaction, *Nippon Juigaku Zasshi.*, 1986, **48**, 1207–1214.
524. N. E. Palumbo, R. S. Desowitz and S. F. Perri, Observations on the adverse reaction to diethylcarbamazine in *Dirofilaria immitis*-infected dogs, *Tropenmed. Parasitol.*, 1981, **32**, 115–118.
525. P. F. Boreham and R. B. Atwell, Adverse drug reactions in the treatment of filarial parasites: haematological, biochemical, immunological and pharmacological changes in *Dirofilaria immitis* infected dogs treated with diethylcarbamazine, *Int. J. Parasitol.*, 1983, **13**, 547–556.
526. D. Brown, Ingestion of equine moxidectin by dogs, *Vet. Rec.*, 2000, **147**, 340.
527. A. K. Gray, Avermectin toxicity in the dog, *Vet. Rec.*, 1997, **140**, 563.
528. S. Eaton, Ingestion of Equest oral gel by dogs, *Vet. Rec.*, 1999, **145**, 236.

529. L. R. Hovda and S. B. Hooser, Toxicology of the newer pesticides for use in dogs and cats, *Vet. Clin. Small Anim. Pract.*, 2002, **32**, 455–467.

530. M. J. Novotny, M. J. Krautmann, J. C. Ehrhart, C. S. Godin, E. I. Evans, J. W. McCall, F. Sun, T. G. Rowan and A. D. Jernigan, Safety of selamectin in dogs, *Vet. Parasitol.*, 2000, **91**, 377–391.

531. P. A. Karns and D. G. Luther, A survey of adverse effects associated with ivermectin use in Louisiana horses, *J. Am. Vet. Med. Assoc.*, 1984, **185**, 782–783.

532. L. M. Godber, F. Derksen, R. Williams and B. Mahmoud, Ivermectin toxicosis in a mule foal, *Austr. Vet. J.*, 1995, **72**, 191–192.

533. T. M. Swor, J. L. Whittenburg and M. K. Chaffin, Ivermectin toxicosis in three adult horses, *J. Am. Vet. Med. Assoc.*, 2009, **235**, 558–562.

534. C. E. Plummer, M. E. Kallberg, F. J. Ollivier, D. E. Brooks and K. N. Gelatt, Suspected ivermectin toxicoses in a miniature mule foal causing blindness, *Vet. Ophthalmol.*, 2006, **9**, 29–32.

535. L. A. Hautekeete, S. A. Khan and W. S. Hales, Ivermectin toxicosis in a zebra, *Vet. Hum. Toxicol.*, 1998, **40**, 29–31.

536. S. A. Khan, D. E. Kuster and S. R. Hansen, A review of moxidectin overdose cases in equines from 1998 through 2000, *Vet. Hum. Toxicol.*, 2002, **44**, 232–235.

537. L. S. Goehring and M. M. Sloet van Oldruitenborgh-Oosterbann, Moxidectin overdose in a foal, *Tijdschr. Diergeneeskd.*, 1999, **124**, 412–414.

538. P. J. Johnson, D. R. Mrad, A. J. Schwarz and L. Kellam, Presumed moxidectin toxicosis in 3 foals, *J. Am. Vet. Med. Assoc.*, 1999, **214**, 678–680.

539. J. K. Thomas, Suspect ivermectin toxicity, *Vet. Rec.*, 1988, **123**, 631–632.

540. C. Button, R. Barton, P. Honey and P. Rickford, Avermectin toxicity in calves and an evaluation of picrotoxin as an antidote, *Austr. Vet. J.*, 1988, **65**, 157–158.

541. J. T. Seaman, J. S. Eagleson, M. J. Carrigan and R. F. Webb, Avermectin B$_1$ toxicity in a herd of Murray Grey cattle, *Austr. Vet. J.*, 1987, **64**, 284–285.

542. J. M. Rose, S. L. Peckham, J. L. Scism and K. L. Audus, Evaluation of the role of P-glycoprotein in ivermectin uptake by primary cultures of bovine brain microvessel endothelial cells, *Neurochem. Res.*, 1998, **23**, 203–209.

543. R. B. Richards and J. R. Edwards, A progressive spinal myelinopathy in beef cattle, *Vet. Pathol.*, 1986, **23**, 35–41.

544. J. R. Edwards, R. B. Richards and M. J. Carrick, Inherited progressive spinal myelinopathy in Murray Grey cattle, *Aust. Vet. J.*, 1988, **5**, 108–109.

545. R. D. Jolly, Mannosidosis and its control in Angus and Murray Gray cattle, *N. Z. Vet. J.*, 1978, **26**, 194–198.

546. F. L. Njoo, C. E. Flack, J. Oosting, J. S. Stilma and A. Kijlstra, Neutrophil activation in ivermectin-treated onchocerciasis patients, *Clin. Exp. Immunol.*, 1993, **94**, 330–333.

547. J. Geyer, S. Klintzsch, K. Meerkamp, A. Wöhle, O. Distl, A. Moritz and E. Petzinger, Detection of the nt230(del4) MDR 1 mutation in White

Swiss Shepherd dogs: case reports of doramectin toxicoses, breed pre-disposition and microsatellite analysis, *J. Vet. Pharmacol. Ther.*, 2007, **30**, 482–485.

548. J. L. Barbet, T. Snook, J. M. Gay and K. L. Mealey, ABCB1-1Δ (MDR1-1Δ) genotype is associated with adverse reactions in dogs treated with milbemycin oxime for generalized demodicosis, *Vet. Dermatol.*, 2009, **20**, 111–114.
549. L. L. Sartor, S. A. Bentjen, L. Trepanier and K. L. Mealey, Loperamide toxicity in a collie with the MDR1 mutation associated with ivermectin sensitivity, *J. Vet. Intern. Med.*, 2004, **18**, 117–118.
550. N. MacDonald and A. Gledhill, Potential impact of the ABCB1 (p-glycoprotein) polymorphisms on avermectin toxicity in humans, *Arch. Toxicol.*, 2007, **81**, 553–563.
551. G. Edwards, Ivermectin: does P-glycoprotein play a role in neurotoxicity? *Filaria J.*, 2003, **2**(1), 58–63.
552. C. N. Burkhart and C. G. Burkhart, Another look at ivermectin in the treatment of scabies and head lice, *Int. J. Dermatol.*, 1999, **36**, 235.
553. M. L. Elgart, A risk-benefit assessment of agents used in the treatment of scabies, *Drug Saf.*, 1996, **14**, 386–393.
554. K. M. Burkhart, C. N. Burkhart and C. G. Burkhart, Comparing topical scabietic treatments will soon be extinct, *Arch. Dermatol.*, 1997, **133**, 1314.
555. M. A. Aziz, S. Diallo, I. M. Diop, M. Larivière and M. Porta, Efficacy and tolerance of ivermectin in human onchocerciasis, *Lancet*, 1982, **2**, 171–173.
556. J.-L. Cartel, N. L. Nguyen, J.-P. Moulia-Pelat, R. Plichart, P. M. V. Martin and A. Spiegel, Mass chemoprophylaxis of lymphatic filariasis with a single dose of ivermectin in a polynesian community with a high *Wucheria bancrofti* infection rate, *Trans. R. Soc. Trop. Med. Hyg.*, 1992, **86**, 537–540.
557. S. Diallo, M. Larivière, L. Diop-Mar, R. N'Diaye, S. Badiane, M. Porta and M. Aziz, Conduct in Senegal of first studies on efficacy and safety of ivermectin (MK 993) in human onchocerciasis, *Bull. Soc. Pathol. Exot. Filiales*, 1984, **77**, 196–205.
558. V. Kumaraswami, E. A. Ottesen, V. Vijayasekaran, U. Deli, M. Swaminathan, M. A. Aziz, G. R. Sarma, R. Prabhakar and S. P. Tripathy, Ivermectin for the treatment of *Wucheria bancrofti* filariasis, *JAMA*, 1988, **259**, 3105–3153.
559. C. Naquira, G. Jiminez, J. G. Guerra, R. Bernal, D. R. Nalin, D. Neu and M. Aziz, Ivermectin for human strongyloidosis and other intestinal helminths, *Am. J. Trop. Med. Hyg.*, 1989, **40**, 304–309.
560. D. Richard-Lenoble, M. Kombila, E. A. Rupp, E. S. Pappayliou, P. Gaxotte, C. Nguiri and M. A. Aziz, Ivermectin in loiasis and concomitant *O. volvulus* and *M. perstans* infections, *Am. J. Trop. Med. Hyg.*, 1988, **39**, 480–483.

561. I. A. Conti Diaz and J. Amaro, Treatment of human scabies with oral ivermectin, *Rev. Inst. Trop. Sao Paolo*, 1999, **41**, 259–261.

562. J. Remme, G. De Sole, K. Y. Dadzie, R. H. Baker, J. D. Hatbema, A. P. Plaisier, G. J. Oortmarssen and E. M. Samba, Large scale ivermectin distribution and its epidemiological consequences, *Acta Leiden.*, 1990, **59**, 177–191.

563. M. C. Pacque, Z. Dukuly, B. M. Greene, E. Munoz, E. Keyvan-Larijani, P. N. Williams and H. R. Taylor, Community-based treatment of onchocerciasis with ivermectin: acceptability and early adverse reactions, *Bull. World Health Organ.*, 1989, **67**, 721–730.

564. J. P. Coulaud, M. Larivière, M. C. Gervias, P. Gaxotte, A. Aziz, A. M. Deluol and J. Cenac, Treatment of human onchocerciasis with ivermectin, *Bull. Soc. Pathol. Exot. Filiales*, 1983, **76**, 681–688.

565. D. A. Hilmarsdottir, R. Mayorga-Sagastume, M. Lyagoubi, P. Gaxotte, S. Biligui, J. Chodakewitz, D. Neu and M. Gentilini, Treatment of *Strongyloides stercoralis* infection with ivermectin compared to albendazole: results of an open study with 60 cases, *Trans. R. Soc. Trop. Med. Hyg.*, 1994, **88**, 344–345.

566. A. González-Canga, A. M. Sahagún Prieto, M. J. Diez Liébana, N. F. Martinez, M. S. Vega and J. J García Vieitez, The pharmacokinetics and interactions of ivermectin in humans – a mini-review, *AAPS J.*, 2008, **10**, 42–46.

567. G. M. Burnham, Adverse reactions to ivermectin treatment for onchocerciasis. Results of a placebo-controlled, double blind-trial in Malawi, *Trans. R. Soc. Trop. Med. Hyg.*, 1993, **87**, 313–317.

568. J. P. Chippaux, N. Gardon-Wendel, J. Gardon and J. C. Ernould, Absence of any adverse effect of inadvertent ivermectin treatment during pregnancy, *Trans. R. Soc. Trop. Med. Hyg.*, 1993, **87**, 318.

569. C. A. Guzzo, C. L. Furtek, A. G. Porras, C. Chen, R. Tipping, C. M. Clineschmidt, D. G. Scibberas, J. Y. Hsieh and K. C. Lasseter, Safety, tolerability and pharmacokinetics of escalating high doses of ivermectin in healthy adult subjects, *J. Clin. Pharmacol.*, 2002, **42**, 1122–1133.

570. Y. F. Sung, C. T. Huang, C. K. Fan, C. H. Lin and S. P. Lin, Avermectin intoxication with coma, myoclonus, and polyneuropathy, *Clin. Toxicol.*, 2009, **47**, 686–688.

571. B. G. Olson and J. B. Domachowske, Mazzotti reaction after presumptive treatment for schistosomiasis and strongyloidiasis in a Liberian refugee, *Pediatr. Infect. Dis. J.*, 2006, **25**, 466–468.

572. J. Gardon, N. Gardon-Wendel, J. Demanga-Ngangue, J. P. Kamgno, Chippaux and M. Boussinesq, Serious reactions after mass treatment of onchocerciasis with ivermectin in an area endemic for *Loa loa* infection, *Lancet*, 1997, **350**, 18–22.

573. J. P. Chippaux, M. Boussinesq, J. Gardon, N. Gardon-Wendel and J. C. Emould, Severe adverse reaction risks during mass treatment with ivermectin in loiasis-endemic areas, *Parasitol. Today*, 1996, **12**, 448–450.

574. G. De Sole, J. Remme, K. Awadzi, S. Accorsi, E. S. Alley, O. Ba, K. Y. Dadzie, J. Giese, M. Karam and F. M. Keita, Adverse reactions after large-scale treatment of onchocerciasis with ivermectin: combined results from eight community trials, *Bull. World Health Org.*, 1989, **67**, 707–719.
575. C. D. Mackenzie, T. G. Geary and J. A. Gerlach, Possible pathogenic pathways in the adverse clinical events seen following ivermectin administration to onchocerciasis patients, *Filaria J.*, 2003, **2**(1), S5.
576. Scientific Working Group on Serious Adverse Events in Loa Loa Endemic Areas, Report of a Scientific Group on Serious Adverse Events following Mectizan® treatment of onchocerciasis in *Loa loa* endemic areas, *Filaria J.*, 2003, **2**(1), S2.
577. D. Shorter, K. Hale and E. Elliot, Mazzotti-like reaction after treatment with praziquantel for schistosomiasis, *Pediatr. Infect. Dis. J.*, 2006, **25**, 1087–1088.
578. H. Francis, K. Awadzi and E. A. Ottesen, The Mazzotti reaction following treatment of onchocerciasis with diethylcarbamazine: clinical severity as a function of infection intensity, *Am. J. Trop. Med. Hyg.*, 1985, **34**, 529–536.
579. P. Stingl and M. Stingl, Leprosy, onchocerciasis, diethylcarbamazine and the Mazzotti reaction, *Lepr. Rev.*, 1982, **53**(4), 317–318.
580. G. M. Ackerman, H. Kephart, K. Francis, G. J. Awadzi, G. J. Gleich and E. A. Ottesten, Eosinophil deregulation. An immunologic determinant in the pathogenesis of the Mazzotti reaction in human onchocerciasis, *J. Immunol.*, 1990, **144**, 3961–3969.
581. N. E. Erondu and J. E. Donelson, Characterization of a myosin-like antigen from *Onchocera volvulus*, *Mol. Biochem. Parasitol.*, 1990, **40**, 213–224.
582. N. A. Y. Twum-Danso, Serious adverse events following treatment with ivermectin for onchocerciasis control: a review of reported cases, *Filaria J.*, 2003, **2**(1), S3.
583. N. A. Y. Twum-Danso, *Loa loa* encephalopathy temporally related to ivermectin administration reported from onchocerciasis mass treatment programs from 1989 to 2001: implications for the future, *Filaria J*, 2003, **2**(1), S7.
584. N. D. E. Alexander, M. J. Bockarie, W. A. Kastens, J. W. Kazura and M. P. Alpers, Absence of ivermectin-associated excess deaths, *Trans. R. Soc. Trop. Med. Hyg.*, 1998, **92**, 342.
585. K. Chung, C.-C. Yang, M.-L. Wu, J.-F. Deng and W.-J. Tsai, Agricultural avermectins: an uncommon but potentially fatal cause of pesticide poisoning, *Ann. Emerg. Med.*, 1999, **34**, 51–57.
586. K. N. Woodward, Toxicity in animals: target species, *Curr. Pharm. Biotechnol.*, 2012, **13**, 952–968.
587. C. C. Yang, Acute human toxicity of macrocyclic lactones, *Curr. Pharm. Biotechnol.*, 2012, **13**, 99–1003.
588. B. Skopets, R. F. Wilson, J. W. Griffith and C. M. Lang, Ivermectin toxicity in young mice, *Lab. Anim. Sci.*, 1996, **46**, 111–112.

589. S. A. Iliff-Sizemore, M. R. Partlow and S. T. Kelley, Ivermectin toxicology in a rhesus macaque, *Vet. Hum. Toxicol.*, 1990, **32**, 530–532.

590. J. S. Kim and E. C. Crichlow, Clinical signs of ivermectin toxicity and efficacy of antigabergic convulsants as antidotes for ivermectin poisoning in epileptic chickens, *Vet. Hum. Toxicol.*, 1995, **37**, 122–126.

591. J. A. Teare and M. Bush, Toxicity and efficacy of ivermectin in chelonians, *J. Am. Vet. Med. Assoc.*, 1983, **183**, 1195–1197.

592. Z. Széll, T. Sréter and I. Varga, Ivermectin toxicosis in a chameleon (*Chamaeleo senegalensis*) infected with *Foleyella furcata*, *J. Zoo Wildl. Med.*, 2001, **32**, 115–117.

593. J. H. DeMarco, D. J. Heard, G. J. Fleming, B. A. Lock and T. J. Scase, Ivermectin toxicosis after topical administration in dog-faced fruit bats (*Cynopterus brachyotis*), *J. Zoo Wildl. Med.*, 2002, **33**, 147–150.

594. M. J. Costello, Review of methods to control sea lice (Caligidae: Crustacea) infestations on salmon (*Salmo salar*) farms in *Pathogens of Wild and Farmed Fish*, ed. G. A. Boxall and D. Defaye, Ellis Horwood Series in Aquaculture and Fisheries Support, London, 1993, pp. 219–252.

595. R. Palmer, H. Rodger, E. Drinan, C. Dwyer and P. R. Smith, Preliminary trials on the efficacy of ivermectin against parasitic copepods of Atlantic salmon, *Bull. Eur. Assoc. Fish Pathol.*, 1987, **7**, 47–54.

596. J. O'Halloran, J. Carpenter, D. Ogden, W. E. Hogans and M. Jansen, Atlantic Canada. *Ergasilus labracis* on Atlantic salmon, *Can. Vet. J.*, 1992, **33**, 75.

597. P. González, F. A. González and K. Ueno, Ivermectin in human medicine, an overview of the current status of its clinical applications, *Curr. Pharm. Biotechnol.*, 2012, **13**, 1103–1109.

CHAPTER 7

Antineoplastic Drugs

7.1 Introduction

Although cancer tends to be thought of as a human disease, it can occur in any species of animal.[1–7] In fact, cancer has been detected in the fossils of various dinosaur species.[8,9] As with humans, cancer in animals may be treated using a variety of modalities including surgery, radiotherapy and chemotherapy and the major species that are treated in this way are cats and dogs. Although there is no medical reason why food animals cannot be treated for cancer, the costs involved probably make this impractical and, furthermore, the nature of anticancer drugs means that the animal would almost certainly be unfit for human consumption. It would be difficult, if not impossible, to establish maximum residue limits or tolerances for the vast majority of substances used in chemotherapy because of their toxicity and, notably, because of their genotoxicity and carcinogenicity.

A variety of drugs has been used in the chemotherapy of cancers in cats and dogs, both of which are susceptible to a range of malignant tumours. These include cyclophosphamide, chlorambucil, melphalan, lomustine, 5-fluorouracil, 6-mercaptopurine, methotrexate, doxorubicin, mitoxantrone, bleomycin, actinomycin D, docetaxel, vinblastine, vincristine, piroxicam, cisplatin and carboplatin.[1,2,6,10–43] They may also be used in the treatment of some immune diseases in dogs and cats.[44]

7.2 Classification of Antineoplastic Drugs

A number of antineoplastic drugs, and notably the older ones or newer versions related to these, act on proliferating cells at different points of the cell cycle. The cell cycle is made up of a number of phases as shown in Figure 7.1. The S-phase

Issues in Toxicology No. 14
Toxicological Effects of Veterinary Medicinal Products in Humans: Volume 1
By Kevin N. Woodward
© The Royal Society of Chemistry 2013
Published by the Royal Society of Chemistry, www.rsc.org

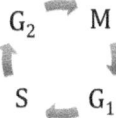

Figure 7.1   Simplified version of the cell cycle showing main phases.

is the period during which DNA is synthesised while the M-phase is the period during which dividing cells undergo mitosis. The G-phases were initially thus termed as they appeared to be gaps in the cycle. However, during these phases, protein synthesis and RNA transcription is occurring along with other events. At around the G_1 phase, cells may leave the cell cycle and become non-cycling. For example, most hepatocytes are in this phase but in the event of liver damage they may re-enter the cell cycle and begin to proliferate again. Despite its apparent simplicity, the cell cycle is extremely complex and depends on a number of factors to control and modulate it including cyclins and associated protein kinase complexes and phosphatases,[45–51] and the various cytotoxic antineoplastic drugs can make use of various sensitive or vulnerable phases.

7.2.1   The Alkylating Agents

In organic chemistry, the alkylating agents are chemicals that can transfer an alkyl (or acyl) group. They are usually either nucleophilic agents that transfer a carbanion or electrophilic agents that transfer a cation. The most well-known example is the reaction of aromatic molecules with alkyl halides in the presence of a Lewis acid that leads to the formation of alkylated aromatic molecules in the Friedel–Crafts reaction. The antineoplastic drugs tend to be relatively simple organic molecules that alkylate DNA or, more specifically, the nitrogenous bases that constitute DNA. Cells affected in this way undergo cell cycle arrest, DNA repair and apoptosis. Some of the alkylating agents used in cancer chemotherapy are highly reactive. Mechlorethamine is unstable and it reacts with other chemicals in the body soon after administration. Cyclophosphamide (Figure 7.2) on the other hand has to be metabolised in the liver to generate the active moieties, phosphoramide mustard and acrolein. Chlorambucil (Figure 7.3) is sufficiently stable to be administered orally. The major alkylating agents used in veterinary oncology are shown in Table 7.1. Dacarbazine was originally considered to be an antimetabolite but its therapeutic activity is now known to be through alkylation.[1,2,10–13,15,16,19,32–34,37] Cyclophosphamide is cell cycle specific at therapeutic doses but may be unspecific at higher doses.

7.2.2   Inhibitors of Mitosis

The inhibitors of mitosis function through their action as spindle poisons, thus disrupting mitosis. This results in arrest of mitosis at metaphase and thus these compounds are cell cycle specific operating at the M phase. Two major drugs

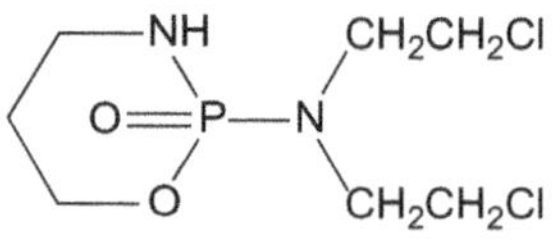

Figure 7.2 Chemical formula of cyclophosphamide.

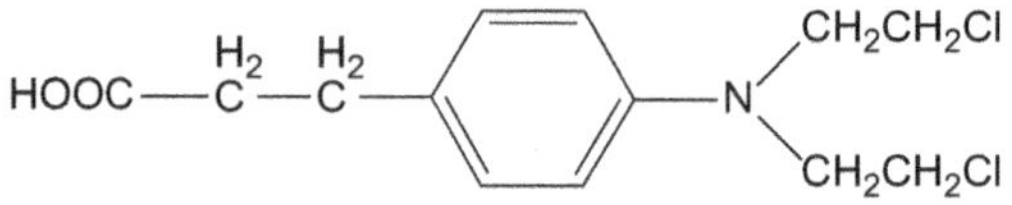

Figure 7.3 Chemical formula of chlorambucil.

Table 7.1 Major alkylating agents used in veterinary oncology.

Agent	Main indications	Side effects
Cyclophosphamide	Several types	Myelosuppression, alopecia in susceptible dogs, haemorrhagic cystitis
Melphalan	Plasma cell tumours	Myelosuppression
Chlorambucil	Chronic lymphocytic leukaemia, small cell lymphoma	Myelosuppression
Nitrosoureas (lomustine, carmustine)	Central nervous system tumours	Nausea, vomiting, myelosuppression
Dacarbazine	Relapsed lymphoma, melanosarcoma	Nausea, vomiting, mild myelosuppression

used in veterinary oncology are vincristine and vinblastine (Figure 7.4), which were originally extracted from the periwinkle, *Vinca rosea*. They have been used in the treatments of lymphomas and leukaemias in companion animals, usually in combination with other drugs. Side effects frequently seen in cats and dogs include neutropenia, anorexia and nausea. Vinblastine, but not vincristine, is myelosuppressive.[1,2,19,23] Other drugs in this group include docetaxel and paclitaxel but these drugs have so far found only limited use in veterinary oncology.

7.2.3 Antimetabolites

The antimetabolites are structural analogues of normal physiological molecules but their chemical structure has been altered in a manner that blocks their normal function. For example, methotrexate (Figure 7.5) is a structural analogue of folic acid. Methotrexate is an inhibitor of dihydrofolate reductase and it inhibits the biosynthesis of folate-dependent enzymes involved in purine and thymidylate synthesis. Hence, the drug interferes with nucleic acid synthesis and acts by killing cells as they enter the S-phase of the cell cycle. Unlike human

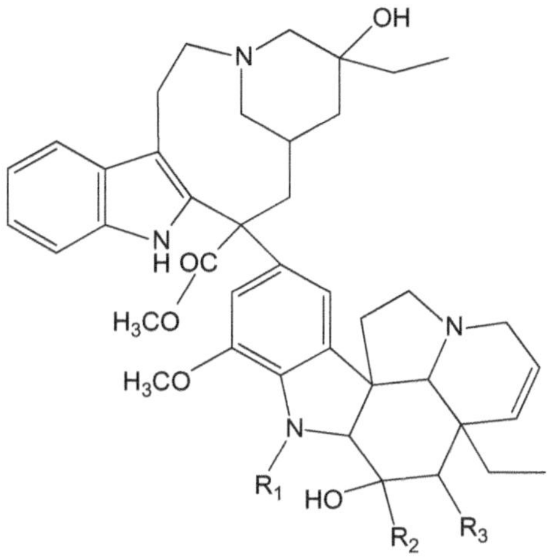

Vinblastine R$_1$ = CH$_3$ R$_2$ = COOCH$_3$ R$_3$ = OCOCH$_3$
Vincristine R$_1$ = CHO R$_2$ = COOCH$_3$ R$_3$ = OCOCH$_3$

Figure 7.4 Chemical formulae of vinblastine and vincristine.

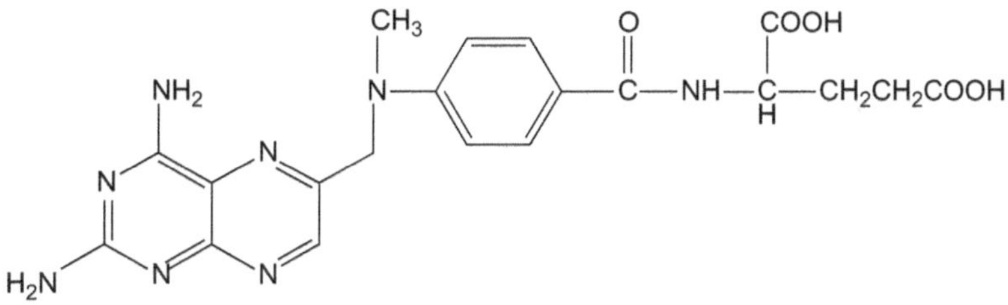

Figure 7.5 Chemical formula of methotrexate.

medicine, methotrexate has not found wide use in veterinary medicine although it has been employed in combination chemotherapy in the treatment of lymphoma. As with human medicine, high-dose methotrexate chemotherapy may require "rescue" with leucovorin (folinic acid, usually as the calcium salt). Methotrexate inhibits normal populations of dividing cells, including those of the gastrointestinal tract and, as a result, one of its major side effects is gastrointestinal toxicity. Myelosuppression is usually mild but it might be increased by co-administration of potentiated sulfonamides, as trimethoprim is a dihydrofolate inhibitor.

The other major antimetabolites used in veterinary oncology are cytosine arabinoside (ara C; Figure 7.6) and 5-fluorouracil (Figure 7.7). The former is a cytidine analogue while the latter is a purine derivative. Hence, both compounds inhibit DNA synthesis. Cytosine arabinoside is highly specific for the S-phase, while 5-fluorouracil acts on cells in G$_1$ and the S-phase. The major

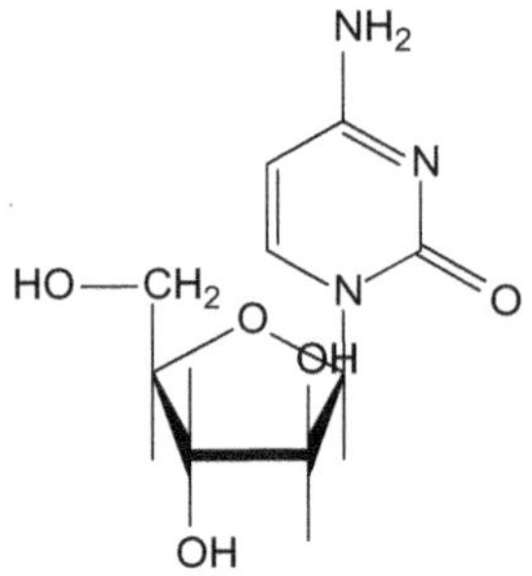

Figure 7.6   Chemical formula of cytosine arabinoside.

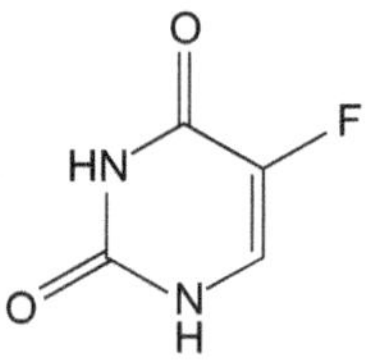

Figure 7.7   Chemical formula of 5-fluorouracil.

$$H_2CONHOH$$

Figure 7.8   Chemical formula of hydroxyurea.

clinical use of cytosine arabinoside is in the treatment of canine and feline lymphomas and for certain leukaemias. The use of 5-fluorouracil is limited by neurotoxicity in cats and dogs but it has found use in the treatment of gastrointestinal carcinomas, as well as in the palliative treatment of certain gastrointestinal tumours in companion animals. Cytosine arabinoside may result in myelosuppression and nausea, while 5-fluorouracil frequently causes adverse central nervous system reactions producing barking and aggressiveness.[1,2,19,38]

A major antimetabolite with utility in veterinary oncology is hydroxyurea (hydroxycarbamide; Figure 7.8), an inhibitor of ribonucleotide reductase, which leads to depletion of cellular DNA and arrest of cells in the S-phase of the cell cycle. It is used in the treatment of chronic myelogenous leukaemia and eosinophilic leukaemia in cats and polycythaemia vera in dogs and cats. It is less toxic than many other antineoplastic drugs but toenail loss may occur in dogs.[1,2]

7.2.4   Antibiotics

A number of antibiotics have been developed based on the anthracycline structure and the naturally occurring compound daunomycin isolated from

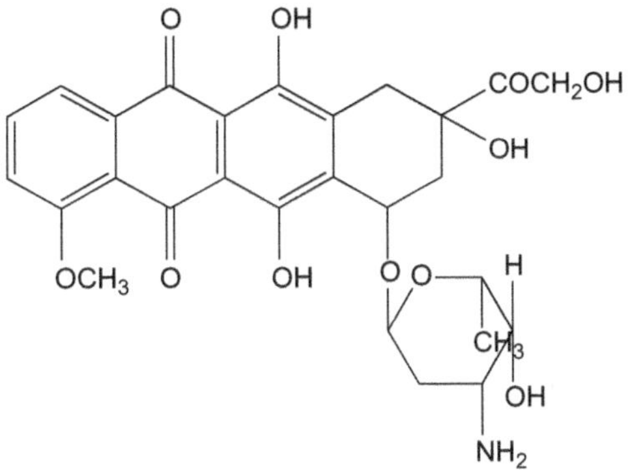

Figure 7.9 Chemical formula of doxorubicin.

strains of *Streptomyces* fungus. They include doxorubicin (Figure 7.9), daunorubicin, actinomycin D (Dactinomycin) and mitoxantrone. These compounds have planar molecules that can intercalate into DNA strands, hence their other name – the intercalating agents. The basic structure of the molecules is related to tetracycline attached by a glycosidic bond to the sugar daunosamine, a deoxy amino hexosamine derivative. In binding to nucleic acids in this way, they exert direct cytotoxicity by preventing synthesis of DNA and RNA and thus adversely affect cells entering the S-phase of the cell cycle. They also inhibit the enzyme topoisomerase II.

Doxorubicin has been used in human and veterinary oncology against a variety of malignant tumours. In the latter, it has been used in the treatment of lymphomas, leukaemias, some sarcomas and various carcinomas. The limiting factor with this group of compounds, or specifically with older members of the group, is severe cardiotoxicity. Although myelosuppression can and does occur along with gastrointestinal effects and, in humans at least, alopecia, the major treatment-limiting effect in humans and dogs is cardiomyopathy. In humans, an acute form of cardiac toxicity results in an abnormal electrocardiogram and changes in the ST-T wave while a chronic form is characterised by congestive heart failure that does not respond to digitalis. The mortality rate in humans exceeds 50%. Similar effects are seen in dogs but cats are less susceptible to these effects.[1,2,10,13,16,17,19,20,24,25,28] Doxorubicin and related drugs are iron chelators and the complexes formed cause free-radical damage, including myocardial damage.

Actinomycin D (Figure 7.10) is also an intercalating agent. It causes single strand breaks and apoptosis. It has been used in the treatment of nephroblastoma and rhabdomyosarcoma in the dog. It lacks the cardiotoxic properties of the anthracycline antibiotics but it is extremely necrotising on extravasation. It may produce nausea, vomiting and myelosuppression.

Bleomycin (Figure 7.11) is a complex glycopeptide antibiotic isolated from *Streptomyces verticillus*. Its therapeutic effects are derived from its ability to bind to DNA, which it then cleaves and fragments. Unlike many other antineoplastic

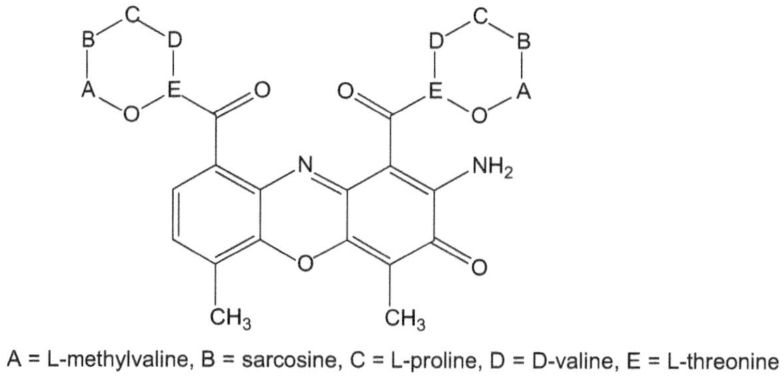

A = L-methylvaline, B = sarcosine, C = L-proline, D = D-valine, E = L-threonine

Figure 7.10 Chemical formula of actinomycin D.

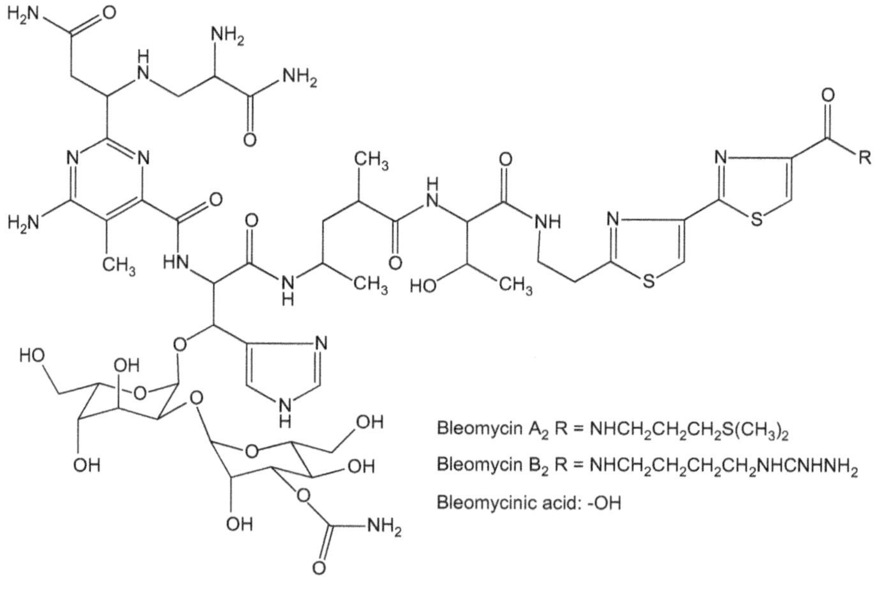

Bleomycin A_2 R = $NHCH_2CH_2CH_2S(CH_3)_2$
Bleomycin B_2 R = $NHCH_2CH_2CH_2CH_2NHCNHNH_2$
Bleomycinic acid: -OH

Figure 7.11 Chemical formula of bleomycin.

drugs, bleomycin seems to be more toxic to non-proliferating cells than it does to proliferating cells. It has been used successfully in the treatment of a number of tumours including squamous cell carcinomas in cats and dogs. It produces only minimal myelosuppression. However, in dogs and humans, a pneumonitis may appear, which progresses to pulmonary fibrosis. In humans, around 5 to 10% of patients treated with bleomycin develop some degree of pulmonary toxicity and around 1% will die from this. The risk appears to be related to total dose administered rather than with any specific acute or subchronic dosage.

7.2.5 Platinum Drugs

The two major platinum-containing drugs used in human and veterinary oncology are cisplatin and carboplatin. Cisplatin (*cis*-diamminedichloroplatinum (II); Figure 7.12) is an inorganic coordination compound. Carboplatin (*cis*-diammine(1,1-cyclobutanedicarboxylato)platinum(II); Figure 7.13) is an organic complex. These platinum complexes can interact with DNA forming interstrand and intrastrand cross-links. This leads to inhibition of DNA replication and transcription, and eventually to breaks and miscoding. The phase of the cell cycle where the platinum compounds exert their effects appears to vary from cell to cell, but the effects are most pronounced during S-phase.

Cisplatin is nephrotoxic in humans and in animals. However, this can be mitigated by hydration and diuresis. However, diuresis and hydration have no protective effects on the ototoxicity due to cisplatin. Mild to moderate mye-losuppression may also occur along with nausea and vomiting. Carboplatin is less reactive than cisplatin and it is generally less toxic. It produces less nausea, vomiting, ototoxicity and nephrotoxicity in human patients but myelosup-pression may be the dose-limiting effect. In veterinary use, carboplatin is also less nephrotoxic and it requires no hydration or diuresis.[20,35,36,38–40]

Cisplatin and carboplatin are used to treat various tumours. Carboplatin is safer for use in cats than cisplatin. It has been used to treat and cure squamous cell carcinomas of the nasal planum in feline patients.

7.3 Toxicity

As described in the preceding sections, all of these drugs can exert various toxic effects when given to human and animal patients therapeutically. Depending on the type of drug administered, these effects may be related to dose, to total dose

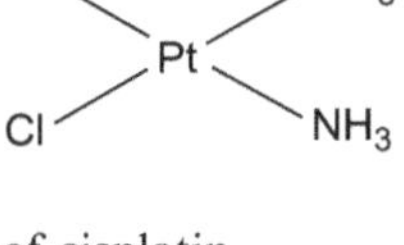

Figure 7.12 Chemical formula of cisplatin.

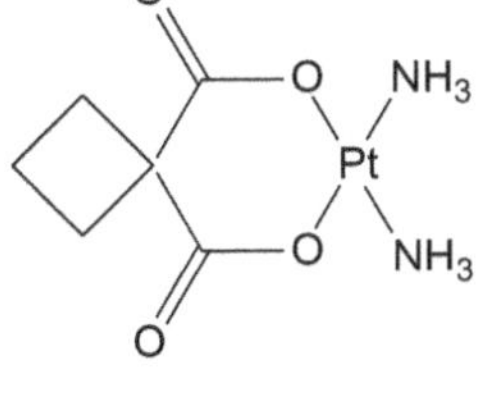

Figure 7.13 Chemical formula of carboplatin.

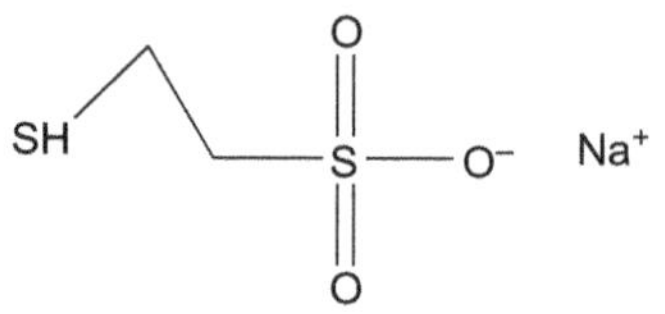

Figure 7.14   Mesna.

or to duration of dosing or due to a combination of these effects. Some of these effects may be severe and life-threatening, and they may lead to drug withdrawal and to a change of therapeutic direction. This is particularly true of patients with other conditions such as renal impairment (platinum) or pulmonary disease (bleomycin). Cyclophosphamide and related drugs (*e.g.* ifosfamide) induce a sterile, haemorrhagic cystitis in both human and veterinary patients. This can be ameliorated with the concomitant administration of mesna (sodium 2-sulfanylethane sulfate; Figure 7.14) or through better hydration of patients.[1,2,15,52–54] However, the majority of these effects are only seen in human or animal patients given therapeutic doses, usually in a repeated manner. They are unlikely to be seen in human users of the drugs treating human or animal oncology patients. Hence, the risk benefit profiles for the patient are clear, and for the forms of toxicity described for each drug or class of drugs above, so are any adverse effects for the user.

The major effects of concern for user safety are not limited to or even associated with the effects already described. The majority of these compounds, almost by virtue of their pharmacodynamic effects, are genotoxic and carcinogenic.[55–92] Indeed, one of the major concerns from the use of these drugs is the occurrence of second cancers after successful treatment for the initial tumour. In humans, several of these drugs are associated with second tumours in surviving patients previously treated for earlier disease. These include patients treated for a variety of malignancies (and occasionally other diseases) with cytotoxic drugs. The diseases include testicular tumours, breast, cervical and ovarian cancers, multiple myeloma, Hodgkin's disease, non-Hodgkin's disease, malignant melanoma, osteosarcoma, hairy cell leukaemia and other leukaemias while the drugs involved include alkylating agents, platinum compounds and antibiotics such as doxorubicin and adriamycin.[93–132] The most common secondary neoplasms described in these articles are leukaemia, usually acute myeloid leukaemia and myelodysplastic syndrome and non-Hodgkin's lymphoma, but occasionally second solid tumours are also reported.[98–100,102,105] A wide range of antineoplastic drugs have been implicated in the aetiology of myeloid malignancies and, in addition to the alkylating agents, antibiotics and antimetabolites, some growth factors and immunomodulators may have been involved.[128,133]

This information confirms that the cytotoxic drugs, as might be expected from their mode of action, are genotoxic and carcinogenic, including carcinogenic in humans. In fact some of these drugs have been reviewed by the International Agency for Research on Cancer (IARC) and it concluded that

Table 7.2 Classification of some cytotoxic drugs by IARC.[134,135]

Drug	Human cancers	Cancers in experimental animals	Genotoxicity	IARC classification[a]
Chlorambucil	Acute myeloid leukaemia; squamous cell carcinoma	Lung, mammary and lymphomas	+	Group 1[b]
Cyclophosphamide	Myeloid leukaemia, bladder cancer	Skin, bladder, leukaemia, mammary, liver	+	Group 1[b]
Hydroxyurea	Acute myeloid leukaemia	None	+	Group 3[c]
Mitoxantrone	Acute myeloid leukaemia, myelodysplastic syndrome	None	+	Group 2B[d]

[a]Group 1 – Carcinogenic to humans; Group 2B – Possibly carcinogenic to humans; Group 3 – not classifiable.
[b]Sufficient evidence in animals; sufficient evidence in humans.
[c]Inadequate evidence in animals; inadequate evidence in humans.
[d]Inadequate evidence in animals; limited evidence in humans.

there is sufficient evidence for the human carcinogenicity of chlorambucil and cyclophosphamide, while mitoxantrone is possibly carcinogenic to humans (Table 7.2). Several are carcinogenic in experimental animals.[134–137] Consequently, those involved in clinical oncology, human or veterinary, are potentially occupationally exposed to genotoxic carcinogens.

As if to emphasise this latter point, there are significant data to indicate that those involved in cancer therapy, including nurses and pharmacists, are often found to have a significant degree of genetic abnormalities. As discussed in Chapter 4, this is often pronounced enough to allow it to be used as a method of biological monitoring in workers exposed to cytotoxic drugs. Higher incidences of DNA damage, sister chromatid exchanges, micronuclei and chromosomal aberrations and exchanges have been reported in these workers.[138–180]

There appear to be no comparable studies for veterinary workers exposed to cytostatic drugs. This may be because many of these agents are used by general practitioners who are only intermittently exposed. With the rise in the numbers of specialist veterinary oncology centres, and the potential for greater or more prolonged exposures, then the similarities with human oncology will be more pronounced. Nevertheless, in the United Kingdom at least, prescription of cytotoxic drugs is significant in small animal practice.[181] Concern has been expressed about the use of cytostatic drugs in veterinary practice because of direct exposure to the drugs or through serum and excreta of treated animals.[182–185]

Clearly, this is a major concern for the physicians and veterinarians and ancillary staff involved in clinical oncology. To make matters worse, there are very few presentations of these drugs available for veterinary use and practitioners are therefore forced to use those available for human treatment. Hence, the safety of the products and their labelling has been developed to suit the human clinical use and conditions of use, and not the veterinary option. These products will not have been considered for user safety in the veterinary context as part of the approval process.

Need this be a major concern? The answer to this has to be *possibly*. In the UK at least, user warnings are not given prominence on oncology products intended for human use in the same manner that they would almost certainly be if they had been authorised through the veterinary regulatory systems. Furthermore, as is evident from the previous paragraphs, there are reasons for concern over the safe use of these products in human medicine. Hence, concerns over their use in veterinary medicine, as described above, are justified.

These concerns have led to recommendations for the safer use of cytostatic drugs in veterinary practice, as well as in human medicine.[186–199] Much of this advice is aimed at the protection of workers in human oncology practice and includes recommendations for equipment to handle drugs remotely, protective clothing, isolation techniques, surface hygiene and advice for dealing with spillages and accidents. For example, one recent report published by an international group of pharmacists made a number of recommendations for the safe use of cytotoxic drugs including those for safe storage, protective clothing, separation of equipment used for cytotoxic drugs and training and competencies for users. It also made recommendations for safe disposal of unwanted drugs and contaminated clothing.[191]

In the US, the Centers for Disease Control and Prevention (CDC) have produced a list of relevant publications, which features articles on protective clothing as well as safe handling of cytotoxic drugs.[200] The CDC's National Institute for Occupational Safety and Health (NIOSH) has produced a list of antineoplastic (and other hazardous) drugs, which includes bleomycin, busulfan, carmustine, chlorambucil, cisplatin, carboplatin, cyclophosphamide, dacarbazine, dactinomycin, daunorubicin, doxorubicin, docetaxel, fluorouracil, hydroxyurea, ifosfamide, mechlorethamine, melphalan, methotrexate, paclitaxel, vinblastine and vincristine, as well as other agents, monoclonal antibodies and antiviral compounds used in human medicine.[201] NIOSH has also published guidance on reducing and preventing occupational exposure to antineoplastic drugs in healthcare environments.[202] This guidance is aimed at both human medicine and veterinary professionals.

The NIOSH guidance reviews situations where exposure can occur. These include:

- Reconstituting powdered or lyophilised drugs and/or diluting them further
- Expelling air from syringes prior to injection
- Administering drugs by intramuscular, subcutaneous or intravenous routes
- Counting out tablets
- Adding tablets to a unit dose machine

- Crushing tablets to make liquid doses
- Compounding powders into custom dose capsules
- Contact with drugs on vials, work surfaces, floors and syringes
- Generating aerosols during product administration
- Priming intravenous infusion sets
- Handling body fluids or material contaminated with body fluids such as dressings
- Intraoperative procedures *e.g.* intraperitoneal chemotherapy
- Handling unused drugs or contaminated waste
- Decontaminating drug preparation or clinical areas
- Transporting contaminated waste
- Removing and disposing of personal protective equipment.

The guidance makes several recommendations for healthcare workers including evaluations of the workplace environment, physical layout, equipment maintenance, decontamination and cleaning, waste handling and likely methods of exposure, for example during administration and cleaning of drug-contaminated surfaces. It makes firm recommendations on the establishment of procedures for handling hazardous drugs safely, removing spills and using personal protective equipment properly. The recommendations for protective clothing include gowns and chemotherapy gloves. Use should be made of closed-system transfer devices, glovebags and needleless systems while drug preparation should be restricted to ventilated cabinets. These cabinets should be monitored for adequate air flow and exhausts should be equipped with high-efficiency particulate air (HEPA) filters. The guidance provides robust advice on cleaning, dealing with spillages and spill control and there is detailed advice on occupational medical surveillance of those involved in chemotherapy at all of its stages from preparation, to administration, to drug and equipment disposal.

In the UK, the agency responsible for occupational safety, the Health and Safety Executive (HSE), has also published detailed guidance on working with cytotoxic drugs, which, like its US counterpart, is aimed at veterinary professionals as well as human health professionals.[203] Its recommendations are very similar to those set out in the NIOSH document and these include an evaluation of the workplace and the potential risks, exposure control and personal protective equipment (Table 7.3). Emphasis is placed on regular training and workplace monitoring. There is also an emphasis on reporting workplace accidents under the Reporting of Injuries and Dangerous Occurrences Regulations 1995 (RIDDOR), which places a legal duty on employers to report incidents and dangerous occurrences. The HSE has also produced a guidance note for occupational health inspectors that draws attention to relevant legislation and the major points for focus during inspections. This circular stresses that cytotoxic drugs should be treated as occupational carcinogens and it details action steps including inspection of protocols for dealing with spillages and provision of training.[204] The UK's agency responsible for the authorisation of veterinary medicinal products has also issued guidance on the safety of

Table 7.3   Recommendations for personal protective equipment issued by the UK's Health and Safety Executive for workers exposed to cytotoxic drugs.

Exposure	*Equipment*
Skin contact	Appropriate gloves
Face and eyes	Face shield, visor, goggles, safety spectacles
Inhalation	Suitable cabinet or pharmaceutical isolator. If not available, respiratory protective equipment. Note: surgical masks are inadequate
General	Gowns, aprons. Note: standard laboratory coats are considered inadequate as solutions of cytotoxic drugs may penetrate them

cytotoxic drugs, including that veterinarians do not require clients to break or crush tablets prior to administration to their animals.[205]

7.4   Conclusions

Cytotoxic drugs must be regarded as genotoxic carcinogens and adequate care must be taken in the workplace environment to prevent exposure and to ensure their safe handling. These drugs have undoubted benefits for animal (and human) patients and, for the patient, adequate benefit-risk profiles. However, they pose hazards to those exposed to them, which will largely be healthcare professionals and any risks must be mitigated by the adoption of appropriate occupational hygiene measures. There is sound and practical advice available in the scientific literature and from government agencies that can be used when working with these agents and, indeed, with other hazardous drugs and che-micals. Biomonitoring of veterinary personnel who handle these materials should be considered, especially as the methodologies concerned are easily at hand and practicable.[206] This will become more important as other therapies become introduced into veterinary oncology. For example, tamoxifen, widely used in the treatment of hormonally responsive human breast cancer, has previously been tested in dogs but it produced too many hormone-related side effects to be considered a useful treatment option.[207] However, more recently, interest has again been shown in the use of this drug and a relatively low dose (0.8 mg/kg bw/day) was found to produce minimal adverse effects in healthy dogs although there was a risk of pyometra, which can be minimised through ovariohysterectomy.[208] As drugs new to veterinary oncology like tamoxifen are introduced there must be careful consideration of the hazards and risks to indi-viduals potentially exposed. However, the most critical issues are monitoring of occupational exposure, and reduction of exposures where this is practicable.[209,210]

References

1. C. L. Barton, Chemotherapy in *Small Animal Clinical Pharmacology and Therapeutics*, ed. D. M. Boothe, W. B. Saunders Company, London, 2001, pp. 330–348.

2. K. S. Rogers and G. L. Coppoc, Chemotherapy of neoplastic diseases in *Veterinary Pharmacology and Therapeutics*, ed. H. R. Adams, Iowa State Press, Ames, 8th edn, 2001, pp. 1064–1083.
3. M. Efron, L. Griner and K. Bernirschke, Nature and rate of neoplasia in captive wild mammals, birds, and reptiles at necropsy, *J. Natl Cancer Inst.*, 1977, **59**, 212–217.
4. E. G. MacEwen, Spontaneous tumors in dogs and cats: Models for the study of cancer in humans, *Cancer Metast. Rev.*, 1990, **9**, 125–136.
5. R. Schneider, The natural history of malignant lymphoma and sarcoma in cats and their associations with cancer in man and dog, *J. Am. Vet. Med. Assoc.*, 1970, **157**, 1753–1758.
6. S. J. Withrow and D. M. Vail (ed.), *Withrow and MacEwen's Small Animal Clinical Oncology*, Saunders Elsevier, St Louis, USA, 4th edn, 2006, pp. 425–454.
7. J. M. Dobson, S. Samuel, H. Milstein, K. Rogers and J. L. N. Wood, Canine neoplasia in the UK: estimates of incidence rates from a population of insured dogs, *J. Small Anim. Pract.*, 2002, **43**, 240–246.
8. B. M. Rothschild, D. H. Tanke, M. Hebling and L. D. Martin, Epidemiology study of tumors in dinosaurs, *Naturwissenschaften*, 2003, **90**, 495–500.
9. L. C. Natarjan, A. C. Melott, B. M. Rothschild and L. D. Martin, Bone cancer rates in dinosaurs compared with modern vertebrates, 2007. Available at: http://arxiv.org/abs/0704.1912.
10. L. G. Barber, K. U. Søenmo, K. L. Cronin and E. S. Shofer, Combined doxorubicin and cyclophosphamide for nonresectable feline fibrosarcoma, *J. Am. Vet. Med. Assoc.*, 2000, **36**, 416–421.
11. R. E. Elmslie, P. Glawe and S. W. Dow, Metronomic therapy with cyclophosphamide and piroxicam effectively delays tumor recurrence in dogs with incompletely resected soft tissue sarcomas, *J. Vet. Intern. Med.*, 2008, **22**, 1373–1379.
12. S. Lana, L. U'ren, S. Plaza, R. Elmslie, D. Gustafson, P. Morley and S. Dow, Continuous low-dose oral chemotherapy for adjuvant therapy of splenic hemangiosarcoma in dogs, *J. Vet. Intern. Med.*, 2007, **21**, 764–769.
13. G. Sylvester, R. L. Page, B. M. Fischer, J. F. Levine and T. M. Gerig, Efficacy and toxicity of doxorubicin/cyclophosphamide in dogs with multicentric lymphosarcoma, *J. Vet. Intern. Med.*, 1991, **5**, 259–262.
14. D. W. Knapp, R. C. Richardson, T. C. K. Chan, G. D. Bottoms, W. R. Widmer, D. B. DeNicola, R. Teclaw, P. L. Bonney and T. Kuczek, Piroxicam therapy in 34 dogs with transitional cell carcinoma of the urinary bladder, *J. Vet. Intern. Med.*, 1994, **8**, 273–278.
15. S. C. Charney, P. J. Bergman, A. E. Hohenhaus and J. A. Knight, Risk factors for sterile hemorrhagic cystitis in dogs with lymphoma receiving cyclophosphamide with or without concurrent administration of furosemide: 216 cases (1990–1996), *J. Am. Vet. Med. Assoc.*, 2003, **222**, 1388–1393.
16. J. C. Lori, T. J. Stein and D. H. Thamm, Doxorubicin and cyclophosphamide for the treatment of canine lymphoma: a randomized, placebo-controlled study, *Vet. Comp. Oncol.*, 2010, **8**, 188–195.

17. L. A. Wittenburg, D. L. Gustafson and D. H. Thamm, Phase I pharmacokinetic and pharmacodynamic study of combined valproic acid/doxorubicin treatment of dogs with spontaneous cancer, *Clin. Cancer Res.*, 2010, **16**, 4832–4842.

18. W. B. Morrison, Cancer chemotherapy: an annotated history, *J. Vet. Intern. Med.*, 2010, **24**, 1249–1262.

19. A. M. Morris and S. J. Withrow, A review of cancer chemotherapy for pet animals, *Can. Vet. J.*, 1984, **25**, 153–157.

20. G. N. Mauldin, R. E. Matus, S. J. Withrow and A. K. Patnaik, Canine osteosarcoma. Treatment by amputation versus amputation and adjuvant chemotherapy using doxorubicin and cisplatin, *J. Vet. Intern. Med.*, 1988, **2**, 177–180.

21. G. K. Ogilvie, Chemotherapy and the surgery patient: principles and recent advances, *Clin. Tech. Small Anim. Pract.*, 1998, **13**, 22–32.

22. M. Clemente, P. J. Andrés, L. Peña and M. D. Pérez-Alenza, Survival of dogs with inflammatory mammary cancer treated with palliative therapy alone or palliative therapy plus chemotherapy, *Vet. Rec.*, 2009, **165**, 78–81.

23. K. R. Vickery, H. Wilson, D. M. Vail and D. H. Thamm, Dose-escalating vinblastine for the treatment of canine mast cell tumours, *Vet. Comp. Oncol.*, 2008, **6**, 111–119.

24. E. O. Bannink, M. L. Sauerbrey, M. N. Mullins, J. G. Hauptman and J. E. Obradovich, Actinomycin D as rescue therapy in dogs with relapsed or resistant lymphoma: 49 cases (1999–2006), *J. Am. Vet. Med. Assoc.*, 2008, **233**, 446–451.

25. D. Simon, D. Schoenrock, W. Baumgärtner and I. Nolte, Postoperative adjuvant treatment of invasive malignant mammary gland tumours in dogs with doxorubicin and docetaxel, *J. Vet. Intern. Med.*, 2006, **20**, 1184–1190.

26. N. R. Gustafson, S. E. Lana, M. N. Mayer and S. M. LaRue, A preliminary assessment of whole-body radiotherapy interposed within a chemotherapy protocol for canine lymphoma, *Vet. Comp. Oncol.*, 2004, **2**, 125–131.

27. D. M. Vail and D. H. Thamm, Cytotoxic chemotherapy: new players, new tactics, *J. Am. Anim. Hosp. Assoc.*, 2005, **41**, 209–214.

28. E. A. Ahaus, C. G. Couto and K. D. Valerius, Hematological toxicity of doxorubicin-containing protocols in dogs with spontaneously occurring malignant tumours, *J. Am. Anim. Hosp. Assoc.*, 2000, **36**, 422–426.

29. C. A. Clifford, A. J. Mackin and C. J. Henry, Treatment of canine hemangiosarcoma: 2000 and beyond, *J. Vet. Intern. Med.*, 2000, **14**, 479–485.

30. M. Karayannapoulou, E. Kaldrymidou, T. C. Constantinidis and A. Dessiris, Adjuvant post-operative chemotherapy in bitches with mammary cancer, *J. Vet. Med. A. Physiol. Pathol. Clin. Med.*, 2001, **48**, 84–96.

31. C. Tripp, J. Fidel, C. L. Anderson, M. Patrick, C. Pratt, R. Sellon and J. N. Bryan, Tolerability of metronomic administration of lomustine in dogs with cancer, *J. Vet. Intern. Med.*, 2011, **25**, 278–284.

32. C. F. Saba, D. M. Vail and D. H. Thamm, Phase II clinical evaluation of lomustine chemotherapy for feline vaccine-associated sarcoma. *Vet. Comp. Oncol.*, 2011, epub ahead of publication.

33. N. C. Northrup, T. L. Geiger, C. E. Kosarek, C. F. Saba, B. E. LeRoy, T. M. Wall, K. R. Hume, M. O. Childress and D. A. Keys, Mechlorethamine, procarbazine and prednisone for the treatment of resistant lymphoma in dogs, *Vet. Comp. Oncol.*, 2009, **45**, 38–45.

34. T. N. Leach, M. O. Childress, A. S. Mohamed, G. E. Moore, D. R. Schrempp, S. R. Lahrman and D. W. Platt, Prospective trial of metronomic chlorambucil chemotherapy in dogs with naturally occurring cancer, *Vet. Comp. Oncol.*, 2012, **10**, 102–112.

35. D. W. Knapp, R. C. Richardson, P. L. Bonney and K. Hahn, Cisplatin therapy in 41 dogs with malignant tumors, *J. Vet. Intern. Med.*, 1988, **2**, 41–46.

36. I. D. Kurzman, G. MacEwen, R. C. Rosenthal, L. E. Fox, E. T. Keller, S. C. Helfand, D. M. Vail, R. R. Dubielzig, B. R. Madewell, C. O. Rodriguez, J. Obradovich, J. Fidel and M. Rosenberg, Adjuvant therapy for osteosarcoma in dogs: results of randomized clinical trials using combined liposome-encapsulated muramyl tripeptide and cisplatin, *Clin. Cancer Res.*, 1995, **1**, 1595–1601.

37. A. T. Daters, G. E. Mauldin, G. N. Mauldin, E. M. Brodsky and G. S. Post, Evaluation of a multidrug chemotherapy protocol with mitoxanthrone based maintenance (CHOP-MA) for the treatment of canine lymphoma, *Vet. Comp. Oncol.*, 2010, **8**, 11–22.

38. R. M. Stancliff and S. D. Gilson, Use of cisplatin, 5-fluorouracil, and second-look laparotomy for the management of gastrointestinal adenocarcinoma in three dogs, *J. Am. Vet. Med. Assoc.*, 2004, **225**, 1412–1417.

39. S. E. Lana, W. S. Dernell, M. H. Lafferty, S. J. Withrow and S. M. LaRue, Use of radiation and a slow-release cisplatin formulation for treatment of canine nasal tumors, *Vet. Radiol. Ultrasound*, 2004, **45**, 577–581.

40. E. P. Spunini, B. Vincenzi, G. Citro, I. Dotsinsky, T. Mudrov and A. Baldi, Evaluation of cisplatin as an electrochemotherapy agent for the treatment of incompletely excised mast cell tumors in dogs, *J. Vet. Intern. Med.*, 2011, **25**, 407–411.

41. L. Marcanato, K. Ruess-Melzer, J. Buchholz and B. Kaser-Hotz, New concepts in human oncology: is it possible to use them in veterinary medicine as well? *Schweiz. Arch. Tierheilkd.*, 2011, **153**, 351–360.

42. D. E. Saam, J. M. Liptak, M. J. Stalker and R. Chun, Predictors of outcome in dogs treated with adjuvant carboplatin for appendicular osteosarcoma: 65 cases (1996–2006), *J. Am. Vet. Med. Assoc.*, 2011, **15**, 195–206.

43. C. Kidd, The many challenges of veterinary oncology, *Can. Vet. J.*, 2008, **49**, 1132–1136.

44. E. Miller, The use of cytotoxic agents in the treatment of immune-mediated diseases of dogs and cats, *Sem. Vet. Med. Surg. (Small Anim.)*, 1997, **12**, 157–160.

45. J. Pines, Four-dimensional control of the cell cycle, *Nat. Cell Biol.*, 1999, **1**, E73–E79.
46. R. T. Abraham, Cell cycle checkpoint signaling through the ATM and ATR kinases, *Genes Dev.*, 2005, **15**, 2177–2196.
47. W. A. Aherne, R. S. Camplejohn and N. A. Wright, *An Introduction to Cell Population Kinetics*, Arnold, London, 1977.
48. M. B. Kastan and J. Bartek, Cell-cycle checkpoints and cancer, *Nature*, 2004, **432**, 316–323.
49. M. Pagano, R. Pepperkok, F. Verde, W. Ansorge and G. Draetta, Cyclin A is required at two points in the human cell cycle, *EMBO J.*, 1992, **11**, 961–971.
50. A. W. Murray, Recycling the cell cycle: cyclins revisited, *Cell*, 2004, **116**, 221–2234.
51. K. Rothkamm, I. Krüger, L. H. Thompson and M. Löbrich, Pathways of DNA double-strand break repair during the mammalian cell cycle, *Molec. Cell. Biol.*, 2003, **23**, 5707–5715.
52. M. P. Goren, L. M. McKenna and T. L. Goodman, Goodman, Combined intravenous and oral mesna in outpatients treated with ifosfamide, *Cancer Chemother. Pharmacol.*, 1997, **40**, 371–375.
53. M. J. Drake, P. M. Nixon and J. P. Crew, Drug-induced bladder and urinary disorders: Incidence, prevention and management, *Drug Saf.*, 1998, **19**, 45–55.
54. N. Brock and J. Pohl, Prevention of urotoxic side effects by regional detoxification with increased selectivity of oxazaphosphorine cytostatics, *IARC Sci. Publ.*, 1986, **78**, 269–279.
55. W. Jiang, Y. Lu, Z. Chen, M. Zhang, L. Jin, J. Lou and J. He, Studying the genotoxicity of vincristine on human lymphocytes using comet assay, micronucleus assay and TCR gene mutation test *in vitro*, *Toxicology*, 2008, **252**, 113–117.
56. S. P. Adams, G. M. Laws, R. D. Storer, J. G. DeLuca and W. W. Nichols, Detection of DNA damage induced by human carcinogens in acellular assays: potential application for determining genotoxic mechanisms, *Mutat. Res.*, 1996, **368**, 235–248.
57. E. W. Vogel and A. T. Natarajan, DNA damage and repair in somatic and germ cells *in vivo*, *Mutat. Res.*, 1995, **330**, 183–208.
58. J. K. Wiencke and J. Wiemels, Genotoxicity of 1,3-bis(2-chloroethyl)-1-nitrosourea (BCNU), *Mutat. Res.*, 1995, **339**, 91–119.
59. R. P. Solana, V. M. Chinchilli, J. D. Wilson, W. H. Carter and R. A. Carchman, Evaluation of the interaction of three genotoxic agents in eliciting sister-chromatid exchanges using response surface methodology, *Fundam. Appl. Toxicol.*, 1987, **9**, 541–549.
60. F. Drabløs, E. Feyzi, P. A. Aas, C. B. Vaagbø, B. Kavli, M. S. Bratlie, J. Peña-Diaz, M. Otterlei, G. Slupphaug and H. E. Krokan, Alkylation damage in DNA and RNA – repair mechanisms and medical significance, *DNA Repair (Amst)*, 2004, **3**, 1389–1407.

61. H. Tinwell and J. Ashby, Activity of the human carcinogen MeCCNU in the mouse bone marrow micronucleus test, *Environ. Mol. Mutagen.*, 1991, **17**, 152–154.

62. B. Kersten, P. Kasper, S. Y. Bentley-Schwaab and L. Müller, Use of the photo-micronucleus assay in Chinese hamster V79 cells to study photo-chemical genotoxicity, *Mutat. Res.*, 2002, **519**, 49–66.

63. R. C. Choudhury, A. K. Palo and A. Padhy, Cytogenetic consequences of vinblastine treatment in mouse bone marrow, *Chemotherapy*, 2004, **50**, 171–177.

64. M. Tiburi, M. L. Reguly, G. Schwartsmann, K. S. Cunha, M. Lehmann and H. H. Rodrigues de Andrade, Comparative genotoxic effects of vincristine, vinblastine and vinorelbine in somatic cells of *Drosophila melanogaster*, *Mutat. Res.*, 2002, **519**, 141–149.

65. S. G. Xing, X. Shi, Z. L. Wu, J. K. Chen, W. Wallace, W. Z. Whong and T. Ong, Transplacental genotoxicity of triethylenemelamine, benzene and vinblastine in mice, *Teratog. Carcinog. Mutagen.*, 1992, **12**, 223–230.

66. L. Migliore and M. Nieri, Evaluation of twelve potential aneuploidogenic chemicals by the *in vitro* human lymphocyte micronucleus assay, *Toxicol. In Vitro*, 1991, **5**, 325–336.

67. S. Padmanabhan, D. N. Tripathi, A. Vikram, P. Ramaraoo and G. B. Jena, Methotrexate-induced cytotoxicity and genotoxicity in germ cells of mice: intervention of folic and folinic acid, *Mutat. Res.*, 2009, **673**, 43–52.

68. A. D. Shahin, M. M. Ismail, A. M. Saleh, H. A. Moustafa, A. A. Aboul-Ella and H. M. Gabr, Protective effect of folinic acid on low-dose methotrexate genotoxicity, *Z. Rheumatol.*, 2001, **60**, 63–68.

69. D. M. Yourtee, L. L. Elkins, E. L. Nalvarte and R. E. Smith, Amplification of doxorubicin mutagenicity by cupric ion, *Toxicol. Appl. Pharmacol.*, 1992, **116**, 57–65.

70. C. C. Danesi, B. C. Bellagamba, R. R. Dihi, H. H. de Andrade, K. S. Cunha and M. Lehman, Evaluation of the genotoxicity of cisplatin, paclitaxel and 5-fluorouracil combined treatment in the *Drosophila* wing-spot test, *Food Chem. Toxicol.*, 2010, **48**, 3120–3124.

71. R. Zounkova, L. Kovalova, L. Blaha and W. Dott, Ecotoxicity and genotoxicity assessment of cytotoxic antineoplastic drugs and their metabolites, *Chemosphere*, 2010, **81**, 253–260.

72. J. M. Flanagan, T. A. Howard, N. Mortier, S. L. Avlasevich, M. P. Smeltzer, S. Wu, S. D. Dertinger and R. Ware, Assessment of genotoxicity associated with hydroxyurea therapy in children with sickle cell anemia, *Mutat. Res.*, 2010, **698**, 38–42.

73. D. L. Ramos, J. F. Gaspar, M. Pingarilho, O. M. Gil, A. S. Fernandes, J. Rueff and N. G. Oliveira, Genotoxic effects of doxorubicin in cultured lymphocytes with different glutathione S-transferase genotypes, *Mutat. Res.*, 2011, **724**, 28–34.

74. H. H. Tan and A. G. Porter, DNA methyltransferase I is a mediator of doxorubicin-induced genotoxicity in human cancer cells, *Biochem. Biophys. Res. Commun.*, 2009, **382**, 462–467.

75. A. A. Tohamy, A. A. El-Ghor, S. M. El-Nahas and M. M. Noshy, Beta-glucan inhibits the genotoxicity of cyclophosphamide, adriamycin and cisplatin, *Mutat. Res.*, 2003, **541**, 45–53.

76. A. Buschini, P. Poli and C. Rossi, *Saccharomyces cerevisiae* as a eukaryotic cell model to assess cytotoxicity and genotoxicity of three anticancer anthraquinones, *Mutagenesis*, 2003, **18**, 25–36.

77. G. Marzue, G. Williams, M. Iatropoulos, A. Newman, U. Sammartini, R. Pulci, S. Catellino, G. Scampini, M. Brughera, A. Imondi and A. Podesta, Anthracyclines, *Int. J. Oncol.*, 1996, **8**, 525–536.

78. R. D. Anderson, M. L. Veigl, J. Baxter and W. D. Sedwick, Excision repair reduces doxorubicin-induced genotoxicity, *Mutat. Res.*, 1993, **294**, 215–222.

79. C. T. Miyamato, J. R. Sant'Anna, C. C. Franco and M. A. Castro-Prado, Genotoxicity (mitotic recombination) of the cancer chemotherapeutic agents cisplatin and cytosine arabinoside in *Aspergillus nidulans*, *Food Chem. Toxicol.*, 2007, **45**, 1091–1095.

80. B. Kosmider, R. Osiecka, E. Zyner and J. Ochocki, Comparison between the genotoxicity of cis-Pt(II) complex of 3-aminoflavone and cis-DDP in lymphocytes evaluated by the comet assay, *Drug Chem. Toxicol.*, 2005, **28**, 231–244.

81. S. M. Cohen and S. J. Lippard, Cisplatin: from DNA damage to cancer chemotherapy, *Prog. Nucleic Acid Res. Mol. Biol.*, 2001, **67**, 93–130.

82. L. J. Bradley, K. J. Yarema, S. J. Lippard and J. M. Essigmann, Mutagenicity and genotoxicity of the major DNA adduct of the antitumor drug cis-diamminedichloroplatinum(II), *Biochemistry*, 1993, **32**, 982–988.

83. H. Vojteková, J. Svorc and S. Miertus, The SOS chromotest study on cisplatin: the genotoxicity evaluation and analytical determination in human urine, *Neoplasma*, 1990, **37**, 667–674.

84. J. Marczewska and J. Koziorowska, Comparison of the induction of SOS repair in *Escherichia coli* PQ37 and PQ243 by antineoplastic agents, *Acta Pol. Pharm.*, 1997, **54**, 35–41.

85. S. Coffing, M. Engel, D. Dickinson, C. Thiffeault, R. Spellman, T. Shutsky and M. Schuler, The rat gut micronucleus assay: a good choice for alternative *in vivo* genetic toxicology testing strategies, *Environ. Mol. Mutagen.*, 2011, **52**, 269–279.

86. P. M. Ecki, S. C. Strom, G. Michalopoulos and R. L. Jirtle, Induction of sister chromatid exchanges in cultured adult rat hepatocytes by directly and indirectly acting mutagens/carcinogens, *Carcinogenesis*, 1987, **8**, 1077–1083.

87. L. Recio, C. Hobbs, W. Caspary and K. L. Witt, Dose-response assessment of four genotoxic chemicals in a combined mouse and rat micronucleus (MN) and Comet assay protocol, *J. Toxicol. Sci.*, 2010, **35**, 149–162.

88. Q. H. Zhang, C. F. Wu, J. Y. Yang, Y. H. Mu, X. X. Chen and Y. Q. Zhao, Reduction of cyclophosphamide-induced DNA damage and apoptosis effects of ginsenoside Rb(1) on mouse bone marrow cells and peripheral blood leucocytes, *Environ. Toxicol. Pharmacol.*, 2009, **27**, 384–389.

89. R. C. Choudhury, B. Das, S. Misra and M. B. Jagdale, Cytogenetic toxicity of vincristine, *J. Environ. Pathol. Toxicol. Oncol.*, 2000, **19**, 347–355.

90. J. M. Gentile, S. Rahimi, J. Zwiesler, G. J. Gentile and L. R. Ferguson, Effect of selected antimutagens on the genotoxicity of antitumor agents, *Mutat. Res.*, 1998, **402**, 289–298.

91. K. J. Schiamenti, W. H. Hanneman and J. C. Schiamenti, Evidence for cyclophosphamide-induced gene conversion and mutation in mouse germ cells, *Toxicol. Appl. Pharmacol.*, 1997, **147**, 343–350.

92. J. Marhan, Mutagenicity of cytostatic drugs in a bacterial system. II. DNA-repair test, *Folia Microbiol (Praha)*, 1995, **40**, 462–466.

93. L. B. Travis, R. E. Curtis, J. D. Boice, C. E. Platz, B. F. Hankey and J. F. Fraumeni, Second malignant neoplasms among long-term survivors of ovarian cancer, *Cancer Res.*, 1996, **56**, 1564–1570.

94. L. B. Traviss, E. J. Holowaty, K. Bergfeldt, C. F. Lynch, B. A. Kohler, T. Wiklund, R. E. Curtis, P. Hall, M. Andersson, E. Pukkala, J. Sturgeon and M. Stovall, Risk of leukemia after platinum-based chemotherapy for ovarian cancer, *N. Engl. J. Med.*, 1999, **340**, 351–357.

95. N. J. Philpott, M. O. Elebute, R. Powless, J. G. Treleaven, M. Gore, M. G. Dainton, T. Min, G. J. Swanbury and D. Catovsky, Platinum agents and secondary myeloid leukaemia: two cases treated only with platinum-based drugs, *Br. J. Haematol.*, 1996, **93**, 884–887.

96. C. Kollmannsberger, J. T. Hartmann, L. Kanz and C. Bokemeyer, Therapy-related malignancies following treatment of germ cell cancer, *Br. J. Cancer*, 1999, **83**, 860–863.

97. L. B. Travis, R. E. Curtis, H. Storm, P. Hall, E. Holowaty, F. E. van Leeuwen, B. A. Kohler, E. Pukkala, C. F. Lynch, M. Andersson, K. Bergfeldt, E. A. Clarke, T. Wiklund, G. Stoter, M. Gospodarowicz, M. Sturgeon, J. F. Fraumeni and J. D. Boice, Risk of second malignant neoplasms among long-term survivors of testicular cancer, *J. Natl. Cancer Inst.*, 1997, **89**, 1429–1439.

98. G. M. Dores, C. Metayer, R. E. Curtis, C. F. Lynch, E. A. Clarke, B. Glimelius, H. Storm, E. Pukkala, F. E. van Leeuwen, E. J. Holowaty, M. Andersson, T. Wikund, T. Joensuu, M. B. van't Veer, M. Stovall, M. Gospodarowicz and L. B. Travis, Second malignant neoplasms among long-term survivors of Hodgkin's disease: a population-based evaluation over 25 years, *J. Clin. Oncol.*, 2002, **20**, 3484–3494.

99. L. B. Travis, Therapy-associated solid tumours, *Acta Oncol.*, 2002, **41**, 323–333.

100. L. B. Travis, S. D. Fosså, S. J. Schonfeld, M. L. McMaster, C. F. Lynch, H. Storm, P. Hall, E. Holowaty, A. Andersen, E. Pukkala, M. Andersson,

M. Kaijser, M. Gospodarowicz, T. Joensuu, R. J. Cohen, J. D. Boice, G. M. Dores and E. S. Gilbert, Second cancers among 40, 576 testicular cancer patients: focus on long-term survivors, *J. Natl. Cancer Inst.*, 2005, **97**, 1354–1365.

101. S. J. Schonfeld, E. S. Gilbert, G. M. Dores, C. F. Lynch, D. C. Hodgson, P. Hall, H. Storm, A. Andersen, E. Pukkala, E. Holowaty, M. Kaijser, M. Andersson, H. Joensuu, S. D. Fosså, J. M. Allan and L. B. Travis, Acute myeloid leukemia following Hodgkin lymphoma: a population-based study of 35,511 patients, *J. Natl. Cancer Inst.*, 2006, **98**, 215–218.

102. L. B. Travis, The epidemiology of second primary cancers, *Cancer Epidemiol. Biomarkers Prev.*, 2006, **15**, 2020–2026.

103. L. M. Brown, B. E. Chen, R. M. Pfeiffer, C. Schairer, P. Hall, E. Pukkala, F. Langmark, M. Kaijser, M. Andersson, H. Joensuu, S. D. Fosså and L. B. Travis, Risk of second non-hematological malignancies among 376, 825 breast cancer survivors, *Breast Cancer Res. Treat.*, 2007, **106**, 439–451.

104. M. Hisada, B. E. Chen, E. S. Jaffe and L. B. Travis, Second cancer incidence and cause-specific mortality among 3104 patients with hairy cell leukaemia: a population-based study, *J. Natl. Cancer Inst.*, 2007, **99**, 215–222.

105. D. C. Hodgson, E. S. Gilbert, G. M. Dores, S. J. Schonfeld, C. F. Lynch, H. Storm, P. Hall, E. Langmark, E. Pukkala, M. Andersson, M. Kaijser, H. Joensuu, S. D. Fosså and L. B. Travis, Long-term solid cancer risk among 5-year survivors of Hodgkin's lymphoma, *J. Clin. Oncol.*, 2007, **25**, 1489–1497.

106. A. K. Chaturvedi, E. A. Englis, E. S. Gilbert, B. E. Chen, H. Storm, C. F. Lynch, P. Hall, F. Langmark, E. Pukkala, M. Kaijser, M. Andersson, S. D. Fosså, H. Joensuu, J. D. Boice, R. A. Kleinerman and L. B. Travis, Second cancers among 104 760 survivors of cervical cancer: evaluation of long-term risk, *J. Natl. Cancer Inst.*, 2007, **99**, 1634–1643.

107. A. K. Chaturvedi, R. A. Kleinerman, A. Hildesheim, E. S. Gilbert, H. Storm, C. F. Lynch, P. Hall, F. Langmark, E. Pukkala, M. Andersson, S. D. Fosså, H. Joensuu, L. B. Travis and E. A. Engels, Second cancers after squamous cell carcinoma and adenocarcinoma of the cervix, *J. Clin. Oncol.*, 2009, **27**, 967–973.

108. R. Howard, E. Gilbert, C. F. Lynch, P. Hall, H. Storm, E. Holowaty, E. Pukkala, F. Langmark, M. Kaijser, M. Andersson, H. Joensuu, S. D. Fosså, J. M. Allen and L. B. Travis, Risk of leukaemia among survivors of testicular cancer: a population-based study of 42, 722 patients, *Ann. Epidemiol.*, 2008, **18**, 416–421.

109. A. K. Ng and L. B. Travis, Subsequent malignant neoplasms in cancer survivors, *Cancer J.*, 2008, **14**, 429–434.

110. A. K. Ng, L. B. Kenney, E. S. Gilbert and L. B. Travis, Secondary malignancies across the age spectrum, *Semin. Radiat. Oncol.*, 2010, **20**, 67–78.

111. R. L. Andersson, G. C. Bagby, K. Richert-Boe, R. L. Magenis and R. D. Koler, Therapy-related preleukemic syndrome, *Cancer*, 1981, **47**, 1867–1871.

112. O. Landgren, A. Thomas and S. Mailankody, Myeloma and second primary cancers, *N. Engl. J. Med.*, 2011, **365**, 2241–2242.

113. M. J. Thirman and R. A. Larson, Therapy-related myeloid leukemia, *Hematol. Oncol. Clin. North Am.*, 1996, **10**, 293–320.

114. D. R. Barnard and W. G. Woods, Treatment-related myelodysplastic syndrome/acute myeloid leukemia in survivors of childhood cancer – an update, *Leuk. Lymphoma*, 2005, **46**, 651–663.

115. S. Mailankody, R. M. Pfeiffer, S. Y. Kristinsson, N. Korde, M. Bjorkholm, L. R. Goldin, I. Turesson and O. Landgren, Risk of acute myeloid leukemia and myelodysplastic syndromes after multiple myeloma and its precursor disease (MGUS), *Blood*, 2011, **118**, 4086–4092.

116. C. G. Valentini, L. Fianchi, M. T. Voso, M. Caira, G. Leone and L. Pagano, Incidence of acute myeloid leukemia after breast cancer, *Mediterr. J. Hematol. Infect. Dis.*, 2011, **3**, e2011069.

117. A. S. Duffield, J. Aoki, M. Levis, K. Cowan, C. D. Gocke, K. H. Burns, M. J. Borowitz and M. Vuica-Ross, Clinical and pathologic features of secondary acute promyelocytic leukemia, *Am. J. Clin. Pathol.*, 2012, **137**, 395–402.

118. F. Ravandi, Therapy-related acute promyelocytic leukemia, *Haematologica*, 2011, **96**, 493–495.

119. A. Abdulwahab, J. Sykes, S. Kamel-Reid, H. Chang and J. M. Brandwein, Therapy-related acute lymphoblastic leukemia is more common than previously recognized and has a poor prognosis, *Cancer*, 2012, **118**, 3962–3967.

120. J. G. Taylor, D. S. Darari, I. Maric, Z. McIver and D. C. Arthur, Therapy-related myelogenous leukemia in a hydroxyurea-treated patient with sickle cell anemia, *Ann. Intern. Med.*, 2011, **155**, 722–724.

121. Y. Zhou, G. Tang, L. J. Medeiros, T. J. McDonnell, M. J. Keating, W. G. Wierda and S. A. Wang, Therapy-related myeloid neoplasms following fludarabine, cyclophosphamide, and rituximab (FCR) treatment in patients with chronic lymphocytic leukemia/small lymphocytic lymphoma, *Mod. Pathol.*, 2012, **25**, 237–245.

122. J. H. Cho, M. Hur, H. W. Moon, Y. M. Yun, Y. S. Ko, W. S. Kim and M. H. Lee, Therapy-related acute leukemia with mixed phenotype and t(9;22)(q32;q11.2): a case report and review of the literature, *Hum. Pathol.*, 2012, **43**, 605–609.

123. G. Leone, L. Fianchi and M. T. Voso, Therapy-related myeloid neoplasms, *Curr. Opin. Oncol.*, 2011, **23**, 672–680.

124. A. Vay, S. Kumar, S. Seward, A. Semaan, C. A. Schiffer, A. R. Munkarah and R. T. Morris, Therapy-related myeloid leukemia after treatment for epithelial ovarian carcinoma: an epidemiological analysis, *Gynecol. Oncol.*, 2011, **123**, 456–460.

125. K. Schmiegelow, Epidemiology of therapy-related myeloid neoplasms after treatment for pediatric acute lymphoblastic leukemia in the Nordic countries, *Mediterr. J. Hematol. Infect. Dis.*, 2011, **3**, e2011020.

126. A. Bagg, Therapy-associated lymphoid proliferations, *Adv. Anat. Pathol.*, 2011, **18**, 199–205.

127. A. Bari, L. Marcheselli, R. Marcheselli, E. V. Liardo, S. Pozzi, P. Ferri and S. Sacchi, Therapy-related myeloid neoplasms in non-Hodgkin lymphoma survivors, *Mediterr. J. Hematol. Infect. Dis.*, 2011, **3**, e2011065.

128. H. Sill, W. Olipitz, A. Zebisch, E. Schulz and A. Wölfer, Therapy-related myeloid neoplasms: pathobiology and clinical characteristics, *Br. J. Pharmacol.*, 2011, **162**, 792–805.

129. H. Shim, H.-S. Chi, S. Jang, E.-J. Seo, C.-J. Park and J.-H. Lee, Therapy-related acute leukemia in breast cancer patients: twelve cases treated with a topoisomerase inhibitor, *Korean J. Hematol.*, 2010, **45**, 177–182.

130. Y. Nitta, T. Ikeya, A. Sakakibara and Y. Tomita, Therapy-related myelodysplastic syndrome developed by dacarbazine, nimustine hydrochloride and vincristine sulphate (DAV) therapy for patient with malignant melanoma, *J. Dermatol.*, 2011, **38**, 164–168.

131. B. Bielorai, C. Meyer, L. Trakhtenbrot, H. Golan, E. Rozner, N. Amariglio, S. Izraeli, R. Marschalek and A. Toren, Therapy-related acute myeloid leukemia with t(2;11)9q37;q23) after treatment for osteosarcoma, *Cancer Genet. Cytogenet.*, 2011, **203**, 288–291.

132. P. Karran, Thiopurines, DNA damage, DNA repair and therapy-related cancer, *Br. Med. Bull.*, 2006, **79/80**, 153–170.

133. M. Czader, Therapy-related neoplasms, *Am. J. Clin. Pathol.*, 2009, **132**, 410–425.

134. International Agency for Research on Cancer, Monographs on the Evaluation of Carcinogenic Risk to Humans, *Some Antiviral and Antineoplastic Drugs, and Other Pharmaceutical Agents*, vol. 76, IARC, Lyon, 2000.

135. International Agency for Research on Cancer, Monographs on the Evaluation of Carcinogenic Risk to Humans, *A Review of Human Carcinogens*, vol. 100A, IARC, Lyon, 2011.

136. M. R. Berger, *Carcinogenicity of Alkylating Cytostatic Drugs in Animals*, IARC Scientific Publications, 1986, **No. 78**, pp. 161–176.

137. G. Eisenbrand and M. Habs, Chronic toxicity and carcinogenicity of cytostatic N-nitroso-(2-chloroethyl) ureas after repeated intravenous application to rats, *Dev. Toxicol. Environ. Sci.*, 1980, **8**, 273–278.

138. P. Møller, L. E. Knudsen, S. Loft and H. Wallin, The comet assay as a rapid test in biomonitoring occupational exposure to DNA-damaging agents and the effect of confounding factors, *Cancer Epidemiol. Biomarkers Prev.*, 2000, **9**, 1005–1015.

139. N. Kopjar and V. Garaj-Vrhovac, Application of the alkaline comet assay in human biomonitoring for genotoxicity: a study on Croatian medical personnel handling antineoplastic drugs, *Mutagenesis*, 2001, **16**, 71–78.

140. T. Cornetta, L. Padua, A. Testa, E. Levoli, F. Festa, G. Tranfo, L. Baccelliere and R. Cozzi, Molecular biomonitoring of nurses handling antineoplastic drugs, *Mutat. Res.*, 2008, **638**, 75–82.
141. R. Turci, C. Sottani, A. Ronchi and C. Minoia, Biological monitoring of hospital personnel occupationally exposed to antineoplastic agents, *Toxicol. Lett.*, 2002, **134**, 57–64.
142. C. L. Ursini, D. Cavallo, A. Colombi, M. Giglio, A. Marinaccio and S. Iavicoli, Evaluation of early DNA damage in healthcare workers handling antineoplastic drugs, *Int. Arch. Occup. Environ. Health*, 2006, **80**, 134–140.
143. P. J. Sessink and R. P. Bos, Drugs hazardous to healthcare workers. Evaluation of methods for monitoring occupational exposure to cytostatic drugs, *Drug Saf.*, 1999, **20**, 347–359.
144. M. Sorsa, K. Hemminki and H. Vainio, Occupational exposure to anticancer drugs – potential and real hazards, *Mutat. Res.*, 1985, **154**, 135–149.
145. M. Sorsa, L. Pyy, S. Salomaa, L. Nylund and J. W. Yager, Biological and environmental monitoring of occupational exposure to cyclophosphamide in industry and hospitals, *Mutat. Res.*, 1988, **204**, 465–479.
146. R. Barale, G. Sozzi, P. Toniolo, O. Borghi, D. Reali, N. Loprieno and G. Della Porta, Sister-chromatid exchanges in lymphocytes and mutagenicity in urine of nurses handling cytostatic drugs, *Mutat. Res.*, 1985, **157**, 235–240.
147. D. Cavallo, C. L. Ursini, B. Perniconi, A. D. Francesco, M. Giglio, F. M. Rubino, A. Marinaccio and S. Iavicoli, Evaluation of genotoxic effects induced by exposure to antineoplastic drugs in lymphocytes and exfoliated buccal cells of oncology nurses and pharmacy employees, *Mutat. Res.*, 2005, **587**, 45–51.
148. D. Cavallo, C. L. Ursini, E. Omodeo-Santé and S. Iavicoli, Micronucleus induction and FISH analysis in buccal cells and lymphocytes of nurses administering antineoplastic drugs, *Mutat. Res.*, 2007, **628**, 11–18.
149. D. Cavallo, C. L. Ursini, B. Rondinone and S. Iavicoli, Evaluation of a suitable DNA damage biomarker for human biomonitoring of exposed workers, *Environ. Mol. Mutagen.*, 2009, **50**, 781–790.
150. N. Kopjar, D. Zeljezić, V. Kasuba and R. Rozgaj, Antineoplastic drugs as a potential risk factor in occupational settings: mechanisms of action at the cell level, genotoxic effects, and their detection using different biomarkers, *Arh. Hig. Rada. Toksikol.*, 2010, **61**, 121–146.
151. V. Kasuba, R. Rozgaj and V. Garaj-Vrhovac, Analysis of sister chromatid exchanges and micronuclei in peripheral blood lymphocytes of nurses handling cytostatic drugs, *J. Appl. Toxicol.*, 1999, **19**, 401–404.
152. G. Thiringer, G. Granung, A. Holmén, B. Högstedt, B. Järvholm, D. Jönnson, L. Persson, J. Wahlström and J. Westin, Comparison of methods for the biomonitoring of nurses handling antitumor drugs, *Scand. J. Environ. Health*, 1991, **17**, 133–138.

153. G. M. Machado-Santelli, E. M. Cerqueira, C. T. Oliveira and C. A. Pereira, Biomonitoring of nurses handling antineoplastic drugs, *Mutat. Res.*, 1994, **322**, 203–208.

154. F. Oesch, J. G. Hengstler, M. Arand and J. Fuchs, Detection of primary DNA damage: application to biomonitoring of genotoxic occupational exposure and in clinical therapy, *Pharmacogenetics*, 1995, **5**, Special No., S118–S122.

155. R. P. Bos and P. J. Sessink, Biomonitoring of occupational exposures to cytostatic anticancer drugs, *Rev. Environ. Health*, 1997, **12**, 43–58.

156. F. Fucic, A. Jazbec, A. Mijic, Đ. Šešo-Šimic and R. Tomec, Cytogenetic consequences after occupational exposure to antineoplastic drugs, *Mutat. Res.*, 1998, **416**, 59–66.

157. A. Suspiro and J. Prista, Biomarkers of occupational health exposure to anticancer drugs: a minireview, *Toxicol. Lett.*, 2011, **207**, 42–52.

158. A. A. El-Ebiary, A. A. Abuelfadi and N. I. Sarhan, Evaluation of genotoxicity induced by exposure to antineoplastic drugs in lymphocytes of oncology nurses and pharmacists, *J. Appl. Toxicol.*, 2011, epub ahead of print.

159. A. B. Boughattas, S. Bouraoui, F. Debbabi, H. El Ghazel, A. Saad and N. Mrizak, Genotoxic risk assessment of nurses handling antineoplastic drugs, *Ann. Biol. Clin. (Paris)*, 2010, **68**, 545–553.

160. P. V. Rekhadevi, N. Sailaja, M. Chandrasekhar, M. Mahboob, M. F. Rahman and P. Grover, Genotoxicity assessment in oncology nurses handling anti-neoplastic drugs, *Mutagenesis*, 2007, **22**, 395–401.

161. H. Waksvik, O. Klepp and A. Brøgger, Chromosome analyses of nurses handling cytostatic drugs, *Cancer Treat. Rep.*, 1981, **65**, 607–610.

162. A. Testa, M. Giachelia, S. Palma, M. Appolloni, L. Padua, G. Tranfo, M. Spagnoli, D. Trindelli and R. Cozzi, Occupational exposure to anti-neoplastic agents induces a high level of chromosome damage, *Toxicol. Appl. Pharmacol.*, 2007, **223**, 46–55.

163. J. Rubeš, S. Kucharová, M. Vozdová, P. Musilová and Z. Zudová, Cytogenetic analysis of peripheral lymphocytes in medical personnel by means of FISH, *Mutat. Res.*, 1998, **412**, 293–298.

164. H. Pohlová, M. Černá and P. Rössner, Chromosomal aberrations, SCE and urine mutagenicity in workers occupationally exposed to cytostatic drugs, *Mutat. Res.*, 1986, **174**, 213–217.

165. A. Pilger, I. Köhler, H. Stettner, R. M. Mader, B. Rizowski, R. Terkola, E. Diem, E. Franz-Hainzi, C. Konnaris, E. Valic and H. W. Rüdiger, Long-term monitoring of sister-chromatid exchanges and micronucleus frequencies in pharmacy personnel occupationally exposed to cytostatic drugs, *Int. Arch. Occup. Environ. Health*, 2000, **73**, 442–448.

166. U. Oestreicher, G. Stephan and M. Glatzel, Chromosome and SCE analysis in peripheral lymphocytes of persons occupationally exposed to cytostatic drugs handled with and without use of safety covers, *Mutat. Res.*, 1990, **242**, 271–277.

167. H. Norppa, M. Sorsa, H. Vainio, P. Gröhn, E. Heinonen, L. Hosti and E. Nordman, Increased sister chromatid exchange frequencies in lymphocytes of nurses handling cytostatic drugs, *Scand. J. Work Environ. Health*, 1980, **6**, 299–301.

168. E. Nikula, K. Kiviniitty, J. Leisti and P. J. Taskinen, Chromosome aberrations in lymphocytes of nurses handling cytostatic agents, *Scand. J. Work Environ. Health*, 1984, **10**, 71–74.

169. S. Milković-Kraus and D. Horvat, Chromosomal abnormalities among nurses occupationally exposed to antineoplastic drugs, *Am. J. Ind. Med.*, 1991, **19**, 771–774.

170. J. J. McDevitt, P. S. J. Lees and M. A. McDiarmid, Exposure of hospital pharmacists and nurses to antineoplastic agents, *J. Occup. Med.*, 1993, **35**, 57–60.

171. S. Izdes, S. Sardas, E. Kadioglu, C. Kaymak and E. Ozcagli, Assessment of genotoxic damage in nurses occupationally exposed to anaesthetic gases or antineoplastic drugs by the comet assay, *J. Occup. Health*, 2009, **51**, 283–286.

172. E. M. Goloni-Bertollo, E. H. Tajara, A. J. Manzato and M. Varella-Garcia, Sister chromatid exchanges and chromosome aberrations in lymphocytes of nurses handling antineoplastic drugs, *Int. J. Cancer*, 1992, **50**, 341–344.

173. W. A. Anwar, S. I. Salama, M. M. El Serafy, S. A. Hemida and A. S. Hafez, Chromosomal aberrations and micronucleus frequency in nurses occupationally exposed to cytotoxic drugs, *Mutagenesis*, 1994, **9**, 315–317.

174. J. Yoshida, H. Kosaka, K. Tomioka and S. Kumagai, Genotoxic risks to nurses from contamination of the work environment with antineoplastic drugs in Japan, *J. Occup. Health*, 2006, **48**, 517–522.

175. K. Szmyd and O. Haus, Cancers among medical personnel exposed to anticancer agents, *Med. Pr*, 2011, **62**, 17–21.

176. T. Raposa and J. Várkonyi, The relationship between sister chromatid exchange induction and leukemogenicity of different cytostatics, *Cancer Detect. Prev.*, 1987, **10**, 141–151.

177. V. Brumen and D. Horvat, Work environment influence on cytostatics-induced genotoxicity in oncologic nurses, *Am. J. Ind. Med.*, 1996, **30**, 67–71.

178. S. Baourai, A. Brahem, F. Tabka, N. Mrizek, A. Saad and H. Elghezal, Assessment of chromosomal aberrations, micronuclei and proliferation rate index in peripheral lymphocytes from Tunisian nurses handling cytotoxic drugs, *Environ. Toxicol. Pharmacol.*, 2011, **31**, 250–257.

179. T. H. Connor, G. DeBord, J. R. Pretty, M. S. Oliver, T. S. Roth, P. S. J. Lees, E. F. Krieg, B. Rogers, C. P. Escalante, C. A. Toennis, J. C. Clark, B. Johnson and M. A. McDiarmid, Evaluation of antineoplastic drug exposure of health care workers at three university-based US cancer centers, *J. Occup. Environ. Med.*, 2010, **52**, 1019–1027.

180. M. A. McDiarmid, M. S. Oliver, T. S. Roth, B. Rogers and C. P. Escalante, Chromosome 5 and 7 abnormalities in oncology personnel handling anticancer drugs, *J. Occup. Environ. Med.*, 2010, **52**, 1028–1034.

181. T. A. Cave, P. Norman and D. Mellor, Cytotoxic drug use in treatment of dogs and cats with cancer by UK veterinary practices (2003 to 2004), *J. Small Anim. Pract.*, 2007, **48**, 371–377.

182. C. H. Pellicaan and E. Teske, Risks of using cytostatic drugs in veterinary medical practice, *Tijdschr. Diergeneeskd.*, 1999, **124**, 210–215.

183. C. Pellicaan, E. Teske, H. Varkamp and T. Willemse, Use of carcinogenic veterinary drugs in the veterinary clinic. Unacceptable risk for people? *Tijdschr. Diergeneeskd.*, 2002, **127**, 734–735.

184. A. Knobloch, S. A. Mohring, N. Eberle, I. Nolte, G. Hamscher and D. Simon, Drug residues in serum of dogs receiving anticancer chemotherapy, *J. Vet. Intern. Med.*, 2010, **24**, 379–383.

185. G. Hamscher, S. A. Mohring, A. Knobloch, N. Eberle, H. Nau, I. Nolte and D. Simon, Determination of drug residues in urine of dogs receiving anti-cancer chemotherapy by liquid chromatography-electrospray ionization-tandem mass spectrometry: is there an environmental or occupational risk? *J. Anal. Toxicol.*, 2010, **34**, 142–148.

186. S. Takada, Principles of chemotherapy safety procedures, *Clin. Tech. Small Anim. Pract.*, 2003, **18**, 73–74.

187. B. W. Chafee, J. A. Armistead, B. E. Benjamin, M. C. Cotugno, R. A. Forey, B. L. Pfeffenberger and J. C. Stevenson, Guidelines for the safe handling of hazardous drugs: consensus recommendations, *Am. J. Health Syst. Pharm.*, 2010, **67**, 1545–1546.

188. M. D. Zoch, S. Soefje and K. Rickabaugh, Evaluation of surface contamination with cyclophosphamide following simulated hazardous drug preparation activities using two closed-system products, *J. Oncol. Pharm. Pract.*, 2011, **17**, 49–54.

189. L. A. Power and M. Polovich, Safe handling of hazardous drugs: reviewing standards for worker protection, *Pharm. Pract. News*, 2011, **March**, 1–12.

190. P. J. M. Sessink, T. H. Connor, J. A. Jorgensson and T. G. Tyler, Reduction in surface contamination with antineoplastic drugs in 22 hospital pharmacies in the US following implementation of a closed-system drug transfer device, *J. Oncol. Pharm. Pract.*, 2011, **17**, 39–48.

191. S. Goodin, N. Griffith, B. Chen, K. Chuk, M. Douphars, C. Doreau, R. A. Patel, R. Schwartz, M. J. Tamés, R. Terkola, B. Vadnais, D. Wright and K. Meier, Safe handling of oral chemotherapeutic agents in clinical practice: recommendations from an international pharmacy panel, *J. Oncol. Pract.*, 2011, **7**, 7–12.

192. E. Green, M. Johnston, M. Trudeau, L. Schwartz, S. Poirier, G. Macartney and D. Milliken, Safe handling of parenteral cytotoxics: Recommendations for Ontario, *J. Oncol. Pract.*, 2009, **5**, 1–5.

193. R. Gonzalez and F. Massomi, Manufacturers' recommendations for handling spilled hazardous drugs, *Am. J. Health Syst. Pharm.*, 2010, **67**, 1985–1986.

194. J. Siderov, S. Kirsa and R. McLauchlan, Reducing workplace cytotoxic surface contamination using a closed-system drug transfer device, *J. Oncol. Pharm. Pract.*, 2010, **16**, 19–25.

195. R. Schierl, A. Bohlandt and D. Nowak, Guidance for surface monitoring of antineoplastic drugs in German pharmacies, *Ann. Occup. Hyg.*, 2009, **53**, 1–9.
196. B. Furlow, How to improve the safety of chemotherapy administration, *Oncol. Nurse Advisor*, 2010, 21–25.
197. R. Turci, C. Minola, C. Sottani, R. Coghi, P. Severi, C. Castriotta, M. Del Bianco and M. Imbriani, Occupational exposure to antineoplastic drugs in seven Italian hospitals: the effect of quality assurance and adherence to guidelines, *J. Oncol. Pharm. Pract.*, 2011, **17**, 320–332.
198. J. O. Jacobsen, M. Polovich, K. K. McNiff, K. B. LeFebvre, C. Cummings, M. Galioto, K. R. Bonelli and M. R. McCorkle, American Society of Clinical Oncology/Oncology Nursing Society chemotherapy administration safety standards, *J. Clin. Oncol.*, 2009, **27**, 5469–5475.
199. T. L. Willemson-McBride and K. Gehan, Safe handling of cytotoxic agents: A team approach, *AORN J.*, 2009, **90**, 731–740.
200. Centers for Disease Control and Prevention, Occupational Exposure to Antineoplastic Agents, Publications, Guidelines, Review Articles and Surveys, http://www.cdc.gov/niosh/topics/antineoplastics/pubs.html.
201. National Institute for Occupational Safety and Health, Centers for Disease Control and Prevention, NIOSH List of Antineoplastic and Other Hazardous Drugs in Healthcare Settings 2010, DHHS (NIOSH) Publication Number 2010-167, CDC, 2010.
202. National Institute for Occupational Safety and Health, Centers for Disease Control and Prevention, NIOSH Alert, Preventing Occupational Exposure to Antineoplastic and Other Hazardous Drugs in Health Care Settings, DHHS (NIOSH) Publication Number 2004-165, 2004.
203. Health and Safety Executive, Safe Handling of Cytotoxic Drugs, HSE Information Sheet MISC615, HSE, 2003. Available from: www.hse.gov.uk.
204. Health and Safety Executive, Operational Circular, OC/285/9, Safe Handling of Cytotoxic Drugs, September 2003. Available from: www.hse.gov.uk.
205. Veterinary Medicines Directorate, Handling cytotoxic drugs under veterinary practice conditions, MAVIS (Medicines Act Veterinary Information Service), edn 43, July, 2002. Available at: http://www.vmd.defra.gov.uk/pdf/mavis/mavis43.pdf.
206. P. B. Farmer and R. Singh, Use of DNA adducts to identify health risk from exposure to hazardous environmental pollutants: The increasing role of mass spectrometry in assessing biologically effective doses of genotoxic carcinogens, *Mutat. Res.*, 2008, **659**, 68–76.
207. J. S. Morris, J. M. Dobson and D. E. Bostock, Use of tamoxifen in the control of canine mammary neoplasia, *Vet. Rec.*, 1993, **133**, 539–542.
208. W. L. F. Tavares, G. E. Lavalle, M. S. Figueiredo, A. G. Souza, A. C. Betagnolli, F. A. B. Viana, P. R. O. Paes, R. A. Carneiro, G. A. O. Cavalcanti, M. M. Melo and G. D. Cassali, Evaluation of adverse effects

of tamoxifen exposed healthy female dogs, *Acta Vet. Scand.*, 2010, **52**, 67.

209. M. Sorsa and D. Anderson, Monitoring of occupational exposure to cytostatic anticancer drugs, *Mutat. Res.*, 1996, **355**, 253–261.

210. B. Kandel-Tschieder, M. Kessler, A. Schwietzer and A. Michel, Reduction of workplace contamination with platinum-containing cytostatic drugs in a veterinary hospital by introduction of a closed system, *Vet. Rec.*, 2010, **166**, 822–825.

CHAPTER 8

Antimicrobial Drugs

8.1 Introduction

Animals suffer from a variety of infectious diseases caused by bacteria and, to a lesser extent, by mycoplasmas. These range from highly infectious respiratory diseases that may affect whole herds or flocks to conditions affecting individual animals. The latter include abscesses, infected wounds or infected ears. As a result, a wide range of antimicrobial drug formulations have been developed for the treatment of disease in farm animals, including poultry and fish, and in companion animals. These drugs are available in a variety of presentations for administration by several routes including tablets and capsules for oral dosing, topical preparations and injectable formulations. However, these formulations may be impractical for administration to large numbers of animals and so these may be treated with antimicrobial drugs incorporated into feed or given in the drinking water.

As a consequence of the routes of administration used, there are a number of ways in which operators, including veterinarians, farmers and members of the pet-owning public, may become exposed. Additionally, with drugs intended for use in food-producing animals, consumers of animal products may be potentially exposed to residues of antimicrobial drugs in food including milk, meat, offal and eggs. Antimicrobial drugs take advantage of the fact that bacteria and mycoplasma have unique metabolic pathways and physiologies that either are absent in animals or differ significantly. Hence, it is possible to target these selectively. In theory, therefore, it should be possible to design antimicrobial drugs that are toxic to their intended targets but are harmless to the patient, to those caring for the patient and to those who might eventually consume products derived from the patient. To a large extent this objective has been achieved. However, many antimicrobial drugs have the capacity for harmful

Issues in Toxicology No. 14
Toxicological Effects of Veterinary Medicinal Products in Humans: Volume 1
By Kevin N. Woodward
© The Royal Society of Chemistry 2013
Published by the Royal Society of Chemistry, www.rsc.org

effects, and these tend to be specific for the class of drugs being considered. This chapter will review these drugs and their potential for adversely affecting human health.

8.2   The β-Lactam Drugs

These can be divided into two major groups, the penicillins and the cephalosporins. They are widely used in the treatment of diseases caused by suitably sensitive organisms. There are other members of the β-lactam group including the carbapenems typified by imipenem and the monobactams, where the β-lactam ring is not fused to another ring. Aztreonam is the representative member of the monobactams but these drugs are currently not used in veterinary medicine. Clavulanic acid is a drug that contains the β-lactam nucleus but the sulfur atom of the fused five-membered ring in penicillins is replaced by an oxygen atom. It has poor antimicrobial activity. However, it is used for its ability to bind irreversibly to β-lactamases, enzymes released by microorganisms that deactivate β-lactam antibiotics, and thus it acts as a suicide inhibitor. It is given with a β-lactam, usually amoxicillin as an oral preparation or tiarcillin as a parenteral dosage form. Clavulanic acid is used in veterinary medicine.

8.2.1   The Penicillins

The penicillins are a group of antibiotics containing the β-lactam ring system fused to a five-membered heterocyclic ring, the thiazolidine ring (Figure 8.1).[1] Chemically, the simplest members of the group are penicillin G and penicillin V. In the former, the substituent is a benzyl group while in the latter it is a phenoxymethyl group (Figure 8.2). The discovery, early development and uses of the penicillins are described in Sir Alexander Fleming's 1946 book, *Penicillin. Its Practical Application*, which, even at that early stage in its use, included a chapter on uses in animal disease.[2,3] They are used in animals to treat a variety of conditions caused by β-lactam sensitive organisms and they may be administered orally, by injection and, in the treatment of clinical mastitis in cattle and other animals, by direct application into the teat canal of the udder. The penicillins and cephalosporins exert their effects by disruption of synthesis of the bacterial cell wall.[4,5]

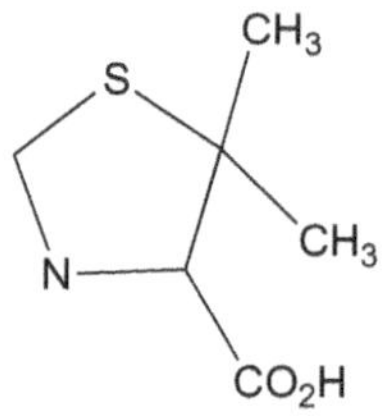

Figure 8.1   Chemical formula of the thiazolidine ring.

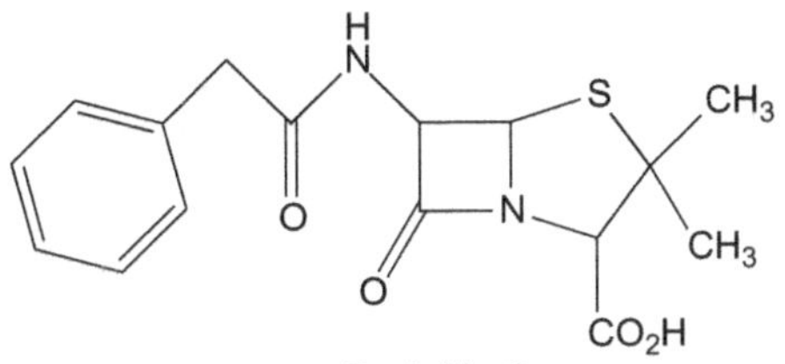

Penicillin G

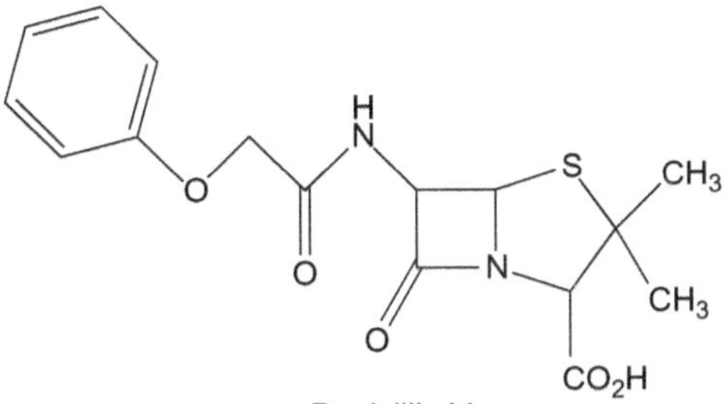

Penicillin V

Figure 8.2 Chemical formulae of penicillin G and penicillin V.

8.2.1.1 Toxicity of the Penicillins

The mode of action of the penicillins is specific for their bacterial targets and consequently, they have no specific ramifications for toxicity in animals, including humans. In fact the penicillins have low toxicity under normal circumstances. The major adverse reactions associated with penicillins (including clavulanic acid) in human patients are of an allergic nature and include maculopapular rash, urticarial rash, bronchospasm, dermatitis, fever, vasculitis, serum sickness, Stevens–Johnson syndrome and anaphylaxis.[1,6–27] These reactions are complex and they include IgE-mediated Type I reactions (*e.g.* anaphylaxis, bronchospasm) and IgG-mediated Type IV reactions (*e.g.* skin rashes, contact dermatitis) as well as Type III immune complex mediated reactions (serum sickness, arthralgia, vasculitis); it is possible for patients to have more than one form of β-lactam related allergy.[8,20,27–31]

Patients are not the only individuals at risk from the penicillins and related compounds. Allergic reactions have been noted in factory personnel and in healthcare workers exposed to these drugs. These reactions have included contact dermatitis, pneumonitis, urticaria, rhinitis and asthma.[32–49] Adverse reactions may also have occurred due to penicillin present in animal feeds and there have been reports of adverse skin reactions and respiratory symptoms in veterinarians exposed to penicillin.[50–53] There have also been a number of adverse reactions, mainly dermal effects, following the consumption of milk and meat containing low concentrations of penicillin, presumably from animals treated with the drug.[54–64] The majority of these reports appeared in the 1950s and 1960s and they are now rare. This may be for several reasons including the partial replacement of penicillins with other less allergenic drugs such as the cephalosporins, the establishment of tolerances and maximum residue limits (MRLs) (see Chapter 3) and milk withdrawal periods, the use of strict residue limits by dairies so that food processing *e.g.* cheese and yoghurt production is not adversely affected, or the wider use of heat treatments of milk, which may deactivate some β-lactams.[65]

It is still difficult to quantify the public health risks from penicillin residues in food.[66] Several factors combine to ensure that the risks are low, including the low doses likely to be received, the oral intake and the low densities of antigenic determinants.[67] Even with the reports cited here, the overall incidence is very low.[68] Nevertheless, the risks cannot be ignored entirely and they have been taken into account during the establishment of tolerances and MRLs. These are usually established on the basis of acceptable daily intake (ADI) values that, in turn, are calculated using no-effect levels (NOELs) from toxicology studies or, for antimicrobial drugs, from studies of their potential effects on the human gut flora (Chapter 3). The latter tend to give generally lower values than do the NOEL values from toxicology studies. In practice this means that MRLs or tolerances are likely to be lower, sometimes substantially lower for antimicrobial drugs than for agents that have comparative toxicity but lack antimicrobial properties. Consequently, the withdrawal periods for antimicrobial products, that is the time that must elapse between treatment and slaughter or between treatments and when milk is permitted to be collected for human consumption, are frequently longer than for other drugs. As is clear from Table 8.1, the majority of β-lactam drugs, or more specifically the cephalosporins (see next section), have ADI values, and hence MRLs, derived from microbiological studies for the reasons mentioned above. The only exception is clavulanic acid, which, as already described, has low microbiological activity. The MRLs for the penicillins are set at the lowest limits practicable, the limits of the analytical assays available, to minimise any potential allergic effects in consumers.

8.2.2   The Cephalosporins

A number of cephalosporin drugs are used in veterinary medicine against a variety of infectious agents in companion and farm animals. Cephalosporins have a similar basic chemical structure to penicillins except that the β-lactam ring is fused to a 6-membered sulfur-containing ring, the dihydrothiazine structure (Figure 8.3). They belong to a wider family of agents called the cephems, a group that also includes the cephamycins. The cephamycins are very similar in chemical structure to the cephalosporins but they contain a methoxy group at the 7-α position. They are not used in veterinary medicine.

Cephalosporins are divided into generations based largely on their antimicrobial activity and similarities in chemical structure. To a limited extent, their year of introduction is also a factor. First-generation cephalosporins are active against a range of Gram-positive organisms but they have limited

Table 8.1 The basis of the Acceptable Daily Intake and Maximum Residue Limits for β-lactam drugs in the European Union.

Drug	ADI value (µg/kg bw)		ADI selected for MRL elaboration
	Toxicological	*Microbiological*	
Penicillins (including benzylpenicillin, ampicillin, amoxicillin, oxacillin, cloxacillin and dicloxacillin)	–[c]	–[d]	MRLs generally, established at lowest practicable level, the limit of quantitation of the analytical method for the tissue/milk
Cefacetrile	–[a]	3.5	Microbiological
Cefalexin	500	54.4	Microbiological
Cefalonium	20	15.3	Food processing[b]
Cefapirin	100	2.54	Microbiological
Cefazolin	100	10	Microbiological
Cefoperazone	750	2.8	Microbiological
Cefquinome	–[a]	3.8	Microbiological
Ceftiofur	300	20	Microbiological
Clavulanic acid	50	90	Toxicological

[a]Toxicity too low to identify NOEL.
[b]The effects on food processing organisms (yoghurt starter cultures) gave a lower value than studies of toxicological or microbiological effects.
[c]For many penicillins there are inadequate conventional toxicity data to identify a suitable NOEL.
[d]For many penicillins there are inadequate microbiological studies to identify a suitable microbiological end-point from which to derive a microbiological ADI.

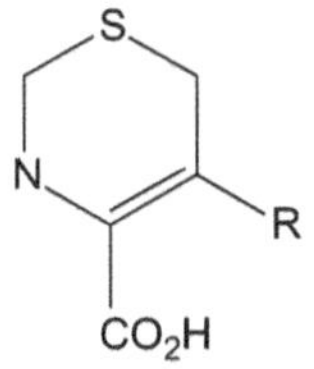

Figure 8.3 Chemical formula of the dihydrothiazine structure.

activity against Gram-negative pathogens, while second-generation cephalosporins have greater activity to Gram-negative bacteria. In human medicine, third- and fourth-generation cephalosporins are more stable against the effects of β-lactamases and are therefore considered essential in the treatment of pathogens that have become resistant to first- and second-generation cephalosporins. The major cephalosporins used in veterinary medicine are shown in Table 8.2, which also shows the generation in which they are included. Cefalonium is an example of a first generation cephalosporin and cefuroxime an example of a second-generation drug (Figure 8.4).

Table 8.2   Some cephalosporins authorised for use as veterinary medicines.

Generation	Cephalosporin	Comments
First	Cefalexin	
	Cefapirin	
	Cefalonium	
	Cefacetrile	
	Cefazolin	
Second	Cefuroxime	EU MRLs could not be established
Third	Cefoperazone	
	Ceftiofur	
	Cefovecin	
Fourth	Cefquinome	Companion-animal use only

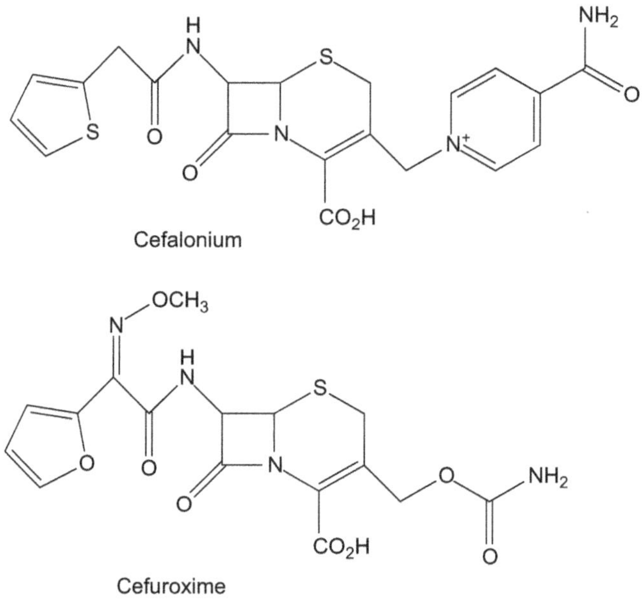

Cefalonium

Cefuroxime

Figure 8.4   Chemical formulae of cefalonium and cefuroxime.

Like the penicillins, their mode of action is specific to their target organisms and they generally show little toxicity. Consequently, their EU MRL values (Table 8.1) have generally been established on the basis of microbiological end-points, rather than on the basis of toxicology and NOEL values from toxicity studies. An EU MRL for cefuroxime could not be established. However, this was due to concerns over residues, and specifically related to questions over the identities of metabolites with respect to the marker residue rather than because of issues relating to toxicity. Studies with ceftiofur demonstrated it to be devoid of genotoxic activity in a range of *in vitro* and *in vivo* mutagenicity assays except for a positive result in an *in vitro* test for chromosomal aberrations.[69] This was unexpected as β-lactams in general give negative results in these tests and there are no structural or other reasons to suppose that they might be genotoxic. Consequently, the mechanism by which ceftiofur produced these effects was intensively investigated. It was found to be extremely cytostatic to the cells used in the study, Chinese hamster ovary cells. Removal of the drug from the cells led to a reversal of the cytostatic effects, and a reduction in the numbers of cells with chromosome aberrations. There was no evidence of cytotoxicity or lethality and the results suggest that the chromosomal effects occurred due to a prolongation of the cell cycle and not because of a true genotoxic effect.[70–72] The third-generation cephalosporin drug cefovecin is currently only available for companion-animal use and therefore has no EU MRL.[73–75]

In human patients treated with cephalosporins, the most common adverse drug reactions are hypersensitivity reactions.[1] Individuals who are sensitive to the effects of penicillins may show cross-reactivity, and similar signs and symptoms, when treated with cephalosporins. However, the situation is far from clear cut. There is cross-reactivity of this type, and the reverse – patients who become sensitised to cephalosporins may show cross-reactivity to penicillins, but some patients may be uniquely sensitive to one group of drugs but not to the other.[9,12,17,28,29,31,76–80] As with the penicillins, reactions may be mediated by IgE or IgG, and the latter group, which includes anaphylaxis, may be severe or life-threatening.[12,17,28,29,31,77,78,80,81] The use of microbiological end-points in the elaboration of MRL values for cephalosporins, which, as already described, are usually much lower than those based on NOEL values from toxicology studies, should ensure an increased margin of safety for consumers who otherwise might be exposed to higher concentrations of these drugs in food of animal origin. As with penicillins, occupational allergy, including asthma, may develop in exposed healthcare workers.[37,46]

The major safety issue associated with the use of cephalosporins in human and veterinary medicine is microbiological rather than toxicological. Third-generation cephalosporins or extended-spectrum cephalosporins such as cefotaxime, ceftazidine and ceftriaxone are recognised as being critical drugs in the treatment of human pathogens that have developed resistance to other antimicrobial agents. The use of these products in humans is thought to have exerted a major selective pressure on the emergence of resistance due to extended-spectrum β-lactamases.[82–89] There is now evidence that similarly resistant organisms are present in companion and farm animals and there is increasing concern that resistance, especially in zoonotic organisms, and its transfer to human pathogens, could have major implications for the treatment of disease in humans.[90–102] Consequently, advice has been issued to ensure their safe use or, more specifically, to ensure that third-generation cephalosporins remain effective in the treatment of critical bacterial diseases in humans. Thus, in the EU, the Scientific Advisory Group on Antimicrobials (SAGAM) has drafted advice, now adopted by the Committee for Medicinal Products for Veterinary Use (CVMP), while in the UK the DEFRA Antimicrobial Resistance Coordination (DARC) Group and the Advisory Committee on Antimicrobial Resistance and Healthcare Associated Infection (ARHAI) have drafted a report that also provides guidance on the use of third-generation cephalosporins.[103,104] Together, this guidance recommends that the emergence of resistance in animal pathogens and indicator bacteria be monitored, that the use of cephalosporins in each EU country be monitored, that EU countries enforce codes of practice on the prudent use of cephalosporins, that cephalosporins should not be advertised directly to animal owners, that cephalosporins should not be used off-label and that prescribing policies should be developed for the use of these drugs in veterinary medicine.

8.2.3   Aminoglycosides

The aminoglycoside antibiotics share a common chemical structural similarity with amino sugars linked to an aminohexose moiety by way of glycosidic bonds. Gentamicin has a structure that is typical of the group (Figure 8.5). The notable forms of toxicity with the aminoglycoside antibiotics are ototoxicity and nephrotoxicity. Apramycin is the only aminoglycoside that is used in veterinary, but not in human, medicine.

8.2.3.1   Ototoxicity

The ototoxicity of aminoglycosides has been well documented. It was discovered in the first clinical trials for streptomycin.[105,106] This drug causes damage to the vestibular organ of the ear while its derivative dihydrostreptomicin produces damage in the cochlea. Neomycin, kanamycin and amikacin also result in toxic effects in the cochlea while gentamicin causes mainly vestibular effects.[106–112] The ototoxic effects begin days or weeks after drug administration commences and they are irreversible. The vestibular effects are typified by loss of equilibrium

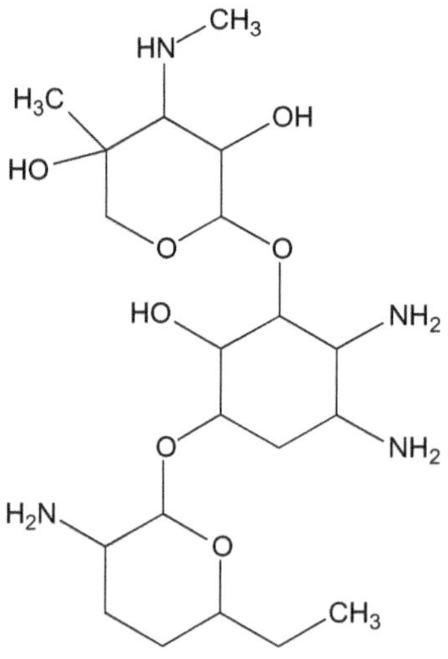

Figure 8.5   Chemical formula of gentamicin.

and dizziness, while the cochlear effects include hearing loss and tinnitus. When hearing loss occurs, high frequency hearing is lost first, and lower frequencies follow with continued drug administration. Aminoglycosides affect the hair cells in the organ of Corti of the cochlea and, as a result of therapeutic treatment, up to 25% of human patients develop hearing loss. Adverse effects in the vestibule occur in around 15% of patients treated.[112,113] Cochlear and vestibular damage is frequent in aminoglycoside-treated patients.[114–124] Factors involved may include the presence of functional hair cell mechanotransducer channels and the presence or otherwise of heat-shock proteins; heat-shock proteins inhibit aminoglycoside-induced ototxicity.[125,126] However, animals are also affected when therapeutically treated with these drugs or when given the drugs experimentally.[4,117,127–140] There are reports of ototoxicity in the children of mothers treated with aminoglycosides during pregnancy.[117,141–146]

Aminoglycosides may reach their targets in the hair cells either by endocytosis or through transport in ion channels. As well as systemic exposure, adverse effects may occur from local application of drug when otic formulations, *e.g.* for the treatment of otitis media, are instilled into the ear.[107,109]

8.2.3.2 Nephrotoxicity

The aminoglycosides are nephrotoxic in experimental animals.[134,147,148] All of the aminoglycosides used in veterinary and human medicine, namely streptomycin, dihydrostreptomycin, gentamicin, neomycin, framycetin, paromomycin (aminosidine), kanamycin, amikacin and gentamicin, are nephrotoxic to some degree as are aminoglycosides, which at present are only used to a very limited extent (or not at all) in animals such as tobramycin and verdamicin, in animal models.[134,147–160] These drugs are also nephrotoxic to animal patients treated therapeutically.[4,161–164] In human patients, around 8 to 25% of those treated will develop mild renal impairment that is usually reversible.[123,165–170] It may be influenced by a number of factors including the dose, the duration of dosing, frequency of dosing, hypotension, volume depletion, concurrent liver disease, diabetes and concurrent use of other nephrotoxic drugs including vancomycin. Once daily regimens appear to be less toxic than multiple regimens or continuous infusions.[123,156,171–179] Neonates may be more susceptible than adults.[180,181]

The precise mechanisms of nephrotoxicity still require elucidation. However, toxicity is preceded by accumulation and retention of aminoglycosides and phospholipids in lysosomes in the proximal tubules of the kidney and initial toxicity is indicated by release of enzymes of the renal tubular brush border. The lysosomes become overloaded and rupture, releasing high concentrations of the drug and phospholipids into the cytoplasm of the cell. Individual aminoglycosides differ quantitatively in their nephrotoxic potential and this may be related to their ability to be taken up by the tubules and in their potential to perturb cell membranes. Tubular dysfunction is usually mild and glomerular filtration rates decrease proportionally with the degree of damage inflicted, usually 5 to 7 days after administration of the drug commenced.[154,182–190]

The damage is reversible and human and animal patients usually fully recover but intensive care unit patients may be at greater risk and mortality may be high.[123,156,171,174,191,192] A number of factors affect toxicity, and several produce a protective effect including some natural oils and a number of drugs, possibly by reducing inflammation and preventing apoptosis.[153,154,193–197]

8.2.3.3   Hypersensitivity Reactions

Contact dermatitis has been reported with some aminoglycoside antibiotics. This has usually followed topical treatments, frequently with neomycin or gentamicin, although there is evidence of cross-sensitisation between different aminoglycosides.[198–213] Occupational dermatitis has been reported, particularly after exposure to streptomycin, including effects in healthcare workers,[214,215,217–222] and in one case in a cattle breeder.[223] Hence, occupational exposure to aminoglycosides in veterinarians and veterinary workers may result in contact dermatitis.

In the EU, the critical ADI values for the aminoglycosides used in food-producing animals were generally derived from the microbiological data with the exception of neomycin where the ADI was based on ototoxicity in the guinea pig (Table 8.3).

8.2.4   Aminocyclitols

Spectinomycin is an antibiotic closely related to the aminoglycosides and some authorities include it in this group. However, the aminoglycosides are generally composed of amino sugar residues whereas spectinomycin possesses a fused ring system[224–226] (Figure 8.6).

Table 8.3   The basis of the Acceptable Daily Intake (ADI) for aminoglycosides in the European Union.

Drug	NOEL for ototoxicity/nephrotoxicity mg/kg bw/day		ADI (µg/kg bw)	
	Ototoxicity	Nephrotoxicity	Toxicological	Microbiological
Apramycin	–[a]	–[a]	250	40
Streptomycin/ Dihydrostreptomycin	250	50–100	25[b]	80
Gentamicin	25	25	100	4
Kanamycin	100	50	–[c]	8
Neomycin[d]	6	10	60	160
Paromomycin	–[e]	3.4[f]	34	25

[a]Only limited evidence for ototoxicity and nephrotoxicity.
[b]Based on body weight reductions in repeat-dose studies.
[c]Definitive NOELs for general toxicity were not identified.
[d]Also applies to framycetin (soframycin).
[e]Vestibular effects noted in cats at 50 mg/kg bw.
[f]Dog was more sensitive than rat; this NOEL is based on a repeat-dose toxicity study in the dogs where the main effects were nephrotoxicity and the induction of cataracts.

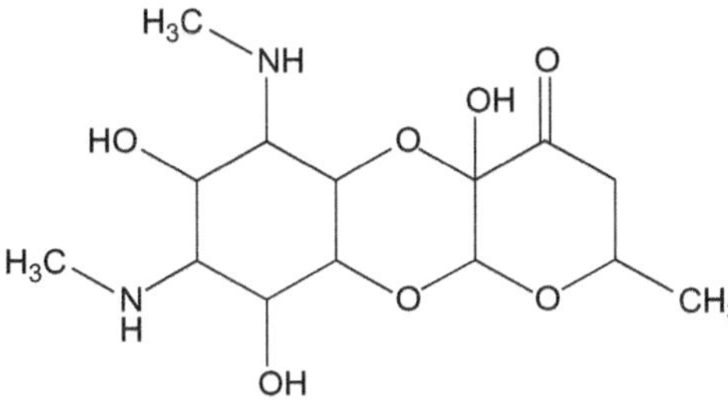

Figure 8.6 Chemical formula of spectinomycin.

The drug has a low order of toxicity. Repeat dose studies in animals provided no evidence of major toxicity and, unlike the aminoglycosides, it is not nephrotoxic or ototoxic in animal studies or in *in vitro* models of ototoxicity, although cochlear and vestibular effects have been reported at very high single and repeat doses.[227-231] In humans, there was no evidence of ototoxicity in healthy male volunteers given 8 g/day for 21 days intramuscularly and the only major effect noted was pain on injection.[232] Urticaria, dizziness, nausea, chills and fever are the main effects reported after single doses of spectinomycin in clinical trials and anaphylactic reactions are rare.[233] There have been rare cases of occupational dermatitis due to spectinomycin or to spectinomycin plus lincomycin.[234,235]

On the basis of the low mammalian toxicity of spectinomycin, the EU MRL was established on the basis of an ADI derived from microbiological data.

8.2.5   The Quinolones

The earliest quinolone drugs are represented by oxolinic acid and nalidixic acid, and later by flumequine. Oxolinic acid (Figure 8.7) and nalidixic acid are non-fluorine containing quinolones, while flumequine (Figure 8.8) has a single fluorine atom. The next generation of quinolones, the fluoroquinolones, is typified by ciprofloxacin and enrofloxacin (Figure 8.9). The most important fluoroquinolones in veterinary medicine are flumequine, enrofloxacin, sarafloxacin, danofloxacin, orbifloxacin, ibafloxacin, marbofloxacin and pradofloxacin.[236-238] Oxolinic acid and flumequine are almost exclusively used in aquaculture for the treatment of bacterial diseases in farmed fish.[239-242]

The most important toxic effects of the fluoroquinolones are on articular cartilages and tendons, and several of the group have been shown to cause juvenile arthropathies in a number of species including rats, dogs, sheep and birds.[243-259] Grepafloxacin has low toxicity in this respect.[260,261] They are also associated with tendonitis and tendon rupture in human patients.[261-270] There appear to be no major effects in paediatric populations, although arthralgias and minor cartilage changes have been reported.[271-275] The mechanism of action for these adverse effects is unknown. Studies with ofloxacin suggest that chondrocyte apoptosis may occur, possibly because of effects on the

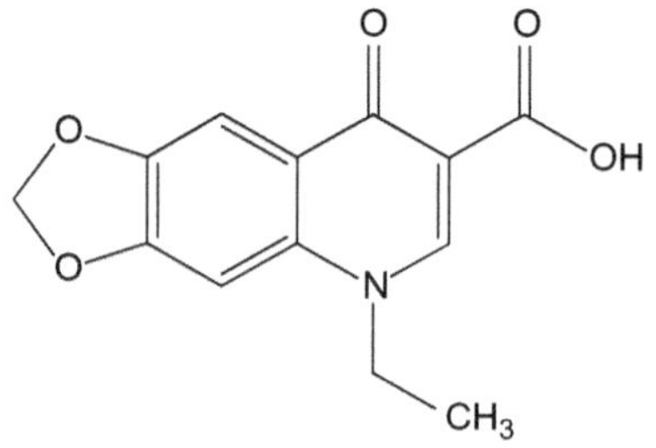

Figure 8.7 Chemical formula of oxolinic acid.

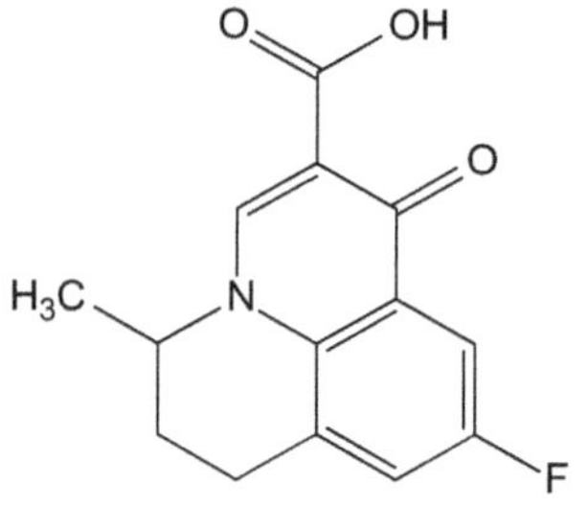

Figure 8.8 Chemical formula of flumequine.

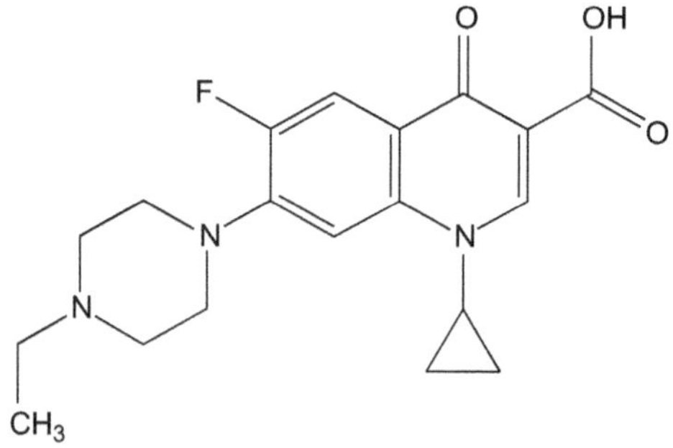

Figure 8.9 Chemical formula of enrofloxacin.

caspase-8-dependent mitochondrial pathway leading to decreases in mito-chondrial activity. Inflammation of cartilage is usually seen. They may affect proteoglycan synthesis in cartilage, including that in the cartilage of tendons, and inhibit tendon cell proliferation and migration.[247,276–282] There is also some evidence that fluoroquinolones may delay or adversely affect cartilage and tendon repair mechanisms.[281,283]

Fluoroquinolones and quinolones also induce neurotoxic effects that may be experienced as mild dizziness or headache. However, other effects can include seizures, which may arise because they antagonise binding of the inhibitory neurotransmitter γ-aminobutyric acid (GABA) to its CNS receptors. Other CNS effects include catatonia, delirium and encephalopathy.[271,284–288] Prolongation of the QT interval has also been reported but severe cardiac toxicity has not been observed in clinical trials or in large cohort studies.[261,271,289]

The fluoroquinolones exert their effects on bacteria by targeting bacterial gyrase, topoisomerase II, an enzyme responsible for maintaining the integrity of DNA and its topological architecture by preventing overwinding or underwinding of the molecule, especially during transcription.[290–295] If bacterial topoisomerases are inhibited, normal DNA duplication cannot proceed, and the tensions caused by overwinding can lead to cessation of replication as well as to DNA breaks, thus inhibiting bacterial growth. Mammalian topoisomerases are the targets of several anticancer drugs including etoposide, mitoxantrone and doxorubicin.[296–299] Hence, drugs or classes of drugs that exert adverse effects on bacterial cells may also exert harmful effects on mammalian cells, especially as the fluoroquinolones can cause mutations in bacteria as their effects on bacterial DNA result in induction of the RecA SOS DNA repair system, which is error prone.[271,294,300,301] Hence, fluoroquinolones may exert mutagenic properties through their pharmacodynamic mode of action and there is evidence for this and, in addition, photoactive fluoroquinolones may induce oxidative DNA damage as a result of the formation of reactive oxygen species.[302–319] However, many of the studies referred to were conducted *in vitro* and some also employed ultraviolet light. In general, the majority of *in vivo* studies with fluoroquinolones produced negative or equivocal results.[271,311,317,320,321] The major concern over positive findings in genotoxicity studies is carcinogenic activity but the fluoroquinolones have given negative results in animal bioassays.[255,271,311,256,322–324] Hence, they are considered to be safe for therapeutic purposes in human and veterinary medicine.

In the EU, MRLs were established for most of the fluoroquinolones and oxolinic acid on the basis of microbiological ADI values. The exception was danofloxacin, where the ADI was based on a toxicological NOEL for arthropathy in the dog.[127] Orbifloxacin, pradofloxacin and ibafloxacin are only authorised for companion-animal uses and have no MRL values.

8.2.6 Macrolides

The macrolides antibiotics, as their class name suggests, are large ring lactones to which are attached one or more deoxy sugars. The group is typified by erythromycin (Figure 8.10), a 14-membered lactone ring structure. In this case, two sugars are attached, L-cladinose and D-decosamine. The other members of the group that are used in veterinary medicine are spiramycin, tilmicosin, tylosin, tylvalosin (acetylisovaleryltylosin), josamycin, gamithromycin and tulathromycin. Tildipirosin, a semisynthetic derivative of tylosin, is a new introduction to the class intended for use in veterinary medicine. In human medicine, the most important macrolides are erythromycin, clarithromycin and

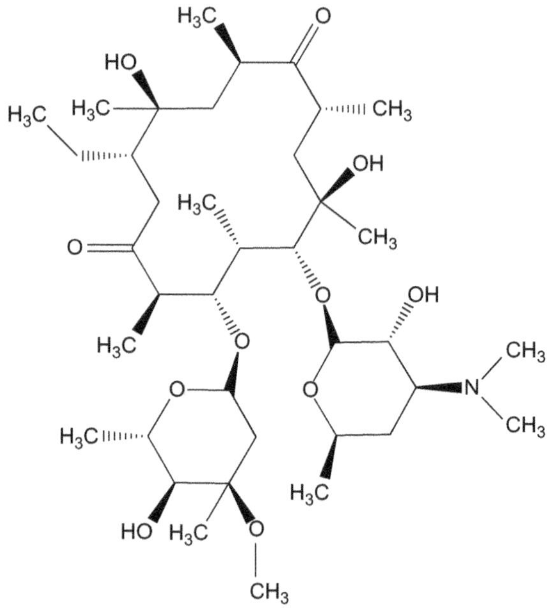

Figure 8.10   Chemical formula of erythromycin.

azithromycin. Clarithromycin differs from erythromycin by the methylation of a single hydroxyl group at the 6 position of the macrocyclic ring, while azithromycin differs from erythromycin by the insertion of a methylated nitrogen into the macrolide ring.[4,325,326]

Spiramycin has low toxicity and lacks teratogenic, genotoxic and carcinogenic activity.[327–331] There are few reports of adverse effects in humans treated with spiramycin. It may have effects on gastric motility, a known side effect of macrolide antibiotics, and there is a report of an ulcerated oesophagus.[332–334] There has been an isolated report of allergic vasculitis following spiramycin use and another of generalised numbness, tingling, a metallic taste and hot flushes.[335,336] Unlike many other macrolides, it has few drug interactions.[337]

There have been reports of dermatitis and bronchial asthma following occupational exposure to spiramycin, including exposures in agricultural workers using the drug in animals, and in workers in the pharmaceutical industry.[338–344]

Tylosin also has very low mammalian toxicity after oral administration and it lacks reproductive toxicity, as well as genotoxic and carcinogenic activity.[345–347] However, like spiramycin, there have been reports of asthma and contact dermatitis following occupational exposure with some of these cases involving veterinarians and farmers, and notably pig farmers handling medicated feed.[340,348–357]

Erythromycin has a good safety profile, although the estolate (dodecyl sulfate) salt was found to be hepatotoxic, and some patients taking the drug for periods in excess of two weeks developed jaundice.[325,358–360]

Hypersensitivity reactions appear to be very rare although there is one report of occupational asthma to erythromycin in a manufacturing plant, and a number of reports of allergic contact dermatitis with the related compound azithromycin.[361–365]

Tilmicosin is structurally related to tylosin (Figure 8.11). However, it appears to have higher acute toxicity when compared with other macrolides, including tylosin, at least under some conditions. Although tilmicosin is of low toxicity for most of the aspects of regulatory toxicology,[366–368] it produces cardiac effects. Dogs given oral doses of tilmicosin for 3 months showed increased heart rates and 50% of animals given 70 mg/kg bw/day died.[369] The NOEL was identified as 6 mg/kg bw/day. Cardiac enlargement occurred in a one-year study in dogs given 36 mg/kg bw/day, while heart rates were increased both at this dose and at 12 mg/kg bw/day. The NOEL was 4 mg/kg.

To date, there have been no reports of occupational asthma or contact dermatitis with tilmicosin. There have been a number of reports of adverse effects in workers who have suffered needlestick injuries on needles contaminated with the drug. The majority of these produced minor local effects resulting from a puncture wound.[370] However, there have been reports of effects on the heart in workers exposed to tilmicosin. These have occurred following accidental self-injection with significant quantities of the drug. Effects have included chest pains, electrocardiographic abnormalities and intraventricular conduction delays.[371,372] There have been reports of fatalities in workers who have self-injected tilmicosin.[371,373] Over 250 cases of human tilmicosin exposure are reported to poison centres each year, and over 250 of these are parenteral, namely self-injection. The majority of cases suffer no ill effects, but fatalities are reported and the case fatality rate with parenteral exposure is ten times that for all human exposures.[374] In the UK, this led to amended labelling for the product concerned, Micotil, while the marketing authorisation was temporarily suspended in France until the safety and labelling issues were resolved a few months later.[375–378]

Experimental studies in dogs have shown that tilmicosin exerts a negative inotropic effect on the heart, thus weakening its contractions, in a manner similar to that noted with β-blocker drugs and verapamil.[366] In fact, similar, though less pronounced, effects have been noted with other macrolides, including erythromycin. These effects have included prolongation of the QT interval and torsades des pointes.[379–388]

There is a paucity of data available for josamycin. That which is available suggests low toxicity.[389,390] There are also few published data on tulathromycin, gamithromycin and tildipirosin. The data that are available suggest low toxicity.[391–393]

All of the macrolides used in human medicine have the capacity for drug–drug interactions. The other drugs involved have included digoxin, statins, carbamazepine, cyclosporine, terfenadine, astemizole and theophylline and some of these interactions may precipitate toxicity while some may also occur in treated animal patients.[394–404]

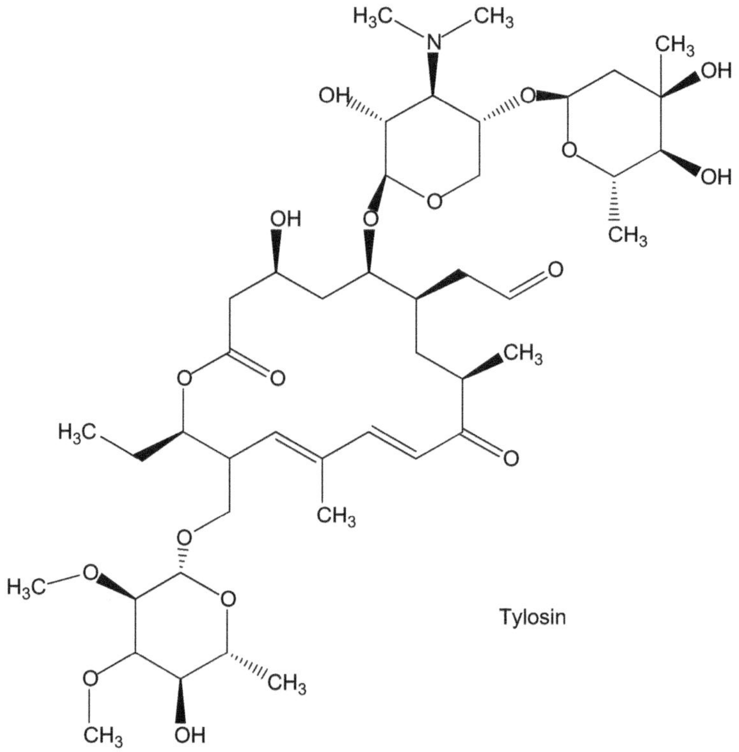

Tylosin

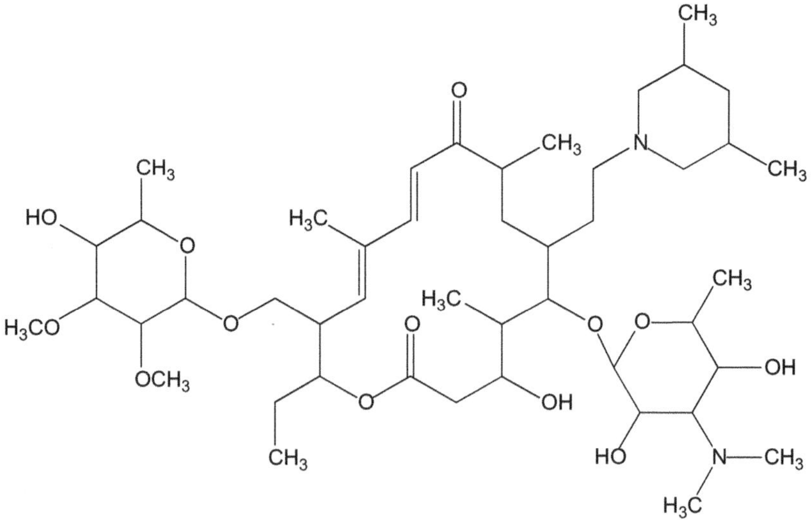

Tilmicosin

Figure 8.11 Chemical formulae of tylosin and tilmicosin.

The EU MRL values for the macrolide antibiotics were based on the microbiological ADI values, as these were lower than those derived from toxicity studies. The exceptions were the MRLs for gamithromycin and tildipirosin where the ADI from toxicity studies was lower than the corresponding values from microbiological assays. Due to lack of information to support the MRL application for josamycin, only provisional MRL values were established. However, as the requested data were not forthcoming, these values have now lapsed and josamycin may no longer be used in food-producing animals in the EU.

8.2.7 The Phenicols

The phenicols are represented by three drugs, chloramphenicol, thiamphenicol and florfenicol, all of which are used in veterinary medicine. Chloramphenicol and thiamphenicol, but not florfenicol, are used in human medicine.

Chloramphenicol was originally isolated from *Streptomyces venezuelae*. It differs from the majority of other antibiotics in that it has a relatively simple chemical structure. In fact it is a derivative of nitrobenzene (Figure 8.12), a functional group that the other two drugs lack (Figure 8.13). It has been widely used in human medicine but its use is now restricted as it causes blood dyscrasias in some human patients treated with the drug. The less serious of these effects is a mild and reversible bone marrow suppression that arises from mitochondrial damage and that results in a mild anaemia.[325,405–408] The more serious effect is irreversible bone marrow aplasia, aplastic anaemia, with pancytopenia and acellular bone marrow. This has been estimated to occur in 1 in 500 to 1 in 100,000 cases treated with chloramphenicol and it is often fatal.[405,409–423] Cases occur in children as well as in adults.[424–428] The effect appears to be independent of dose although total doses may be high (4–80 g), but aplastic anaemia has been reported after topical administration where the total systemic dose was probably low and after the application of ophthalmic eye drops where the systemic dose would be low.[429–437] The risk associated with these uses is thought to be very low.[438,439] There has been a report of aplastic anaemia in a shepherd exposed to an aerosol spray containing the drug.[440]

The mechanism of toxicity is not well understood. There appears to be a lack of correlation with dose and the duration of dosing, and its occurrence in

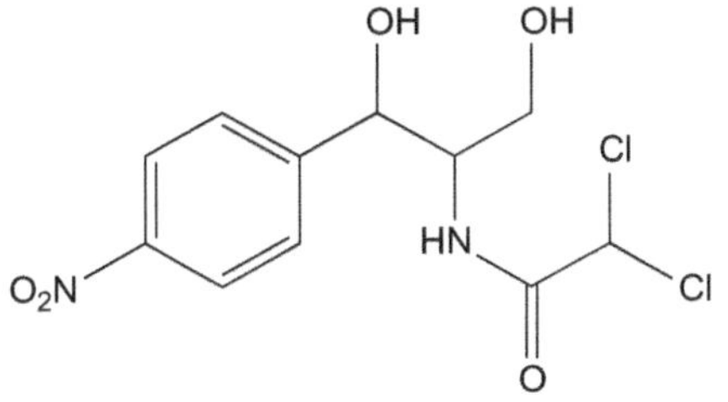

Figure 8.12 Chemical formula of chloramphenicol.

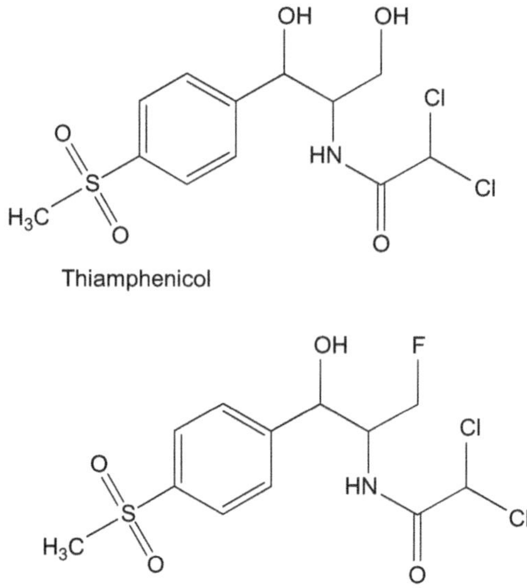

Figure 8.13   Chemical formulae of thiamphenicol and florfenicol.

populations appears to be random. It occurs in identical twins and all of these factors point to an idiosyncratic reaction with a genetic link.[441–443] It has been possible to develop animal models of reversible bone marrow depression, and bone marrow depression is observed in animal studies; a model of chloramphenicol-induced aplastic anaemia has not been found.[444–451] Thiamphenicol and florfenicol induce reversible bone marrow depression in animals.[452–462] The most likely, or at least most plausible, difference between chloramphenicol, and thiamphenicol and florfenicol, is that the chloramphenicol possesses the *p*-nitro group, which the other two drugs lack. This is converted to a toxic nitroso group in susceptible individuals, which then precipitates aplastic anaemia.[441–443,463] However, this remains unproven and the exact mechanism remains unclear.[408,464]

Aplastic anaemia can be treated successfully with supportive care, bone marrow transplant, stem cell therapy, immunosuppressive treatments and a number of drugs.[465–474] However, it may progress to leukaemia in some patients.[441,475,476] Leukaemia has been reported in patients who recovered from chloramphenicol-associated aplastic anaemia.[475–486] The US National Toxicology Program classified chloramphenicol as *reasonably anticipated to be a human carcinogen*.[487]

As a result of these findings, chloramphenicol has been prohibited for use in food animals in several countries, including the EU countries. This was largely on the grounds that the effects of chloramphenicol were serious and that no NOEL could be established for the induction of aplastic anaemia. The possibility that residues of chloramphenicol might induce aplastic anaemia in persons who were uniquely sensitive to its adverse effects could therefore not be excluded. MRLs have been established in the EU for thiamphenicol and florfenicol. For thiamphenicol and florfenicol, these were based on a microbiological ADI values.

8.2.8 Tetracyclines

The major tetracyclines used in veterinary medicine are tetracycline, oxytetracycline, chlortetracycline and doxycycline (Figure 8.14). A further

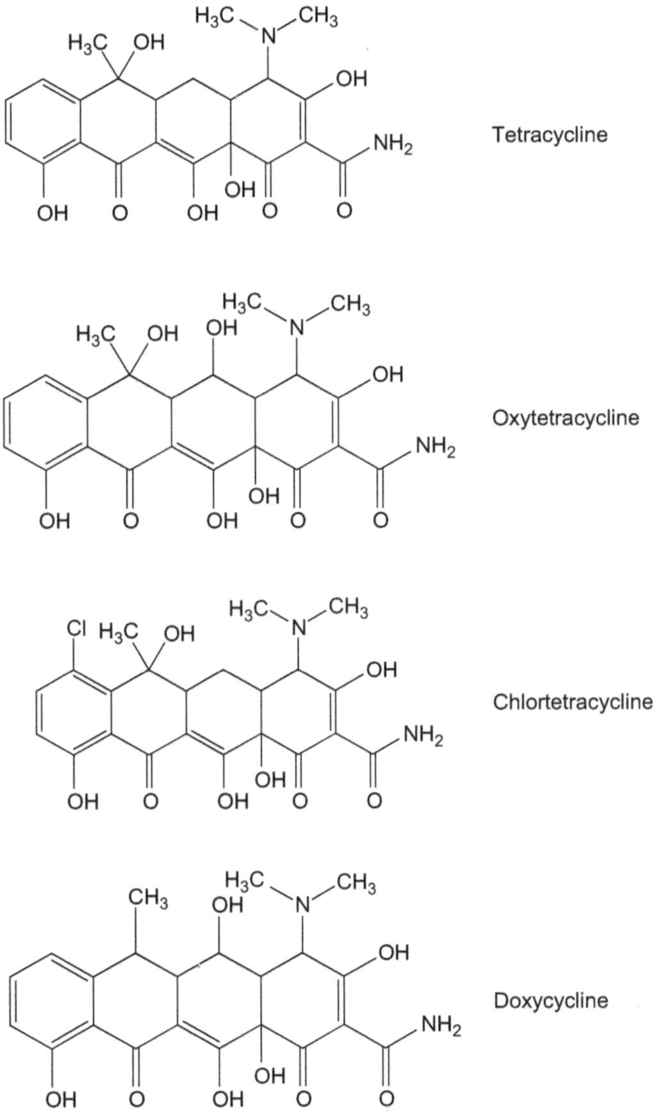

Figure 8.14 Chemical formulae of tetracycline, oxytetracycline, chlortetracycline and doxycycline.

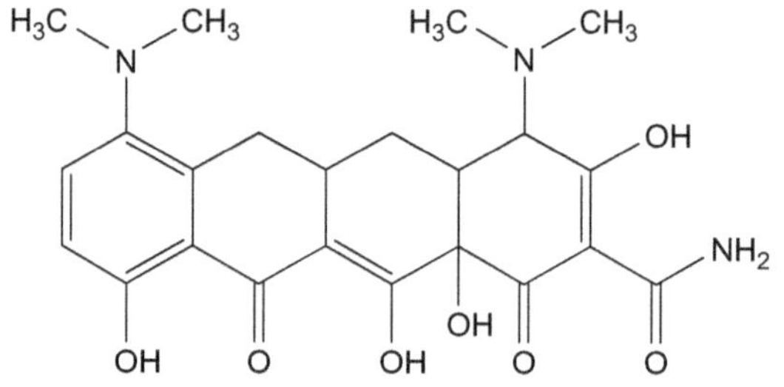

Figure 8.15   Chemical formula of minocycline.

tetracycline, minocycline, is authorised for use in some countries, largely for the treatment of diseases in companion animals.[4,488]

Oxytetracycline, tetracycline, chlortetracycline and doxycycline have low toxicity in laboratory animals.[489–491] However, they may induce hypersensitivity reactions in patients and in occupationally exposed individuals.[492–496] The major adverse effects of these drugs in human patients are the production of teeth staining and bone deposition in children. Patients who are pregnant and are treated with tetracyclines may give birth to children with discoloured teeth. The deposition of the drugs in bone may result in reductions in the rate of bone growth and enamel hypoplasia.[497–509]

Studies in animals showed minocycline (Figure 8.15) to have a similar spectrum of toxicity to tetracycline.[510] However, it has produced adverse effects in patients treated with the drug, not seen with other tetracyclines, or not seen to such a degree or frequency.

8.2.8.1   Autoimmune Hepatitis and Systemic Lupus Erythematosus-like Syndrome

There have been a number of reports of hepatitis, possibly with an autoimmune mechanism, in human patients treated with minocycline. By April 1994, 11 cases of systemic lupus erythematosus (SLE) and 16 cases of autoimmune hepatitis had been reported to the Committee on Safety of Medicines in the UK.[511] A literature review from 1997 to 2001 revealed 76 articles associated with adverse events to acne drug therapy and minocycline was the most widely incriminated drug with 72 cases of autoimmune disorders, mainly lupus-like syndromes; some of these cases also involved autoimmune hepatitis.[512] Another review revealed 57 cases of lupus associated with minocycline therapy. All patients showed symptoms of polyarthralgia and polyarthritis, often accompanied by hepatic abnormalities; it may exacerbate pre-existing SLE.[513] Minocycline-induced autoimmune disease may develop after a short duration of dosing (3 days) or up to 6 years after commencement of treatment.[514–516] Some of these cases are briefly reviewed in Table 8.4. The hepatotoxicity of minocycline has been investigated in mice, including mice pre-treated with

Table 8.4 Reports of cases of autoimmune hepatitis and systemic lupus erythematosus (SLE) and other auto-immune disorders in patients treated with minocycline.

Description	Reference
SLE in Japanese female treated with minocycline	518
Acute hepatitis in a 16-year-old boy (with exfoliative dermatitis); fatal hepatitis in a 17-year-old girl	519
Acute hepatic failure in 39-year-old woman. She recovered after 3 weeks	520
Periarteritis nodosa in two women; resolved on cessation of therapy	521
Serum-sickness-like syndrome in 19-year-old male – urticaria, fever, lymphadenopathy and arthralgia. Recovered after 9 days	522
Review of literature: over 60 cases of SLE associated with minocycline and 24 cases of autoimmune hepatitis. All recovered	523
SLE and serum sickness in 16-year-old girl given minocycline for 3 months	524
Serum sickness in patient treated with minocycline	525
Serum sickness, hepatitis and exfoliative dermatitis in 17-year-old female. Recovered	526
Report of six cases of serum sickness and one with SLE in patients given minocycline. All eventually recovered	527
Lymphadenopathy, fever and other effects similar to serum sickness in a 16-year-old patient, with interstitial nephritis. Eventually recovered	528
Serum sickness in 35-year-old patient treated with minocycline. Patient recovered	529
Serum sickness in five adolescents treated with minocycline. All recovered after 5 days to 5 weeks	530
Serum sickness in two female patients (15 and 30 years old). Both recovered	531
Report of 23 patients who developed SLE during treatment	532
SLE in a patient treated with minocycline	533
Asthma and eosinophilia in 28-year-old patient	534
Autoimmune hepatitis in three adolescent patients. All recovered after 5 weeks to 9 months	535
Autoimmune hepatitis in a 42-year-old patient treated with minocycline. She recovered 3 months after treatment was stopped	536
Case-control study of patients (27,688) with acne, aged 15–29 years, treated with tetracyclines, taken from GPRD, for the period January 1991 to February 1996	537
Risks and 95% confidence intervals (CIs) for SLE were: 32.7 (14.9–62.1) per 100,000 prescriptions for females and 2.3 (1.0–13.0) per 100,000 prescriptions for females, for any tetracycline. The risks for oxytetracycline were 17.2 (2.1–62.1) per 100,000 prescriptions, and for minocycline 52.8 (19.4–115.0) per 100,000 prescriptions. The odd ratios were 3.5 (95% CI, 1.3–7.0) for any tetracycline and 8.5 (95% CI 2.1–35.0) for minocycline	
The data suggest that the risk of SLE is increased by a factor of around 8.5 for young women being treated for acne and this effect is strongest for longer-term users	
Pericardial effusion and hepatic injury in 39-year-old woman treated with minocycline	538
In a review of the literature covering the period up to December 1998, 65 cases of liver damage caused by minocycline, 20 had insufficient information to classify them, but the other 45 were autoimmune in origin	539

phenobarbital. Although liver enzymes and bilirubin were elevated, there was no evidence of the hepatotoxicity noted in humans.[517]

8.2.8.2 Sweet's Syndrome

Sweet's syndrome, first described in 1964, is characterised by an acute onset of non-pruritic, painful reddish nodules on the head, neck, chest and upper limbs, accompanied by fever, general malaise and leucocytosis.[540] Although rare, it has been associated with a number of drugs including furosemide, celecoxib and hydralazine.[541,542] Typical cases occurring with minocycline are described in Table 8.5.

8.2.8.3 Hyperpigmentation

Hyperpigmentation of the skin has been reported after minocycline therapy. It has also been reported in bone. Some typical cases are described in Table 8.6.

Hyperpigmentation due to minocycline is rare in patients taking minocycline for less than 1 year, but it becomes more common in those taking the drug for longer. It may also occur in bone; around 10% of patients taking the drug for more than 1 year developed bone pigmentation while around 20% of those taking it for more than 4 years were affected. It may also affect the buccal mucosal, conjunctiva, sclera, nail beds, cardiac valves, cartilage, thyroid and teeth. In some cases, pigmentation may be permanent.[512,555,556]

Blackening of the thyroid has been seen in rats given minocycline.[557] Studies *in vitro* suggest that the pigmentation and some of the toxicity of minocycline may be due to the formation of a reactive benzoquinone iminium ion.[558]

Table 8.5 Minocycline-induced Sweet's syndrome.

Description	Reference
Patient (25-year-old male) treated with oral minocycline for acne. One week later painful nodules developed on his neck. He recovered after 2 weeks with topical corticosteroid treatment. Similar lesions developed after doxycycline and tetracycline treatment. These also resolved after cessation of treatment. The condition occurred again after re-challenge with doxycycline	541
Sweet's syndrome developed in a 32-year-old man 10 days after treatment commenced. Condition resolved rapidly after cessation of treatment and prednisone treatment	543
Patient (29-year-old female) developed skin lesions and fever 1 week after minocycline treatment started. The condition rapidly resolved following cessation of treatment and corticosteroid treatment. However, it returned in a severe form on re-challenge with minocycline; this resolved within 10 days after treatment with cephadroxil and methylprednisolone. After a further 4 weeks, the condition reappeared within 4 hours following a further treatment with minocycline	544

Table 8.6   Reports of hyperpigmentation following minocycline treatment.

Description	Reference
Patient (18-year-old female) had taken minocycline for 14 months. She then reported "bruises" on her skin. This resolved 16 months after cessation of treatment	545
Review of 77 cases of skin hyperpigmentation reported to manufacturer between 1 January 1976 and 1 January 1983. Pigmentation possibly due to oxidation product of minocycline	546
Review of the nature of hyperpigmentation caused by minocycline. Three types recognised: dark blue macules in areas of depressed acne scarring, circumscribed hyperpigmented macules or a diffuse pigmentation and "muddy skin" syndrome – a generalised darkening of the skin	547
Patient (69-year-old woman) developed hyperpigmentation after 3 months of treatment with minocycline. Improvement occurred 2 months after cessation of treatment	548
Hyperpigmentation, neutrophilic alveolitis and erythema nodosum developed in a 32-year-old woman after approximately 4 months of treatment. The erythema and alveolitis resolved 2 weeks after cessation of treatment but the hyperpigmentation persisted for more than a year	549
Patient, a 62-year-old woman, developed hyperpigmentation of the skin in February 1996 after beginning minocycline treatment in 1990. Minocycline treatment was stopped and she was treated with hydroquinone cream but there was no change in hyperpigmentation after 6 months. The pigmentation finally responded to treatment with a Q-switched neodymium:YAG laser. In a similar report, four cases of minocycline-induced hyperpigmentation resolved after treatment with a Q-switched ruby laser	550
Hyperpigmentation occurred in 65-year-old man given minocycline over a 2.5 year period. Condition resolved over "several years"	551
Hyperpigmentation developed on the lips of a patient treated with minocycline. Resolved several weeks after treatment ceased	552
Two patients developed hyperpigmentation during minocycline treatment. In one patient, this developed on the face after 3 years of treatment while in the other it developed on the lower legs after 6 months of drug administration. The latter patient was treated with a Q-switched ruby laser and the condition rapidly resolved	553
Hyperpigmentation developed in a patient treated post-operatively with minocycline for 8 months	554

8.2.8.4   *Hypersensitivity*

Several cases of hypersensitivity have been reported as described in Table 8.7. The evidence for cross-sensitivity between minocycline and other tetracyclines is ambiguous.[569,570]

8.2.8.5   *Vestibular Reactions*

Vestibular toxicity of minocycline is a relatively common effect, and one that is not seen with other tetracyclines. In some studies, it has been seen in up to 90% of patients treated. Main signs include nausea, vomiting and vertigo. It is reversible, usually within 48 hours of cessation of treatment.[571–576]

Table 8.7   Reports of hypersensitivity to minocycline.

Description	Reference
Erythematous eruption, nausea and vomiting in a 26-year-old woman given minocycline	559
Stevens–Johnson syndrome in a 36-year-old man	560
Necrotising vasculitis of skin and uterine cervix in 35-year-old patient	561
Severe erythematous reaction in young adult male given minocycline	562
Hypersensitivity pneumonitis in a patient given minocycline	563
Exanthematous pustulosis in a patient treated with minocycline	564
Pustulous eruption in 16-year-old female given minocycline	565
A 15-year-old boy and a 17-year-old girl developed skin eruptions in the form of pustular nodules. The boy eventually died and *post mortem* revealed myocardial necrosis with eosinophilic infiltrates. The girl had tachycardia and peripheral, interstitial infiltrates. She recovered after treatment with prednisone	566
Eosinophilic cellulites and eosinophilic pustular folliculitis in a patient treated with minocycline	567
Eosinophilic pneumonia, with acute respiratory failure	568
Hypersensitivity seen in three patients	533

It is difficult to make quantitative estimates of comparative risks between tetracyclines because the numbers of patients presenting and the total numbers of patients treated is unavailable. However, a study in Toronto has compared adverse drug reactions to tetracycline, doxycycline and minocycline.[577] Their findings are summarised in Table 8.8.

While by no means normalised, and lacking in quantitative power, the data suggest that adverse reactions due to tetracyclines are similar in nature and possibly even in incidence (from the limited data available), but that auto-immune disease, including autoimmune hepatitis, and hypersensitivity and hyperpigmentation are largely restricted to minocycline. The mild disorders, rash, urticaria *etc.*, appear to be shared by all three drugs. Other authors note that the incidence of autoimmune disorders, hyperpigmentation and hyper-sensitivity associated with minocycline are low in proportion to the numbers of prescriptions issued, the effects are generally reversible (although some may need treatment) and they are usually not life-threatening once the drug has been discontinued.[577–581] In the United Kingdom, some 6.5 million patients were treated for an average of 9 months with minocycline over the 25-year period until 1996 and yet over the period up until 1994, only 26 cases of minocycline-induced SLE or autoimmune hepatitis had been reported to the UK's Com-mittee on Safety of Medicines; in 1996, around 28 million minocycline tablets were taken.[511,577,582] As the SLE syndrome is uncommon, and the effects reversible on cessation of treatment, it has been suggested that the increased risks should only marginally affect the risk/benefit balance for the use of minocycline.[537] The onset of acute conditions such as non-autoimmune hepa-titis usually occurs after 1–3 months of treatment, while the autoimmune dis-orders generally occur after prolonged treatment (1–6 years).[583] The incidence of Sweet's syndrome is exceptionally rare.[541]

Table 8.8 Comparative adverse reaction data for tetracycline, doxycycline and minocycline (based on data from[577]).

	Tetracycline			Doxycycline			Minocycline		
	Drug Safety Clinic	Health Protection Branch	Literature	Drug Safety Clinic	Health Protection Branch	Literature	Drug Safety Clinic	Health Protection Branch	Literature
Numbers[a]	166	976	–	39	145	–	17	160	–
Mild	66	406	0	15	38	0	1	52	0
Rash	35	138	0	11	0	0	6	7	0
Urticaria	11	8	0	3	1	0	1	8	0
Photosensitivity	4	10	0	3	4	0	0	0	0
Vomiting/diarrhoea	23	159	0	3	17	0	2	53	0
Severe									
Hypersensitivity	0	1	1	0	0	1	2	4	13
Serum sickness	0	3	0	1	1	0	2	4	5
SLE	0	0	0	0	0	0	1	0	32
Single organ dysfunction[b]	2	26	9	0	3	3	0	14	26
Severe cutaneous reaction	1	9	1	0	1	0	0	2	1
Hepatitis	1	7	0	0	0	0	0	7	4
Pneumonitis	0	0	1	0	0	0	0	0	17
Pancreatitis	0	3	4	0	1	0	0	1	1
Nephritis	0	2	0	0	1	0	0	0	1
Haematological	0	4	2	0	0	0	0	4	0
Parotitis	0	1	0	0	0	0	0	0	0
Myocarditis	0	0	1	0	0	0	0	0	0
Arthritis	0	0	0	0	0	0	0	0	2
Hyperpigmentation[c]	–	–	–	–	–	–	+	+	+

[a] Numbers referred.
[b] Single organ dysfunction attributed by the authors.
[c] Not included by the authors, added by this author, where – indicates no effects and + indicates effects noted in patients.

Although two deaths have been reported with minocycline,[511] one of these was due to pancytopenia, a condition not associated with minocycline therapy, and the other was in a patient taking multiple therapies and was probably due to an antimalarial agent.[584]

In the EU, the MRLs for doxycycline, oxytetracycline, chlortetracycline and tetracycline were based on ADI values derived from microbiological studies. Minocycline has not been considered for use in food animals and hence no EU MRL has been considered.

8.2.9   Polyether Ionophore Antibiotics

These are represented by salinomycin, monensin, lasolocid, maduramycin, semduramicin and narasin. These drugs are widely used as coccidiostats in a range of species including poultry. However, they have very narrow therapeutic indices and they are often toxic if the recommended doses, which are frequently low, are exceeded. Ionophore toxicity has been reported in a wide number of animal species including rabbits, dogs, cats, pigeons, quail, ostriches, goats, pigs, sheep, cattle, camels, turkeys and horses. They produce a positive inotropic effect and a cardiomyopathy characterised by a dilated heart and petechial and ecchymotic haemorrhages.[585] Toxicity in humans has not been reported but, based on effects in other species, they can be expected to produce toxic effects should exposure occur. The safety of these drugs, and the establishment of MRL values, is discussed in Chapter 9.

8.2.10   Lincosamides

The lincosamides are used for the treatment of appropriate bacterial diseases in companion and food animals.[4,326] The major ones used in veterinary medicine are clindamycin, lincomycin and pirlimycin (Figure 8.16). Only clindamycin is widely used in human medicine.[325] These drugs are regarded as being safe in humans, and their toxicity is low. The major adverse effect of clindamycin in humans is diarrhoea, which is reported to occur in between 2 and 20% of patients. A number of patients develop pseudomembranous colitis, with abdominal pain, diarrhoea, fever and faeces containing blood and mucus. It is caused by the bacteria *Clostridium difficile*. White to yellow plaques are seen on the mucosa of the colon on proctoscopic examination. This syndrome can be fatal but recovery occurs when the drug is discontinued, although treatment with metronidazole or vancomycin may be required.[325,586–588] The toxicity of these drugs in laboratory animals is low and, consequently, NOEL values tend to be correspondingly high.[589–594] Systemic toxicity is rarely seen in human patients, although it may occur in patients with HIV/AIDS.[595,596] However, a syndrome similar to pseudomembranous colitis seen in humans has been noted in hamsters given the lincomycin or clindamycin, and this too seems to be associated with clostridial toxins and is rapidly fatal.[597–601] Similar effects have also been reported in guinea pigs.[602,603] In guinea pigs given lincomycin orally,

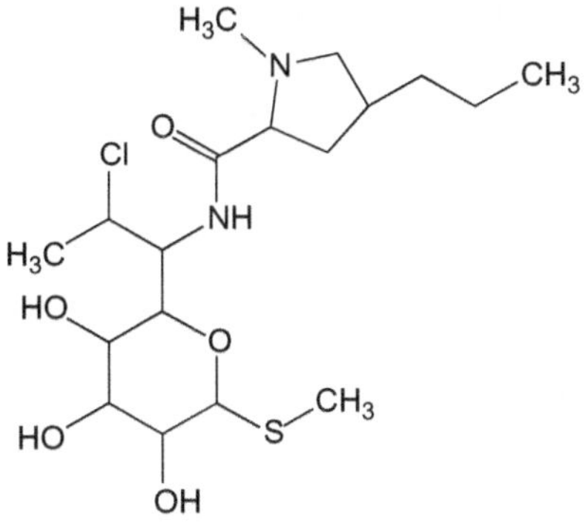

Clindamycin

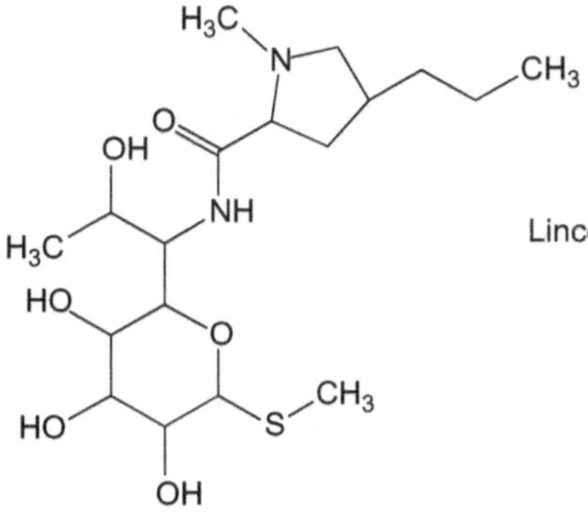

Lincomycin

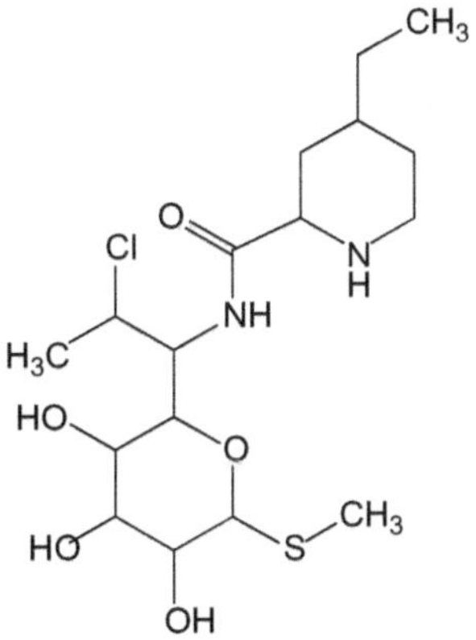

Pirlimycin

Figure 8.16 Chemical formulae of clindamycin, lincomycin and pirlimycin.

the main effects were an increase in the renewal of epithelial cells in the gall bladder, cholecystitis and gallstones composed mainly of calcium and bilirubin.[604]

Skin reactions to clindamycin are rare but they have been reported after topical and oral treatments.[605,606]

The EU MRLs for lincomycin and pirlimycin were established on the basis of microbiological end-points that were lower than NOEL values from toxicology studies.

8.2.11   Polymixins

The polymixins are a class of polypeptide drugs of which polymixin B and colistin (polymixin E) are the major examples used in veterinary medicine. They are composed of a cycloheptapeptide ring made up of D- and L- amino acids with a tripeptide side chain. This is in turn covalently bound to an acyl fatty acid group, α, γ-diaminobutyric acid. Colistin and polymixin B differ in only one of the amino acid residues of the cycloheptapeptide ring. In polymixin B one of these components is D-phenylalanine whereas in colistin this is replaced by D-leucine. Polymixin B is a mixture of two compounds, polymixin B_1 and polymixin B_2. The former has a 6-methyloctanoyl moiety on the fatty acyl group, while the latter possesses a 6-methylheptanoyl group in this position.

In human medicine, polymixin B and colistin are used to treat similar conditions for otic, ocular and dermal infections.[607] Polymixin B is poorly absorbed after oral administration so it may be given by parenteral routes for other infections. Colistin may be given orally or parenterally.[325,608] In veterinary medicine, polymixin B and colistin are used topically for dermal infections in farm and companion animals. Colistin is also used as an oral solution for the treatment of intestinal infections in poultry and pigs.[4,609]

The polymixins are amphipathic surface active agents that behave as detergents. They interact with phospholipids and disrupt bacterial cell membranes. Consequently, bacterial sensitivity depends on the phospholipid content of the cell wall.[610–612] In humans, polymixin B has a high volume of distribution, suggesting extensive distribution.[613,614] When given by the intramuscular route in rabbits, free and bound polymixin B was found in the liver, kidney muscle and brain.[609] There is extensive binding to plasma proteins.[615]

The toxicity of polymixin B is generally poorly documented. However, there are more data available for colistin, and this shows the drug to have a low order of toxicity. The major changes noted in repeat dose studies in rats were minor changes in organ weights. It was not mutagenic in several genotoxicity assays but it produced some evidence of foetotoxicity in the form of delayed ossification.[616]

In humans and other animals, the polymixins including colistin have been found to be nephrotoxic.[617–621] This toxicity was thought to be severe but other studies suggest that this may have been exaggerated.[612,622–624] In humans, nephrotoxicity is unrelated to total dose or to duration of administration, but it may be related to patient age. In a retrospective study of the outcome of treatments with polymixin B, nephrotoxicity was associated with increasing age (76 years *versus* 59 years).[607] In another retrospective study that investigated patients aged between 18 and 79 years, given therapeutic doses of intravenous colistin for periods longer than 4 weeks, there was no evidence of toxicity, including nephrotoxicity.[625] High doses of colistin given intramuscularly to rats for 15 days produced no evidence of nephrotoxicity.[626]

A small number of patients treated with polymixin B or colistin have developed neurotoxicity. This was apparent as diplopia, ptosis and nystagmus and respiratory paralysis has also occurred. These effects occur at a low incidence with between 0 and 5% of patients being affected.[612,614,617] Neurotoxicity is more frequent in patients with compromised renal function and with increasing doses of drug.[612] No evidence of neuromuscular blockade was noted in a retrospective study of patients given colistin at a therapeutic dose for periods in excess of 4 weeks.[625] It is thought that the neurotoxic effects of these drugs may be due to the neurolathyrogenic effects of the α, γ-diaminobutyric acid moiety.[627,628]

The EU MRL values for colistin were based on a microbiological ADI. No MRL was established for polymixin B because of the paucity of data on this drug.

8.2.12 Pleuromutilins

The pleuromutilins are represented by tiamulin and valnemulin, which are mainly used in the treatment of swine dysentery. They are diterpene compounds with the main structure being an 8-membered carbocyclic ring (Figure 8.17). There is little information in the open literature on the safety of these drugs.

The acute oral toxicity of tiamulin is low after oral administration (LD$_{50}$ 2740 and 1830 mg/kg bw for male and female rats). It is much higher after intravenous administration to rats and mice (LD$_{50}$ 20 and 50 mg/kg bw, respectively). Toxicity was generally low in repeat dose studies. The main finding was prolongation of the QT interval in a dog study and an increase in double peaked T-waves in the electrocardiogram after daily doses of 10 mg/kg bw/day or higher. Tiamulin had no adverse effects on reproductive performance in rats and pigs and it produced no evidence of teratogenic effects in rabbits. It was not genotoxic and it showed no evidence of carcinogenic effects in rats and mice.[629] Valnemulin was also of low oral toxicity in rats and it produced no major signs of toxicity in repeat dose studies in rats, mice or dogs. Effects on the electrocardiogram were not investigated. It had no effects on reproductive performance in rats, and it was not teratogenic in mice. However, severe toxicity was seen in treated rabbits and a teratogenicity study could not be conducted in this species. It was not genotoxic.[630] The data suggest that both substances are of low toxicity, but that tiamulin (and possibly valnemulin) may give rise to cardiac effects.

This is of interest because, in combination with ionophores, tiamulin causes severe toxicity. This included severe muscle effects including those on the cardiac muscle. Cardiac toxicity was pronounced.[631–637] Although tiamulin (and presumably valnemulin) may produce a variety of effects on hepatic drug metabolising enzymes, some of these effects may arise from the cardiac effects of tiamulin combined with the known effects of the ionophores, especially their positive inotropic effects and ability to produce cardiomyopathy (see Section

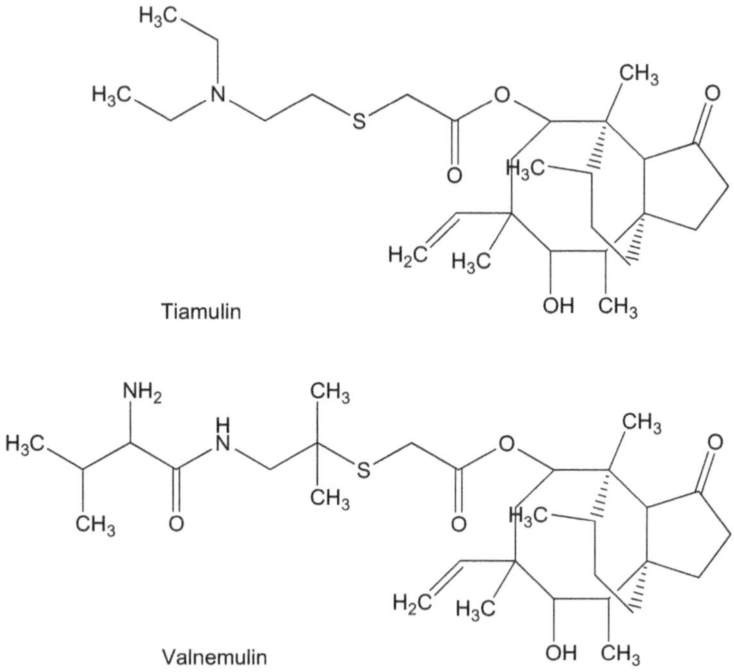

Figure 8.17   Chemical formulae of tiamulin and valnemulin.

8.2.9 and Chapter 9). Valnemulin has produced adverse drug reactions in treated pigs with signs of lethargy, depression, erythema, oedema, pyrexia, ataxia, anorexia and pain; death occurred in some animals.[638-640]

There are no experiences to draw on from use in human medicine, as the pleuromutilins have not been used in human patients. However, this may change with the increase in antibiotic resistance to many existing antibacterial drugs, and a recognition that the pleuromutilins may have a role in the therapy of human infectious diseases.[641,642] The European Medicines Agency has recently published a concept paper on the current use of pleuromutilins because of the rise of the numbers of resistant organisms that potentially threaten the treatment of porcine bacterial gastrointestinal disease.[643] This may have some bearing on the development of resistance in human pathogens and the future utility of the pleuromutilins in treating disease in humans.

The EU MRLs for both drugs were established on the basis of micro-biological ADI values.

8.2.13   Bacitracin

Bacitracin is a peptide antibiotic that is used in human and veterinary medicine. As it is not absorbed after oral administration it is widely used to treat gastrointestinal infection or as a topical treatment. It is also used for wound irrigation, especially during surgery.[4,325,644]

Bacitracin has a low order of toxicity in animal studies.[645] Parenteral use of bacitracin in human medicine may result in severe nephrotoxicity.[325] However, the major problem arising from the use of bacitracin in human medicine is sensitisation. Bacitracin frequently produces a delayed eczematous contact dermatitis, an immediate urticarial reaction and in some cases anaphylaxis after topical use.[646] There have been several cases of anaphylaxis reported after the use of bacitracin during surgery or from the use of topical bacitracin products and some of these have been near fatal.[646-664] IgE antibodies to bacitracin have been detected in a patient who experienced anaphylaxis after application of a bacitracin-containing ointment.[665] Skin reactions are frequent.[666-680]

The EU MRLs for bacitracin were established on the basis of a microbiological ADI value.

8.2.14 Avilamycin

Avilamycin is a member of the orthosomycin group of antibiotics. It is a mixture of oligosaccharides of orthosomycins, and possesses a heptasaccharide chain, at the end of which is a dichloroisoeverninic acid group. It is structurally related to the everninomycins.[681,682] It is used in veterinary medicine for the control of enteric diseases in poultry, rabbits and pigs.

It has extremely low oral toxicity in rodents (LD_{50} values usually in excess of 5000 mg/kg bw) and is only marginally toxic after intraperitoneal administration (LD_{50} 1000–3000 mg/kg bw) although one study in mice produced much higher toxicity ($LD_{50} > 157$ mg/kg bw). The effects after intraperitoneal administration were due to an inflammatory response to unabsorbed avilamycin in the body cavity rather than to frank toxicity. It was of low toxicity in a range of studies in mice, rats, dogs and some farm animal species. It was not mutagenic in a battery of *in vitro* and *in vivo* genotoxicity studies and produced no evidence of carcinogenicity in long-term studies in mice and rats. It gave negative results in reproduction studies and in developmental toxicity studies. There were no indications of sensitising potential in a local lymph node assay or in a modified Buehler assay, and no evidence of neurobehavioral effects in a study that used mice and rabbits. The evidence overall suggests that avilamycin has very low toxic potential.[683,684] As the drug is not used in human medicine, there are no reports of adverse reactions in humans.

The EU MRLs were established on the basis of a toxicological ADI (from an NOEL where increased liver weights were observed in the offspring of rats in a three-generation reproduction study) despite the microbiological ADI value being lower. This was because residues of avilamycin in food animals showed no antimicrobial properties and so the toxicological effects were considered more relevant than microbiological effects.

8.2.15 Trimethoprim, Baquiloprim and Sulfonamides

Trimethoprim and the related compound baquiloprim are inhibitors of bacterial dihydrofolate reductase and thus they inhibit bacterial cell division.

Trimethoprim (Figure 8.18) has been widely used in human and veterinary medicine, while baquiloprim was used in veterinary medicine but the drug has largely disappeared from use, mainly for commercial reasons. Ormetoprim is also used in human and veterinary medicine, but it is not used widely in the latter. Trimethoprim may be used alone on in combination with sulfonamide drugs (potentiated sulfonamides). They then operate synergistically. The sulfonamides are structurally related to *p*-aminobenzoic acid, and they block the normal utilisation of this compound by bacteria. They are competitive inhibitors of dihydropteroate synthase, an enzyme responsible for the incorporation of *p*-aminobenzoic acid into dihydropteroic acid, the precursor of dihydrofolic acid. Trimethoprim blocks the next stage in the process, the conversion of dihydrofolic acid into folic acid.[4,685–694]

In animal studies, trimethoprim and baquiloprim have low toxicity.[695,696] the major effects of trimethoprim, but not baquiloprim, were on bone marrow in repeat-dose studies in rats and monkeys where bone marrow hypoplasia with reductions in erythrocyte, leucocyte and neutrophil counts occurred.[696] These effects are probably related to antifolate activity and are similar, at least qualitatively, to those seen with methotrexate (see Chapter 7).

In fact, trimethoprim can cause bone marrow depression in humans, or it can exacerbate it in patients being treated with other drugs that depress bone marrow such as the antineoplastic drugs, and notably methotrexate, when being used either in anticancer therapy or as an immunosuppressant drug.[697–703] Trimethoprim can inhibit potassium secretion in the distal tubule and so may cause hyperkalaemia.[704,705] Combinations of trimethoprim and a sulfonamide drug, and notably sulfamethoxazole, may produce hepatotoxicity in treated humans and animals, especially in dogs, and a range of other adverse effects, including severe skin reactions such as Stevens–Johnson syndrome.[706–723] Trimethoprim and sulfamethoxazole may be specifically toxic in HIV/AIDS patients.[724–727]

The first commercially available sulfonamide drug was Prontosil (4-(2,4-diaminophenyl)azobenzenesulfonamide), which was developed in Germany

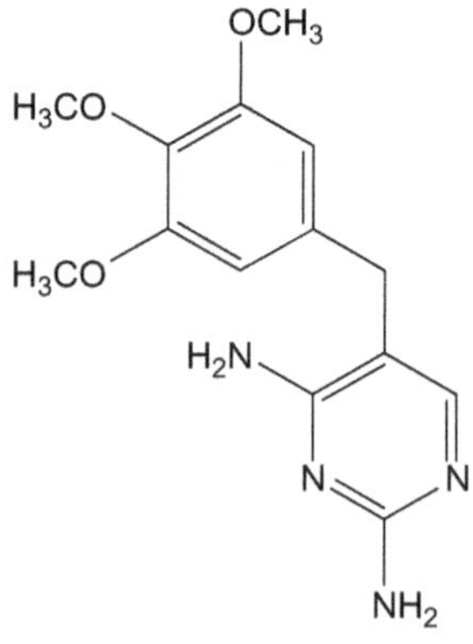

Figure 8.18   Chemical formula of trimethoprim.

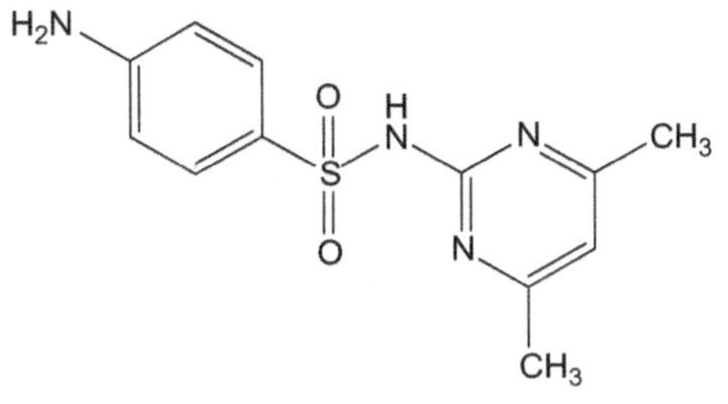

Figure 8.19   Chemical formula of sulfamethazine.

during the 1930s. It was later discovered that Prontosil was in fact a prodrug that is metabolised to *p*-aminobenzenesulfonamide, or sulfanilamide. This became the basis of the development of the whole class of sulfonamide drugs.[728] One of the most widely used sulfonamides in veterinary medicine is sulfamethazine (sulfadimidine, sulphadimidine, Figure 8.19), although sulfadimethoxine, sulfamerazine, sulfaquinoxaline, sulfadiazine and others are also employed.[4,686] In human medicine, the major sulfonamides are sulfamethoxazole, sulfadiazine and sulfisoxazole. Sulfacetamide is used for topical administration, while sulfasalazine, a poorly absorbed sulfonamide, is used to treat gastrointestinal conditions and notably ulcerative colitis.[685]

Some of the adverse effects of sulfonamides have been discussed already, at least in so far as they occur when given in potentiated form with trimethoprim. In animal studies, they have a low order of toxicity and they are not genotoxic.[729,730] However, when administered to rats, but not to mice, for prolonged periods, sulfamethazine induces thyroid hyperplasia.[731–734] Administration to mice for 24 months resulted in follicular cell adenomas of the thyroid, while similar administration to rats in a two-generation study resulted in adenocarcinomas of the thyroid.[735,736] Thus, there is evidence that sulfamethazine is possibly carcinogenic to mice, and is carcinogenic to rats.

Sulfamethazine has been shown to be goitrogenic to rodents, resulting in a constant stimulation of the thyroid by thyroid stimulating hormone (TSH) during drug administration and this leads to reductions in thyroid hormones.[737–745] Fluctuating TSH levels may have a similar outcome.[746] Similar effects have been observed in pigs but not in primates.[729] Sulfanilamidoindazole, a sulfonamide that induces an acute arthritis in rats, and sulfamethoxazole also induce thyroid follicular hyperplasia in rodents.[747,748] Sulfadimethoxine is also a thyroid carcinogen.[749–755] When given at high therapeutic doses, disruption of thyroid function also occurs in dogs.[756,757]

Thus, the sulfonamides are non-genotoxic carcinogens that produce thyroid tumours through perturbations in TSH, and subsequently in thyroid hormones. Humans are insensitive to this mechanism of thyroid-induced neoplasia. Hence, the tumours noted in rodents have no relevance to human risk assessment. The International Agency for Research on Cancer (IARC) has concluded that sulfamethazine and sulfamethoxazole are not classifiable as to their carcinogenicity to humans. However, it notes that evidence from epidemiology studies and from animal studies provides "compelling evidence that rodents are substantially more sensitive than humans" to the effects of sulfonamide on the thyroid.[758,759] Hence, it is possible to identify suitable NOEL values for these drugs, so that ADI values can be calculated and MRLs established.[742,760–762]

The EU MRL value for sulfonamides was established at 100 μg/kg as this took into account the toxicological ADI value but also potential allergic and microbiological effects. The MRL for trimethoprim was based on microbiological effects, while that for baquiloprim was based on toxicological effects.

8.2.16   Quinoxaline-N-Oxides

The main members of this group of drugs are carbadox, olaquindox, cyadox and quindoxin. Of these, the two most important members are carbadox and olaquindox. They have been used for therapeutic purposes but their main uses were as growth promoters, especially in pigs.[763–772] In the EU, they were approved under Directive 70/524/EEC as feed additives.[773]

The most notable aspects of the toxicology of these drugs is the genotoxic activity and, in the case of carbadox, its carcinogenic activity. Carbadox (methyl (2E)-2-[(1,4-dioxido-2-quinoxalinyl)methylene]hydrazinecarboxylate; Figure 8.20) has been subject to a number of studies in rats, and in doses of 1 mg/kg bw/day it has resulted in the induction of tumours. In fact, tumours occurred even in a severely limited study of only 11 months' duration and in another where rats were dosed by the intraperitoneal route prior to weaning for 8 to 20 days, and in the feed at 300 ppm for 1 year.[774,775] The drug was genotoxic in a wide range of *in vitro* and *in vivo* studies with a range of end-points.[776–787]

A genotoxic, carcinogenic drug would not normally be permitted for use in food animals because of obvious concerns over consumer safety. However, the major metabolites of carbadox in the pig are methyl carbazate, the quinoxaline-2-carboxylic acid and desoxycarbadox, and these gave negative results in genotoxicity and carcinogenicity studies, indicating that they did not pose risks to the consumer, but the metabolism of carbadox is complex and a number of other metabolites are also produced.[774,788,789] Relay toxicity studies have

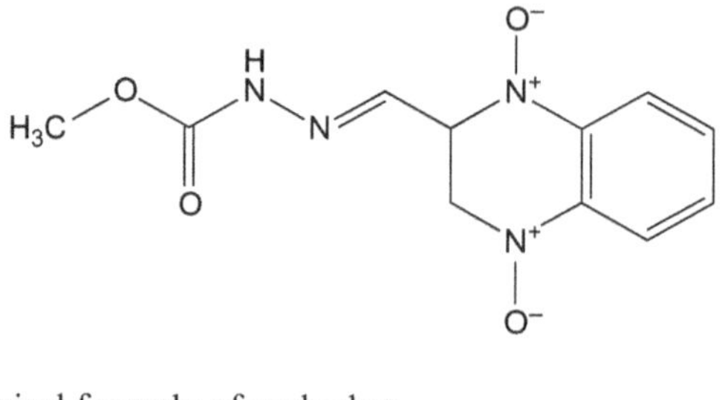

Figure 8.20   Chemical formula of carbadox.

therefore been used to try and determine the safety of carbadox residues. In relay toxicity studies, food commodities containing residues of the drug are fed to experimental animals, rather than administration of the parent drug itself. The tissues of the food animal therefore serve as a proxy for the drug in toxicity studies, including carcinogenicity studies.[790–806]

This approach is undoubtedly useful in demonstrating the lability of drug residues covalently bound to cellular macromolecules.[807–812] However, its utility is more doubtful in toxicity testing because the doses given are very low, and in carcinogenicity studies the doses are far below the maximum tolerated dose and the metabolites of drug actually present are unknown.[800,801,803] Despite this, it can be argued that the residues present in the tissues used in the study are representative of what is actually present as residues in food of animal origin and that the concentrations found are towards the lower end of the dose-response curve for carcinogenicity. Hence, the relay toxicity approach is a valid methodology to complement conventional toxicity studies but not to replace them.[800,801] Relay carcinogenicity studies were conducted with carbadox over 2 years in rats and 7.5 years in dogs, and no evidence was seen suggesting a carcinogenic effect.[788,813–815] Thus, there is compelling evidence that residues of carbadox in food of animal origin lack carcinogenic potential.

Olaquindox, cyadox and quindoxin are also genotoxic.[776,778,783,784,786,816–824] Olaquindox (Figure 8.21) has been tested in carcinogenicity studies in rats and mice and there was no evidence for a carcinogenic effect.[774] Studies with cyadox in rats for 13 weeks and for 78 weeks produced no evidence of neoplastic precursor lesions or of carcinogenicity.[825,826] The major effects noted were fatty degeneration of hepatocytes and changes in renal proximal tubule epithelial cells.[775,776] There is no convincing evidence of teratogenicity, but these drugs may be foetotoxic.[774,827–829]

Olaquindox, and to a lesser extent carbadox, has produced contact dermatitis and photoallergic dermatitis in farm workers exposed to it occupationally. The latter usually has increased UV-A and UV-B sensitivity.[830–842] Experimental studies have also demonstrated these effects,[843,844] and quindoxin was withdrawn commercially because of these effects.[843]

Toxicity due to carbadox and olaquindox has also been reported in pigs during treatments and, notably, after overdosing. The adverse effects noted were mainly on the adrenals and kidneys. There were abnormalities in renal

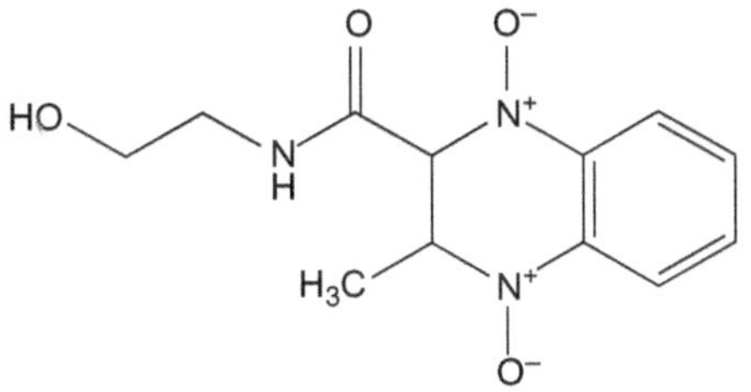

Figure 8.21 Chemical formula of olaquindox.

function, hypoaldosteronism, hyponatraemia, hyperkalaemia and haemo-concentration.[845–848] Experimental studies with pigs revealed adrenal toxicity with carbadox, cyadox and olaquindox. The glomerular cells in the adrenal cortex were swollen with hydropic changes and there were degenerative changes. Necrosis was seen in the medulla and pelvis of the kidney. The severity of the lesions increased with dose and, with high doses of carbadox, the adrenal lesions were persistent and the hypoaldosteronism slow to resolve.[849–859] Inhibition of aldosterone production has been demonstrated *in vitro* using pig adrenal preparations.[860] Adrenal degeneration has also been observed in rats given high doses of carbadox but there were no adverse effects on kidneys. Adrenal atrophy occurred in rats given high doses of olaquindox. Olaquindox led to fatty degeneration of the kidneys in dogs. No adverse effects were produced in monkeys administered carbadox but rhesus monkeys given olaquindox for up to 19 days showed evidence of minor kidney and adrenal toxicity.[774,762]

The European Commission believed it to be impractical to suggest protective methods and equipment to protect workers from the toxic effects of these substances and prohibited the use of carbadox and olaquindox in 1998.[861] Quindoxin had already been withdrawn as mentioned earlier, while cyadox had not been approved. Since that time, other countries have prohibited these drugs, although they are still used in some territories.

8.2.17   Other Antibiotic Growth Promoters

In addition to the quinoxaline-N-oxides discussed in the previous section, other antibiotics have been used as growth promoters. In the EU, these were spiramycin, avoparcin, flavomycin (bambermycin, flavophospholipol), bacitracin, tylosin and virginiamycin, which were all approved under Directive 70/524/EEC. Unlike carbadox and olaquindox, these substances, some of which have already been discussed in this chapter, are not significantly toxic, especially under normal conditions of use but, nevertheless, they were banned in the EU for growth-promoting purposes, although bacitracin, tylosin and spiramycin are still available for therapeutic purposes. The reasons for the prohibition were nominally public health issues, and notably because of fears over the induction of antibiotic resistance, as well as opposition from public and political opinion.[862] Other countries have also eliminated or significantly restricted their uses.[862–866] In fact the only significant effect of these drugs reported in humans is contact dermatitis.[867–869] The immediate benefits from these prohibitions are yet to become obvious but it seems likely that they will increase the cost of food, especially food derived from pigs, and lead to the more extensive use of therapeutic antibiotics.[870]

8.2.18   Nitrofurans

The nitrofurans are a group of heterocyclic antimicrobial drugs that have been widely used in veterinary medicine. The major examples of the group that are

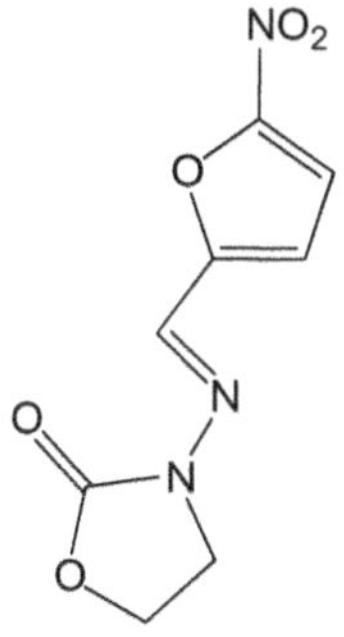

Figure 8.22 Chemical formula of furazolidone.

used in veterinary medicine are furazolidone (Figure 8.22) and nitrofurazone (nitrofural).

These drugs are toxic in some animal patients, and may cause a congestive cardiomyopathy in poultry.[871–877] In human patients the main effects are nausea and vomiting, abdominal pain, anorexia, diarrhoea and heartburn.[878] There may also be skin reactions, leukopenia and, occasionally, adverse hepatic and renal reactions. Nitrofurazone and furazolidone have caused contact dermatitis, including after occupational exposure to furazolidone.[879–883] However, the main concern is due to their genotoxicity and carcinogenicity. These drugs are genotoxic in numerous studies.[884–925] They have also been tested in animal bioassays or in more specialised studies for carcinogenic activity and they have produced evidence of carcinogenic potential.[926–931] Nitrofurazone was unusual in National Toxicology Program studies in that, along with four other chemicals, it only produced benign tumours.[932] Several other nitrofurans have produced malignant tumours in animal studies.[933,934]

The carcinogenicity of nitrofurazone and the related compound, nitrofurantoin, has been reviewed by the International Agency for Research on Cancer. It concluded that there was inadequate evidence for the carcinogenicity of nitrofurazone in humans, but there was limited evidence in animals. It reached similar conclusions on the carcinogenicity of nitrofurantoin.[935,936]

As with carbadox discussed previously, some attempt was made to assess whether the metabolites of nitrofurans in food-producing animals were likely to pose a human consumer risk. Some of the residues were found to be bound to macromolecules and there was concern that these could be released as potentially toxic materials on digestion in the human gut. The major questions concerned the bioavailability of these residues and whether they were toxic, genotoxic and carcinogenic. Unfortunately, with this group of drugs, relay toxicity and other relevant studies described earlier for carbadox proved equivocal and inconclusive. There is significant binding of furazolidone residues to macromolecules, notably to protein, and, while some data suggested that these bound residues are likely to be converted to non-toxic metabolites, the evidence was not convincing.[811,937–942]

As a result of these considerations, and the activity of the nitrofurans in genotoxicity tests and carcinogenicity studies, the drugs were prohibited in the EU for use in food animals, and no MRLs were established.

8.2.19 Fusidic Acid

Fusidic acid (Figure 8.23) is an antimicrobial drug with a chemical structure that is related to those of the steroids. It is not widely used in human medicine, and even less so in veterinary medicine, where its main use is in ophthalmic products, mainly for use in dogs.[644] It has no major uses in food animal treatment.

Its introduction into human medicine was noted not to be accompanied by "extensive studies on toxicity and side effects".[943] Its main side effects in humans are hepatotoxicity and immune suppression, but these are rare and the most common effects are gastrointestinal disturbances after oral administration.[943–947] There has been a case of rhabdomyolysis following co-administration with atorvastatin, suggesting that it may inhibit cytochrome P450 3A4 and, subsequently, the metabolism of atorvastatin.[947] Its use in veterinary medicine is unlikely to pose any realistic threat to human health.

8.2.20 Novobiocin

Novobiocin (Figure 8.24) is an aminocoumarin derivative that is thought to exert its effects on bacteria by inhibiting DNA gyrase, but at a different site on the enzyme from that targeted by the quinolones (see Section 8.2.1.5).[948–952] It is not widely used in human medicine as an antibiotic but there has been renewed interest in the drug in cancer chemotherapy, as it may be able to

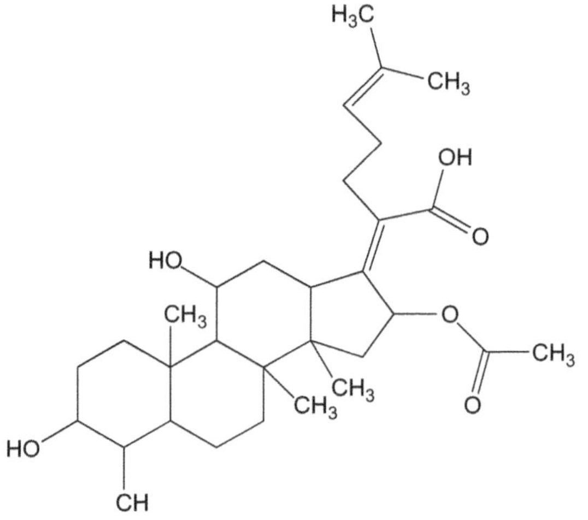

Figure 8.23   Chemical formula of fusidic acid.

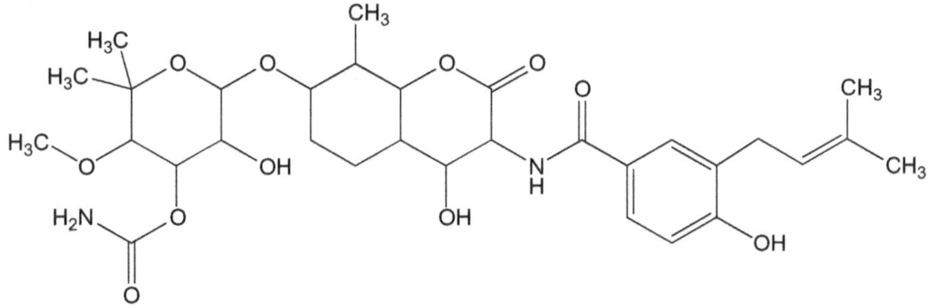

Figure 8.24 Chemical formula of novobiocin.

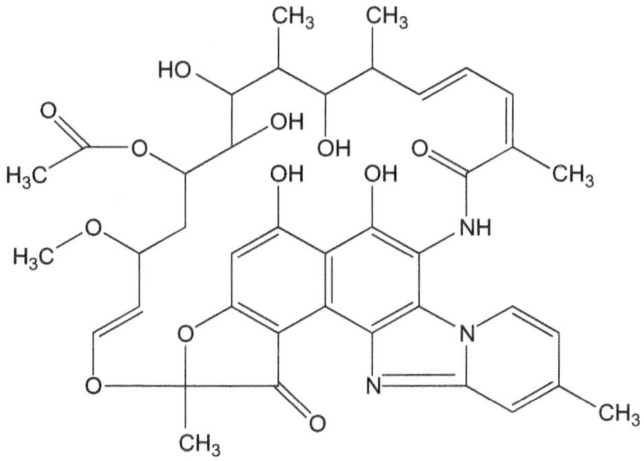

Figure 8.25 Chemical formula of rifaximin.

overcome resistance to the therapeutic effects of other antineoplastic drugs such as the alkylating agents and the epipodophyllotoxins such as etoposide. This may be through its interference with topoisomerase II or through pharmacological effects.[953–959]

In animal studies it has low toxicity. In genotoxicity studies, it showed evidence of interacting with DNA, which in view of its known pharmacological effects is not surprising. It was not carcinogenic in a long-term feeding study in rats.[960] It has occasionally produced haemolysis and jaundice in humans.[961–963]

In the EU, the MRL values for novobiocin were established on the basis of microbiological studies.

8.2.21 Rifaximin

Rifaximin (Figure 8.25) is a drug that is included in the ansamycin group and it has structural similarities with rifampin (rifampicin). In human medicine it is mainly used in the treatment of travellers' diarrhoea and it may be useful in the treatment of irritable bowel syndrome and for hepatic encephalopathy.[964–966] In veterinary medicine it is used in cattle for the treatment of bacterial mastitis using the intramammary route and for the treatment of *post-partum* metritis by the intrauterine route. It has relatively low toxicity in animals, although it may cause neutropenia in humans.[967–971] The microbiological ADI is about 100 times lower than the toxicological ADI and so this formed the basis of the EU MRL.

Rifampin is not authorised in the EU for veterinary use but it is used elsewhere, notably for the treatment of certain diseases in horses. In humans it has been used for many years, usually in combination with isoniazid, for the treatment of tuberculosis.[972] Its therapeutic use in humans is associated with hepatotoxicity, sometimes in combination with isoniazid, which is also hepatotoxic, nephritis and nephrotoxicity and skin reactions, which may be severe; rifampicin is also hepatotoxic in animal models.[973–986]

8.2.22   Dapsone

Dapsone (4,4′-sulfonyldianiline; Figure 8.26) is a sulfone drug that in human medicine has been one of the major drugs used in the treatment of leprosy (Hansen's disease).[972] In veterinary medicine it is used for its anti-inflammatory effects in certain dermatological conditions of companion animals.[987] It has also been used for the treatment of bovine mastitis where there is a possibility of producing drug residues in milk, and for bovine coccidiosis and intrauterine treatment of endometritis.[988]

One of the major adverse effects is the dapsone syndrome or dapsone hypersensitivity syndrome. This is a potentially fatal condition that usually presents with fever, skin eruption and major effects in internal organs including the lung, liver and other systems. These may be accompanied by fever, hepatitis, cholangitis, exfoliative dermatitis, adenopathy and haemolytic anaemia. The reaction usually begins after 7 to 10 days of treatment or it may be delayed until as late as 6 months. The mechanism is unknown. It is an idiosyncratic reaction that may involve a reactive metabolite, slow acetylator status and possibly a viral infection.[989–994] It also induces a number of other idiosyncratic reactions including Stevens–Johnson syndrome, toxic epidermal necrolysis, cholestasis, nephritis, pneumonitis and hypothyroidism.[989]

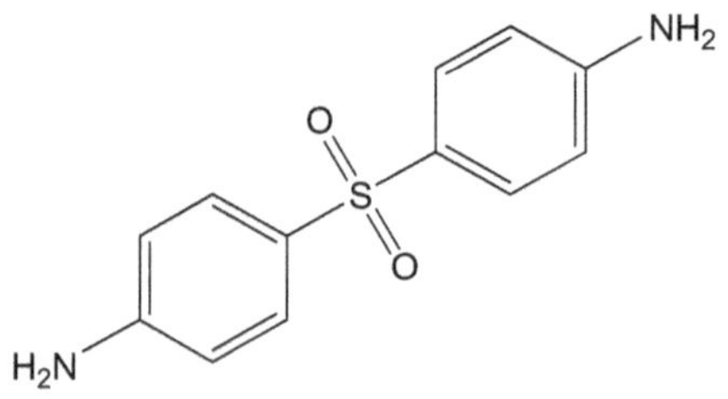

Figure 8.26   Chemical formula of dapsone.

One of the predictable, as opposed to idiosyncratic, effects of dapsone is the induction of haemolysis, with methaemoglobinaemia. This tends to be dose related and duration of treatment related.[995–999] Agranulocytosis may also occur.[1000–1002]

The haemolytic effects of dapsone are almost certainly related to the formation of a metabolite, probably through N-hydroxylation, followed by acetylation to a non-toxic product. There may be species differences in the toxicity of dapsone in this respect, as male rats and humans appear to be more susceptible to the haemolytic effects than female rats and male and female mice and this is possibly associated with the formation of the hydroxylamine metabolite.[1003–1009]

The sulfonyl group is thought to be at least partly responsible for the haemotoxicity of dapsone.[1010] However, perhaps these effects should come as no surprise as many aniline derivatives, or substances that are metabolised to aniline-containing products, cause methaemoglobinaemia. Examples include *p*-chloroaniline, indoxacarb and the benzoylureas (see Chapter 6).[1011]

In long-term studies in mice and rats, dapsone produced only limited evidence of carcinogenicity in rats and no evidence in mice. The tumours in rats were unusual in that they were sarcomas of the spleen that are rarely seen in animal carcinogenicity studies.[1012]

EU MRLs were not established for dapsone. Provisional MRL values had been established but further data were required on teratogenicity and reproductive toxicity before full MRLs could be established. However, these data were not forthcoming and the provisional MRLs expired in January 1994.[1013] Consequently, dapsone may not be used in food-producing animals in the EU.

8.2.23 Chlorhexidine

Chlorhexidine is a bis-biguanide cationic chemical antiseptic (Figure 8.27), which is effective against Gram-positive and Gram-negative bacteria. It is widely used in mouthwashes and skin cleansers for human use but it also has medical and dental applications as a general disinfectant. It is also available for use against acne and athlete's foot. In animal husbandry it is used as a general disinfectant for cleaning animal housing and dairy units, while in some countries, including the UK, it is available in authorised veterinary medicinal products for use as teat dips as aids in the prevention of bovine mastitis and for

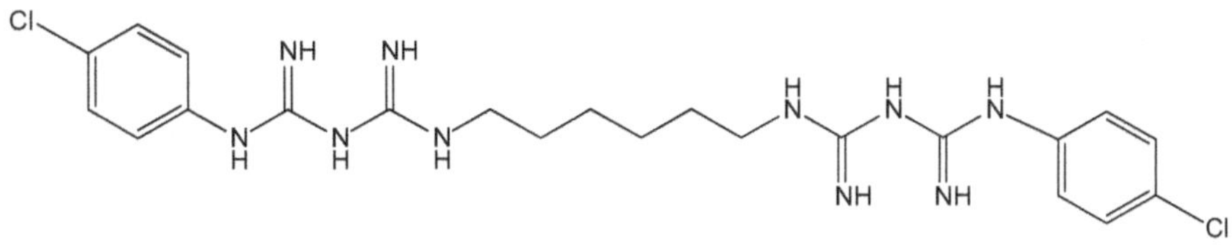

Figure 8.27 Chemical formula of chlorhexidine.

cleaning wounds, and in medicated shampoo formulations for companion animal dermatological treatmets.[1014–1020]

Chlorhexidine has low mammalian toxicity in the usual tests for medicinal products.[1021,1022] It is not genotoxic although it has only been tested in a limited number of tests.[1023,1024] Oral consumption of 20% chlorhexidine, approximately equal to 100 standard mouthwash doses, resulted in headache, euphoria, dizziness, blurred vision and stomach ache. The patient recovered after gastric lavage with demulcents but there was a complete lack of taste for 48 hours.[1025] In children, accidental ingestion of chlorhexidine (0.06 mg/kg bw) and lignocaine (2.7 mg/kg bw) resulted in no major adverse effects.[1026] Pulmonary instillation in rats induced inflammatory changes with intra-alveolar oedema and haemorrhages.[1027]

The major toxicological effect of chlorhexidine in treated animal patients is ototoxicity. This has occurred in cats and dogs after its use in ear surgery.[1028,1029] It has been replicated in experimental studies in guinea pigs.[1030,1031] It has also been shown to be ototoxic in humans.[1032,1033] It seems that the substance is likely to be ototoxic in humans and animals if it reaches the inner ear, usually during ear surgery.

Chlorhexidine is often encountered as a dilute solution through dermal exposure when cleaning medical and veterinary medical areas *e.g.* operating rooms and tables, or when cleansing wounds or body areas prior to surgery. Dermal exposure in users has resulted in occupational allergic dermatitis.[1034–1038] It has given positive results in the local lymph node assay for allergic potential.[1039] Concentrated solutions may be severe eye irritants and two patients accidentally exposed to a 4% solution developed severe and permanent corneal opacification.[1040,1041]

In the EU it was considered that as chlorhexidine has low absorption after oral administration and in view of its low toxicity, MRL values were not required on public health grounds when used on food-producing animals.[1042]

8.3   Conclusions

As the antimicrobial drugs are represented by a wide variety of chemical structures and biological properties, it is not surprising that, as a group, they display a wide range of toxicities. The vast majority of these agents, or at least their close relatives, are used in human medicine, and most have a high safety profile, although many also display a range of idiosyncratic reactions that may be at best uncomfortable and at worst fatal in human patients.

The use of these drugs in veterinary medicine means that humans may be exposed occupationally or through residues in food of animal origin. However, in the latter case at least, this exposure is but a fraction of the dose humans might take therapeutically. Hence, any exposure resulting from residues is low and consumers are protected by legislation to ensure that residues are controlled. For occupational exposure, the main adverse effects with a number of classes of antimicrobial drug are allergic and include contact dermatitis and asthma. Some antibiotics like carbadox, chloramphenicol and the nitrofurans, which may be seen as posing unacceptable occupational or consumer risks, have been prohibited in many countries, at least for use in food animals. Others, such as the growth-promoting antibiotics, have also been prohibited, again ostensibly to protect human health and specifically to help prevent the development and spread of antimicrobial resistance.

Despite these restrictions and prohibitions, there is still a wide variety of suitable antimicrobial drugs available for use in companion and food animal veterinary medicine.

References

1. G. L. Mandell and W. A. Petri, Penicillins, cephalosporins, and other β-lactam antibiotics in *Goodman and Gilman's The Pharmacological Basis of Therapeutics*, ed. J. G. Hardman, L. E. Limbird, P. B. Molinoff, R. W. Ruddon and A. G. Goodman, McGraw-Hill, London, 9th edn, 1996, pp. 1073–1101.
2. A. Fleming (ed.), *Penicillin. Its Practical Application*, Butterworth & Co., London, 1946.
3. R. Lovell, Penicillin in animal diseases in *Penicillin. Its Practical Application*, ed. A. Fleming, Butterworth & Co., London, 1946, pp. 337–349.
4. D. M. Boothe, Antimicrobial drugs in *Small Animal Clinical Pharmacology and Therapeutics*, ed. D. M. Boothe, W. B. Saunders Company, London, pp. 150–173.
5. S. L. Vaden and J. E. Riviere, Penicillins and related β-lactams in *Veterinary Pharmacology and Therapeutics*, ed. H. R. Adams, Iowa State Press, Ames, 8th edn, pp. 818–840.
6. A. L. de Weck, Penicillins and cephalosporins in *Handbook of Experimental Pharmacology*, ed. A. L. de Weck and H. Bundgaard, Springer, New York, 1982, vol. 63, pp. 423–482.
7. J. P. Griffin, Drug-induced allergic and hypersensitivity reactions in *Iatrogenic Diseases*, ed. P. F. D'Arcy and J. P. Griffin, Oxford Medical Publications, Oxford, 3rd edn, 1986, pp. 82–92.
8. K. N. Woodward, Hypersensitivity in humans and exposure to veterinary drugs, *Vet. Hum. Toxicol.*, 1991, **33**, 168–172.
9. F. Hasdenteufel, S. Luyasu, N. Haugardy, M. Fisher, M. Boisbrun, P. M. Mertes and G. Kanny, Structure-activity relationships and drug allergy, *Curr. Clin. Pharmacol.*, 2012, **7**, 15–27.
10. C. Ponvert, Y. Perrin, A. Bados-Albiero, M. Le Bourgeois, C. Karila, C. Delacourt, P. Scheinmann and J. De Blic, Allergy to betalactam antibiotics in children: results of a 20-year study based on clinical history, skin and challenge tests, *Pediatr. Allergy Immunol.*, 2011, **22**, 411–418.
11. A. Chaabane, K. Aouam, N. A. Boughatttas and M. Chakroun, Allergy to beta lactams: myths and realities, *Med. Mal. Infect.*, 2009, **39**, 278–287.
12. P. Lagacé-Wiens and E. Rubinstein, Adverse reactions to β-lactam antimicrobials, *Expert Opin. Drug Saf.*, 2012, **11**, 381–399.

13. S. Caimmi, D. Caimmi, E. Lombardi, G. Crisafulli, F. Franceschini, G. Ricci and G. L. Marseglia, Antibiotic allergy, *Int. J. Immunopathol. Pharmacol.*, 2011, **24**(3), S47–S53.

14. D. T. O'Keefe and R. Cooke, Serum sickness like reaction in an 11-year-old boy, *Ir. J. Med. Sci.*, 2011, **180**, 605–606.

15. A. J. Tatum, A. M. Ditto and R. Patterson, Severe serum sickness-like reaction to oral penicillin drugs: three case reports, *Ann. Allergy Asthma Immunol.*, 2001, **86**, 330–334.

16. C. Chang, M. M. Mahmood, S. S. Teuber and M. E. Gershwin, Overview of penicillin allergy, *Clin. Rev. Allergy Immunol.*, 2012, **43**, 84–97.

17. X. D. Liu, N. Gao and H. L. Qiao, Cephalosporin and penicillin cross-reactivity in patients allergic to penicillin, *Int. J. Clin. Pharmacol. Ther.*, 2011, **49**, 206–216.

18. M. Blanca, M. Jose Torres, N. Blanca-Lopez and M. Gabriela Canto, Penicillin determinants in the diagnosis of immediate hypersensitivity reactions to β-lactams, *Int. Arch. Allergy Immunol.*, 2011, **155**, 187–188.

19. J. C. Caubet, L. Kaiser, B. Lemaître, B. Fellay, A. Gervaix and P. A. Eigenmann, The role of penicillin in benign skin rashes in childhood: a prospective study based on drug rechallenge, *J. Allergy Clin. Immunol.*, 2011, **127**, 218–222.

20. S. Battacharya, The facts about penicillin allergy: a review, *J. Adv. Pharm. Technol. Res.*, 2010, **1**, 11–17.

21. M. Gallego Segovia and A. M. Garcia Dumpiérrez, Systemic reactions in anamnestic responses during penicillin allergy study, *J. Invest. Allergol. Clin. Immunol.*, 2009, **19**, 240–241.

22. P. Lee and D. Shanson, Results of a UK survey of fatal anaphylaxis after oral amoxicillin, *J. Antimicrob. Chemother.*, 2007, **60**, 1172–1173.

23. S. B. Meropol, K. A. Chan, Z. Chen, J. A. Finkelstein, S. Hennessy, E. Lautenbach, R. Platt, S. D. Schech, D. Shatin and J. P. Metlay, Adverse events associated with prolonged antibiotic use, *Pharmacoepidemiol. Drug Saf.*, 2008, **17**, 523–532.

24. A. L. Kedward and K. McKenna, A fatal case of toxic epidermal necrolysis with extensive intestinal involvement, *Clin. Exp. Dermatol.*, 2009, **34**, e484.

25. Y. H. Kim, J. Y. Ko, Y. S. Kim and Y. S. Ro, A case of contact dermatitis to clavulanic acid, *Contact Dermatitis*, 2008, **59**, 378–379.

26. N. Longo, P. M. Gambao, G. Gastaminza, M. T. Audicana, I. Antepara, I. Jaúre-gui and M. L Sanz, Diagnosis of clavulanic acid allergy using basophil activation and leukotriene release by basophils, *J. Invest. Allergol. Clin. Immunol.*, 2008, **18**, 473–475.

27. M. Fernandez-Rivas, C. Perez Carral, M. Cuevas, C. Marti, A. Moral and C. J. Senent, Selective allergic reactions to clavulanic acid, *J. Allergy Clin. Immunol.*, 1995, **95**, 748–750.

28. M. J. Torres and M. Blanca, The complex clinical picture of beta-lactam hypersensitivity: penicillins, cephalosporins, monobactams, carbapenems, and clavams, *Med. Clin. North Am.*, 2010, **94**, 805–820.

29. R. Warrington and F. Silviu-Dan, Drug allergy, *Allergy Asthma Clin. Immunol.*, 2011, **7**(1), S10.
30. S. Macy and N. J. Ho, Adverse reactions associated with therapeutic antibiotic use after penicillin testing, *Perm. J.*, 2011, **15**, 31–37.
31. A. Romano, F. Gaeta, R. L. Valluzzi, C. Caruso, G. Rumi and P. J. Bousquet, IgE-mediated hypersensitivity to cephalosporins: cross-reactivity and tolerability of penicillins, monobactams and carbapenems, *J. Allergy Clin. Immunol.*, 2010, **126**, 994–999.
32. I. Jiménez, E. Antón, I. Picáns, I. Sánchez, M. D Quiñomes and J. Jerez, Occupational asthma specific to amoxicillin, *Allergy*, 1998, **53**, 104–105.
33. G. Moscato, E. Gaidl, J. Scibilia, A. Dellablanca, P. Omodeo, G. Vittadini and G. P. Biscaldi, Occupational asthma, rhinitis and urticaria due to piperacillin sodium in a pharmaceutical worker, *Eur. Resp. J.*, 1995, **8**, 467–469.
34. A. de Hoyos, D. L. Holness and S. M. Tarlo, Hypersensitivity pneumonitis and airways hyperreactivity induced by occupational exposure to penicillin, *Chest*, 1993, **103**, 202–204.
35. N. E. Møller and K. von Würden, Hypersensitivity to semisynthetic penicillins and cross-reactivity with penicillin, *Contact Dermatitis*, 1992, **26**, 351–352.
36. N. E. Møller, B. Nielsen and K. von Würden, Changes in penicillin contamination and allergy in factory workers, *Contact Dermatitis*, 1990, **22**, 106–107.
37. I. S. Choi, E.-R. Han, S.-W. Lim, S.-R. Lim, J.-N. Kim, S.-Y. Park, S.-K. Chae, H.-H. Lim, Y.-A. Seol and Y.-H. Won, Beta-lactam antibiotic sensitization and its relationship to allergic diseases in tertiary hospital nurses, *Allergy Asthma Immunol. Res.*, 2010, **2**, 114–122.
38. E. R. Gomes and P. Demoly, Epidemiology of hypersensitivity drug reactions, *Curr. Opin. Allergy Clin. Immunol.*, 2005, **5**, 309–316.
39. K. Tondoro, N. Niimi, T. Ohtoshi, K. Nakajima, S. Takafuji, K. Onodera, S. Suzuki and M. Muranaka, Cefotiam-induced IgE-mediated occupational contact anaphylaxis of nurses; case reports, RAST analysis, and a review of the literature, *Clin. Exp. Allergy*, 1994, **24**, 127–133.
40. S. Shimizu, K. R. Chen and S. Miyakawa, Cefotiam-induced contact urticarial syndrome: an occupational condition in Japanese nurses, *Dermatology*, 1996, **192**, 174–176.
41. K. Y. Shin, J. Y. Lee, C. W. Park and C. H. Lee, A case of cefotiam-induced contact urticarial syndrome, *Korean J. Dermatol.*, 1998, **36**, 1092–1095.
42. P. M. Jang, H. J. Kim, Y. S. Kim, Y. S. Cho, J. W. Lee, K. W. Yu and H. Lim, Two cases of contact urticarial syndrome from cefotiam in nurses, *J. Korean Soc. Clin. Toxicol.*, 2006, **4**, 65–68.
43. J. Jeong, K. You, S. Nahm and E. Kim, Anaphylaxis after epidermal contact with cefotiam hydrochloride, *J. Allergy Clin. Immunol.*, 2006, **117**, S227.
44. F. Cetinkaya, A. O. Ozturk, G. Kutluk and E. Erdem, Penicillin sensitivity among hospital nurses without a history of penicillin allergy, *J. Adv. Nurs.*, 2006, **58**, 126–129.

45. L. Condé-Salazar, D. Guimaraens, M. A. González and E. Mancebo, Occupational allergic contact urticarial from amoxicillin, *Contact Dermatitis*, 2001, **45**, 109.

46. J. Sastre, S. Quirce, A. Novalbos, M. Lluch-Bernal, C. Bombin and A. Umpiérrez, Occupational asthma induced by cephalosporins, *Eur. Respir. J.*, 1999, **13**, 1189–1191.

47. R. E. Reisman and C. E. Arbesman, Systemic allergic reactions due to inhalation of penicillin, *J. Am. Med. Assoc.*, 1968, **203**, 986–987.

48. J. P. Girard, Recurrent angioneurotic oedema and contact dermatitis due to penicillin, *Contact Dermatitis*, 1978, **4**, 309.

49. E. Rudski and P. Rebandel, Occupational contact urticaria from penicillin, *Contact Dermatitis*, 1985, **13**, 192.

50. P. Mauranges, Antibiotics and animal feeds. Allergic reactions to residues, *Econ. Med. Anim.*, 1972, **13**, 131–135.

51. K. H. Nelder, Contact dermatitis from animal feed additives, *Arch. Dermatol.*, 1972, **106**, 722–723.

52. W. Becker, On the possibility of sensitisation and allergic reactions after the oral absorption of medicated feedingstuffs (literature review), *Arch. Lebenmittelhyg.*, 1976, **27**, 161–196.

53. E. S. Falk, H. Hektoen and P. O. Thune, Skin and respiratory tract symptoms in veterinary surgeons, *Contact Dermatitis*, 1985, **12**, 274–278.

54. D. Erskine, Dermatitis caused by penicillin in milk, *Lancet*, 1958, **i**, 431–432.

55. H. R. Vickers, L. Bagratuni and S. Alexander, Dermatitis caused by penicillin in milk, *Lancet*, 1958, **i**, 351–352.

56. H. R. Vickers, Dermatological hazards of penicillin in milk, *Proc. R. Soc. Med.*, 1964, **57**, 1091–1092.

57. M. C. Zimmerman, Chronic penicillin urticaria from dairy products, proved by penicillinase cures, *Arch. Dermatol.*, 1959, **79**, 1–6.

58. P. Borrie and J. Barrett, Dermatitis caused by penicillin in milk, *Lancet*, 1961, **i**, 1267.

59. G. T. Stewart, Allergenic residues in penicillins, *Lancet*, 1967, **i**, 1177–1183.

60. W. Minkin and P. J. Lynch, Allergenic reaction to penicillin in milk, *J. Am. Med. Assoc.*, 1969, **209**, 1089–1090.

61. K. Wicher, R. E. Reisman and C. E. Arbesman, Allergic reaction to penicillin present in milk, *J. Am. Med. Assoc.*, 1969, **208**, 143–145.

62. J. C. Olson and A. C. Sanders, Penicillin in milk and milk products: some regulatory and public health considerations, *J. Milk Food Technol.*, 1975, **38**, 630–63.

63. J. Cany, A hidden source of allergic reactions by sensitisation to penicillin, *Rev. Franc. Allergol.*, 1977, **17**, 133–136.

64. H. Lindemayr, R. Knobler, D. Kraft and W. Baumgartner, Challenge of penicillin-allergic volunteers with penicillin-contaminated meat, *Allergy*, 1981, **36**, 471–478.

65. M. Roca, L. Villegas, M. L. Kortabitarte, R. L. Althaus and M. P. Molina, Effects of heat treatments on stability of β-lactams in milk, *J. Dairy Sci.*, 2011, **94**, 1155–1164.

66. J. M. Dewdney and R. G. Edwards, Penicillin hypersensitivity – is milk a significant hazard? *Proc. R. Soc. Med.*, 1984, **77**, 866–867.

67. J. M. Dewdney, L. Maes, J. P. Raynaud, F. Blanc, J. P. Scheid, T. Jackson, S. Lens and C. Verscheuren, Risk assessment of beta-lactams and macrolides in food products with regard to immune-allergic potential, *Food Chem. Toxicol.*, 1991, **29**, 477–483.

68. A. D. Dayan, Allergy to antimicrobial residues in food: assessment of the risk to man, *Vet. Microbiol.*, 1993, **35**, 213–226.

69. C. S. Aaron, R. L. Yu, P. R. Harbach, J. M. Mazurek, D. H. Svenson, D. Kirkland, R. Marshall and S. McEnaney, Comparative mutagenicity testing of ceftiofur sodium: 1. Positive results in *in vitro* cytogenetics, *Mutat.Res.*, 1995, **345**, 27–35.

70. C. S. Aaron, R. L. Yu, J. A. Bacon, D. Kirkland, S. McEnany and R. Marshall, Comparative mutagenicity testing of ceftiofur sodium: II. Cytogenetic damage induced *in vitro* by ceftiofur is reversible and is due to cell cycle delay, *Mutat.Res.*, 1995, **345**, 37–47.

71. C. S. Aaron, R. L. Yu, P. S. Jaglan, R. D. Roof, C. Hamilton, R. Sorg, R. Gudi and A. Thilagar, Comparative mutagenicity testing of ceftiofur sodium: III. Ceftiofur sodium is not an *in vitro* mutagen, *Mutat. Res.*, 1995, **345**, 49–56.

72. Joint FAO/WHO Expert Committee on Food Additives, Toxicological Evaluation of Certain Veterinary Drug Residues in Food, The Forty-Fifth Meeting of the Joint FAO/WHO Expert Committee on Food Additives (JECFA), International Programme on Chemical Safety, World Health Organization, Geneva, 1996, pp. 61–84.

73. M. R. Stegemann, C. A. Passmore, J. Sherington, C. J. Lindeman, G. Papp, D. Weigel and T. L. Skogerboe, Antimicrobial activity and spectrum of Cefovecin, a new extended-spectrum cephalosporin, against pathogens collected from dogs and cats in Europe and North America, *Antimicrob. Agents Chemother.*, 2006, **50**, 2286–2292.

74. R. Six, D. M. Cleaver, C. J. Lindeman, J. Cherni, R. Cheeseborough, G. Papp, T. L. Skogerboe, D. J. Weigel, J. F. Boucher and M. R. Stegemann, Effectiveness and safety of Cefovecin sodium, an extended-spectrum injectable cephalosporin, in the treatment of cats with abscesses and infected wounds, *J. Am. Vet. Med. Assoc.*, 2009, **234**, 81–87.

75. R. Six, J. Cherni, R. Cheeseborough, D. Cleaver, C. J. Lindeman, G. Papp, T. L. Skogerboe, D. J. Weigel, J. F. Boucher and M. R. Stegemann, Efficacy and safety of Cefovecin in treating bacterial folliculitis, abscesses, or infected wounds in dogs, *J. Am. Vet. Med. Assoc.*, 2008, **233**, 433–439.

76. L. Fonacier, R. Hirschberg and S. Gerson, Adverse drug reactions to cephalosporins in hospitalized patients with a history of penicillin allergy, *Allergy Asthma Proc.*, 2005, **26**, 135–141.

77. C. Antunez, N. Blanca-Lopez, M. J. Torres, C. Mayorga, E. Perez-Inestrosa, M. I. Montañez, T. Fernandez and M. Blanca, Immediate allergic reactions to cephalosporin: evaluation of cross-reactivity with a panel of penicillins and cephalosporins, *J. Allergy Clin. Immunol.*, 2006, **117**, 404–110.

78. J. D. Campagna, M. C. Bond, E. Schabelman and B. D. Hayes, The use of cephalosporins in penicillin-allergic patients: A literature review, *J. Emerg. Med.*, 2012, **42**, 612–620.

79. A. Romano, R. M. Guéant-Rodriguez, M. Viola, R. Pettinato and J. L. Guéant, Cross-reactivity and tolerability of cephalosporins with immediate hypersensitivity to penicillins, *Ann. Intern. Med.*, 2004, **14**, 16–22.

80. A. Madaan and J. T. Li, Cephalosporin allergy, *Immunol. Allergy Clin. North Am.*, 2004, **24**, 463–476.

81. R. Somech, E. A. Weber and S. Lavi, Evaluation of immediate allergic reactions to cephalosporins in non-penicillin-allergic patients, *Int. Arch. Allergy Immunol.*, 2009, **150**, 205–209.

82. R. Bonnet, Growing group of extended-spectrum beta-lactamases: the CTX-M enzymes, *Antimicrob. Agents Chemother.*, 2004, **48**, 1–14.

83. N. P. Brenwald, G. Jevons, J. M. Andrews, J. H. Jong, P. M. Hawkey and R. Wise, An outbreak of a CTX-M-type beta-lactamase producing *Klebsiella pneumoniae*: the importance of using cefpodoxime to detect extended-spectrum beta-lactamases, *Antimicrob. Agents Chemother.*, 2003, **51**, 195–196.

84. P. M. Hawkey and A. Jones, The changing epidemiology of resistance, *J. Antimicrob. Chemother.*, 2009, **64**(1), 3–10.

85. L. C. Hibbert-Rogers, J. Heritage, D. M. Gascoyne-Binzi, P. M. Hawkey, N. Todd, I. J. Lewis and C. Bailey, Molecular epidemiology of ceftazidime resistant *Enterobacteriaceae* from patients on a paediatric oncology ward, *J. Antimicrob. Chemother.*, 1995, **35**, 65–82.

86. H. Knothe, P. Shah, V. Kremery, M. Antal and S. Mitsuhashi, Transferable resistance to cefotaxime, cefoxitin, cefamandole and cefuroxime in clinical isolates of *Klebsiella pneumoniae* and *Serratia marcescens*, *Infection*, 1983, **11**, 315–317.

87. D. M. Livermore, R. Canton, M. Gniadkowski, P. Nordmann, G. M. Rossolini, G. Arlet, J. Ayala, T. M. Coque, I. Kern-Zdanowicz, F. Luzzaro, L. Poirel and N. Woodford, CTX-M: changing the face of ESBLs in Europe, *J. Antimicrob. Chemother.*, 2007, **59**, 165–174.

88. C. T. Moore, S. A. Roberts, G. Simmons, S. Briggs, A. J. Smith, J. Smith and H. Hefferman, Extended beta-lactamase (ESBL)-producing enterobacteria: factors associated with infection in the community setting, *J. Hosp. Infect.*, 2008, **68**, 355–362.

89. D. L. Paterson and R. A. Bonomo, Extended-spectrum beta-lactamases: a clinical update, *Clin. Microbiol. Rev.*, 2005, **18**, 657–686.

90. A. Caratolli, Animal reservoirs for extended spectrum beta-lactamase producers, *Clin. Microbiol. Infect.*, 2008, **14**(1), 117–123.

91. G. Chiaretto, P. Zavagnin, F. Bettini, M. Mancin, C. Minorello, C. Saccardin and A. Ricci, Extended spectrum beta-lactamase SHV-12-producing *Salmonella* from poultry, *Vet. Microbiol.*, 2008, **128**, 406–413.

92. D. Girlich, L. Poirel, A. Carotti, I. Kempf, M. F. Lartigue, A. Bertini and P. Nordmann, Extended-spectrum beta-lactamase CTX-M-1 in *Escherichia coli* isolates from healthy poultry in France, *Appl. Environ. Microbiol.*, 2007, **73**, 4681–4685.

93. H. Hasman, D. Mevius, K. Veldman, I. Olesen and F. M. Aarestrup, Beta-lactamases among extended-spectrum beta-lactamase (ESBL)-resistant *Salmonella* from poultry, poultry products and human patients in The Netherlands, *J. Antimicrob. Chemother.*, 2005, **56**, 115–121.

94. S. Lavilla, J. J. Gonzalez-Lopez, E. Miro, P. H. Edelstein and N. O. Fishman, Extended-spectrum beta-lactamase-producing *Escherichia coli* and *Klebsiella pneumoniae*: risk factors for infection and impact of resistance on outcomes, *Clin. Infect. Dis.*, 2008, **32**, 1244–1251.

95. E. Liebana, M. Batchelor, K. L. Hopkins, F. A. Clifton-Hadley, C. J. Teale, A. Foster, E. J. Threlfall and R. H. Davies, Longitudinal farm study of extended-spectrum beta-lactamase-mediated resistance, *J. Clin. Microbiol.*, 2006, **44**, 1630–1634.

96. W. Machado, T. Coque, R. Canton, F. Baquero, J. Silva, J. C. Sousa and L. Peixe, ESBL-producing *Enterobacteriaceae* from non-human sources (poultry and swine) in Portugal, *Int. J. Antimicrob. Agents*, 2007, **29**(2), S277–S278.

97. J. Y. Madec, C. Lazizzera, P. Chatre, D. Meunier, S. Martin, G. Lepage, M. F. Menard, P. Lebreton and T. Rambaud, Prevalence of fecal carriage of acquired expanded-spectrum cephalosporin resistance in *Enterobacteriaceae* from cattle in France, *J. Clin. Microbiol.*, 2008, **46**, 1566–1567.

98. I. Phillips, M. Casewell, T. Cox, B. de Groot, C. Friis and R. Jones, C. Nightingale, R. Preston and J. Waddell, Does the use of antibiotics in food animals pose a risk to human health? A critical review of published data, *J. Antimicrob. Chemother.*, 2004, **53**, 28–52.

99. L. P. Randall, C. Clouting, R. A. Horton, N. G. Coldham, G. Wu, F. A. Clifton-Hadley, R. H. Davies and C. J. Teale, Prevalence of *Escherichia coli* carrying extended-spectrum β-lactamases (CTX-M and TEM-52) from broiler chickens and turkeys in Great Britain between 2006 and 2009, *J. Antimicrob. Chemother.*, 2011, **66**, 86–95.

100. D. L. Smith, J. Dushoff and J. G. Morris, Agricultural antibiotics and human health, *PLoS Med.*, 2005, **2**, e232.

101. C. J. Teale, L. Barker, A. P. Foster, E. Liebana, M. Batchelor, D. M. Livermore and E. J. Threlfall, Extended-spectrum beta-lactamase detected in *E. coli* recovered from calves in Wales, *Vet. Rec.*, 2005, **156**, 186–187.

102. C. J. Teale, ESBLs in animals, *J. Antimicrob. Chemother.*, 2010, **65**(1), 13–17.

103. Committee for Medicinal Products for Veterinary Use (CVMP), Revised reflection paper on the use of 3rd and 4th generation cephalosporins in food producing animals in the European Union: development of resistance and impact on human health, 2009, EMEA/CVMP/SAGAM/81730/2006-Rev.1. Available at: http://.www.ema.europa.eu/docs/en_GB/document_library/Scientific-guidelines/2009/10/WC00004307.pdf.

104. Report by the Joint Working Group of DARC and ARHAI. ESBLs – a threat to human and animal health? 2012. Available from: http://vmd.defra.gov.uk/pdf/ESBL_report.pdf.

105. R. A. Hettig and J. D. Adcock, Studies on the toxicity of streptomycin for man: a preliminary report, *Science*, 1946, **103**, 355–357.

106. H. C. Hinshaw, W. H. Feldman and K. H. Pfuetze, Treatment of tuberculosis with streptomycin: a summary of observations on a hundred cases, *J. Am. Med. Assoc.*, 1946, **132**, 778–782.

107. G. Matz, L. Rybak, P. S. Roland, M. Hannley, R. Friedman, S. Manolidis, M. G. Stewart, P. Weber and F. Owens, Ototoxicity of ototopical antibiotic drops in humans, *Otolarngol. Head Neck Surg.*, 2004, **130**(3), S79–S82.

108. M. D. Rizzi and K. Hirose, Aminoglycoside ototoxicity, *Curr. Opin. Otolaryngol. Head Neck Surg.*, 2007, **15**, 352–357.

109. G. J. Matz, Aminoglycoside cochlear ototoxicity, *Otolaryngol. Clin. North Am.*, 1993, **26**, 705–712.

110. W. E. Heck, H. G. Hinshaw and H. Parsons, Auditory ototoxicity in tuberculosis patients treated with dihydrostreptomycin: a report of the incidence of hearing loss in 1,150 cases, *J. Am. Med. Assoc.*, 1963, **86**, 1–19.

111. W. E. Fee, Aminoglycoside ototoxicity in the human, *Laryngoscope*, 1980, **90**, 1–19.

112. M. Mulheran, C. Degg, S. Burr, D. W. Morgan and D. E. Stableforth, Occurrence and risk of cochleotoxicity in cystic fibrosis patients receiving high-dose aminoglycoside therapy, *Antimicrob. Agents Chemother.*, 2001, **45**, 2502–2509.

113. M. E. Huth, A. J. Ricci and A. G. Cheng, Mechanisms of aminoglycoside ototoxicity and targets of hair cell protection, *Int. J. Otolaryngol.*, 2011, article ID 937861, p. 19.

114. B. A. Waisbren and W. W. Spink, A clinical appraisal of neomycin, *Ann. Intern. Med.*, 1950, **33**, 1099–1119.

115. J. R. Lindsay, L. R. Proctor and W. P. Work, Histopathological inner ear changes in deafness due to neomycin in a human, *Laryngoscope*, 1960, **70**, 382–392.

116. E. B. Halpern and M. F. Heller, Ototoxicity of orally administered neomycin, *Arch. Otolaryngol.*, 1961, **73**, 675–677.

117. P. Erlanson and A. Lundgren, Ototoxic side effects following treatment with streptomycin, dihydrostreptomycin and kanamycin. Connection with dosage and renal function: preventative medicine, *Acta Med. Scand*, 1964, **176**, 147–163.

118. L. H. Greenberg and H. Momary, Audiotoxicity and nephrotoxicity due to orally administered neomycin, *J. Am. Med. Assoc.*, 1965, **194**, 827–828.
119. R. M. Meyers, Ototoxic effects of gentamicin, *Arch. Otolaryngol.*, 1970, **92**, 160–162.
120. P. Gailiunas, M. Dominguez-Moreno, M. Lazarus, E. G. Lowrie, M. N. Gottlieb and J. P. Merrill, Vestibular toxicity of gentamicin. Incidence in patients receiving long-term haemodialysis, *Arch. Intern. Med.*, 1978, **138**, 1621–1624.
121. V. S. Dayal, G. E. Chait and S. S. Fenton, Gentamicin vestibulotoxicity. Long-term disabilities, *Ann. Otol. Rhinol. Laryngol.*, 1979, **88**, 36–39.
122. S. A. Lerner, B. A. Schmitt, R. Seligsohn and G. J. Matz, Comparative study of ototoxicity and nephrotoxicity in patients randomly assigned to treatment with amikacin or gentamicin, *Am. J. Med.*, 1986, **80**, 98–104.
123. H. F. Chambers and M. A. Sande, Antimicrobial agents. The aminoglycosides in *Goodman and Gilman's The Pharmacological Basis of Therapeutics*, ed. J. G. Hardman, L. E. Limbird, P. B. Molinoff, R. W. Ruddon and A. G. Goodman, McGraw-Hill, London, 9th edn, 1996, pp. 1103–1121.
124. O. W. Guthrie, Aminoglycoside induced ototoxicity, *Toxicology*, 2008, **249**, 91–96.
125. A. Alharazneh, L. Luk, M. Huth, A. Monfared, P. S. Steyger, A. G. Cheng and A. J. Ricci, Functional hair cell mechanotransducer channels are required for aminoglycoside ototoxicity, *PLoS One*, 2011, **6**, e22347.
126. S. P. Francis, I. I. Kramarenko and C. S. Brandon, F.-S. Lee, T. G. Baker and L. L. Cunningham, Celastrol inhibits aminoglycoside-induced ototoxicity via heat shock protein 32, *Cell Death Dis.*, 2011, **2**, e195.
127. K. N. Woodward, Preclinical safety testing and assessment of veterinary pharmaceuticals and pharmacovigilance in *Veterinary Pharmacovigilance. Adverse Reactions to Veterinary Medicinal Products*, ed. K. N. Woodward, Wiley-Blackwell, Chichester, 2009, pp. 297–345.
128. E. Christensen, H. Hertz, N. Riskaer and G. Vra-Tensen, Histological investigations in chronic streptomycin poisoning in guinea-pigs, *Ann. Otol. Rhinol. Laryngol.*, 1951, **60**, 343–349.
129. N. Riskaer, E. Christensen and H. Hertz, The toxic effects of streptomycin and dihydrostreptomycin in pregnancy, illustrated experimentally, *Acta Tuberc. Scand.*, 1952, **27**, 211–216.
130. N. Riskaer, E. Christensen, E. Petersen and H. Weidman, The ototoxicity of neomycin, *Acta Oto-Laryngol.*, 1956, **46**, 137–152.
131. J. E. Hawkins and M. H. Lurie, The ototoxicity of dihydrostreptomycin and neomycin in the cat, *Ann. Otol. Rhinol. Laryngol.*, 1953, **62**, 1128–1148.
132. T. M. McGee and J. Olszewski, Streptomycin sulphate and dihydrostreptomycin toxicity, *Arch. Otolaryngol.*, 1962, **75**, 295–311.
133. Y. C. Tsang and T. C. Chin, Neurotoxicity of streptomycin, *Sci. Sin.*, 1963, **12**, 1019–1040.

134. J. A. Waitz, E. L. Moss and M. J. Weinstein, Aspects of the chronic toxicity of gentamicin sulfate in cats, *J. Infect. Dis.*, 1971, **124**(Suppl.), S125–S129.

135. R. E. Brummett, Ototoxicity resulting from the combined administration of potent diuretics and other agents, *Scand. Audiol.*, 1981, **14**(Suppl.), 214–224.

136. R. E. Brummett, Effects of antibiotic-diuretic interactions in the guinea-pig model of ototoxicity, *Rev. Infect. Dis.*, 1981, **3**(Suppl.), S216–S223.

137. M. Yakota, U. Takeda, K. Sakamoto, N. Seto and M. Igarashi, The comparative ototoxicities of panimycin and gentamicin in cynomolgus monkeys (*Maccaca fascicularis*), *Chemother.*, 1984, **30**, 248–254.

138. G. R. Hodges, I. S. Watanabe, P. Singer, S. Rengachary, R. E. Brummett, D. Reeves, D. R. Justesen, S. E. Worley and E. P. Gephardt, Ototoxicity of intraventricularly administered gentamicin in adult rabbits, *Res. Commun. Chem. Pathol. Pharmacol.*, 1985, **50**, 337–347.

139. A. Ernst, G. Reuter, U. Zimmerman and H. P. Zeneer, Acute gentamicin ototoxicity in cochlear cells of the guinea-pig, *Brain Res.*, 1994, **636**, 153–156.

140. P. A. Leake, A. L. Kuntz, C. M. Moore and P. L. Chambers, Cochlear pathology induced by aminoglycoside ototoxicity during maturation in cats, *Hearing Res.*, 1997, **113**, 117–132.

141. C. G. Robinson and K. G. Cambon, Hearing loss in infants of tuberculous mothers treated with streptomycin during pregnancy, *N. Engl. J. Med.*, 1964, **271**, 949–951.

142. E. Varpela, J. Hietlahti and M. J. T. Aro, Streptomycin and dihydrostreptomycin during pregnancy and their effect on the child's inner ear, *Scand. J. Resp. Dis.*, 1969, **50**, 101–109.

143. J. Warkany, Antituberculous drugs, *Teratology*, 1979, **20**, 133–138.

144. D. E. Snider, P. M. Layde, M. W. Johnson and M. A. Lyle, Treatment of tuberculosis during pregnancy, *Am. Rev. Resp. Dis.*, 1980, **122**, 65–79.

145. D. M. Davies, *Textbook of Adverse Drug Reactions*, Oxford University Press, Oxford, 1991, p. 51.

146. G. J. Matz, Aminoglycoside cochlear ototoxicity, *Otolaryngol. Clin. North Am.*, 1993, **26**, 705–712.

147. H. Molitor, O. E. Graessle, S. Kuna, C. W. Mushett and R. H. Silber, Some toxicological and pharmacological properties of streptomycin, *J. Pharmacol. Exp. Ther.*, 1946, **86**, 151–173.

148. A. A. Nelson, J. L. Radowski and E. C. Hagan, Renal and other lesions in dogs and rats from intramuscular injection of neomycin, *Fed. Proc.*, 1951, **10**, 366–367.

149. P. M. Tulkens, Nephrotoxicity of aminoglycoside antibiotics, *Toxicol. Lett.*, 1989, **46**, 107–123.

150. R. A. Parker, W. H. Bennett and G. A. Porter, Animal models in the study of aminoglycoside nephrotoxicity in *The Aminoglycosides: Microbiology, Clinical Use and Toxicology*, ed. A. Whelton and H. C. Neu, Marcel Dekker, New York, 1982, pp. 235–267.

151. D. N. Gilbert, D. C. Houghton, W. M. Bennett, C. E. Plamp, K. Reger and G. A. Porter, Reversibility of gentamicin nephrotoxicity in rats: recovery during continued drug administration, *Proc. Soc. Exp. Biol. Med.*, 1978, **160**, 199–103.

152. D. C. Houghton, D. Lee, D. N. Gilbert and W. M. Bennett, Chronic gentamicin nephrotoxicity. Continued tubular injury with preserved glomerular filtration function, *Am. J. Pathol.*, 1986, **123**, 183–194.

153. B. H. Ali, M. Za'abi, G. Blunden and A. Nemmar, Experimental gentamicin nephrotoxicity and agents that modify it: a mini-review of recent research, *Basic Clin. Pharmacol. Toxicol.*, 2011, **109**, 225–232.

154. Y. Quiros, L. Vicente-Vicente, A. I. Morales, J. López-Novoa and F. J. López-Hernández, An integrative overview on mechanisms underlying the renal cytotoxicity of gentamicin, *Toxicol. Sci.*, 2011, **199**, 245–256.

155. M. Sieber, D. Hoffmann, M. Adler, V. S. Vaidya, M. Clement, M. Bonventre, N. Zidek, E. Rached, A. Amberg, J. J. Callanan, W. Dekant and A. Mally, Comparative analysis of novel noninvasive changes in a rat model of gentamicin nephrotoxicity, *Toxicol. Sci.*, 2009, **109**, 336–349.

156. F. Rougier, D. Claude, M. Maurin, A. Sedoglavic, M. Ducher, S. Corvaisier, R. Jelliffe and P. Maire, Aminoglycoside nephrotoxicity: modeling, simulation and control, *Antimicrob. Agents Chemother.*, 2003, **47**, 1010–1016.

157. M.-P. Mingeot-Leclercq and P. M. Tulkens, Aminoglycosides: nephrotoxicity, *Antimicrob. Agents Chemother.*, 1999, **43**, 1003–1012.

158. M. Kandeel, I. Abdelaziz, N. Elhabashy, H. Hegazy and Y. Tolba, Nephrotoxicity and oxidative stress of single large dose or two divided doses of gentamicin to rats, *Pak. J. Biol. Sci.*, 2011, **14**, 627–633.

159. International Programme on Chemical Safety, Toxicological Evaluation of Certain Veterinary Drug Residues in Food, The Forty-Third Meeting of the Joint FAO/WHO Expert Committee on Food Additives (JECFA), WHO Food Additives Series 34, WHO, Geneva, 1995, pp. 11–60, 85–112 and 113–142.

160. International Programme on Chemical Safety, Toxicological Evaluation of Certain Veterinary Drug Residues in Food, The Forty-Seventh Meeting of the Joint FAO/WHO Expert Committee on Food Additives (JECFA), WHO Food Additives Series 38, WHO, Geneva, 1996, pp. 79–81.

161. J. E. Riviere and J. W. Spoo, Aminoglycoside antibiotics in *Veterinary Pharmacology and Therapeutics*, ed. H. R. Adams, Iowa State Press, Ames, 8th edn, 2001, pp. 841–867.

162. R. H. Cowan, A. F. Jukkola and B. S. Arant, Pathophysiologic evidence of gentamicin nephrotoxicity in neonatal puppies, *Pediatr. Res.*, 1980, **14**, 1204–1211.

163. C. H. Hsu, T. W. Kurtz, R. E. Easterling and J. M. Weller, Potentiation of gentamicin nephrotoxicity by metabolic acidosis, *Proc. Soc. Exp. Biol. Med.*, 1974, **146**, 894–897.

164. D. L. Frazier, D. P. Aucoin and J. E. Riviere, Gentamicin pharmaco-kinetics and nephrotoxicity in naturally acquired and experimentally induced disease in dogs, *J. Am. Vet. Med. Assoc.*, 1988, **192**, 57–63.

165. W. L. Hewitt, Gentamicin: toxicity in perspective, *Postgrad. Med. J.*, 1974, **50**(7), 55–59.

166. H. Masur, P. K. Whelton and A. Whelton, Neomycin toxicity revisited, *Arch. Surg.*, 1976, **111**, 822–825.

167. P. Noone, D. F. Beale, S. S. Pollock, M. R. Perrera, I. D. Amirak, O. N. Fernando and J. F. Moorhead, Monitoring aminoglycoside use in patients with severely impaired renal function, *BMJ*, 1978, **ii**, 470–473.

168. L. W. Powell and J. W. Hooker, Neomycin nephropathy, *J. Am. Med. Assoc.*, 1956, **160**, 557–560.

169. W. B. Pratt and R. Fekety, Bactericidal inhibitors of protein synthesis, the aminoglycosides, in *The Antimicrobial Drugs*, Oxford University Press, Oxford, 1986, pp. 153–183.

170. L. Solgaard, J. L. Tuxoe, M. Mafi, S. Due Olsen and T. Toftgaard Jensen, Nephrotoxicity by dicloxacillin and gentamicin in 163 patients with intertrochanteric hip fractures, *Int. Orthop.*, 2000, **24**, 155–157.

171. E. J. Begg and M. L. Barclay, Aminoglycosides – 50 years on, *Br. J. Clin. Pharmacol.*, 1995, **39**, 597–603.

172. G. L. Drusano, P. G. Ambrose, S. M. Bhavani, J. S. Bertino, A. N. Nafziger and A. Louie, Back to the future: using aminoglycosides again and how to dose them optimally, *Clin. Infect. Dis.*, 2007, **45**, 753–760.

173. P. R. Ingram, D. C. Lye, P. A. Tambyah, W. P. Goh, V. H. Tam and D. A. Fisher, Risk factors for nephrotoxicity associated with continuous vancomycin infusion in outpatient parenteral antibiotic therapy, *J. Antimicrob. Chemother.*, 2008, **62**, 168–171.

174. J. F. P. Oliveira, C. A. Silva, C. D. Barbieri, G. M. Oliveira, D. M. T. Zanetta and E. A. Burdmann, Prevalence and risk factors for amino-glycoside nephrotoxicity in intensive care units, *Antimicrob. Agents Chemother.*, 2009, **53**, 2887–2891.

175. V. Tzovaras, V. Tsimihodimos, C. Kostara, Z. Mitrogianni and M. Elisaf, Aminoglycoside-induced nephrotoxicity studied by proton magnetic resonance spectroscopy of urine, *Nephrol. Dial. Transplant.*, 2011, **26**, 3219–3224.

176. S. Croes, A. H. Koop, S. A. van Gils and C. Neef, Efficacy, nephro-toxicity and ototoxicity of aminoglycosides, mathematically modelled for modelling supported drug monitoring, *Eur. J. Pharm. Sci.*, 2012, **45**, 90–100.

177. A. T. Gerlach, S. P. Stawicki, C. H. Cook and C. Murphy, Risk factors for aminoglycoside-associated nephrotoxicity in surgical intensive care unit patients, *Int. J. Crit. Care Illn. Inj. Sci.*, 2011, **1**, 17–21.

178. R. K. Tang and R. K. Tse, Acute renal failure after topical fortified gentamicin and vancomycin eyedrops, *J. Ocul. Pharmacol. Ther.*, 2011, **27**, 411–413.

179. M. L. Barclay and E. J. Begg, Aminoglycoside toxicity and relation to dose, *Adverse Drug React. Toxicol. Rev.*, 1994, **13**, 207–234.

180. G. Heimann, Renal toxicity of aminoglycosides in the neonatal period, *Pediatr. Pharmacol.*, 1983, **3**, 251–257.

181. B. J. Khoory, V. Fanos, A. Dall'Agnola and L. Cataldi, Aminoglycosides, risk factors and the neonatal kidney, *Pediatr. Med. Chir.*, 1996, **18**, 495–499.

182. R. A. Giuliano, G. A. Verpoten, L. Verbist, R. P. Wedeen and M. E. DeBroe, *In vivo* uptake kinetics of aminoglycosides in the kidney cortex of rats, *J. Pharmacol. Exp. Ther.*, 1986, **236**, 470–475.

183. G. J. Kaloanides, Aminoglycoside nephrotoxicity in ed. R. W. Schrier and C. W. Gottschalk, *Diseases of the Kidney,* Little, Brown and Co., Boston, 1992, pp. 1131–1164.

184. C. Josepovitz, R. Levine, T. Farrugella and G. J. Kaloyanides, Comparative effects of aminoglycosides on renal cortical and urinary phospholipids in the rats, *Proc. Soc. Exp. Biol. Med.*, 1986, **182**, 1.

185. G. B. Appel, Aminoglycoside nephrotoxicity, *Am. J. Med.*, 1990, **88**(3c), 16S–20S.

186. P. C. Luft, R. Bloch, R. S. Sloan, M. N. Yum, R. Costello and D. R. Maxwell, Comparative nephrotoxicity of aminoglycoside antibiotics in rats, *J. Infect. Dis.*, 1978, **138**, 541–545.

187. P. D. Williams, D. B. Bennett, C. R. Gleason and G. H. Hottendorf, Correlation between renal membrane binding and nephrotoxicity of aminoglycosides, *Antimicrob. Agents Chemother.*, 1987, **31**, 570–574.

188. R. J. Anderson, S. L. Linas, A. S. Bern, W. L. Henrich, T. R. Miller, P. A. Gabow and R. W. Schrier, Nonoliguric acute renal failure, *N. Engl. J. Med.*, 1977, **296**, 1134–1138.

189. J. H. Schwartz and P. Schein, Fanconi syndrome associated with cephalosporin and gentamicin therapy, *Cancer*, 1978, **41**, 769–772.

190. P. S. Lietman and C. R. Smith, Aminoglycoside nephrotoxicity in humans, *Rev. Infect. Dis.*, 1983, **5**, S284.

191. F. C. Luft, Clinical significance of renal changes engendered by aminoglycosides in man, *J. Antimicrob. Chemother.*, 1984, **13**, 23–30.

192. J. P. Fillastre, B. Moulin and S. Josse, Aetiology of nephrotoxic damage to the renal interstitium and tubuli, *Toxicol. Lett.*, 1989, **46**, 45–54.

193. G. Bledsoe, S. Crickman, J. Mao, C.-F. Xia, H. Murakami, L. Chao and J. Chao, Kallikrein/kinin protects against gentamicin-induced nephrotoxicity by inhibition of inflammation and apoptosis, *Nephrol. Dial. Transplant.*, 2006, **21**, 624–623.

194. S. Raju, S. Kavimani, V. U. Maheshwara Rao, K. S. Reddy and G. V. Kumar, Floral extract of *Tecoma stans*: a potent inhibitor of gentamicin-induced nephrotoxicity in vivo, *Asian Pac. J. Trop. Med.*, 2011, **4**, 680–685.

195. Y. C. Chen, C. H. Chen, Y. H. Hsu, T. H. Chen and Y. M. Sue, C, Y. Cheng and T. W. Chen, Leptin reduces gentamicin-induced apoptosis in

rat renal tubular cells via the P13-Akt signalling pathway, *Eur. J. Pharmacol.*, 2011, **658**, 213–218.

196. S. I. Al-Azzam, K. K. Abdul-Razzak and M. W. Jaradat, The nephroprotective effects of pioglitazone and glibenclamide against gentamicin-induced nephrotoxicity in rats: a comparative study, *J. Chemother.*, 2010, **22**, 88–91.

197. E. Ozbek, M. Cekman, Y. O. Ilbey, A. Simsek, E. C. Polat and A. Somay, Atorvastatin prevents gentamicin-induced renal damage in rats through the inhibition of p38-MAPK and NF-kappaB pathways, *Ren. Fail.*, 2009, **31**, 382–392.

198. R. L. Baer and J. S. Ludwig, Allergic eczematous sensitization to neomycin, *Ann. Allergy*, 1952, **10**, 136–137.

199. S. Epstein, Neomycin sensitivity and atopy, *Dermatologica*, 1965, **130**, 280–286.

200. S. Epstein and F. J. Wenzel, Cross-sensitivity to various 'mycins', *Arch. Dermatol.*, 1962, **86**, 183–194.

201. C. D. Calnan and I. Sarkany, Contact dermatitis from neomycin, *Br. J. Dermatol.*, 1958, **70**, 435–445.

202. M. Hannuksela, R. Suhonene and L. Fröström, Delayed contact dermatitis in patients with photosensitivity dermatitis, *Acta Derm. Venereol.*, 1981, **61**, 303–306.

203. R. Ghadially and C. A. Ramsay, Gentamicin: systemic exposure to a contact allergen, *Am. Acad. Dermatol.*, 1988, **19**, 428–430.

204. M. Bigby, R. S. Stern and K. A. Arndt, Allergic cutaneous reactions to drugs, *Prim. Care*, 1989, **16**, 713–727.

205. C. L. Goh, Contact sensitivity to topical medications, *Int. J. Dermatol.*, 1989, **28**, 25–28.

206. M. T. Gette, J. G. Marks and M. E. Maloney, Frequency of post-operative allergic contact dermatitis to topical antibiotics, *Arch. Dermatol.*, 1992, **128**, 365–367.

207. C. A. de Pádua, A. Schnuch, K. Nink, A. Pfahlberg and W. Uter, Allergic contact dermatitis to topical drugs – epidemiological risk assessment, *Pharmacoepidemiol. Drug Saf.*, 2008, **17**, 813–821.

208. A. B. Patel and R. Katta, Neomycin, *Dermatitis*, 2008, **19**, E7–E8.

209. J. Liippo and K. Lammintausta, Positive reactions to gentamicin show sensitization to aminoglycoside from topical therapies, bone cements and from systemic medication, *Contact Dermatitis*, 2008, **59**, 268–272.

210. S. E. Jacob, C. Barland and M. L. ElSaie, Patch-test-induced "flare-up" reactions to neomycin at prior biopsy sites, *Dermatitis*, 2008, **19**, E46–E48.

211. B. Añibarro and F. J. Seoane, Immediate allergic reaction due to neomycin, *J. Investig. Allergol. Clin. Immunol.*, 2009, **19**, 64–65.

212. B. Gorgievska Sukarovska, P. Turcić, D. Marasović and J. Lipozencić, Allergic contact dermatitis to antibacterial agents, *Acta Dermatovenereol. Croat.*, 2009, **17**, 70–76.

213. D. Sasseville, Neomycin, *Dermatitis*, 2010, **21**, 3–7.

214. K. Gielen and A. Goossens, Occupational allergic contact dermatitis from drugs in healthcare workers, *Contact Dermatitis*, 2001, **45**, 273–279.

215. L. Kanerva, P. Miettinen, K. Alanko, T. Estlander and R. Jolanki, Occupational allergic contact dermatitis from glyoxal, glutaraldehyde and neomycin sulphate in a dental nurse, *Contact Dermatitis*, 2000, **42**, 116–117.

216. W. G. van Ketel and D. P. Bruynzeel, Sensitization to gentamicin alone, *Contact Dermatitis*, 1989, **20**, 303–304.

217. A. A. Fisher, Allergic contact dermatitis to penicillin and streptomycin, *Cutis*, 1983, **32**, 314, 318, 324.

218. G. Hovding and L. Utne, Streptomycin allergy in nurses, *Nord. Med.*, 1955, **54**, 1750–1753.

219. G. Paparopoli, Occupational dermatitis due to streptomycin; case report, *Med. Lav.*, 1954, **45**, 386–391.

220. A. Chierici, Occupational dermatosis due to streptomycin, *Minerva Med.*, 1951, **42**, 230–233.

221. B. Zaffi, Case of extreme intolerance to streptomycin of occupational origin, *Arch. Ital. Dermatol. Sifilogr. Venereol.*, 1952, **25**, 193–198.

222. G. Leoncini, Occupational allergic dermatitis due to streptomycin, *G. Ital. Della Tuberc.*, 1950, **4**, 451–455.

223. R. Gauchia, M. Rodriguez-Serna, J. F. Silvestre, J. J. Linana and A. Aliaga, Allergic contact dermatitis from streptomycin in a cattle breeder, *Contact Dermatitis*, 1996, **35**, 374–375.

224. G. E. Burrows, Aminocyclitol antibiotics, *J. Am. Vet. Med. Assoc.*, 1980, **176**, 1280–1281.

225. W. Rosenbrook, Chemistry of spectinomycin, *Jpn. J. Antibiot.*, 1979, **32**(Suppl.), S211–S227.

226. W. J. Holloway, Spectinomycin, *Med. Clin. North Am.*, 1982, **66**, 169–173.

227. Joint FAO/WHO Expert Committee on Food Additives, Toxicological Evaluation of Certain Veterinary Drug Residues in Food, The Forty-Second Meeting of the Joint FAO/WHO Expert Committee on Food Additives (JECFA), International Programme on Chemical Safety, World Health Organization, Geneva, 1994, pp. 59–89.

228. B. Kotecha and G. P. Richardson, Ototoxicity in vitro: effects of neomycin, gentamicin, dihydrostreptomycin, amikacin, spectinomycin, neamine, spermine and poly-L-lysine, *Hear. Res.*, 1994, **73**, 173–184.

229. M. Akiyoshi, S. Yano and T. Ikeda, Ototoxicity of spectinomycin, *Jpn. J. Antibiot.*, 1976, **29**, 771–782.

230. I. Umezawa, H. Ogawa, K. Komiyama, Y. Kawakubo and T. Morino, Studies on acute and subacute toxicity of spectinomycin dihydrochloride pentahydrate, *Jpn. J. Antibiot.*, 1976, **29**, 43–54.

231. I. Umezawa, H. Ogawa, K. Komiyama, Y. Kawakubo and T. Morino, Studies on chronic toxicity of spectinomycin dihydrochloride pentahydrate, *Jpn. J. Antibiot.*, 1976, **29**, 55–60.

232. E. Novak, J. E. Gray and R. T. Pfeiffer, Animal and human tolerance of high-dose intramuscular therapy with spectinomycin, *J. Infect. Dis.*, 1974, **130**, 50–55.

233. C. Dollery, Spectinomycin in *Therapeutic Drugs*, Churchill-Livingstone, London, vol. 2, 1998, S78–S80.
234. J. Vilaplana, C. Romaguerra and F. Grimault, Contact dermatitis from lincomycin and spectinomycin, *Contact Dermatitis*, 1991, **24**, 225–226.
235. A. Dalmonte, G. Laffe and G. Mancini, Occupational contact dermatitis due to spectinomycin, *Contact Dermatitis*, 1994, **31**, 204–205.
236. L. A. Mitscher, P. Devasthale and R. Zavod, Structure activity relationships in *Quinolone Antimicrobial Agents*, ed. D. C. Hooper and J. S. Wolfson, American Society for Microbiology, Washington DC, 1993, pp. 3–51.
237. D. E. Greene and S. C. Budsberg, Veterinary use of quinolones in *Quinolone Antimicrobial Agents*, ed. D. C. Hooper and J. S. Wolfson, American Society for Microbiology, Washington DC, 1993, pp. 473–488.
238. S. A. Brown, Fluoroquinolones in animal health, *J. Vet. Pharmacol. Ther.*, 1996, **19**, 1–14.
239. N. Stuart, Common skin diseases of farmed and pet fish, *In Practice*, 1988, **March**, 47–53.
240. J. H. Brown, Antibiotics in aquaculture: their use and abuse in aquaculture, *World Aquacult.*, 1989, **20**, 34–43.
241. D. J. Alderman and T. S. Hastings, Antibiotic use in aquaculture: development of antibiotic resistance – a potential consumer health risk, *Int. J. Food Sci. Technol.*, 1998, **33**, 139–155.
242. J. F. Burka, K. L. Hammell, T. E. Horsberg, G. R. Johnson, D. J. Rainnie and D. J. Speare, Drugs in salmonid aquaculture – A review, *J. Vet. Pharmacol. Ther.*, 1997, **20**, 333–349.
243. J. E. Burkhardt, M. A. Hill, W. W. Carlton and J. W. Kesterton, Ultrastructural changes in articular cartilages of immature beagle dogs dosed with difloxacin, a fluoroquinolone, *Vet. Pathol.*, 1990, **29**, 230–238.
244. W. Crist, T. Lehert and E. Ulbrich, Specific toxicologic aspects of the quinolones, *Rev. Infect. Dis.*, 1988, **10**(Suppl.), 141–146.
245. G. Hayem, and C. Carbon, A reappraisal of quinolone tolerability. The experience of the musculoskeletal effects, *Drug Saf.*, 1995, **13**, 338–342.
246. E. M. Kappel, M. Shakibaei, A. Bello and R. Stahlman, Effects of des-F(6)-quinolone garenoxacin on joint articular cartilage in immature rats, *Antimicrob. Agents Chemother.*, 2002, **46**, 3320–3322.
247. Y. Kashida and M. Kato, Characterization of fluoroquinolone induced Achilles tendon toxicity in rats. Comparison of toxicities in 10 fluoroquinolones and effects of anti-inflammatory compounds, *Antimicrob. Agents Chemother.*, 1997, **41**, 2389–2393.
248. A. Nagai, M. Miyazaki, T. Morita, S. Furobo, K. Kizawa, H. Fukomoto, T. Sanzen, H. Hayakawa and Y. Kawamura, Comparative articular cartilage of garenoxacin, a novel quinolone antimicrobial agent, in juvenile beagle dogs, *J. Toxicol. Sci.*, 2002, **27**, 219–228.
249. D. R. Patterson, Quinolone toxicity, *Am. J. Med.*, 1991, **91**(6A), 35–37.

250. T. L. Peters, R. M. Fulton, K. D. Robertson and M. W. Orth, Effects of antibiotics on in vitro and in vivo avian cartilage degradation, *Avian Dis.*, 2002, **46**, 75–86.

251. G. Schluter, Ciprofloxacin: Review of potential toxicologic effects, *Am. J. Med.*, 1987, **82**(4A), 91–93.

252. R. Stahlman, Safety profile of the quinolones, *J. Antimicrob. Chemother.*, 1990, **26**(D), 31–34.

253. R. Stahlman and H. Lode, Toxicity of quinolones, *Drugs*, 1999, **58**(2), 37–42.

254. R. Stahlman, S. Kuhner, M. Shakibaei, R. Schwabe, J. Flores, S. A. Evander and D. C. Van Sickle, Chondrotoxicity of ciprofloxacin in immature beagle dogs. Immunohistochemistry, electron microscopy and drug plasma concentrations, *Arch. Toxicol.*, 2000, **73**, 564–572.

255. Joint FAO/WHO Expert Committee on Food Additives, Toxicological Evaluation of Certain Veterinary Drug Residues in Food, The Forty-Third Meeting of the Joint FAO/WHO Expert Committee on Food Additives (JECFA), International Programme on Chemical Safety, World Health Organization, Geneva, 1995, pp. 61–84.

256. Joint FAO/WHO Expert Committee on Food Additives, Toxicological Evaluation of Certain Veterinary Drug Residues in Food, The Forty-Eighth Meeting of the Joint FAO/WHO Expert Committee on Food Additives (JECFA), International Programme on Chemical Safety, World Health Organization, Geneva, 1997, pp. 13–38.

257. T. Takizawa, K. Hashimoto, T. Minami, S. Yamashita and K. Owen, The comparative arthropathy of fluoroquinolones in dogs, *Hum. Exp. Toxicol.*, 1999, **18**, 392–399.

258. J. M. Sansone, N. J. Wilsman, E. M. Leiferman, J. Conway, P. Hutson and K. J. Noonan, The effect of fluoroquinolone antibiotics on growing cartilage in the lamb model, *J. Pediatr. Orthop.*, 2009, **29**, 189–195.

259. E. Olcay, O. Beytemur, F. Kaleagasioglu, T. Gulmez, Z. Mutlu and V. Olgac, Oral toxicity of pefloxacin, norfloxacin, ofloxacin and ciprofloxacin: comparison of biomechanical and histopathological effects on Achilles tendon in rats, *J. Toxicol. Sci.*, 2011, **36**, 339–345.

260. T. Takizawa, K. Hashimoto, N. Itoh, S. Yamashita and K. Owen, A comparative study of the repeat dose toxicity of grepafloxacin and a number of other fluoroquinolones in rats, *Hum. Exp. Toxicol.*, 1999, **18**, 38–45.

261. R. Leone, M. Venegoni, D. Motola, U. Moretti, V. Piazetta, A. Cocci, D. Resi, F. Mozzo, G. Velo, L. Burzilleri, N. Montanaro and A. Conforti, Adverse drug reactions to the use of fluoroquinolone anti-microbials: an analysis of spontaneous reports and fluoroquinolone consumption data from three Italian regions, *Drug Saf.*, 2003, **26**, 109–203.

262. F. Muzi, G. Gravante, E. Tati and G. Tati, Fluoroquinolones-induced tendinitis and tendon rupture in kidney transplant recipients: 2 cases and a review of the literature, *Transplant. Proc.*, 2007, **39**, 1673–1675.

263. L. Strobbe, R. J. M. Brüggermann, P. J. Donnelly and N. M. A. Blijlevens, A rare case of supraspinatus tendon rupture, *Ann. Hematol.*, 2012, **91**, 131–132.

264. A. Karstinos and L. E. Paulos, Ciprofloxacin-induced bilateral rectus femoris tendon rupture, *Clin. J. Sports Med.*, 2007, **17**, 406–407.

265. Y. Khaliq and G. G. Zhanel, Fluoroquinolone-associated tendinopathy: a critical review of the literature, *Clin. Infect. Dis.*, 2003, **36**, 1404–1410.

266. W.-C. Tsai and Y.-M. Yang, Fluoroquinolone-associated tendinopathy, *Chang Gung Med. J.*, 2011, **34**, 461–467.

267. A. Durey, Y. S. Baek, J. S. Park, K. Lee, J. S. Ryu, J. S. Lee and M. H. Cheong, Levofloxacin-induced Achilles tendinitis in a young adult in the absence of predisposing conditions, *Yonsei Med. J.*, 2010, **51**, 454–456.

268. G. K. Kim and J. Q. Del Rosso, The risk of fluoroquinolone-induced tendinopathy and tendon rupture. What does the clinician need to know? *J. Clin. Aesthet. Dermatol.*, 2010, **3**, 49–54.

269. D. J. Stinner, J. D. Orr and J. R. Hsu, Fluoroquinolone-associated bilateral tendon rupture: a case report and review of the literature, *Mil. Med.*, 2010, **175**, 457–459.

270. P. D. Van der Linden and E. P. van Puijenbroek, Tendon disorders attributable to fluoroquinolones: a study on spontaneous reports in the period 1988 to 1998, *Arthritis Rheum.*, 2001, **45**, 235–239.

271. D. C. Hooper and J. S. Wolfson, Adverse effects in *Quinolone Antimicrobial Agents*, ed. D. C. Hooper and J. S. Wolfson, American Society for Microbiology, Washington DC, 1993, pp. 489–512.

272. K. A. Camp, S. L. Miyagi and D. J. Schroeder, Potential quinolone-induced cartilage toxicity in children, *Ann. Pharmacother.*, 1994, **28**, 336–338.

273. S. Jick, Ciprofloxacin safety in a paediatric population, *Pediatr. Infect. Dis. J.*, 1997, **16**, 130–133.

274. R. W. Warren, Rheumatologic aspects of pediatric cystic fibrosis patients treated with fluoroquinolones, *Pediatr. Infect. Dis. J.*, 1997, **16**, 118–122.

275. D. Gendrel, and F. Moulin, Fluoroquinolones in paediatrics, *Paediatr. Drugs*, 2001, **3**, 365–377.

276. Z. Sheng, X. Cao, S. Peng, C. Wang, Q. Li, Y. Wang and M. Li, Ofloxacin induces apoptosis in microencapsulated juvenile rabbit chondrocytes by caspase-8-dependent mitochondrial pathway, *Toxicol. Appl. Pharmacol.*, 2008, **226**, 119–127.

277. M. A. Simonin, P. Gegout-Pottie, A. Minn, P. Gillet, P. Netter and B. Terlain, Pefloxacin-induced Achilles tendon toxicity in rodents: biochemical changes in proteoglycan synthesis and oxidative damage to collagen, *Antimicrob. Agents Chemother.*, 2000, **44**, 867–872.

278. R. J. Williams, E. Attia, T. L. Wickiewicz and J. A. Hannafin, The effects of ciprofloxacin on tendon, paratendon and capsular fibroblast metabolism, *Am. J. Sports Med.*, 2000, **28**, 364–369.

279. R. L. Harrell, Fluoroquinolone-induced tendinopathy: what do we know? *South. Med. J.*, 1999, **92**, 622–625.

280. A. N. Corps, R. L. Harrell, V. A. Curry, S. A. Fenwick, B. L. Hazleman and G. P. Riley, Ciprofloxacin enhances the stimulation of matrix metalloproteinase 3 expression by interleukin-1β in human tendon-derived cells: a potential mechanism of fluoroquinolone-induced tendinopathy, *Arthritis Rheum.*, 2002, **46**, 3034–3040.

281. W. C. Tsai, C. C. Hsu, C. P. Cheng, H. N. Chang, A. M. Wong, M. S. Lin and J. H. Pang, Ciprofloxacin up-regulates tendon cells to express matrix metalloproteinase-2 with degradation of type-I collagen, *J. Orthop. Res.*, 2011, **29**, 67–73.

282. W. C. Tsai, C. C. Hsu, F. T. Tang, A. M. Wong, Y. C. Chen and J. H. Pang, Ciprofloxacin mediated cell proliferation inhibition and G2/M cell cycle arrest in rat tendons cells, *Arthritis Rheum.*, 2008, **58**, 1657–1663.

283. W. C. Tsai, C. C. Hsu, H. C. Chen, Y. H. Hsu, M. S. Lin, C. W. Wu and J. H. Pang, Ciprofloxacin-mediated inhibition of tenocyte migration and down-regulation of focal adhesion kinase phosphorylation, *Eur. J. Pharmacol.*, 2009, **607**, 23–26.

284. M. J. Barrett and I. S. Login, Gemifloxacin-associated neurotoxicity presenting as encephalopathy, *Ann. Pharmacother.*, 2009, **43**, 782–784.

285. B. Kiangkitiwan, A. Doppalapudi, K. Solberg and B. Bohner, Levofloxacin-induced delirium with psychotic features, *Gen. Hosp. Psychiatry*, 2008, **30**, 381–383.

286. E. O. Guven, D. Balbay and M. Kilciler, Unexpected, severe central nervous system toxicity of ofloxacin: report of two cases, *Int. Urol. Nephrol.*, 2007, **39**, 647–649.

287. L. Denysenko and S. E. Nicolson, Cefoxitin and ciprofloxacin neurotoxicity and catatonia in a patient on hemodialysis, *Psychosomatics*, 2011, **52**, 379–383.

288. I. Kocyigit, S. Dortdudak, M. Sipahioglu, A. Unal, H. E. Yucel, B. Tokgoz, E. Eroglu, O. Oymak and C. Utas, Levofloxacin-induced delirium: is it a dangerous drug in patients with renal dysfunction? *Ren. Fail.*, 2012, **34**, 634–636.

289. F. Van Bambeke and P. M. Tulkens, Safety profile of the respiratory fluoroquinolone moxifloxacin: comparison with other fluoroquinolones and other antibacterial classes, *Drug Saf.*, 2009, **32**, 359–378.

290. J. C. Wang, DNA topoisomerases: Why so many? *J. Biol. Chem.*, 1991, **266**, 6659–6662.

291. S. J. Froelich-Ammon and N. Osheroff, Topoisomerase poisons: harnessing the dark side of enzyme mechanisms, *J. Biol. Chem.*, 1995, **270**, 21429–21432.

292. L. F. Liu, T. C. Rowe, L. Yang, K. M. Tewey and G. L. Chen, Cleavage of DNA by mammalian topoisomerase II, *J. Biol. Chem.*, 1983, **258**, 15365–15370.

293. J. M. Berger, S. J. Gamblin, S. C. Harrison and J. C. Wang, Structure and mechanism of DNA topoisomerase II, *Nature*, 1996, **379**, 225–232.

294. D. C. Hooper and J. S. Wolfson, Mechanisms of quinolone action and bacterial killing in *Quinolone Antimicrobial Agents*, ed. D. C. Hooper and J. S. Wolfson, American Society for Microbiology, Washington DC, 1993, pp. 53–75.

295. L. L. Shen, Quinolone-DNA interaction in *Quinolone Antimicrobial Agents*, ed. D. C. Hooper and J. S. Wolfson, American Society for Microbiology, Washington DC, 1993, pp. 77–95.

296. J. A. Holden, Human deoxyribonucleic acid topoisomerases: molecular targets of anticancer drugs, *Ann. Clin. Lab. Sci.*, 1997, **27**, 402–412.

297. C. Sissi and M. Palumbo, The quinolone family: from antibacterial to anticancer agents, *Curr. Med. Chem. Anticancer Agents*, 2003, **3**, 439–450.

298. Y. Pommier, E. Leo, H. Zhang and C. Marchland, DNA topoisomerases and their poisoning by anticancer and antibacterial drugs, *Chem. Biol.*, 2010, **17**, 421–433.

299. B. S. Dwarakanath, D. Khaitan and R. Mathur, Inhibitors of topo-isomerases as anticancer drugs: problems and prospects, *Indian J. Exp. Biol.*, 2004, **42**, 649–659.

300. I. Phillips, Bacterial mutagenicity and the 4-quinolones, *J. Antimicrob. Agents Chemother.*, 1986, **20**, 771–782.

301. E. G. Powell and I. Phillips, Correlation between umuC induction and Salmonella mutagenicity assay for quinolone antimicrobial agents, *FEMS Microbiol. Lett.*, 1993, **112**, 251–254.

302. C. E. Perrone, K. C. Takahashi and G. M. Williams, Inhibition of human topoisomerase IIα by fluoroquinolones and ultraviolet A irradiation, *Toxicol. Sci.*, 2002, **69**, 16–22.

303. J. E. Rosen, D. Chen, A. K. Prahalad, T. E. Spratt, G. Schlüter and G. M. Williams, A fluoroquinolone antibiotic with a methoxy group at the 8 position yields reduced generation of 8-oxo-7,8-dihydro-2'-deoxyguanosine after ultraviolet irradiation, *Toxicol. Appl. Pharmacol.*, 1997, **145**, 361–367.

304. J. E. Rosen, A. K. Prahalad, G. Schlüter, D. Chen and G. M. Williams, Quinolone antibiotic photodynamic production of 8-oxo-7, 8-dihydro-2'-deoxyguanosine in cultured liver epithelial cells, *Photochem. Photo-biol.*, 1997, **65**, 990–996.

305. T. E. Spratt, S. S. Schultz, D. Levy, D. Chen, G. Schlüter and G. M. Williams, Different mechanisms for the photoinduced production of oxidative DNA damage by fluoroquinolones differing in photostability, *Chem. Res. Toxicol.*, 1999, **12**, 809–815.

306. L. K. Verna, D. Chen, G. Schlüter and G. M. Williams, Inhibition by singlet oxygen quenchers of the oxidative damage to DNA produced in cultured cells by exposure to a quinolone antibiotic and ultraviolet irradiation, *Cell Biol. Toxicol.*, 1998, **14**, 237–242.

307. W. E. Kohlbrenner, N. Wideburg, S. Weigl, A. Saldivar and D. T. Chu, Induction of calf thymus topoisomerase II-mediated DNA breakage by the antibacterial isothiazoloquinolones, A-65281 and A-65282, *Anti-microb. Agents Chemother.*, 1992, **36**, 81–86.

308. M. J. Robinson, B. A. Martin, T. D. Gootz, P. R. McGuirk, M. Moynihan, J. A. Sutcliffe and N. Osterhoff, Effects of quinolone derivatives on eukaryotic topoisomerase II. A novel mechanism for enhancement of enzyme-mediated DNA cleavage, *J. Biol. Chem.*, 1991, **266**, 14585–14592.

309. A. Belicová, L. Krizková, M. Nagy, J. Krajovic and L. Erbinger, Phenolic acids reduce the genotoxicity of acridine orange and ofloxacin in Salmonella typhimurium, *Folia Microbiol. (Praha)*, 2001, **46**, 511–514.

310. E. Gocke, Photochemical mutagenesis: examples and toxicological relevance, *J. Environ. Pathol. Toxicol. Oncol.*, 2001, **20**, 285–292.

311. B. A. Herbold, S. Y. Brendler-Schwaab and H. J. Ahr, Ciprofloxacin: in vivo genotoxicity, *Mutat. Res.*, 2001, **498**, 193–205.

312. E. Gocke, S. Albertini, A. A. Chételat, S. Kirchner and W. Muster, The photomutagenicity of fluoroquinolones and other drugs, *Toxicol. Lett.*, 1998, **102–103**, 375–381.

313. D. P. Gibson, X. Ma, A. G. Switzer, V. A. Murphy and M. J. Aardema, Comparative genotoxicity of quinolone and quinolonyl-lactam antibacterials in the in vitro micronucleus assay in Chinese hamster ovary cells, *Environ. Mol. Mutagen.*, 1998, **31**, 345–351.

314. A.-A. Chételet, S. Albertini and E. Gocke, The photomutagenicty of fluoroquinolones in tests for gene mutation, gene conversion and DNA breakage (Comet assay), *Mutagenesis*, 1996, **11**, 497–504.

315. S. Albertini, A. A. Chételet, B. Miller, W. Muster, E. Pujadas, R. Strobel and E. Gocke, Genotoxicity of 17 gyrase- and four mammalian topoisomerase II-poisons in prokaryotic and eukaryotic test systems, *Mutagenesis*, 1995, **10**, 343–351.

316. A. Mukherjee, S. Sen and K. Agarwal, Ciprofloxacin: mammalian DNA topoisomerase type II poison *in vivo*, *Mutat. Res.*, 1993, **301**, 87–92.

317. D. J. Smart and A. M. Lynch, Evaluating the genotoxicity of topoisomerase-targeted antibiotics, *Mutagenesis*, 2012, **27**, 359–365.

318. S. Thomé, C. R. Bizarro, M. Lehmann, B. R. de Abreu, H. H. de Andrade, K. S. Cunha and R. R. Dihl, Recombinagenic and mutagenic activities of fluoroquinolones in *Drosophila melanogaster*, *Mutat. Res.*, 2012, **742**, 43–47.

319. A. C. Singh, M. Kumar and A. M. Jha, Genotoxicity of lomefloxacin – an antibacterial drug in somatic and germ cells of Swiss albino mice in vivo, *Mutat. Res.*, 2003, **535**, 35–42.

320. C. A. McQueen, B. M. Way, S. M. Queener, G. Schlüter and G. M. Williams, Study of potential *in vitro* and *in vivo* genotoxicity in hepatocytes of quinolone antibiotics, *Toxicol. Appl. Pharmacol.*, 1991, **111**, 255–262.

321. W. Kullich, P. Brugger and G. Klein, Assessment of the genotoxic risk caused by the gyrase inhibitor ofloxacin using sister chromatid exchange rate analysis, *Wien. Med. Wochenschr*, 1988, **138**, 107–109.

322. P. Ball, Adverse reactions and interactions of fluoroquinolones, *Clin. Invest. Med.*, 1989, **12**, 28–34.

323. W. Christ, T. Lehnert and B. Ulbrich, Specific toxicologic aspects of the quinolones, *Rev. Infect. Dis.*, 1988, **10**(1), S141–S146.

324. M. L. Corrado, W. E. Struble, C. Peter, V. Hoagland and J. Sabbaj, Norfloxacin: review of safety studies, *Am. J. Med.*, 1987, **82**(6B), 22–26.

325. J. E. Kapusnik-Uner, M. A. Sande and H. F. Chambers, Antimicrobial Agents. Tetracyclines, erythromycin, and miscellaneous antibacterial agents, in *Goodman and Gilman's The Pharmacological Basis of Therapeutics*, ed. J. G. Hardman, L. E. Limbird, P. B. Molinoff, R. W. Ruddon and A. G. Goodman, McGraw-Hill, London, 9th edn, 1996, pp. 1123–1153.

326. M. G. Papich and J. E. Riviere, Chloramphenicol and derivatives, macrolides, lincosamides and miscellaneous antimicrobials in *Veterinary Pharmacology and Therapeutics*, ed. H. R. Adams, Iowa State Press, Ames, 8th edn, pp. 868–897.

327. E. M. Boyd, The acute oral toxicity of spiramycin, *Can. J. Biochem. Physiol.*, 1958, **36**, 103–110.

328. E. M. Boyd and M. A. Price Jones, The comparative oral acute toxicity of spiramycin adipate in mice, rats, guinea-pigs and rabbits, *Antibiot. Chemother.*, 1960, **10**, 273–284.

329. E. M. Boyd, S. Jarzylo, C. E. Body and W. A. Cassell, The chronic oral toxicity of spiramycin in dogs, *Arch. Int. Pharmacodyn.*, 1958, **CVX**, 360–371.

330. P. Dubost, R. Ducrot and M. Kolsky, Chronic toxicity and local tolerance of spiramycin, *Therapie*, 1956, **ii**, 329–336.

331. Joint FAO/WHO Expert Committee on Food Additives, Toxicological Evaluation of Certain Veterinary Drug Residues in Food, The Thirty-Eighth Meeting of the Joint FAO/WHO Expert Committee on Food Additives (JECFA), International Programme on Chemical Safety, World Health Organization, Geneva, 1991, pp. 109–138.

332. X. Qin, M. Pilot, H. Thomson and J. Maskell, Effects of spiramycin on gastrointestinal motility, *Chemoterapia*, 1987, **2**(Suppl.), 319–320.

333. M. A. Pilot and X. Y. Qin, Macrolides and gastrointestinal motility, *J. Antimicrob. Chemother.*, 1988, **22**(B), 201–206.

334. M. Perreard and F. Klotz, Ulcerated oesophagus after taking spiramycin, *Ann. Gastroenterol. Hepatol.*, 1989, **25**, 313–314.

335. M. C. Galland, F. Rodor and J. Jouglard, Spiramycin causing toxic skin reaction and allergic vasculitis, *Therapie*, 1987, **42**, 227–229.

336. B. Juliac, H. Théophile, M. Begorre, B. Richez and F. Haramburu, Side effects of spiramycin masquerading as local anesthetic toxicity during labor epidural analgesia, *Int. J. Obstet. Anesth.*, 2010, **19**, 331–332.

337. J. Descotes, T. Vial, D. Delattre and J. C. Evreux, Spiramycin: safety in man, *J. Antimicrob. Chemother.*, 1988, **22**(B), 207–210.

338. R. J. Davies and J. Pepys, Asthma due to chemical agents – the macrolide antibiotic spiramycin, *Clin. Allergy*, 1975, **1**, 99–107.

339. P. L. Paggiaro, A. M. Loi and G. Toma, Bronchial asthma and dermatitis due to spiramycin in a chick breeder, *Clin. Allergy*, 1979, **9**, 571–574.

340. N. K. Veien, T. Hattel, O. Justensen and A. Nordholm, Occupational contact dermatitis due to spiramycin and/or tylosin among farmers, *Contact Dermatitis*, 1980, **6**, 410–413.
341. N. K. Veien, T. Hattel, O. Justensen and A. Nordholm, Patch testing with substances not included in the standard series, *Contact Dermatitis*, 1983, **9**, 304–308.
342. G. Moscato, L. Naldi and F. Candura, Bronchial asthma due to spiramycin and adipic acid, *Clin. Allergy*, 1984, **14**, 355–361.
343. J.-L. Malo and A. Cartier, Occupational asthma in workers of a pharmaceutical company, *Thorax*, 1988, **43**, 371–377.
344. C. Nava, Work risks from antibiotics: contribution to the study of occupational disease from spiramycin, *Securitas*, 1976, **61**, 275–280.
345. K. Aiso, M. Kanisawa, T. Okamoto, M. Okita and T. Chujo, Chronic oral toxicity of tylosin, *Nippon Eiseigaku Zasshi*, 1966, **20**, 383–397.
346. R. C. Anderson, H. M. Worth, R. M. Small and P. N. Harris, Toxicological studies on tylosin: its safety as a food additive, *Food Cosmet. Toxicol.*, 1966, **4**, 1–15.
347. Joint FAO/WHO Expert Committee on Food Additives, Toxicological Evaluation of certain Veterinary Drug Residues in Food, The Thirty-Eighth Meeting of the Joint FAO/WHO Expert Committee on Food Additives (JECFA), International Programme on Chemical Safety, World Health Organization, Geneva, 1991, pp. 139–163.
348. H. D. Jung, Occupationally-induced contact eczema by tylosin (Tylan), *Dermatol. Monatsschr.*, 1983, **169**, 235–237.
349. J. Verbov, Tylosin dermatitis, *Contact Dermatitis*, 1983, **9**, 325–326.
350. E. Barbera and J. de la Cuadra, Occupational airborn allergic contact dermatitis from tylosin, *Contact Dermatitis*, 1989, **20**, 308–309.
351. W. J. F. Gollins, Occupational asthma to tylosin, *Br. J. Occup. Med.*, 1989, **46**, 894.
352. H. S. Lee, Y. T. Wang, C. T. Yeo, K. T. Tan and K. V. Ratnam, Occupational asthma due to tylosin tartrate, *Br. J. Ind. Med.*, 1989, **46**, 498–499.
353. S. Caraffini, D. Assalve, L. Stingeni and P. Lisi, Tylosin, an airborne contact allergen in veterinarians, *Contact Dermatitis*, 1994, **31**, 327–328.
354. P. Danese, A. Zanca and M. G. Bertazzoni, Occupational contact dermatitis from tylosin, *Contact Dermatitis*, 1994, **30**, 122–123.
355. J. E. Pirkiss, K. O'Regan and R. Bailie, Contact dermatitis and in-feed exposure to antibiotics among pig feed handlers, *Aust. J. Rural Health*, 1997, **5**, 76–79.
356. M. L. Tuomi and L. Räsänen, Contact allergy to tylosin and cobalt in a pig-farmer, *Contact Dermatitis*, 1995, **33**, 285.
357. K. H. Kraemer, V. Torres and G. D. Weinstein, Contact allergy to tylosin, *Arch. Dermatol.*, 1976, **112**, 561.
358. Committee for Veterinary Medicinal Products, Erythromycin, EMEA/MRL/720/99-FINAL. Available from: http://www.ema.europa.eu.
359. R. W. Lacey, A new look at erythromycin, *Postgrad. Med. J.*, 1977, **53**, 195–200.

360. C. M. Ginsburg, G. H. McCracken, S. D. Crow, B. R. Dildy, G. Morchower, J. B. Steinberg and K. Lancaster, Erythromycin therapy for group A streptococcal pharyngitis. Results of a comparative study of the estolate and ethyl succinate formulations, *Am. J. Dis. Child.*, 1984, **138**, 536–539.

361. S. D. Angulo, J. Szram, J. Welch, J. Cannon and P. Cullinan, Occupational asthma in antibiotic manufacturing workers: case reports and systematic review, *J. Allergy*, 2011, **2011**, article ID 365683, p. 9.

362. S. Milković-Kraus and B. Kanceljak-Macan, Occupational airborne allergic contact dermatitis from azithromycin, *Contact Dermatitis*, 2001, **45**, 184.

363. S. Mimesh and M. Pratt, Occupational airborne allergic contact dermatitis from azithromycin, *Contact Dermatitis*, 2004, **51**, 151.

364. S. Milković-Kraus, J. Macan and B. Kanceljak-Macan, Occupational allergic contact dermatitis from azithromycin in pharmaceutical workers: a case series, *Contact Dermatitis*, **56**, 99–102.

365. I. López-Lerma, C. Romaguera and J. Vilaplana, Occupational airborne contact dermatitis from azithromycin, *Clin. Exp. Dermatol.*, 2009, **34**, e358–e359.

366. Joint FAO/WHO Expert Committee on Food Additives, Toxicological Evaluation of Certain Veterinary Drug Residues in Food, The Forty-Seventh Meeting of the Joint FAO/WHO Expert Committee on Food Additives (JECFA), International Programme on Chemical Safety, World Health Organization, Geneva, 1996, pp. 109–130.

367. W. H. Jordan, R. A. Byrd, M. S. Cochrane, G. K. Hanasomo, J. A. Hoyt, B. W. Main, R. D. Meterhoff and R. D. Sarazan, A review of the toxicology of the antibiotic Micotil 300, *Vet. Hum. Toxicol.*, 1993, **35**, 151–158.

368. V. Altunok, E. Yazar, M. Elmas, B. Tras, A. L. Bas and R. Col, Investigation of the haematological and biochemical side effects of tilmicosin in healthy New Zealand rabbits, *J. Vet. Med. B. Infect. Dis. Public Health*, 2002, **49**, 68–70.

369. B. W. Main, J. R. Mears, L. E. Rinkema, W. C. Smith and R. D. Sarazan, Cardiovascular effects of the macrolide antibiotic tilmicosin, administered alone and in combination with propranolol or dobutamine, in conscious unrestrained dogs, *J. Vet. Pharmacol. Ther.*, 1996, **19**, 225–232.

370. M. A. McGuigan, Human exposures to tilmicosin (Micotil), *Vet. Hum. Toxicol.*, 1994, **36**, 306–308.

371. S. Von Essen, J. Spencer, B. Haas, P. List and S. A. Seifert, Unintentional human exposure to tilmicosin (Micotil 300), *Clin. Toxicol.*, 2003, **41**, 229–233.

372. L. A. Crown and R. B. Smith, Accidental veterinary antibiotic injection into a farm worker, *Tenn. Med.*, 1999, **92**, 339–340.

373. E. K. Kuffner and R. C. Dart, Death following intravenous injection of Micotil 300, *J. Toxicol. Clin Toxicol.*, 1996, **34**, 574.

374. J. Oakes and S. Seifert, American association of poison control centers database characterization of human tilmicosin exposures, 2001–2005, *J. Med. Toxicol.*, 2008, **4**, 225–231.

375. K. Lawrence, Change to user warning for Micotil, *Vet. Rec.*, 2004, **154**, 703.

376. Agence Francais de Securité des Aliments, Communiqué de Presse, Suspension du MICOTIL 300, Fougères, France, 7 May 2004.

377. Anon, France suspends Micotil after human deaths in US, *Animal-Pharm*, 2004, **541**, 1.

378. Anon, France lifts Micotil ban, *AnimalPharm*, 2004, **545**, 4.

379. T. J. Regan, M. I. Khan, H. A. Oldewurtel and A. J. Passannante, Antibiotic effect on myocardial K^+ transport and the production of ventricular tachycardia, *J. Clin. Invest.*, 1969, **48**, 68a.

380. S. Nattel, S. Ranger, M. Talijic, R. Lemery and D. Roy, Erythromycin-induced long QT syndrome: concordance with quinidine and underlying cellular electrophysiologic mechanism, *Am. J. Med.*, 1990, **89**, 235–238.

381. H. C. Farrar, M. C. Walsh-Sukys, K. Kyllonen and J. L. Blumer, Cardiac toxicity associated with intravenous erythromycin lactobionate: two case reports and a review of the literature, *Pediatr. Infect. Dis.*, 1993, **12**, 688–691.

382. M. W. Brandriss, W. S. Richardson and S. S. Barold, Erythromycin-induced QT prolongation and polymorphic ventricular tachycardia (torsades de pointes): case report and review, *Clin. Infect. Dis.*, 1994, **18**, 995–998.

383. Z. Orban, L. L. MacDonald, M. A. Peters and B. Guslits, Erythromycin-induced cardiac toxicity, *Am. J. Cardiol.*, 1995, **75**, 859–861.

384. P. Periti, T. Mazzei, E. Mini and A. Novelli, Adverse effects of macrolide antibacterials, *Drug Saf.*, 1993, **9**, 346–364.

385. R. C. Owens, QT prolongation with antimicrobial agents: understanding the significance, *Drugs*, 2004, **64**, 1091–1124.

386. N. Goldschmidt, T. Azaz-Livshits, I. Gotsman, R. Nir-Paz, A. Ben-Yuhuda and M. Muszkat, Compound cardiac toxicity of oral erythromycin and verapamil, *Ann. Pharmacother.*, 2001, **35**, 1396–1399.

387. V. B. Pai and M. C. Nahata, Cardiotoxicity of chemotherapeutic agents: incidence, treatment and prevention, *Drug Saf.*, 2000, **22**, 263–302.

388. D. Guo, Y. Cai, D. Chai, B. Liang, N. Bai and R. Wang, The cardio-toxicity of macrolides: a systematic review, *Pharmazie*, 2010, **65**, 631–640.

389. K. Kasahara, A. Nishikawa, F. Furukawa, F. Ikezaki, Z. Tanakamaru, I.-S. Lee, T. Imazawa and M. Hirose, A chronic toxicity study of josa-mycin in F344 rats, *Food Chem. Toxicol.*, 2002, **40**, 1017–1022.

390. Committee for Veterinary Medicinal Products, Josamycin (Chicken), EMEA/MRL/011/95. Available from: http://www.ema.europa.eu.

391. Committee for Veterinary Medicinal Products, Tulathromycin, EMEA/MRL/894/04-FINAL. Available from: http://www.ema.europa.eu.

392. Committee for Medicinal Products for Veterinary Use, European MRL Assessment Report, Gamithromycin, EMEA/CVMP/567075/2008. Available from: http://www.ema.europa.eu.

393. Committee for Medicinal Products for Veterinary Use, European MRL Assessment Report, Tildipirosin, EMA/CVMP/709377/2009. Available from: http://www.ema.europa.eu.

394. I. Ewings and W. White, Statins and pneumonia. Beware statins with macrolides, *BMJ*, 2011, **342**, d2703.

395. A. L. Chang, M. T. Wang, C. Y. Su and F. H. Tsai, Risk of digoxin intoxication caused by clarithromycin-digoxin interactions in heart failure patients: a population-based study, *Eur. J. Clin. Pharmacol.*, 2009, **65**, 1237–1243.

396. S. P. Nordt, S. R. Williams, A. S. Manoguerra and R. F. Clark, Clarithromycin induced digoxin toxicity, *J. Accid. Emerg. Med.*, 1998, **15**, 194–195.

397. R. Santucci, H. Fothergill, V. Laugel, A. Perville, A. De Saint Martin, A. C. Gerout and M. Fischbach, The onset of oxcarbazepine toxicity to prescription of clarithromycin in a child with refractory epilepsy, *Br. J. Clin. Pharmacol.*, 2010, **69**, 314–331.

398. T. Gomes, M. M. Mamdani and D. N. Juurlink, Macrolide-induced digoxin toxicity: a population-based study, *Clin. Pharmacol. Ther.*, 2009, **86**, 383–386.

399. J. Baillargeon, H. M. Holmes, Y. L. Lin, M. A. Raji, G. Sharma and Y. F. Kuo, Concurrent use of warfarin and antibiotics and the risk of bleeding in older adults, *Am. J. Med.*, 2012, **125**, 183–189.

400. L. E. Hines and J. E. Murphy, Potentially harmful drug-drug interactions in the elderly: a review, *Am. J. Geriatr. Pharmacother.*, 2011, **9**, 364–377.

401. C. Y. Lee, F. Marcotte, G. Giraldeau, G. Koren, M. Juneau and J. C. Tardiv, Digoxin toxicity precipitated by clarithromycin use: case presentation and concise review of the literature, *Can. J. Cardiol.*, 2011, **27**, e15–e16.

402. N. A. von Rosensteil and D. Adam, Macrolide antibacterials. Drug interactions of clinical significance, *Drug Saf.*, 1995, **13**, 105–122.

403. T. J. Pallasch, Macrolide antibiotics, *Dent. Today*, 1997, **16**(72), 74–75.

404. A. Anadón and L. Reeve-Johnson, Macrolide antibiotics, drug interactions and microsomal enzymes: implications for veterinary medicines, *Res. Vet. Sci.*, 1999, **66**, 197–203.

405. G. Keiser and U. Bucheggar, Haematological side effects of chloramphenicol and thiamphenicol, *Helv. Med. Acta*, 1973, **37**, 265–278.

406. W. Nijhof and A. M. Kroon, The interference of chloramphenicol and thiamphenicol with the biogenesis of mitochondria in animal tissues. A possible clue to toxic action, *Postgrad. Med. J.*, 1974, **50**(5), 53–59.

407. S. Chaplin, Bone marrow depression due to mianserin, phenylbutazone, oxyphenazone and chloramphenicol, *Adverse Drug React. Acute Poisoning Rev.*, 1986, **3**, 181–196.

408. D. Holt, D. Harvey and R. Hurley, Chloramphenicol toxicity, *Adverse Drug React. Toxicol. Rev.*, 1993, **12**, 83–95.
409. A. A. Sharp, Chloramphenicol-induced blood dyscrasias. Analysis of 40 cases, *BMJ*, 1963, **284**, 1331.
410. R. O. Wallerstein, P. K. Candit, C. K. Casper, J. W. Brown and F. R. Morrison, Statewide study of chloramphenicol therapy and fatal aplastic anemia, *J. Am. Med. Assoc.*, 1969, **208**, 2045–2050.
411. B. P. C. Polak, H. Wesseling, D. Schut, A. Herxheimer and L. Meyler, Blood dyscrasias attributable to chloramphenicol. A review of 576 published and unpublished cases, *Acta Med. Scand.*, 1972, **192**, 409–414.
412. K. Hausman and G. Skrandies, Aplastic anaemia following chloramphenicol therapy in Hamburg and surrounding districts, *Postgrad. Med. J.*, 1974, **50**, 136–142.
413. B. Modan, S. Segal, M. Sham and C. Sheba, Aplastic anaemia in Israel: evaluation of the etiological role of chloramphenicol on a community-wide basis, *Am. J. Med. Sci.*, 1975, **270**, 441–445.
414. H. A. B. Al-Moudhiry, Aplastic anaemia in Iraq. A prospective study, *Haematologica*, 1978, **12**, 159–164.
415. H. B. Benestad, Drug mechanisms in marrow aplasia in *Aplastic Anaemia*, ed. G. C. Geary, Ballière Tindall, London, 1979, pp. 26–42.
416. L. E. Bottinger, Epidemiology and aetiology of aplastic anaemia, *Haematol. Blood Transfus.*, 1979, **24**, 27–37.
417. R. P. Perez, M. L. Puig, J. L. A. Sanchez and E. L. Torres, Aplastic anaemia and drugs as causal agents, *Rev. Farm. Cuba*, 1981, **15**, 97–103.
418. E. Bamelou and Y. Najean, Why still prescribe chloramphenicol in 1983? *Blut*, 1983, **47**, 317–320.
419. G. R. Venning, Identification of adverse reactions to new drugs. II – How were 18 important adverse reactions discovered and with what delays, *BMJ*, 1983, **286**, 289–292.
420. Widayat, Sunarto, M. Sutaryo, Zurghiban and Ismangoen, Aplastic anaemia in children, *Paediatr. Indones.*, 1983, **23**, 183–191.
421. M. Aksoy, S. Erdem, G. Dinkol, I. Bakioglu and A. Kutlar, Aplastic anaemia due to chemicals and drugs, *Sex. Transm. Dis.*, 1984, **11**, 347–350.
422. Y. Najean and E. Baumelou, Toxic epidemiology of aplastic anaemia, *Sex. Transm. Dis.*, 1984, **11**, 343–346.
423. D. W. Kaufman, J. P. Kelly, J. M. Jurgelon, T. Anderson, S. Issaragrisil, B. E. Wiholm, N. S. Young, P. Leaverton, M. Levy and S. Shapiro, Drugs in the aetiology of agranulocytosis and aplastic anaemia, *Eur. J. Haematol.*, 1996, **60**(Suppl.), 23–30.
424. S. L. Leiken, H. Welch and G. H. Guin, Aplastic anemia due to chloramphenicol, *Clin. Proc. Child. Hosp. Dist. Columbia*, 1961, **17**, 171–180.
425. S. Awaad, A. S. Khalifa and K. Kamel, Vacuolization of leukocytes and bone-marrow aplasia due to chloramphenicol toxicity, *Clin. Pediatr.*, 1975, **14**, 499–506.

426. L. W. Young, J. S. Mitnick, W. A. Jankus and N. B. Genieser, Radiological case of the month, *Am. J. Dis. Child.*, 1979, **133**, 545–546.
427. M. L. Lepow, Aplastic anemia following chloramphenicol therapy still happens! *Pediatrics*, **77**, 932–933.
428. M. P. White, H. W. Haboush and L. G. Alroomi, Fatal bone marrow aplasia due to chloramphenicol in a baby, *Lancet*, 1986, **i**, 555–556.
429. R. Hodgkinson, Infectious hepatitis and aplastic anaemia, *Lancet*, 1971, **i**, 1014.
430. K. P. Hellriegel and R. Cross, Follow-up studies in chloramphenicol-induced aplastic anaemia, *Postgrad. Med. J.*, 1974, **50**(5), 136–142.
431. R. L. Rosenthal and A. Blackman, Bone marrow hypoplasia following the use of chloramphenicol eye drops, *J. Am. Med. Assoc.*, 1965, **191**, 148–149.
432. G. Carpenter, Chloramphenicol eye-drops and marrow aplasia, *Lancet*, 1975, **i**, 326–327.
433. S. M. Abrams, T. J. Degnan and V. Vinciguerra, Marrow aplasia following topical treatment application of chloramphenicol eye ointment, *Arch. Intern. Med.*, 1980, **140**, 576–577.
434. E. T. Fraunfelder and G. C. Bagby, Fatal aplastic anemia following topical administration of ophthalmic chloramphenicol, *Am. J. Ophthalmol.*, 1982, **93**, 356–360.
435. M. E. Plaut and W. R. Best, Aplastic anemia after parenteral chloramphenicol: warning renewed, *N. Engl. J. Med.*, 1982, **306**, 1486.
436. S. Issaragisil and A. Piankijagum, Aplastic anaemia following topical administration of ophthalmic chloramphenicol: report of a case and review of the literature, *J. Med. Assoc. Thai.*, 1985, **88**, 309–312.
437. G. W. Korting and H. Kifle, Systemic side-effects from external application of chloramphenicol, *Hautartz*, 1985, **36**, 181–183.
438. T. Lancaster, A. M. Swart and H. Jick, Risk of serious haematological toxicity with use of chloramphenicol eye drops in British general practice database, *BMJ*, 1998, **316**, 667.
439. S. Walker, C. J. M. Diaper, R. Bowman, G. Sweeney, D. V. Seal and C. M. Kirkness, Lack of evidence for systemic toxicity following topical chloramphenicol use, *Eye*, 1998, **12**, 875–879.
440. G. S. Del Giacco, M. T. Petrini, S. Jannelli and U. Carcasi, Fatal bone marrow hypoplasia in a shepherd using chloramphenicol spray, *Lancet*, 1981, **i**, 945.
441. A. A. Yunis and G. R. Bloomberg, Chloramphenicol toxicity: clinical features and pathogenesis, *Prog. Hematol.*, 1964, **4**, 138–159.
442. A. A. Yunis, Differential in vitro toxicity of chloramphenicol, nitrosochloramphenicol, and thiamphenicol, *Sex. Transm. Dis.*, 1984, **11**, 340–342.
443. A. A. Yunis, Chloramphenicol toxicity: 25 years of research, *Am. J. Med.*, 1989, **87**, 3–44N-3-48N.
444. D. E. Holt, T. A. Ryder, A. Fairburn, R. Hurley and D. Harvey, The myelotoxicity of chloramphenicol in vitro and in vivo studies. I. In vitro effects on cells in culture, *Hum. Exp. Toxicol.*, 1997, **16**, 570–576.

445. D. E. Holt, C. M. Andrews, J. P. Payne, T. C. Williams and J. A. Turton, The myelotoxicity of chloramphenicol in vitro and in vivo studies. II. In vivo myelotoxicity in the B3C3F$_1$ mouse, *Hum. Exp. Toxicol.*, 1998, **17**, 8–17.

446. J. A. Turton, D. Yallop, C. M. Andrews, R. Fagg, M. York and T. C. Williams, Haematotoxicity of chloramphenicol succinate in the CD-1 mouse and Wistar Hanover rat, *Hum. Exp. Toxicol.*, 1999, **18**, 566–576.

447. J. A. Turton, A. C. Havard, S. Robinson, D. E. Holt, C. M. Andrews, R. Fagg and T. C. Williams, An assessment of chloramphenicol and thiamphenicol in the induction of aplastic anaemia in the BALB/c mouse, *Food Chem. Toxicol.*, 2000, **38**, 925–938.

448. J. A. Turton, C. M. Andrews, A. C. Havard and T. C. Williams, Studies on the haematotoxicity of chloramphenicol succinate in the Dunkin Hartley guinea pig, *Int. J. Exp. Pathol.*, 2002, **83**, 225–238.

449. M. F. W. Festing, P. Diamanti and J. A. Turton, Strain differences in haematological response to chloramphenicol succinate in mice: implications for toxicological research, *Food Chem. Toxicol.*, 2001, **39**, 375–383.

450. J. A. Turton, Characterisation of the myelotoxicity of chloramphenicol succinate in the B6C3F$_1$ mouse, *Int. J. Exp. Pathol.*, 2006, **87**, 101–112.

451. Joint FAO/WHO Expert Committee on Food Additives, Toxicological Evaluation of Certain Veterinary Drug Residues in Food, The 32nd Meeting of the Joint FAO/WHO Expert Committee on Food Additives (JECFA), International Programme on Chemical Safety, Cambridge University Press, Cambridge, 1988, pp. 1–71.

452. Committee for Veterinary Medicinal Products, Thiamphenicol, EMEA/MRL/256/97-FINAL. Available from: http://www.ema.europa.eu.

453. Committee for Veterinary Medicinal Products, Florfenicol. Available at: http://www.ema.europa.eu.

454. J. Ando, R. Ishiwara, S. Imai, T. Kitamura, M. Takahashi, M. Yoshida and A. Maekawa, Thirteen-week subchronic toxicity study of thiamphenicol in F344 rats, *Toxicol. Lett.*, 1997, **91**, 137–146.

455. M. Loeffler, B. Bungart, H. Goris, S. Schmitz and W. Nijhof, Haematopoiesis during thiamphenicol treatment. II. A theoretical analysis shows consistency of new data with a previously hypothesized model of stem cell regulation, *Exp. Haematol.*, 1989, **17**, 962–967.

456. V. Ferrari, Salient features of thiamphenicol: review of clinical pharmacokinetics and toxicity, *Sex. Transm. Dis.*, 1984, **11**(Suppl.), 336–339.

457. J. P. Ryckelynck, J. Potier and P. Beuve-Mery, Bone marrow toxicity of a combination of thiamphenicol and trimethoprim-sulfamethoxole, *Nouv. Presse. Med.*, 1979, **8**, 3839.

458. J. J. Sotto, P. Simon, P. Subtil, A. Rozenbaum, Y. Najean and A. Pecking, Hematologic toxicity of thiophenicol, *Nouv. Presse. Med.*, 1976, **5**, 2163.

459. J. P. Kaltwasser, E. Werner, B. Simon, U. Bellenberg and H. J. Becker, The effect of thiamphenicol on normal and activated erythropoiesis in the rabbit, *Postgrad. Med. J.*, 1974, **50**(5), 118–122.

460. A. D. Tuttle, M. G. Papich and B. A. Wolfe, Bone marrow hypoplasia secondary to florfenicol toxicity in a Thomson's gazelle (*Gazella thomsonii*), *J. Vet. Pharmacol. Ther.*, 2006, **29**, 317–319.

461. Joint FAO/WHO Expert Committee on Food Additives, Toxicological Evaluation of Certain Veterinary Drug Residues in Food, The Forty-Seventh Meeting of the Joint FAO/WHO Expert Committee on Food Additives (JECFA), International Programme on Chemical Safety, World Health Organization, Geneva, 1996, pp. 83–107.

462. J. A. Turton, C. M. Andrews, A. C. Havard, S. Robinson, M. York, T. C. Williams and F. M. Gibson, Haematotoxicity of thiamphenicol in the BALB/c mouse and Wistar Hanover rat, *Food Chem. Toxicol.*, 2002, **40**, 1849–1861.

463. A. A. Yunis, Chloramphenicol: relation of structure to activity and toxicity, *Ann. Rev. Pharmacol. Toxicol.*, 1988, **28**, 83–100.

464. D. Malkin, G. Koren and E. F. Saunders, Drug-induced aplastic anaemia: pathogenesis and clinical aspects, *Am. J. Pediatr. Haematol. Oncol.*, 1990, **12**, 402–410.

465. A. Pilai, C. Hartford, C. Wang, D. Pei, J. Yang, A. Srinivasan, B. Triplett, M. Dallas and W. Yeung, Favorable preliminary results using the TLI/ATG-based immunomodulatory condition for matched unrelated donor allogenic hematopoietic stem cell transplantation in pediatric severe aplastic anemia, *Pediatr. Transplant.*, 2011, **15**, 628–634.

466. A. M. Ristano and F. Perna, Aplastic anemia: immunosuppressive therapy in 2010, *Pedtr. Rep.*, 2011, **22**(2), e7.

467. A. E. DeZern and E. C. Guinan, Therapy for aplastic anemia, *Haematology Am. Soc. Haematol. Educ. Program*, 2011, **2011**, 82–83.

468. E. C. Guinan, Diagnosis and management of aplastic anemia, *Haematology Am. Soc. Haematol. Educ. Program*, 2011, **2011**, 76–81.

469. J. H. Kwon, I. Kim, Y. G. Lee, Y. Koh, H. C. Park, E. Y. Song, H. K. Kim, S. S. Yoon, D. S. Lee, S. S. Park, H. Y. Shin, S. Park, M. H. Park, H. S. Ahn and B. K. Kim, Clinical course of non-severe aplastic anemia in adults, *Int. J. Hematol.*, 2010, **91**, 770–775.

470. D. M. Mintzer, S. N. Billet and L. Chmielewski, Drug-induced hematologic syndromes, *Adv. Hematol.*, 2009, **2009**, article ID 495863, p. 11.

471. R. Gurion, A. Gafter-Gvili, M. Paul, L. Vidal, I. Ben-Bassat, M. Yeshurun, O. Shpilberg and P. Raanani, Hematopoietic growth factors in aplastic anemia patients treated with immunosuppressive therapy – systematic review and meta-analysis, *Haematologica*, 2009, **94**, 712–719.

472. S. Samarasinghe and D. K. Webb, How I manage aplastic anaemia in children, *Br. J. Haematol.*, 2012, e-pub ahead of print.

473. S. Samarasinghe, C. Steward, P. Hiwarkar, M. A. Saif, R. Hough, D. Webb, A. Norton, S. Lawson, A. Qureshi, P. Connor, P. Carey, R. Skinner, A. Vora, B. Gibson, G. Stewart, S. Keogh, N. Golden, D. Bonney, M. Stubbs, P. Amrolia, K. Rao, S. Meyer, R. Wynn and P. Veys, Excellent outcome of matched unrelated donor transplantation in

paediatric aplastic anaemia following failure with immunosuppressive therapy: a United Kingdom multicentre retrospective experience, *Br. J. Haematol.*, 2012, **157**, 339–346.

474. N. S. Young, A. Bacigalupo and J. C. Marsh, Aplastic anemia: pathophysiology and treatment, *Biol. Blood Marrow Transplant.*, 2010, **16**(1), S119–S125.

475. I. H. Krakoff, D. A. Karnofsky and J. H. Burchenal, Effects of large doses of chloramphenicol on human subjects, *N. Engl. J. Med.*, 1955, **253**, 7–10.

476. J. L. Scott, S. M. Finegold, G. A. Belkin and J. S. Lawrence, A controlled double blind study of the hematologic toxicity of chloramphenicol, *N. Engl. J. Med.*, 1965, **272**, 1137–1142.

477. M. J. Brauer and W. Dameshek, Hypoplastic anemia and myeloblastic leukemia following chloramphenicol therapy, *N. Engl. J. Med.*, 1967, **277**, 1003–1005.

478. J. F. Fraumeni, Bone-marrow depression induced by chloramphenicol or phenylbutazone, *J. Am. Med. Assoc.*, 1967, **201**, 150–156.

479. K. R. Humphries, Acute myelomonocytic leukaemia following chloramphenicol therapy, *N. Z. Med. J.*, 1968, **68**, 248–249.

480. A. J. Seaman, Sequels to chloramphenicol aplastic anemia: acute leukemia and paroxysmal nocturnal hemoglobinuria, *Northwest Med.*, 1969, **68**, 831–834.

481. H. Gadner, U. Gethmann, K. Jessenberger and H. Riehm, Acute leukaemia following exposure to chloramphenicol? Three case reports and review of the literature, *Monatsschr. Kinderheilkd.*, 1973, **121**, 590–594.

482. J. S. Meyer and M. Boxer, Leukemic thrombi in pulmonary blood vessels. Subleukemic myelogenous leukaemia following chloramphenicol-induced aplastic anaemia, *Cancer*, 1973, **32**, 363–372.

483. A. Forni and E. C. Vigliani, Chemical leukemogenesis in man, *Haematologica*, 1974, **7**, 211–213.

484. L. Meyler, B. C. P. Polak, D. Schut, H. Wesseling and A. Herxheimer, Blood dyscrasias attributed to chloramphenicol. A review of 64 published and unpublished cases, *Postgrad. Med. J.*, 1974, **50**(5), 123–126.

485. A. Schmitt-Graf, Chloramphenicol-induced aplastic anemia terminating with acute nonlymphocytic leukaemia, *Acta. Haematol.*, 1981, **66**, 267–268.

486. J. M. J. C. Scheres, T. W. J. Hustinx, J. P. M. Geraedts, C. H. W. Leeksma and P. S. Meltzer, Translocation 1:7 in hematologic disorders. A brief review of 22 cases, *Cancer Genet. Cytogenet.*, 1985, **18**, 207–213.

487. National Toxicology Program, Chloramphenicol, *Rep. Carcinog.*, 2011, **12**, 92–94.

488. J. E. Riviere and J. W. Spoo, Tetracycline antibiotics in *Veterinary Pharmacology and Therapeutics*, ed. H. R. Adams, Iowa State Press, Ames, 8th edn, 2001, pp. 828–840.

489. Joint FAO/WHO Expert Committee on Food Additives, Toxicological Evaluation of Certain Veterinary Drug Residues in Food, The Forty-

Fifth Meeting of the Joint FAO/WHO Expert Committee on Food Additives (JECFA), International Programme on Chemical Safety, World Health Organization, Geneva, 1996, pp. 85–116.

490. Committee for Veterinary Medicinal Products, Oxytetracycline, Tetracycline, Chlortetracycline. Available from: http://www.ema.europa.eu.

491. Committee for Veterinary Medicinal Products, Doxycycline, EMEA/MRL/270/97-FINAL. Available from: http://www.ema.europa.eu.

492. M. P. Menon and A. K. Das, Tetracycline asthma – a case report, *Clin. Allergy*, 1977, **7**, 285–290.

493. H. H. Schwarting, Occupational tetracycline allergy, *Derm. Beruf. Umwelt.*, 1983, **31**, 130.

494. E. Rudzki, Contact sensitivity to systemically administered drugs, *Dermatol. Clin.*, 1990, **8**, 177–180.

495. E. Rudzki and P. Rebandel, Sensitivity to oxytetracycline, *Contact Dermatitis*, 1997, **37**, 136.

496. E. M. Ory, The tetracyclines, *Med. Clin. North Am.*, 1970, **54**, 1173–1186.

497. American Academy of Pediatrics, Committee on Drugs. Requiem for tetracyclines, *Pediatrics*, 1975, **55**, 142–143.

498. J. J. Cloud and B. Weibling, Whitening challenges: tetracycline staining and fluorosis, *Dent. Today*, 2009, **28**, 84–85.

499. A. S. Kashvap and H. S. Shrama, Discolouration of permanent teeth and enamel hypoplasia due to tetracycline, *Postgrad. Med. J.*, 1999, **75**, 772.

500. P. Fleming, C. J. Witkop and W. H. Kuhlmann, Staining and hypoplasia of enamel caused by tetracycline: case report, *Pediatr. Dent.*, 1987, **9**, 245–246.

501. H. C. Skinner and J. Nalbandian, Tetracyclines and mineralized tissues: review and perspectives, *Yale J. Biol. Med.*, 1975, **48**, 377–397.

502. H. A. McIntosh and E. Storey, Tetracycline-induced tooth changes. 4. Discolouration and hypoplasia induced by tetracycline analogues, *Med. J. Aust.*, 1970, **1**, 114–119.

503. K. L. Baker, Tetracycline-induced tooth changes. Part 5. Incidence in extracted first permanent teeth: a resurvey after four years, *Med. J. Aust.*, 1975, **2**, 301–304.

504. M. T. Golan, H. P. Golan, P. J. Porter and E. H. Kass, Effect of administration of tetracycline in pregnancy on the primary dentition of the offspring, *J. Oral Med.*, 1970, **25**, 75–79.

505. N. D. Martin and P. D. Barnard, The prevalence of tetracycline staining in erupted teeth, *Med. J. Aust.*, 1969, **1**, 1286–1289.

506. S. E. Hamp, The tetracyclines and their effect on teeth. A clinical study, *Odontol. Tidskr.*, 1967, **75**, 33–49.

507. R. H. Johnson and D. F. Mitchell, The effects of tetracycline on teeth and bones, *J. Dent. Res.*, 1966, **45**, 86–93.

508. R. H. Johnson, The tetracyclines: a review of the literature – 1948 through 1963, *J. Oral Ther. Pharmacol.*, 1964, **46**, 190–217.

509. S. Q. Cohlan, G. Bevelander and T. Tiamsic, Growth inhibition of prematures receiving tetracycline: clinical and laboratory investigation, *Am. J. Dis. Child.*, 1963, **105**, 453–461.

510. J. F. Noble, L. A. Kanegis and D. W. Hallesy, Short-term toxicity and observations on certain aspects of the pharmacology of a unique tetracycline – minocycline, *Toxicol. Appl. Pharmacol.*, 1967, **11**, 128–149.

511. A. Gough, S. Chapman, K. Wagstaff, P. Emery and E. Elias, Minocycline induced autoimmune hepatitis and systemic lupus erythematosus-like syndrome, *BMJ*, 1996, **312**, 169–172.

512. L. Grasset, C. Guy and M. Ollagnier, Cyclines and acne: pay attention to adverse drug reactions! A recent review of the literature, *Rev. Med. Interne*, 2003, **24**, 305–316.

513. R. G. Schlienger, A. J. Bircher and C. R. Meier, Minocycline-induced lupus. A systematic review, *Dermatology*, 2000, **200**, 223–231.

514. O. Elkayam, M. Yaron and D. Caspi, Minocycline-induced autoimmune syndromes: An overview, *Sem. Arthritis Rheum.*, 1999, **28**, 392–397.

515. Z.-X. Liu and N. Kaplowitz, Immune-mediated drug-induced liver disease, *Clin. Liver Dis.*, 2002, **6**, 467–486.

516. T. Vial, B. Nicolas and J. Descotes, Drug-induced autoimmunity: experience of the French pharmacovigilance system, *Toxicology*, 1997, **119**, 23–27.

517. R. Bocker, C.-J. Estler and D. Ludewig-Sandig, Evaluation of the hepatotoxic potential of minocycline, *Antimicrob. Agents Chemother.*, 1991, **35**, 1434–1436.

518. T. Matsuura, Y. Shimizu, H. Fujimoto, T. Miyazaki and S. Kano, Minocycline-related lupus, *Lancet*, 1992, **340**, 1553.

519. M. G. Davies and P. J. Kersey, Acute hepatitis and exfoliative dermatitis associated with minocycline, *BMJ*, 1989, **298**, 1523–1524.

520. D. I. Min, P. A. Burke, D. Lewis and R. L. Jenkins, Acute hepatic failure associated with oral minocycline: A case report, *Pharmacother.*, 1992, **12**, 68–71.

521. J. V. Schaffer, D. M. Davidson, J. M. McNiff and J. L. Bolognia, Perinuclear antineutrophilic cytoplasmic antibody-positive cutaneous polyarteritis nodosa associated with minocycline therapy for acne vulgaris, *J. Am. Acad. Dermatol.*, 2001, **44**, 198–206.

522. J. Puyana, V. Ureña, S. Quirge, M. Fernandez-Rivas, M. Cuevas and J. Fraj, Serum sickness-like syndrome associated with minocycline, *Allergy*, 1990, **45**, 313–315.

523. J. M. Angulo, L. H. Sigal and L. R. Espinoza, Coexistent minocycline-induced systemic lupus erythematosus and autoimmune hepatitis, *Sem. Arthritis Rheum.*, 1998, **28**, 187–192.

524. R. Somech, R. Arav-Boger, A. Assia, Z. Spirer and U. Jurgenson, Complications of minocycline therapy for acne vulgaris: case reports and review of the literature, *Pediatr. Dermatol.*, 1999, **16**, 469–472.

525. M. Landau, E. Shachr and S. Brenner, Minocycline-induced serum sickness-like reaction, *J. Eur. Acad. Dermatol. Venereol.*, 2000, **14**, 67–68.

526. M. MacNeil, D. A. Haase, R. Tremaine and T. J. Marrie, Fever, lymphadenopathy, eosinophilia, hepatitis and dermatitis: a severe reaction to minocycline, *J. Am. Acad. Dermatol.*, 1997, **38**, 347–350.

527. S. R. Knowles, L. Shapiro and N. H. Shear, Serious adverse reactions influenced by minocycline. Report of 13 patients and review of the literature, *Arch. Dermatol.*, 1996, **132**, 934–939.

528. S. P. Wilkinson, W. K. Stewart, E. M. Spiers and J. Pears, Protracted systemic illness and interstitial nephritis due to minocycline, *Postgrad. Med. J.*, 1996, **65**, 53–56.

529. D. Kaufmann, W. Pichler and J. H. Beer, Severe episode of high fever with rash, lymphadenopathy, neutropenia, and eosinophilia after minocycline therapy for acne, *Arch. Intern. Med.*, 1994, **154**, 1983–1984.

530. L. Harel, J. Amir, E. Livni, R. Straussberg and I. Varsano, Serum-like sickness associated with minocycline therapy in adolescents, *Ann. Pharmacother.*, 1996, **30**, 481–483.

531. T. Levenson, D. Masood and R. Patterson, Minocycline-induced serum sickness, *Allergy Asthma Proc.*, 1996, **17**, 79–81.

532. T. M. Lawson, N. Amos, D. Bulgen and B. D. Williams, Minocycline induced lupus: clinical features and response to rechallenge, *Rheumatol.*, 2001, **40**, 329–335.

533. A. M. Piette, J. Ramanoelina, P. Gepner, C. Larroche and O. Blétry, Systemic reactions induced by minocycline treatment: a report of four patients and a review of the literature, *Rev. Med. Interne*, 1999, **20**, 869–874.

534. C. Parc, A. P. Brézin, I. Nataf, D. Dusser, L. Moachon and F. D'Hermies, Presumed hypersensitivity to minocycline and conjunctival infiltration, *Br. J. Ophthalmol.*, 2002, **86**, 1313–1314.

535. J. E. Teitelbaum, A. R. Perez-Atayde, M. Cohen, A. Bousvaros and M. M. Jonas, Minocycline-related autoimmune hepatitis, *Arch. Pediatr. Adolesc. Med.*, 1998, **152**, 1132–1136.

536. C. M. Hardman, J. N. Leonard, H. C. Thomas and R. Goldin, Minocycline and hepatitis, *Clin. Exp. Derm.*, 1996, **21**, 244–245.

537. M. C. J. M. Sturkenboom, C. R. Meier, H. Jick and B. H. C. Stricker, Minocycline and lupus like syndrome in acne patients, *Arch. Intern. Med.*, 1999, **159**, 493–497.

538. C. Christe, F. Ricou, R. Stoller and N. Vogt, Minocycline-induced pericardial effusion, *Ann. Pharmacother.*, 2000, **34**, 875–877.

539. R. A. Lawrenson, H. E. Seaman, A. Sundstrom, T. J. Williams and R. D. T. Farmer, Liver damage associated with minocycline use in acne, *Drug Saf.*, 2000, **23**, 333–349.

540. R. D. Sweet, An acute febrile neutrophilic dermatosis, *Br. J. Dermatol.*, 1964, **76**, 349–356.

541. B. Khan Durani and U. Jappe, Drug-induced Sweet's syndrome in acne caused by different tetracyclines: a case report and review of the literature, *Br. J. Dermatol.*, 2002, **147**, 558–562.

542. E. Gilmour, R. J. G. Chalmers and D. J. Rowlands, Drug-induced Sweet's syndrome (acute febrile neutrophilic dermatosis) associated with hydralazine, *Br. J. Dermatol.*, 1995, **133**, 490–491.

543. M.-J. Thibault, R. Billick and H. Srolovitz, Minocycline-induced Sweet's syndrome, *J. Am. Acad. Dermatol.*, 1992, **27**, 801–804.

544. H. Mensing and L. Kowalzick, Acute febrile neutrophilic dermatosis (Sweet's Syndrome) caused by minocycline, *Dermatologica*, 1991, **182**, 43–46.

545. P. S. Karofsky and G. P. Williams, Minocycline-induced rash in an 18-year-old patient, *Arch. Pediatr. Adolesc. Med.*, 1995, **149**, 217–218.

546. G. Gordon, B. M. Sparano and M. J. Iatropoulos, Hyperpigmentation of the skin associated with minocycline therapy, *Arch. Dermatol.*, 1985, **121**, 618–623.

547. R. S. Basler, Minocycline-related hyperpigmentation, *Arch. Dermatol.*, 1985, **121**, 606–608.

548. N. R. Wassel, E. H. Schloss and A. N. Lin, Minocycline-induced cutaneous pigmentation, *J. Cutan. Med. Surg.*, 1998, **3**, 105–108.

549. A. J. Bridges, F. M. Graziano, W. Calhoun and G. T. Reizner, Hyperpigmentation, neutrophilic alveolitis, and erythema nodosum resulting from minocycline, *J. Am. Acad. Dermatol.*, 1990, **22**, 959–962.

550. P. Collins and J. A. Cotterhill, Minocycline-induced pigmentation resolves after treatment with the Q-switched ruby laser, *Br. J. Dermatol.*, 1996, **135**, 317–319.

551. M. Pepine, F. P. Flowers and F. A. Ramos-Caro, Extensive cutaneous hyperpigmentation caused by minocycline, *J. Am. Acad. Dermatol.*, 1993, **28**, 292–295.

552. P. Chu, S. L. Van, T. S. Yen and T. G. Berger, Minocycline hyperpigmentation localised to the lips: an unusual fixed drug reaction, *J. Am. Acad. Dermatol.*, 1994, **30**, 802–803.

553. S. Karrer, R. M. Szeiies, A. Pfau, J. Schroder, W. Stolz and M. Landthaler, Minocycline-induced hyperpigmentation, *Hautarzt.*, 1998, **49**, 219–223.

554. T. A. Chave, P. M. Collier and W. B. Campbell, Postoperative minocycline pigmentation, *Ann. R. Coll. Surg. Engl.*, 2000, **82**, 348–349.

555. J. M. Cockings and N. W. Savage, Minocycline and oral pigmentation, *Aust. Dent. J.*, 1998, **43**, 14–16.

556. D. Eisen, Minocycline-induced oral hyperpigmentation, *Lancet*, 1997, **349**, 400.

557. M. Kurosumi and H. Fujita, Fine structural aspects on the fate of rat black thyroids induced by minocycline, *Virch. Archiv.*, 1986, **51**, 207–213.

558. D. R. Doerge, R. L. Divi, J. Deck and A. Taurog, Mechanism for the anti-thyroid action of minocycline, *Chem. Res. Toxicol.*, 1997, **10**, 49–58.

559. B. D. Clayton, M. G. Hitchcock and P. M. Williford, Minocycline hypersensitivity with respiratory failure, *Arch. Dermatol.*, 1999, **135**, 139–140.

560. A. Shoji, Y. Someda and T. Hamada, Stevens-Johnson syndrome due to minocycline therapy, *Arch. Dermatol.*, 1987, **123**, 18–20.

561. B. J. Schrodt, C. L. Kulp-Shorten and J. P. Callen, Necrotizing vasculitis of the skin and uterine cervix associated with minocycline therapy for acne vulgaris, *South. Med. J.*, 1999, **92**, 502–504.

562. S. de Paz, A. Perez, M. Gomez, A. Trampal and A. Dominguez-Lazaro, Dominguez-Lazaro. Severe hypersensitivity reaction to minocycline, *J. Invest. Allergol. Clin. Immunol.*, 1999, **9**, 403–404.

563. M. Kloppenburg, B. A. Dijkmans and F. C. Breedveld, Hypersensitivity pneumonitis during minocycline treatment, *Neth. J. Med.*, 1994, **44**, 210–213.

564. T. Yamamoto and K. Minatohara, Minocycline-induced acute generalised exanthematous pustulosis in a patient with generalised pustular psoriasis showing elevated level of sELAM-1, *Acta Derm. Venereol.*, 1997, **77**, 168–169.

565. A. Antunes, A. Davril, P. Tréchot, M. Grandidier, F. Truchetet and J. F Cuny, Hypersensitivity syndrome with minocycline, *Ann. Dermatol. Venereol.*, 1999, **126**, 518–521.

566. A. Parneix-Spake, S. Bastuji-Garin, J.-B. Lobut, J. Erner, P. Guyet-Rousset, J. Revuz and J.-C. Roujeau, Minocycline as a possible cause of severe and protracted hypersensitivity drug reaction, *Arch. Dermatol.*, 1995, **131**, 490–491.

567. J. M. Andreano, G. R. Kantor, W. F. Bergfeld, R. J. Tuthill and J. S. Taylor, Eosinophilic cellulitis and eosinophilic pustular folliculitis, *J. Am. Acad. Dermatol.*, 1989, **20**, 934–936.

568. M. Oddo, L. Liaudet, M. Lepori, A. F. Broccard and M.-D. Schaller, Relapsing acute respiratory failure induced by minocycline, *Chest*, 2003, **123**, 2146–2148.

569. H. Bargman, Lack of cross-sensitivity between tetracycline, doxycycline, and minocycline with regard to fixed drug sensitivity to tetracycline, *J. Am. Acad. Dermatol.*, 1984, **11**, 900–901.

570. O. Correia, L. Delgado and J. Polónia, Genital fixed drug eruption: cross-reactivity between doxycycline and minocycline, *Clin. Exp. Dermatol.*, 1999, **24**, 137.

571. R. Altman, Epidemiologic notes and reports: vestibular reactions to minocycline after meningococcal prophylaxis, *Morbid. Mortal.*, 1975, **24**, 9–11.

572. R. Garnier and A. Castot, Ph. Louboutin, D. Muzard and F. Conso, Vestibular like reactions associated with minocycline, *Thérapie*, 1981, **36**, 313–317.

573. W. L. Fanning and D. W. Gump, Vestibular reactions to minocycline – follow-up, *Morbid. Mortal.*, 1975, **24**, 55–56.

574. J. A. Jacobson and B. Daniel, Vestibular reactions associated with minocycline, *Antimicrob. Agents Chemother.*, 1975, **8**, 453–456.

575. C. S. Nicol and J. D. Oriel, Minocycline: possible vestibular side-effects, *Lancet*, 1974, **2**, 1260.

576. D. N. Williams, L. W. Laughlin and Y. H. Lee, Minocycline: possible vestibular side-effects, *Lancet*, 1974, **ii**, 744–746.

577. L. E. Shapiro, S. R. Knowles and N. H. Shear, Comparative safety of tetracycline, minocycline, and doxycycline, *Arch. Dermatol.*, 1997, **133**, 1224–1230.

578. R. Corona, Editorial Comment, *Arch. Dermatol.*, 2000, **136**, 1144–1145.

579. M. J. Ellison, Vancomycin, metronidazole, and tetracyclines, *Clin. Podiatr. Med. Surg.*, 1992, **9**, 425–442.

580. J. J. Hoefnagel, R. L. van Leeuwen, H. Mattie and M. T Bastiaens, Adverse effects of minocycline in the treatment of acne vulgaris, *Ned. Tijdschr. Geneeskd.*, 1997, **19**, 1424–1427.

581. S. Malakar, S. Dhar and R. S. Malakar, Is serum sickness an uncommon adverse effect of minocycline treatment, *Arch. Dermatol.*, 2001, **137**, 100–101.

582. A. H. Eichenfield, Minocycline and autoimmunity, *Curr. Opin. Pediatr.*, 1999, **11**, 447–456.

583. N. H. Shear, Delayed systemic toxicity from minocycline for acne, *J. Watch Dermatol.*, 1996, **301**, 1.

584. W. J. Cunliffe, Doctors should not change the way they prescribe for acne, *BMJ*, 1996, **312**, 1101.

585. K. N. Woodward, Adverse effects of veterinary pharmaceutical products in animals in *Veterinary Pharmacovigilance. Adverse Reactions to Veterinary Medicinal Products*, ed. K. N. Woodward, Wiley-Blackwell, Chichester, 2009, pp. 393–421.

586. G. D. Rifkin, F. R. Fekety and J. Silva, Antibiotic-induced colitis: implication of a toxin neutralised by *Clostridium sordellii* antitoxin, *Lancet*, 1977, **2**, 1103–1106.

587. A. J. Scott, G. I. Nicholson and A. R. Kerr, Lincomycin as a cause of pseudomembranous colitis, *Lancet*, 1973, **2**, 1232–1234.

588. R. I. Frankel, Clindamycin – efficacy and toxicity, *West. J. Med.*, 1975, **122**, 526–530.

589. Committee for Veterinary Medicinal Products, Pirlimycin, EMEA/MRL/719/99-FINAL. Available from: http://www.ema.europa.eu.

590. Committee for Veterinary Medicinal Products, Lincomycin, EMEA/MRL/497/98-FINAL. Available from: http://www.ema.europa.eu.

591. J. E. Gray, A. Purmalis and E. S. Feenstra, Animal toxicity studies of a new antibiotic, lincomycin, *Toxicol. Appl. Pharmacol.*, 1964, **6**, 476–496.

592. J. E. Gray, R. N. Weaver, J. A. Bollert and E. S. Feenstra, The oral toxicity of clindamycin in laboratory animals, *Toxicol. Appl. Pharmacol.*, 1972, **21**, 516–531.

593. J. E. Gray, R. N. Weaver, J. Moran and E. S. Feenstra, The parenteral toxicity of clindamycin 2-phosphate in laboratory animals, *Toxicol. Appl. Pharmacol.*, 1974, **27**, 308–321.

594. J. A. Bollert, J. E. Gray, J. D. Highstreete, J. Moran, B. P. Purmalis and R. N. Weaver, Teratogenicity and neonatal toxicity of clindamycin 2-phosphate in laboratory animals, *Toxicol. Appl. Pharmacol.*, 1974, **27**, 322–329.

595. L. Dorrell, A. Fife, M. H. Snow and E. L. Ong, Toxicity of clindamycin in HIV-infected persons, *Scand. J. Infect. Dis.*, 1992, **24**, 689.

596. N. Smith, C. Blanshard, D. Smith and B. Gazzard, Toxicity of clindamycin and primaquine treatment of AIDS-related *Pneumocystis carinii* pneumonia, *AIDS*, 1993, **7**, 749–750.

597. R. H. Lusk, R. Fekety, J. Silva, R. A. Browne, D. H. Ringler and G. D. Abrams, Clindamycin-induced enterocolitis in hamsters, *J. Infect. Dis.*, 1978, **137**, 464–475.

598. G. D. Rifkin, J. Silva and R. Fekety, Gastrointestinal and systemic toxicity of fecal extracts from hamsters with clindamycin-induced colitis, *Gastroenterology*, 1978, **74**, 52–57.

599. J. D. Small, Fatal enterocolitis in hamsters given lincomycin, *Lab. Anim. Care*, 1968, **18**, 411–420.

600. A. B. Price, H. E. Larson and J. Crow, Morphology of experimental antibiotic-associated enterocolitis in the hamster: a model for human pseudomembranous colitis and antibiotic-associated diarrhoea, *Gut*, 1979, **20**, 467–475.

601. A. B. Onderdonk, T. F. Broasky and B. Bannister, Comparative effects of clindamycin and clindamycin metabolites in the hamster model of antibiotic-associated colitis, *J. Antimicrob. Chemother.*, 1981, **8**, 383–393.

602. F. C. Knoop, Clindamycin associated enterocolitis in guinea pigs: evidence for a bacterial toxin, *Infect. Immun.*, 1979, **23**, 31–33.

603. P. F. Brophy and F. C. Knoop, *Bacillus pumilus* in the induction of clindamycin-associated enterocolitis in guinea pigs, *Infect. Immun.*, 1982, **35**, 289–295.

604. A. J. Scott, Lincomycin-induced cholecystitis and gallstones in guinea pigs, *Gastroenterology*, 1976, **71**, 814–820.

605. K. Lammintausta, R. Tokola and K. Kalimo, Cutaneous adverse reactions to clindamycin: results of skin tests and oral exposure, *Br. J. Dermatol.*, 2002, **146**, 643–648.

606. J. Vicente and J. L. Fontela, Delayed reaction to oral treatment with clindamycin, *Contact Dermatitis*, 1999, **41**, 221.

607. J. P. Ouderkirk, J. A. Nord, G. S. Turett and J. W. Kislak, Polymyxin B nephrotoxicity and efficacy against nosocomial infections caused by multiresistant-Gram negative bacteria, *Antimicrob. Agents Chemother.*, 2003, **47**, 2659–2662.

608. A. Kwa, S. K. Kasiakou, V. H. Tam and M. E. Falagas, Polymyxin B: similarities to and differences from colistin (polymyxin E), *Exp. Rev. Anti-Infect. Ther.*, 2007, **5**, 811–821.

609. J. E. Riviere and J. W. Spoo, Dermatopharmacology: drugs acting locally on the skin in *Veterinary Pharmacology and Therapeutics*, ed. H. R. Adams, Iowa State Press, Ames, 8th edn, 2001, pp. 1084–1104.

610. M. R. Brown and S. M. Wood, Relationship between cation and lipid content of cell walls of *Pseudomonas aeruginosa, Proteus vulgaris* and *Klebsiella aerogenes* and their sensitivity to Polymyxin B and other antibacterial agents, *Pharm. Pharmacol.*, 1972, **24**, 215–218.

611. C. M. Kunin and A. Bugg, Binding of polymyxin antibiotics to tissues: The major determinant of distribution and persistence in the body, *J. Infect. Dis.*, 1971, **124**, 394–400.

612. W. E. Sanders and C. C. Sanders, Toxicity of antibacterial agents: mechanism of action on mammalian cells, *Ann. Rev. Pharmacol. Toxicol.*, 1979, **19**, 53–83.

613. A. Kwa, T.-P. Lim, J. G. H. Low, J. G. Hou, A. Kurup, R. A. Prince and V. H. Tam, Pharmacokinetics of polymixin B₁ in patients with multi-drug-resistant Gram-negative bacterial infections, *Diagn. Microbiol. Infect. Dis.*, 2008, **60**, 163–167.

614. D. Landman, C. Georgescu, D. A. Martin and J. Quale, Polymyxins revisited, *Clin. Microbiol. Rev.*, 2008, **21**, 449–465.

615. C. M. Kunin, The pharmacokinetics of polymixin B are dependent on binding and release from deep-tissue compartments, *Clin. Infect. Dis.*, 2009, **48**, 842–843.

616. Committee for Veterinary Medicinal Products, Colistin, EMEA/MRL/815/02-FINAL. Available from: http://www.ema.europa.eu.

617. D. A. Duncan, Colistin toxicity. Neuromuscular and renal manifestations, *Minn. Med.*, 1973, **56**, 31–35.

618. J. H. Moyer, L. C. Mills and E. M. Yow, Toxicity of polymixin B. I. Animal studies with particular reference to evaluation of renal function, *AMA Arch. Intern. Med.*, 1953, **92**, 238–247.

619. P. N. Swift and S. R. M. Bushby, Clinical aspects of the toxicity of polymyxins A, B, and E., *Lancet*, 1953, **i**, 110–112.

620. S. J. Wallace and J. Li, R. L. Nation, C. R. Rayner, D. Taylor, D. Middleton, R. W. Milne, K. Coulthard and J. D. Turnidge, Subacute toxicity of colistin methanesulfonate in rats: comparison of various intravenous dosage regimens, *Antimicrob. Agents Chemother.*, 2008, **52**, 1159–1161.

621. E. M. Yow and J. H. Moyer, Toxicity of polymyxin B, *AMA Archiv. Intern. Med.*, 1953, **92**, 248–257.

622. M. E. Evans, D. J. Feola and R. P. Rapp, Polymyxin B sulphate and colistin: Old antibiotics for emerging multiresistant Gram-negative bacteria, *Ann. Pharmacother.*, 1999, **33**, 960–967.

623. M. E. Falagas and S. K. Kasiakou, Toxicity of polymyxins: a systematic review of the evidence from old and recent studies, *Crit. Care*, 2006, **10**, http://ccforum.com/content/10/R27.

624. M. E. Sobieszczyk, E. Y. Furuya, C. M. Hay, P. Pancholi, P. Della-Latta, S. M. Hammer and C. J. Kubin, Combination Therapy with polymyxin B for the treatment of multidrug-resistant Gram-negative respiratory tract infections, *J. Antimicrob. Chemother.*, 2004, **54**, 566–569.

625. M. E. Falagas, M. Rizos, I. A. Bliziotis, K. Rellos, S. K. Kasiakou and A. Michalopoulos, Toxicity after prolonged (more than four weeks) administration of intravenous colistin, *BMC Infect. Dis.*, 2005, **5**. http://www.biomedcentral.com/1471-2334-5-1.

626. A. Hakim, H. Kallel, Z. Sahnoun, K. Badraoui, M. Bouaziz, K. M. Zeghal and T. Rebaii, Lack of nephrotoxicity following 15-day therapy with high doses of colistin in rats, *Med. Sci. Monit.*, 2008, **14**, BR74–77.

627. C. H. Chen, W. Flory and R. E. Koeppe, Variation of neurotoxicity of L- and D-2,4-diaminobutyric acid with route of administration, *Toxicol. Appl. Pharmacol.*, 1972, **23**, 334–338.

628. R. M. O'Neal, C. H. Chen, C. S. Reynolds, S. K. Meghal and R. E. Koeppe, The 'neurotoxicity' of L-2,4-diaminobutyric acid, *Biochem. J.*, 1968, **23**, 334–338.

629. Committee for Veterinary Medicinal Products, Tiamulin, EMEA/MRL/578/99-FINAL. Available from: http://www.ema.europa.eu.

630. Committee for Veterinary Medicinal Products, Valnemulin, EMEA/MRL/339/98-FINAL. Available from: http://www.ema.europa.eu.

631. G. Szücs, V. Tamási, P. Laczay and K. Monostory, Biochemical background of toxic interaction between tiamulin and monensin, *Chem. Biol Interact.*, 2004, **147**, 151–161.

632. G. Szücs, P. Laczay, J. Bajnógel and Z. Móra, Studies on the toxic interaction between monensin and tiamulin in rats, *Acta Vet. Hung.*, 2000, **48**, 361–368.

633. G. Szücs, J. Bajnógel, A. Varga, Z. Móra and P. Laczay, Studies on the toxic interaction between monensin and tiamulin in rats: toxicity and pathology, *Acta Vet. Hung.*, 2000, **48**, 209–219.

634. G. Szücs, J. Bajnógel, A. Varga, Z. Móra and P. Laczay, Studies on the interaction between monensin and tiamulin in rats, *Cent. Eur. J. Public Health*, 2000, **8**(Suppl.), 82–83.

635. D. J. Miller, J. J. O'Connor and N. L. Roberts, Tiamulin/salinomycin interactions in pigs, *Vet. Rec.*, 1986, **118**, 73–75.

636. T. Umemura, A. Kawaminami, M. Goryo and C. Itakura, Enhanced myotoxicty and involvement of both type 1 and II fibres in monensin-tiamulin toxicosis in pigs, *Vet. Pathol.*, 1985, **22**, 409–414.

637. N. E. Horrox, Monensin-tiamulin interaction risk to poultry, *Vet. Rec.*, 1980, **106**, 278.

638. K. N. Woodward, Veterinary pharmacovigilance – the UK experience in *Veterinary Pharmacovigilance. Adverse Reactions to Veterinary Medicinal Products*, ed. K. N. Woodward, Wiley-Blackwell, Chichester, 2009, pp. 91–117.

639. R. Macgregor, Suspected adverse reaction to valnemulin in pigs: suspension of the marketing authorisation, *Vet. Rec.*, 2000, **147**, 492.

640. A. Gray, Suspected adverse reactions to valnemulin in pigs, *Vet. Rec.*, 2000, **147**, 372.

641. R. Novak, Are pleuromutilin antibiotics fit for human use? *Ann. N. Y. Acad. Sci.*, 2011, **1241**, 71–81.

642. R. Novak and D. M. Shlaes, The pleuromutilin antibiotics: a new class for human use, *Curr. Opin. Investig. Drugs*, 2010, **11**, 182–191.

643. European Medicines Agency, Concept paper on use of pleuromutilins in food-producing animals in the European Union: development of

resistance and impact on human and animal health, EMA/CVMP/ SAGAM/435644/2011. Available from: http://ema.europa.eu.

644. C. P. Moore, Ophthalmic pharmacology in *Veterinary Pharmacology and Therapeutics*, ed. H. R. Adams, Iowa State Press, Ames, 8th edn, pp. 1120–1148.

645. Committee for Veterinary Medicinal Products, Bacitracin, EMEA/ MRL/768/00-FINAL. Available from: http://ema/europa.eu.

646. B. E. Katz and A. A. Fisher, Bacitracin: a unique topical sensitizer, *J. Am. Acad. Dermatol.*, 1987, **17**, 1016–1024.

647. S. Damm, Intraoperative anaphylaxis associated with bacitracin, *Am. J. Health Syst. Pharm.*, 2011, **68**, 323–327.

648. H. Cronin and C. Mowad, Anaphylactic reaction to bacitracin ointment, *Cutis*, 2009, **83**, 127–129.

649. K. Greenberg, J. Espinosa and V. Scali, Anaphylaxis to topical bacitracin ointment, *Am. J. Emerg. Med.*, 2007, **25**, 95–96.

650. M. Blas, K. S. Briesacher and E. B. Lobato, Bacitracin irrigation: a cause of anaphylaxis in the operating room, *Anesth. Analg.*, 2000, **91**, 1027–1028.

651. E. D. Carver, R. M. Broade, A. R. Atkinson and G. M. Gold, Anaphylaxis during insertion of a ventriculoperitoneal shunt, *Anesthesiology*, 2000, **93**, 578–579.

652. R. Gall, B. Blakley, R. Warrington and D. D. Bell, Intraoperative anaphylactic shock from bacitracin nasal packing after septorhinoplasty, *Anesthesiology*, 1999, **91**, 1545–1547.

653. J. A. Servan, T. C. Dammin and A. E. Bouras, Anaphylaxis to topical bacitracin zinc ointment, *Am. J. Emerg. Med.*, 1998, **16**, 512–513.

654. E. D. Dyck and P. Vadas, Anaphylaxis to topical bacitracin, *Allergy*, 1997, **52**, 870–871.

655. S. R. Knowles and N. H. Shear, Anaphylaxis from bacitracin and polymixin B (Polysporin) ointment, *Int. J. Dermatol.*, 1995, **34**, 572–573.

656. K. A. Fox, Anaphylaxis caused by polymixin B sulfate and zinc bacitracin ointment, *J. Emerg. Nurs.*, 1994, **20**, 262–264.

657. J. Sprung, H. K. Schedewie and J. P. Kampine, Intraoperative anaphylactic shock after bacitracin irrigation, *Anesth. Analg.*, 1990, **71**, 430–433.

658. D. J. Eedy, J. C. McMillan and E. A. Bingham, Anaphylactic reactions to topical antibiotic combinations, *Postgrad. Med. J.*, 1990, **66**, 858–859.

659. C. L. Goh, Anaphylaxis from topical neomycin and bacitracin, *Australas. J. Dermatol.*, 1986, **27**, 125–126.

660. J. F. Schecter, R. D. Wilkinson and J. Del Carpio, Anaphylaxis following the use of bacitracin ointment. Report of a case and review of the literature, *Arch. Dermatol.*, 1984, **120**, 909–911.

661. M. A. Vale, A. Connolly, A. M. Epstein and M. R. Vale, Bacitracin-induced anaphylaxis, *Arch. Dermatol.*, 1978, **114**, 800.

662. G. Roupe and O. Strannegård, Anaphylactic shock elicited by topical administration of bacitracin, *Arch. Dermatol.*, 1969, **100**, 450–452.

663. S. B. Greenberg, M. Deshur, Y. Khavin, E. Karaikovic and J. Vender, Successful resuscitation of a patient who developed cardiac arrest from pulsed saline bacitracin lavage during thoracic laminectomy and fusion, *J. Clin. Anesth.*, 2008, **20**, 294–296.

664. F. L. Lin, D. Woodmansee and R. Patterson, Near-fatal anaphylaxis to topical bacitracin ointment, *J. Allergy Clin. Immunol.*, 1998, **101**, 136–137.

665. S. Sharif and B. Goldberg, Detection of IgE antibodies to bacitracin using a commercially available streptavidin-linked solid phase in a patient with anaphylaxis to triple antibiotic ointment, *Ann. Allergy Asthma Immunol.*, 2007, **98**, 563–566.

666. J. Sowa, D. Tsuruta, H. Kobayashi and M. Ishii, Allergic contact dermatitis caused by colistin sulfate and bacitracin, *Contact Dermatitis*, 2005, **53**, 175–176.

667. J. Lipozencić, Bacitracin contact allergy in Zagreb, *Acta Dermatovenereol. Croat.*, 2007, **15**, 45.

668. J. Y. Yoo, M. Al Naami, O. Markowitz and S. M. Hadi, Allergic contact dermatitis: patch testing results at Mount Sinai Medical Center, *Skinmed.*, 2010, **8**, 257–260.

669. V. Pirlä and S. Rouhunkoski, On sensitivity to neomycin and bacitracin, *Acta Derm. Venereol.*, 1959, **39**, 470–476.

670. V. Pirl, J. Saukkonen and I. M. Santaoja, Hypersensitivity to bacitracin. The influence of degradation upon its eczematogenic effect, *J. Invest. Dermatol.*, 1964, **42**, 137–140.

671. V. Pirlä, L. Förström and S. Rouhunkoski, Twelve years of sensitization to neomycin in Finland. Report of 1760 cases of sensitivity to neomycin and-or bacitracin, *Acta Derm. Venereol.*, 1967, **47**, 419–425.

672. A. A. Fisher, Topical medicants which are common sensitizers, *Ann. Allergy*, 1982, **49**, 97–100.

673. A. A. Fisher, Adverse reactions to bacitracin, polymixin, and gentamicin sulfate, *Cutis*, 1983, **32**, 510–512.

674. A. Hätinen, M. Teräsvirta and J. E. Fräki, Contact allergy to components in topical ophthalmologic preparations, *Acta Ophthalmol. (Copenh.)*, 1985, **63**, 424–426.

675. P. Palungwachira, Contact urticaria syndrome and anaphylactoid reaction from topical clioquinol and bacitracin (Banocin): a case report, *J. Med. Assoc. Thai.*, 1991, **74**, 43–46.

676. I. Zaki, L. Shall and K. L. Dalziel, Bacitracin: a significant sensitizer in leg ulcer patients? *Contact Dermatitis*, 1994, **31**, 92–94.

677. A. A. Fisher, Lasers and allergic contact dermatitis to topical antibiotics, with particular reference to bacitracin, *Cutis*, 1996, **58**, 252–254.

678. L. J. Wright, N. Tomlinson and L. Dy, Antibiotic-associated maculopapular reaction, *Ann. Pharmacother.*, 2002, **36**, 1969.

679. A. Sood and J. S. Taylor, Bacitracin: allergen of the year, *Am. J. Contact Dermat.*, 2003, **14**, 3–4.

680. S. E. Jacob and W. D. James, From road rash to top allergen in a flash: bacitracin, *Dermatol. Surg.*, 2004, **30**, 521–524.

681. S. Nakashio, H. Iwasawa, F. Y. Dun, K. Kanemitsu and J. Shimada, Everninomycin, a new oligosaccharide antibiotic: its antimicrobial activity, post-antibiotic effect and synergistic bactericidal activity, *Drugs Exp. Clin. Res.*, 1995, **21**, 7–16.

682. R. Bool, C. Hoffmann, B. Heitmann, G. Hauser, S. Glaser, T. Koslowski, T. Friedrich and A. Bechtold, The conformation of Avilamycin A is conferred by AviX12, a radical AdoMet enzyme, *J. Biol. Chem.*, 2006, **28**, 14756–14763.

683. Committee for Medicinal Products for Veterinary Use, Avilamycin, EMEA/CVMP/102152/2007-FINAL. Available from: http://www.ema. europa.eu.

684. Joint FAO/WHO Expert Committee on Food Additives, Toxicological Evaluation of Certain Veterinary Drug Residues in Food, The Seventieth Meeting of the Joint FAO/WHO Expert Committee on Food Additives (JECFA), International Programme on Chemical Safety, World Health Organization, Geneva, 2009, pp. 3–36.

685. G. L. Mandell and W. A. Petri, Sulfonamides, trimethoprim-sulphamethoxazole, quinolones, and agents for urinary tract infections in *Goodman and Gilman's The Pharmacological Basis of Therapeutics*, ed. J. G. Hardman, L. E. Limbird, P. B. Molinoff, R. W. Ruddon and A. G. Goodman, McGraw-Hill, London, 9th edn, 1996, pp. 1057–1072.

686. J. W. Spoo and J. E. Riviere, Sulfonamides in *Veterinary Pharmacology and Therapeutics*, ed. H. R. Adams, Iowa State Press, Ames, 8th edn, pp. 796–817.

687. R. J. Bywater, Sulphonamides and other antibacterials in *Veterinary and Applied Pharmacology and Therapeutics*, ed. G. C. Brander, D. M. Pugh and R. J. Bywater, Ballière Tindall, London, 1982, 422–433.

688. O. Sköld, Sulfonamides and trimethoprim, *Expert Rev. Anti Infect. Ther.*, 2010, **8**, 1–6.

689. D. Chan and A. Anderson, Towards species specific antifolates, *Curr. Med. Chem.*, 2006, **13**, 377–398.

690. S. Hawser, S. Luciuro and K. Islam, Dihydrofolate reductase inhibitors as antibacterial agents, *Biochem. Pharmacol.*, 2006, **71**, 941–948.

691. J. Liu, D. B. Bolstad, E. S. D. Bolstad, D. L. Wright and A. C. Anderson, Towards new antifolates targeting eukaryotic opportunistic infections, *Eukaryot. Cell*, 2009, **8**, 483–486.

692. W. Brumfitt and J. M. Hamilton-Miller, Use of trimethoprim alone or in combination with drugs other than sulfonamides, *Rev. Infect. Dis.*, 1982, **4**, 402–410.

693. G. White, S. M. Daluge, C. W. Sigel, R. Ferone and H. R. Wilson, Baquiloprim, a new antifolate antibacterial: *in vitro* activity and pharmacokinetic properties in cattle, *Rev. Vet. Sci.*, 1993, **54**, 372–378.

694. A. S. van Miert, The sulfonamide-diaminopyrimidine story, *J. Vet. Pharmacol. Ther.*, 1994, **17**, 309–316.

695. Committee for Veterinary Medicinal Products, Trimethoprim, EMEA/ MRL/255/97-FINAL. Available from: http://www.ema.europa.eu.
696. Committee for Veterinary Medicinal Products, Baquiloprim, EMEA/ MRL/199/97-FINAL. Available from: http://www.ema.europa.eu.
697. J. Sheehan, The sulfonamide-diaminopyrimidine story, *Lancet*, 1981, **ii**, 692.
698. J. Sheehan, Trimethoprim marrow toxicity, *Lancet*, 1981, **ii**, 1294.
699. R. Danesi and M. Del Tacca, Hematologic toxicity of immunosuppressive treatment, *Transplant. Proc.*, 2004, **36**, 703–704.
700. J. Blatt, D. L. Howrie, M. R. Wollman, C. Phebus and J. Mirro, Toxicity following concurrent intrathecal and moderate-dose intravenous methotrexate, *Leukemia*, 1993, **7**, 1734–1737.
701. M. H. Thomas and L. A. Gutterman, Methotrexate toxicity in a patient receiving trimethoprim-sulfamethoxazole, *J. Rheumatol.*, 1986, **13**, 440–441.
702. R. W. Lacy, P. M. Hawkey, S. K. Devaraj, M. R. Millar, T. J. J. Inglis and P. G. R. Goodwin, Co-trimoxazole toxicity, *BMJ*, 1985, **291**, 481.
703. D. H. Lawson and B. J. Paice, Adverse reactions to trimethoprim-sulfamethoxazole, *Rev. Infect. Dis.*, 1982, **4**, 429–433.
704. S. Elam-Ong, N. A. Kurtzman and S. Sabatini, Studies on the mechanism of trimethoprim-induced hyperkalaemia, *Kidney Int.*, 1996, **49**, 1372–1378.
705. M. A. Marinella, Case report: reversible hyperkalemia associated with trimethoprim-sulfamethoxazole, *Am. J. Med. Sci.*, 1985, **10**, 115–117.
706. T. L. Bell, J. N. Foster and M. L. Townsend, Trimethoprim-sulfamethoxazole-induced hepatotoxicity in a pediatric patient, *Pharmacotherapy*, 2010, **30**, 539.
707. E. Karpman and E. A. Kurzrock, Adverse reactions of nitrofurantoin, trimethoprim and sulfamethoxazole in children, *J. Urol.*, 2004, **172**, 448–453.
708. R. E. Mainra and S. E. Card, Trimethoprim-sulfamethoxazole-associated hepatotoxicity – part of a hypersensitivity syndrome, *Can. J. Clin. Pharmacol.*, 2003, **10**, 175–178.
709. D. C. Twedt, K. J. Diehl, M. R. Lappin and D. M. Getzy, Association of hepatic necrosis with trimethoprim sulfonamide administration in 4 dogs, *J. Vet. Intern. Med.*, 1997, **11**, 20–23.
710. K. N. Woodward, Adverse drug reactions in dogs – toxic hepatic responses in *Veterinary Pharmacovigilance. Adverse Reactions to Veterinary Medicinal Products*, ed. K. N. Woodward, Wiley-Blackwell, Chichester, 2009, pp. 423–452.
711. M. L. Hautekeete, Hepatotoxicity of antibiotics, *Acta Gastroenterol. Belg.*, 1995, **58**, 290–296.
712. M. K. Stamatakis, M. I. Sorkin and A. H. Moss, Toxicity following IP trimethoprim-sulfamethoxazole in a CAPD patient, *Perit. Dial. Int.*, 1995, **15**, 180–181.
713. M. Epstein and J. M. Wright, Severe multisystem disease caused by trimethoprim-sulfamethoxazole: possible role of an *in vitro* lymphocyte assay, *J. Allergy Clin. Immunol.*, 1990, **86**, 416–417.

714. J. B. Frain, Methotrexate toxicity in a patient receiving trimethoprim-sulfamethoxazole, *J. Rheumatol.*, 1987, **14**, 176–177.

715. J. C. Bartlett, H. Park and R. Moe, Hepatic toxicity associated with trimethoprim-sulfamethoxazole: report of a case, *J. Am. Osteopath. Assoc.*, 1985, **85**, 381–382.

716. M. J. Kraemer, R. Kendall, R. O. Hickman, J. E. Haas and C. W. Bierman, A generalized allergic reaction with acute interstitial nephritis following trimethoprim-sulfamethoxazole use, *Ann. Allergy*, 1982, **49**, 323–325.

717. H. Jick, Adverse reactions to trimethoprim-sulfamethoxazole in hospitalized patients, *Rev. Infect. Dis.*, 1982, **4**, 426–428.

718. W. Brumfitt and J. M. Hamilton-Miller, Combinations of sulphonamides with diaminopyrimidines: how, when and why? *J. Chemother.*, 1995, **7**, 136–139.

719. W. Brumfitt and J. M. Hamilton-Miller, Limitations of and indications for the use of co-trimoxazole, *J. Chemother.*, 1994, **6**, 3–11.

720. W. Brumfitt and J. M. Hamilton-Miller, Reassessment of the rationale for the combinations of sulphonamides with diaminopyrimidines, *J. Chemother.*, 1993, **5**, 465–469.

721. T. Harr and L. E. French, Toxic epidermal necrolysis and Stevens-Johnson syndrome, *Orphanet. J. Rare Dis.*, 2010, **5**, 39.

722. C. H. Yang, L. J. Yang, T. H. Yaing and H. L. Chan, Toxic epidermal necrolysis following combination of methotrexate and trimethoprim-sulfamethoxazole, *Int. J. Dermatol.*, 2000, **39**, 621–623.

723. A. J. Salter, The toxicity profile of trimethoprim-sulphamethoxazole after four years of widespread use, *Med. J. Aust.*, 1973, **1**(Suppl.), 70–76.

724. J. W. Kelly, D. P. Dooley, C. P. Lattuada and C. E. Smith, A severe, unusual reaction to trimethoprim-sulfamethoxazole in patients infected with human immunodeficiency virus, *Clin. Infect. Dis.*, 1992, **14**, 1034–1039.

725. A. Pozniak, J. Weinberg and G. Macleod, HIV and co-trimoxazole toxicity, *Lancet*, 1991, **338**, 760–761.

726. F. M. Gordin, G. L. Simon, C. B. Wofsy and J. Mills, Adverse reactions to trimethoprim-sulfamethoxazole in patients with the acquired immunodeficiency syndrome, *Ann. Intern. Med.*, 1984, **100**, 495–499.

727. M. A. Floris-Moore, M. I. Amodio-Groton and M. T. Catalano, Adverse reactions to trimethoprim/sulfamethoxazole in AIDS, *Ann. Pharmacother.*, 2003, **37**, 1810–1813.

728. J. E. Lesch, Prontosil, in *The First Miracle Drugs: How the Sulfa Drugs Transformed Medicine*, Oxford University Press, Oxford, 2007, pp. 51–70.

729. Joint FAO/WHO Expert Committee on Food Additives, Toxicological Evaluation of Certain Veterinary Drug Residues in Food, The 34th Meeting of the Joint FAO/WHO Expert Committee on Food Additives (JECFA), International Programme on Chemical Safety, World Health Organization, Geneva, 1990, pp. 79–93 and 95–98.

730. Joint FAO/WHO Expert Committee on Food Additives, Toxicological Evaluation of Certain Veterinary Drug Residues in Food, The Forty-Second Meeting of the Joint FAO/WHO Expert Committee on Food Additives (JECFA), International Programme on Chemical Safety, World Health Organization, Geneva, 1994, pp. 91–103.
731. E. B. Astwood, J. Sullivan, A. Bissell and R. Tyslowitz, Action of certain sulphonamides and thiourea upon the thyroid gland of rats, *Endocrinol.*, 1943, **32**, 210–225.
732. C. G. MacKenzie and J. B. MacKenzie, Effects of sulphonamides and thiourea on thyroid gland and basal metabolism, *Endocrinol.*, 1943, **32**, 185–209.
733. J. E. Heath and N. A. Littlefield, Effects of subchronic oral sulfamethazine administration on Fischer 344 rats and B6C3F1 mice, *J. Environ. Pathol. Toxicol. Oncol.*, 1984, **5**, 201–214.
734. J. E. Heath and N. A. Littlefield, Morphological effects of subchronic oral sulfamethazine administration on Fischer 344 rats and B6C3F1 mice, *Toxicol. Pathol.*, 1984, **12**, 3–9.
735. N. A. Littlefield, D. W. Gaylor, B. N. Blackwell and R. R. Allen, Chronic toxicity/carcinogenicity studies of sulphamethazine in B6C3F1 mice, *Food Chem. Toxicol.*, 1989, **27**, 455–463.
736. N. A. Littlefield, W. G. Sheldon, R. R. Allen and D. W. Gaylor, Chronic toxicity/carcinogenicity studies of sulphamethazine in Fischer 344/N rats: two-generation exposure, *Food Chem. Toxicol.*, 1990, **28**, 156–167.
737. S. Nishikawa, Effects of sulfonamide on the pituitary-thyroid gland. 1. morphological changes of thyroid gland and variation in plasma thyroxine and triiodothyronine, *J. Toxicol. Sci.*, 1983, **8**, 47–59.
738. S. Nishikawa, Effects of sulfonamide on the pituitary-thyroid gland. 2. morphological changes of thyrotrophs in anterior pituitary gland, *J. Toxicol. Sci.*, 1983, **8**, 61–70.
739. F. R. Fullerton, R. J. Kushmaul, R. L. Suber and N. A. Littlefield, Influence of oral administration of sulfamethazine on thyroid hormone levels in Fischer 344 rats, *J. Toxicol. Environ. Health*, 1983, **22**, 175–185.
740. A. Gupta, M. C. Eggo, J. P. Uetrecht, A. E. Cribb, D. Daneman, M. J. Rieder, N. H. Shear, M. Cannon and S. P. Spielberg, Drug-induced hypothyroidism: the thyroid as a target organ in hypersensitivity to anticonvulsants and sulfonamides, *Clin. Pharmacol. Ther.*, 1992, **51**, 56–67.
741. I. C. Shaw and H. B. Jones, Mechanisms of non-genotoxic carcinogenesis, *Trends Pharmacol. Sci.*, 1994, **15**, 89–93.
742. R. M. McClain, Mechanistic considerations for the relevance of animal data on thyroid neoplasia to human risk assessment, *Mutat. Res.*, 1995, **333**, 131–142.
743. R. N. Hill, T. M. Crisp, P. M. Hurley, S. L. Rosenthal and D. V. Singh, Thyroid follicular cell carcinogenesis, *Fundam. Appl. Toxicol.*, 1996, **12**, 627–697.
744. L. A. Poirier, D. R. Doerge, D. W. Gaylor, M. A. Miller, R. J. Lorentzen, D. A. Casciano, F. F. Kadlubar and B. A. Schwetz, An FDA

review of sulfamethazine toxicity, *Regul. Toxicol. Pharmacol.*, 1999, **30**, 217–222.

745. L. Y. Altholtz, K. M. La Perle and F. W. Quimby, Dose-dependent hypothyroidism in mice induced by commercial trimethoprim-sulfamethoxazole rodent feed, *Comp. Med.*, 2006, **56**, 395–401.

746. H. Onodera, K. Mitsumori, M. Yakahashi, T. Shimo, K. Yasuhara, K. Kitaura, M. Takahashi and Y. Hayashi, Thyroid proliferative lesions induced by anti-thyroid drugs in rats are not always accompanied by sustained increases in serum TSH, *J. Toxicol. Sci.*, 1994, **19**, 227–234.

747. Y. Ohmachi, W. Torium, K. Takashima and K. Doi, Systemic histopathology of rats treated with 6-sulfanilamidoindazole, a novel arthritogenic sulfonamide, *Toxicol. Pathol.*, 1998, **28**, 262–270.

748. M. Torii, F. Itoh, K. Yabuuchi, K. Ohno, G. Kominami, K. Hirano, T. Tasaki and H. Nara, Twenty-six-week carcinogenicity study of sulfamethoxazole in CB6F1-Tg-rasH2 mice, *J. Toxicol. Sci.*, 2001, **26**, 61–63.

749. R. L. Swarm, G. K. S. Roberts, A. C. Levy and L. R. Hines, Observations on the thyroid gland in rats following the administration of sulfamethoxazole and trimethoprim, *Toxicol. Appl. Pharmacol.*, 1973, **24**, 351–363.

750. T. Shimo, Y. Takahara, Y. Noguchi, A. Mukawa, H. Kato and Y. Ito, Comparative toxicity test of dexamethasone valerate (DV-17) and other steroid ointments in rats, *J. Toxicol. Sci.*, 1982, **7**, 15–33.

751. T. Shimo, K. Mitsumori, H. Onodera, M. Takahashi, Y. Ueno, J. Katayama, A. Saito and M. Takahashi, Effect of rat thyroid proliferative development by intermittent treatment with sulfadimethoxine, *Cancer Lett.*, 1995, **96**, 209–218.

752. T. Shimo, K. Mitsumori, M. Takahashi, J. Katayama, A. Saito, H. Yoshida, Y. Aoki, H. Onodera and M. Takahashi, Comparison of ultrastructural changes in thyrotrophs of rat pituitary between intermittent and continuous treatments with sulfadimethoxine, *Toxicol. Pathol.*, 1997, **25**, 177–185.

753. T. Imai, J. Onose, M. Hasumura, M. Ueda, T. Takizawa and M. Hirose, Sequential analysis of development of invasive thyroid follicular cell carcinomas in inflamed capsular regions of rats treated with sulfadimethoxine after N-bis(2-hydroxypropyl)nitrosamine induction, *Toxicol. Pathol.*, 2004, **32**, 229–236.

754. T. Imai, M. Hasumura, J. Onose, M. Ueda, T. Takizawa, Y. M. Cho and M. Hirose, Development of invasive follicular cell carcinomas in a rat thyroid carcinogenesis model: biological impact of capsular inflammation and reduced cyclooxygenase-2 expression, *Cancer Sci.*, 2005, **96**, 31–37.

755. K. Mitsumori, H. Onodera, M. Takahashi, T. Shimo, K. Yasuhara, K. Kitaura, M. Takahashi and Y. Hayashi, Effect of thyroid stimulating hormone on the development and progression of rat thyroid follicular cell tumors, *Cancer Lett.*, 1995, **92**, 193–202.

756. S. Daminet and D. C. Ferguson, Influence of drugs on thyroid function in dogs, *J. Vet. Intern. Med.*, 2003, **17**, 463–472.

757. L. A. Trepanier, R. Danhof, J. Toll and D. Watrous, Clinical findings in 40 dogs with hypersensitivity associated with administration of potentiated sulfonamides, *J. Vet. Intern. Med.*, 2003, **17**, 647–652.

758. International Agency for Research on Cancer, Sulfamethazine and its sodium salt, IARC Monographs on the Evaluation of Carcinogenic Risks to Humans, *Some Thyrotropic Agents*, IARC, Lyon, 2001, vol. 79, pp. 341–359.

759. International Agency for Research on Cancer, Sulfamethoxazole. IARC Monographs on the Evaluation of Carcinogenic Risks to Humans, *Some Thyrotropic Agents*, IARC, Lyon, 2001, vol. 79, pp. 361–378.

760. K. N. Woodward, The regulation of carcinogenic veterinary drugs: the carcinogenicity of sulphadimidine – risk assessment for veterinary use in food-producing animals, *Hum. Exp. Toxicol.*, 1991, **10**, 84.

761. K. N. Woodward, Carcinogenicity of sulphadimidine, *Hum. Exp. Toxicol.*, 1992, **11**, 60–61.

762. K. N. Woodward, Concordance between results from animal toxicology studies and adverse reactions in animals in *Veterinary Pharmacovigilance. Adverse Reactions to Veterinary Medicinal Products*, ed. K. N. Woodward, Wiley-Blackwell, Chichester, 2009, pp. 715–748.

763. G. W. Thrasher, J. E. Shively, C. E. Askelson, W. E. Babcock and R. R. Chalquest, Effects of feeding carbadox upon the growth and performance in young pigs, *J. Anim. Sci.*, 1969, **28**, 208–215.

764. J. C. Downing, Carbadox for control of swine dysentery, *Mod. Vet. Pract.*, 1974, **55**, 167–168.

765. K. Bronsch, D. Schneider and F. Rigal-Antonelli, Olaquindox – a new growth promoting feed additive. I. Effectiveness in raising piglets, *Z. Tierphysiol. Tierernähr. Futtermittelkd.*, 1976, **36**, 211–221.

766. G. C. Brander, Growth promoters in *Veterinary and Applied Pharmacology and Therapeutics*, ed. G. C. Brander, D. M. Pugh and R. J. Bywater, Ballière Tindall, London, 1982, pp. 434–450.

767. J. M. Holder and A. N. Sinclair, Carbadox: a new feed additive for pigs, *Aust. Vet. J.*, 1972, **48**, 579.

768. E. T. Kornegay, J. W. Davis and H. R. Thomas, Evaluation of carbadox in prevention of swine dysentery, *Vet. Med. Small Anim. Clinic*, 1968, **63**, 1076–1077.

769. M. J. A. Nabuurs and E. R. van der Molen, Clinical signs and performance of pigs during the administration of different levels of carbadox and after withdrawal, *J. Vet. Med.*, 1989, **36A**, 209–217.

770. M. J. Nabuurs, E. J. van der Molen, G. J. de Graaf and L. P. Jager, Clinical signs and performance of pigs treated with different doses of carbadox, cyadox and olaquindox, *Zentralbl. Veterinarmed. Reihe A*, 1990, **37**, 68–76.

771. R. H. Rainier, R. R. Chalquest, W. E. Babcock and G. W. Thrasher, Therapeutic efficiency of carbadox in field outbreaks of swine dysentery, *Vet. Med. Small Anim. Clinic.*, 1973, **68**, 272–276.

772. D. Schneider, K. Bronsch and L. Richter, Olaquindox – a new growth promoting feed additive. II. Effects on the performance in swine fattening, *Z. Tierphysiol. Tierernähr. Futtermittelkd.*, 1976, **36**, 241–248.

773. K. N. Woodward, The toxicity of particular veterinary drug residues in *Pesticide, Veterinary and Other Residues in Food*, ed. D. H. Watson, CRC Press/Woodhead Publishing, Boca Raton/Cambridge, 2004, pp. 175–223.

774. Joint FAO/WHO Expert Committee on Food Additives, Toxicological Evaluation of Certain Veterinary Drug Residues in Food, The Thirty-Sixth Meeting of the Joint FAO/WHO Expert Committee on Food Additives (JECFA), International Programme on Chemical Safety, World Health Organization, Geneva, 1991, pp. 141–173 and 175–210.

775. I. Sykora and V. Vortel, Post-natal study of the carcinogenicity of cyadox and carbadox, *Biol. Chem. Ziv. Vyrob. Vet. (Praha)*, 1986, **22**, 52–62.

776. L. Beutin, E. Preller and B. Kowalski, Mutagenicity of quindoxin, its metabolites, and two substituted quinoxaline-di-N-oxides, *Antimicrob. Agents Chemother.*, 1981, **20**, 336–343.

777. R. Cihak and V. Srb, Cytogenetic effects of quinoxaline-1,4-dioxide-type growth promoting agents. I. micronucleus test in rats, *Mutat. Res.*, 1983, **116**, 129–135.

778. R. Cihak and M. Vontorkova, Cytogenetic effects of quinoxaline-1,4-dioxide-type growth promoting agents. II. Metaphase analysis in mice, *Mutat. Res.*, 1983, **117**, 311–316.

779. R. Cihak and M. Vontorkova, Cytogenetic effects of quinoxaline-1,4-dioxide-type growth promoting agents. III. Transplacental micronucleus test in rats, *Mutat. Res.*, 1985, **144**, 81–84.

780. T. Negishi, K. Tanaka and H. Hayatsu, Mutagenicity of carbadox and several quinoxaline 1,4-dioxide derivatives, *Chem. Pharm. Bull.*, 1980, **28**, 1347–1349.

781. T. Ohta, M. Moriya, Y. Kaneda, K. Watanabe, T. Miyazawa, F. Sugiyama and Y. Shirasu, Mutagenicity screening of feed additives in the microbial system, *Mutat. Res.*, 1980, **77**, 21–30.

782. J. L. Oud, A. H. Reutlinger and J. Branger, An investigation into the cytogenetic damage induced by the coccidiostatic agents amprolium, carbadox, dimetridazole and ronidazole, *Mutat. Res.*, 1979, **68**, 179–182.

783. M. Scheutwinkel-Reich and W. Hude, Sister-chromatid exchange in Chinese hamster V79 cells exposed to quindoxin, carbadox and olaquindox, *Mutat. Res.*, 1984, **139**, 199–202.

784. C. F. Voogd, J. J. van der Stel and J. J. Jacobs, The mutagenic action of quindoxin, carbadox, olaquindox and some other N-oxides on bacteria and yeast, *Mutat. Res.*, 1980, **78**, 233–242.

785. H. Yoshimura, M. Nakamura, T. Koeda and K. Yoshikawa, Muta-genicities of carbadox and olaquindox – growth promoters for pigs, *Mutat. Res.*, 1981, **90**, 49–55.

786. Q. Chen, Y. Chen, Y. Qi, L. Hao, S. Tang and X. Xiao, Characterization of carbadox-induced mutagenesis using a shuttle vector pSP189 in mammalian cells, *Mutat. Res.*, 2008, **638**, 11–16.

787. Q. Chen, S. Tang, X. Jin, J. Zou, K. Chen, T. Zhang and X. Xiao, Investigation of quinocetone, carbadox and olaquindox in vitro using Vero cells, *Food Chem. Toxicol.*, 2009, **47**, 328–334.

788. R. Truhaut, R. Ferrando, J. M. Faccini and A. M. Monro, Negative results of carcinogenicity bioassay of methyl carbazate in rats: significance for the toxicological evaluation of carbadox, *Toxicology*, 1981, **22**, 219–221.

789. Z. Y. Liu, Y. F. Tao, D. M. Chen, X. Wang and Z. H. Yuan, Identification of carbadox metabolites formed by liver microsomes from rats, pigs and chickens using high-performance liquid chromatography combined with hybrid ion trap/time-of-flight mass spectrometry, *Rapid Commun. Mass Spectrom.*, 2011, **30**, 341–348.

790. R. Truhaut and R. Ferrando, General principles for a new methodological approach for the toxicologic evaluation of additives to food of animal origin, *Toxicology*, 1975, **3**, 361–368.

791. K. M. Orsted, S. A. Dubay, M. F. Raisbeck, R. S. Siemion, D. A. Sanchez and E. S. Williams, Lack of relay toxicity in ferret hybrids fed carbaryl-treated prairie dogs, *J. Wildl. Dis.*, 1998, **34**, 362–364.

792. E. Craine, Relay toxicity studies: a modification of the relay toxicity approach, *J. Toxicol. Environ. Health*, 1977, **2**, 905–907.

793. H. Gallo-Torres, Methodology for the determination of bioavailability of labelled residues, *J. Toxicol. Environ. Health*, 1977, **2**, 827–845.

794. H. Gallo-Torres, The rat as a drug residue bioavailability model, *Drug Metab. Rev.*, 1990, **22**, 707–751.

795. P. S. Jaglan, M. W. Glenn and A. W. Neff, Experiences in dealing with drug-related bound residues, *J. Toxicol. Environ. Health*, 1977, **2**, 815–826.

796. R. Ferrando and R. Truhaut, General aspects of relay toxicity: its applications, *Toxicol. Eur. Res.*, 1982, **IV**, 221–228.

797. P. Evrard and G. Maghuin-Rogister, In vitro metabolism of trenbolone: study of the formation of covalently bound residues, *Food Addit. Contam.*, 1987, **5**, 59–65.

798. A. Y. H. Lu, P. G. Wislocki, S.-H. L. Chiu and G. T. Miwa, Tissue drug residues and their toxicological significance, *Drug Metab. Rev.*, 1987, **18**, 363–378.

799. A. Y. H. Lu, G. T. Miwa and P. G. Wislocki, Toxicological significance of covalently bound drug residues, *Rev. Biochem. Toxicol.*, 1988, **9**, 1–27.

800. D. Arnold, EEC perspectives on relay toxicity and bioavailability studies, *Drug Metab. Rev.*, 1990, **22**, 699–705.

801. J. Boisseau, Relay toxicity, *Drug Metab. Rev.*, 1990, **22**, 685–697.

802. J. M. Frazier, Application of the basic toxicological screening process to problems in bound residue toxicity, *Drug Metab. Rev.*, 1990, **22**, 821–827.
803. G. B. Guest and S. C. Fitzpatrick, Overview on bound residue issue – regulatory aspects, *Drug Metab. Rev.*, 1990, **22**, 595–599.
804. G. Weiss, The integration of pharmacological and toxicological testing of tissue residues in the evaluation of their human food safety, *Drug Metab. Rev.*, 1990, **22**, 829–848.
805. M. S. Yong, Potential use of isolated organ or tissue preparations in the assessment of biological activities of bound residues, *Drug Metab. Rev.*, 1990, **28**, 753–763.
806. D. M. Galer and A. Monro, Veterinary drugs no longer need testing for carcinogenicity in rodent bioassays, *Regul. Toxicol. Pharmacol.*, 1998, **28**, 115–123.
807. W. G. Huber, S. R. Becker and B. P. Archer, Bioavailability of residues: current status, *J. Exp. Pathol. Toxicol.*, 1980, **3**, 45–63.
808. K. Mitsumori, Scientific basis in the setting of residue limits for veterinary drugs in food of animal origin taking into account the presence of their metabolites, *Eisei Shikenjo Hokuku*, 1993, **111**, 148–149.
809. J. L. Stevens and A. Wallin, Is the toxicity of cysteine conjugates formed during mercapturic acid biosynthesis relevant to the toxicity of covalently bound drug residues? *Drug Metab. Rev.*, 1990, **22**, 617–635.
810. P. Wislocki and A. Y. Lu, Formation and biological evaluation of ronidazole bound residues, *Drug Metab. Rev.*, 1990, **22**, 649–661.
811. S. Klee, I. Baumung, K. Kluge, F. R. Ungemach, E. Horne, M. O'Keefe, I. De Angelis, A. L. Vignoli, F. Zucco and A. Stammati, A contribution to safety assessment of veterinary drug residues: in vivo/ex vivo studies on the intestinal toxicity and transport of covalently bound residues, *Xenobiotica*, 1999, **29**, 641–654.
812. D. Maume, Y. Deceuninck, K. Pouponneua, A. Paris, B. Le Bizec and F. André, Assessment of estradiol and its metabolites in meat, *Acta Pathol. Microbiol. Immunol. Scand.*, 2001, **109**, 32–38.
813. R. Ferrando, R. Truhaut, J.-P. Raynaud and J.-P. Spanoghe, A method for the assessment of safety to human consumers of carbadox, a growth promoting additive to the feed of slaughter pigs, *Toxicology*, 1975, **3**, 369–398.
814. R. Ferrando, R. Truhaut and J.-P. Raynaud, Principles of a full relay toxicity experiment and results conducted with carbadox a feed additive used as a growth promoter for growing swine, *Folia Vet. Lat.*, 1977, **7**, 333–340.
815. R. Ferrando, R. Truhaut, J.-P. Raynaud and J.-P. Spanogue, Safety in use for the human consumer of carbadox, a feed additive for swine, as estimated by a 7 year relay toxicity on dogs, *Toxicology*, 1978, **11**, 167–183.
816. W. Suter, A. Rosselet and F. Knusel, Mode of action of quindoxin and substituted quinoxaline-di-N-oxides on Escherichia coli, *Antimicrob. Agents Chemother.*, 1978, **13**, 770–783.

817. D. Pokorna, Cytogenetic analysis of bone marrow cells in Chinese hamster after the administration of cyadox and olaquindox, *Biol. Chem. Ziv. Vyrob. Vet. (Praha)*, 1986, **22**, 23–28.

818. R. J. Sram, S. F. Fernandez Rodriguez and J. Kocisova, Chromosomal aberration in the bone marrow of mice after long-continued administration of cyadox and olaquindox, *Biol. Chem. Ziv. Vyrob. Vet. (Praha)*, 1986, **22**, 17–22.

819. R. J. Sram, S. F. Fernandez Rodriguez and J. Kocisova, Effect of long-term oral administration of cyadox and olaquindox on the frequency of dominant lethal mutations and sperm abnormalities in mice, *Biol. Chem. Ziv. Vyrob. Vet. (Praha)*, 1986, **22**, 37–45.

820. R. J. Sram, S. F. Fernandez Rodriguez and J. Kocisova, Dominant lethal mutation in female mice following the oral application of cyadox and olaquindox, *Biol. Chem. Ziv. Vyrob. Vet. (Praha)*, 1986, **22**, 29–35.

821. W. von der Hude, C. Behm, R. Gurtler and A. Basler, Evaluation of the SOS chromotest, *Mutat. Res.*, 1988, **203**, 81–94.

822. T. Nunoshiba and H. Nishioka, Genotoxicity of quinoxaline 1,4-dioxide derivatives in Escherichia coli and Salmonella typhimurium, *Mutat. Res.*, 1989, **217**, 23–28.

823. L. Hao, Q. Chen and X. Xiao, Molecular mechanism of mutagenesis by olaquindox using a shuttle vector pSP189/mammalian cell system, *Mutat. Res.*, 2006, **599**, 21–25.

824. J. Zou, Q. Chen, S. Tang, X. Jin, K. Chen, T. Zhang and X. Xiao, Olaquindox-induced genotoxicity and oxidative DNA damage in hepatoma G2 (HepG2) cells, *Mutat. Res.*, 2009, **676**, 27–33.

825. G. Fang, Q. He, S. Zhou, D. Wang, Y. Zhang and Z. Yuan, Subchronic feeding study with cyadox in Wistar rats, *Food Chem. Toxicol.*, 2006, **44**, 36–41.

826. X. Wang, G. J. Fang, Y. L. Wang, A. Ihsan, L. L. Huang, W. Zhou, Z. L. Liu and Z. H. Yuan, Two generation reproduction and teratogenicity studies of feeding cyadox in Wistar rats, *Food. Chem. Toxicol.*, 2011, **49**, 1068–1079.

827. X. Wang, Q. H. He, Y. L. Wang, A. Ihsan, L. L. Huang, W. Zhou, S. J. Su, Z. L. Liu and Z. H. Yuan, A chronic toxicity study of cyadox in Wistar rats, *Regul. Toxicol. Pharmacol.*, 2011, **59**, 324–333.

828. V. Bilá and V. Kren, Teratogenicity testing based on interaction with mutant allele, *Folia Biol. (Praha)*, 1992, **38**, 40–47.

829. H. Yoshimura, Teratogenic assessment of carbadox in rats, *Toxicol. Lett.*, 2002, **129**, 115–118.

830. S. Schauder, W. Schröder and J. Geier, Olaquindox-induced airborne photoallergic contact dermatitis followed by transient or persistent light reactions in 15 pig breeders, *Contact Dermatitis*, 1996, **35**, 344–354.

831. S. Francalanci, M. Gola, S. Giorgini, A. Muccinelli and A. Sertoli, Occupational photocontact dermatitis from Olaquindox, *Contact Dermatitis*, 1986, **15**, 112–114.

832. P. G. Bordello, M. Goitre, D. Cane and G. Roncarolo, Allergic contact dermatitis to Bayo-N-ox-1, *Contact Dermatitis*, 1985, **12**, 284.

833. J. Sánchez-Pérez, M. P. López and A. Garcia-Diez, Airborne allergic contact dermatitis from olaquindox in a rabbit breeder, *Contact Dermatitis*, 2002, **46**, 185.

834. R. Hochsattel, H. Gall, L. Weber and R. Kaufmann, Photoallergic dermatitis to olaquindox, *Hautarzt.*, 1991, **42**, 233–236.

835. C. Willa-Craps, P. Eisner and G. Burg, Olaquindox-induced persistent light reaction treated by Escherichia coli filtrate (Colobiogene), *Dermatology*, 1995, **191**, 343–344.

836. B. Eberlein, T. Bergner and B. Przybilla, Demonstration of olaquindox photosensitivity in vitro, *Photodermatol. Photoimmunol. Photomed.*, 1992, **9**, 63–66.

837. J. Fewings and J. Horton, Photoallergic dermatitis to a pig feed additive, *Australas. J. Dermatol.*, 1995, **36**, 99.

838. A. Kumar and S. Freeman, Photoallergic contact dermatitis in a pig farmer caused by olaquindox, *Contact Dermatitis*, 1996, **35**, 249–250.

839. S. Schauder, Photoallergy, chronic dermatitis and extreme increased photosensitivity in the human, hypoaldosteronism in swine, *Derm. Beruf. Umwelt.*, 1989, **37**, 183–185.

840. J. Lonceit, B. Sassolas and G. Guillet, Photoallergic reactions to olaquindox in swine raisers: role of growth promotors used in feed, *Ann. Dermatol. Venereol.*, 2001, **128**, 46–48.

841. P. Sánchez-Pedreño, J. Frias, J. Martinez-Escribano, M. Rodriguez and S. Hernández-Carrasco, Occupational photoallergic contact dermatitis to olaquindox, *Am. J. Contact Derm.*, 2001, **12**, 236–238.

842. H. Belhadjali, M. V. Marguerry, F. Journé, F. Giordano-Labadie, H. Lefebvre and J. Bazex, Allergic and photoallergic contact dermatitis to Olaquindox in a pig breeder with prolonged photosensitivity, *Photodermatol. Photoimmunol. Photomed.*, 2002, **18**, 52–53.

843. H. de Vries, J. Bojarski, A. A. Donker, A. Bakri and G. M. Beyersbergen van Henegouwen, Photochemical reactions of quindoxin, olaquindox, carbadox and cyadox with protein, indicating photoallergic properties, *Toxicology*, 1990, **63**, 85–95.

844. Q. He, G. Fang, Y. Wang, Z. Wei, D. Wang, S. Zhou, S. Fan and Z. Yuan, Experimental evaluation of cyadox phototoxicity to Balb/c mouse skin, *Photodermatol. Photoimmunol. Photomed.*, 2006, **22**, 100–104.

845. F. W. van Schie, A case of carbadox poisoning, *Tijdschr. Diergeneeskd.*, 1982, **107**, 428.

846. S. B. Power, W. J. C. Donnelly, J. G. McLaughlin, M. C. Walsh and M. F. Dromey, Accidental carbadox overdosage in pigs in an Irish weaner-producing herd, *Vet. Rec.*, 1989, **124**, 367–370.

847. K. H. Waldmann, D. Kikovic and N. Stockhofe, Clinical and haematological changes after olaquindox poisoning in fattening pigs, *Zentralbl. Veterinarmed. Reihe A*, 1989, **36**, 676–686.

848. L. P. Jager, A. S. van Miert and L. H. Vroomen, Chronic furazolidone poisoning in swine? Practical problems and legal consequences, *Tijdschr. Diergeneeskd.*, 1984, **109**, 922–927.

849. A. S. J. P. A. M. van Miert, L. H. M. Vroomen and L. P. Jager, Pharmacology and toxicology of furazolidone and carbadox, *Tijdschr. Diergeneeskd.*, 1984, **109**, 928–933.

850. P. van de Kerk, Drug toxicity in piglets following long-term consumption of medicated feed, *Tijdschr. Diergeneeskd.*, 1985, **110**, 181–184.

851. E. J. van der Molen, Pathological effects of carbadox in pigs with special emphasis on the adrenal, *J. Comp. Pathol.*, 1988, **98**, 55–67.

852. E. J. van der Molen, M. J. A. Nabuurs and L. P. Lager, Pathological and clinical changes related to toxicity of carbadox in weaned pigs, *Zentralbl. Veterinarmed. Reihe A*, 1985, **32**, 540–550.

853. E. J. van der Molen, G. J. de Graaf, A. J. Baars and W. Schopman, Carbadox induced changes in aldosterone, sodium and potassium levels in the blood of weaned pigs, *J. Vet. Med.*, 1986, **33**, 617–623.

854. E. J. van der Molen, G. J. Graaf, T. J. Spierenburg, M. J. A. Nabuurs, A. J. Baars and L. P. Jager, Hypoaldosteronism in piglets induced by carbadox, *Experientia*, 1986, **42**, 1247–1249.

855. E. J. van der Molen, F. H. M. Derkx, A. P. M. Lamers, J. H. L. M. van Lieshout, M. J. A. Nabuurs and A. M. Michelakis, Changes in plasma rennin activity and renal immunohistochemically demonstrated rennin in carbadox treated pigs, *Res. Vet. Sci.*, 1989, **46**, 401–405.

856. E. J. van der Molen, G. J. de Graaf and A. J. Baars, Persistence of carbadox-induced adrenal lesions in pigs following drug withdrawal and recovery of aldosterone plasma concentrations, *J. Comp. Pathol.*, 1989, **100**, 295–304.

857. E. J. van der Molen, A. J. Baars, G. J. de Graaf and L. P. Jager, Comparative study of carbadox, olaquindox and cyadox on aldosterone, sodium and potassium levels in weaned pigs, *Res. Vet. Sci.*, 1989, **47**, 11–16.

858. M. J. A. Nabuurs and E. J. van der Molen, Clinical signs and performance of pigs during the administration of different levels of carbadox and after withdrawal, *J. Vet. Med.*, 1989, **36A**, 209–217.

859. M. J. A. Nabuurs, E. J. van der Molen, G. J. de Graaf and L. P. Jager, Clinical signs and performance of pigs treated with different levels of carbadox, cyadox and olaquindox, *Zentralbl. Veterinarmed. Reihe A*, 1990, **37**, 68–76.

860. T. J. Spierenburg, A. J. Baars, G. J. de Graaf and L. P. Jager, Carbadox-induced inhibition of aldosterone production in porcine adrenals in vitro, *Toxicol. In Vitro*, 1988, **2**, 141–143.

861. European Commission, Commission Regulation (EC) No. 2788/98 of 22 December 1998 amending Council Directive 70/524/EEC concerning additives in feedingstuffs as regards the withdrawal of authorisation for certain growth promoters, *Offic. J. Eur. Commun.*, 1998, **L347**, 31–32.

862. M. Casewell, C. Friis, E. Marco, P. McMullin and I. Phillips, The European ban on growth-promoting antibiotics and emerging consequences for human and animal health, *J. Antimicrob. Chemother.*, 2003, **52**, 159–161.

863. J. J. Dibner and J. D. Richards, Antibiotic growth promoters in agriculture: History and mode of action, *Poultry Sci.*, 2005, **84**, 634–643.

864. R. J. Bywater, Benefits and microbiological risks of food additive antibiotics, *Cahiers Options Mediterran.*, 1999, **37**, 77–82.

865. F. M. Aarestrup, Effects of termination of AGP use on antimicrobial resistance in food animals in *Beyond Antimicrobial Growth Promoters in Food Animal Production*, Foulum, Denmark, November 2002.

866. S. Holtz, Reducing and phasing out the use of antibiotics and hormone growth promoters in Canadian agriculture, Canadian Institute for Environmental Law and Policy, Toronto, 2009.

867. D. Tennstedt, M. Dumont-Fruytier and J. M. Lachapelle, Occupational allergic contact dermatitis to virginiamycin, an antibiotic used as a food additive for pigs and poultry, *Contact Dermatitis*, 1978, **4**, 133–134.

868. J. M. Lachapelle and F. Lamy, On allergic contact dermatitis to virginiamycin, *Dermatologica*, 1973, **146**, 320–322.

869. A. Barriga, C. Romaguera and J. Vilaplana, Contact dermatitis from avoparcin, *Contact Dermatitis*, 1992, **27**, 115.

870. D. J. Hayes, H. H. Jensen, L. Backstrom and J. Fabiosa, Economic impact of a ban on the use of over the counter antibiotics in U.S. swine rations, *Int. Food Agribus. Manag. Rev.*, 2001, **4**, 81–97.

871. B. H. Ali, Plasma and histological changes in furazolidone treated chickens, *Res. Vet. Sci.*, 1984, **37**, 290–292.

872. J. A. Frankhauser, B. Bien and R. Cottingham, Nitrofurazone toxicity in dairy calves, *Vet. Med. Small. Anim. Clinic.*, 1981, **76**, 861–862.

873. J. W. Finnie, Two clinical manifestations of furazolidone toxicity in calves, *Aust. Vet. J.*, 1992, **69**, 21.

874. E. E. Lister and L. J. Fisher, Establishment of the toxic level of nitrofurazone for young liquid-fed calves, *J. Dairy Sci.*, 1970, **53**, 1490–1495.

875. P. J. O'Brien, M. O'Grady, J. H. Lumsden, D. L. Holmberg, H. Shen, J. E. Weller, R. D. Horn, S. M. Mirsalimi and R. J. Julian, Clinical pathologic profiles of dogs and turkeys with congestive heart failure, either noninduced or induced by ventricular pacing, and turkeys with furazolidone toxicosis, *Am. J. Vet. Res.*, 1993, **54**, 60–68.

876. J. D. Taylor, J. A. Gibson and C. Yeates, Furazolidone toxicity in dairy calves, *Aust. Vet. J.*, 1991, **68**, 182–183.

877. J. F. van Vleet and V. J. Ferrans, Myocardial diseases of animals, *Am. J. Pathol.*, 1986, **124**, 98–178.

878. A. Altamirano and A. Bondani, Adverse reactions to furazolidone and other drugs. A comparative review, *Scand. J. Gastroenterol.*, 1989, **169**(Suppl.), 70–80.

879. A. Ancona, Allergic contact dermatitis to nitrofurazone, *Contact Dermatitis*, 1985, **13**, 35.

880. A. C. de Groot and M. H. Conemans, Contact allergy to furazolidone, *Contact Dermatitis*, 1990, **22**, 202–205.

881. S. Burge and A. Bransbury, Allergic contact dermatitis due to furazolidone in a piglet medication, *Contact Dermatitis*, 1994, **31**, 199–200.

882. A. K. Bajaj and S. C. Gupta, Contact hypersensitivity to topical antibacterial agents, *Int. J. Dermatol.*, 1986, **25**, 103–105.

883. J. S. Low, J. S. Taylor and H. Oriba, Occupational allergic contact dermatitis to airborne nitrofurazone, *Dermatologic. Clin.*, 1990, **8**, 165–168.

884. P. L. Olive and D. R. McCalla, Cytotoxicity and DNA damage to mammalian cells by nitrofurans, *Chem. Biol. Interact.*, 1977, **16**, 223–233.

885. S. N. Chatterjee, S. K. Bannerjee, A. K. Pal and J. Basak, DNA damage, prophage induction and mutation by furazolidone, *Chem. Biol. Interact.*, 1983, **45**, 315–326.

886. Y. C. Ni, R. H. Heflich, F. F. Kadlubar and P. P. Fu, Mutagenicity of nitrofurans in *Salmonella typhimurium* TA98, TA98NR and TA98/1,8-DNP6, *Mutat. Res.*, 1987, **192**, 15–22.

887. A. K. Pal, M. S. Rahman and S. N. Chatterjee, On the induction of umu gene expression in *Salmonella typhimurium* strain TA1535/pSK1002 by some nitrofurans, *Mutat. Res.*, 1992, **280**, 67–71.

888. E. Madrigal-Bujaidar, J. C. Ibañez, M. Cassani and G. Chamorro, Effect of furazolidone on sister-chromatid exchanges, cell proliferation kinetics, and mitotic index *in vivo* and *in vitro*, *J. Toxicol. Environ. Health*, 1997, **51**, 89–96.

889. X. Jin, S. Tang, Q. Chen, J. Zou, T. Zhang, F. Liu, S. Zhang, C. Sun and X. Xiao, Furazolidone induced oxidative DNA damage via upregulating ROS that caused cell cycle arrest in human hepatoma G2 cells, *Toxicol. Lett.*, 2011, **201**, 205–212.

890. W. G. H. Blijleven, M. J. H. Kortselius and P. G. N. Kramers, Mutagenicity testing of H-193, AF-2 and furazolidone in *Drosophila melanogaster*, *Mutat. Res.*, 1977, **56**, 95–100.

891. D. W. Bryant and D. R. McCalla, Nitrofuran induced mutagenesis and error prone repair in *Escherichia coli*, *Chem. Biol. Interact.*, 1980, **31**, 151–166.

892. A. Carere, L. Conti, R. Crebelli and A. Macri, Quantitative data on urinary recovery of mutagenicity in furazolidone-treated rats, *Mutat. Res.*, 1982, **97**, 461–462.

893. S. N. Chatterjee, M. Maiti and S. Ghosh, Interaction of furazolidone with DNA, *Biochim. Biophys. Acta*, 1975, **402**, 161–165.

894. M. M. Cohen and M. Sagi, The effects of nitrofurans on mitosis, chromosome breakage and sister-chromatid exchange in human peripheral lymphocytes, *Mutat. Res.*, 1979, **59**, 139–142.

895. R. Crebelli, A. Carere, E. Falcone and A. Macri, A study of urinary and fecal excretion of furazolidone in rats by means of mutagenicity assays, *Ecotoxicol. Environ. Saf.*, 1982, **6**, 448–456.

896. N. Gao, Y. C. Ni, J. R. Thornton-Manning, P. P. Fu and R. H. Heflich, Mutagenicity of nitrofurantoin and furazolidone in Chinese hamster ovary cells, *Mutat. Res.*, 1989, **225**, 181–187.

897. P. G. Kramers, Studies on the induction of sex-linked recessive lethal mutations in *Drosophila melanogaster* by nitroheterocyclic compounds, *Mutat. Res.*, 1982, **101**, 209–326.

898. C. Lu, D. R. McCalla and D. W. Bryant, Action of nitrofurans on *E. coli*. Mutation and induction and repair of daughter-strand gaps in DNA, *Mutat. Res.*, 1979, **67**, 133–144.

899. D. R. McCalla and D. Voutsinos, On the mutagenicity of nitrofurans, *Mutat. Res.*, 1974, **16**, 3–16.

900. T. Ohta, N. Nakamura, M. Moriya, Y. Shirasu and T. Kada, The SOS-function-inducing activity of chemical mutagens in *Escherichia coli*, *Mutat. Res.*, 1984, **131**, 101–109.

901. S. G. Paik, Micronucleus induction in mouse bone marrow cells of nitrofurans, 5-nitroimidazole and nitrothiazole derivatives used as trichomonacides in Korea, *Environ. Mutagen. Carcinogen.*, 1985, **5**, 61–72.

902. D. R. Goodman, P. J. Hakkinen, J. H. Nemenzo and M. Vore, Mutagenic evaluation of nitrofurans derivatives in *Salmonella typhimurium*, by the micronucleus test, and by *in vivo* cytogenetics, *Mutat. Res.*, 1977, **48**, 295–305.

903. G. S. Probst, R. E. McMahon, L. E. Hill, C. Z. Thompson, J. K. Epp and S. B. Neal, Chemically-induced unscheduled DNA synthesis in primary rat hepatocyte cultures: a comparison with bacterial mutagenicity using 218 compounds, *Environ. Mutagen.*, 1981, **3**, 11–32.

904. G. Queinnec, R. Babile, R. Darre, H. M. Berland and J. Espinasse, Induction of abnormalities in chromosomes (of cattle and swine) by furazolidone and chloramphenicol, *Vet. Bull.*, 1975, **46**, 330.

905. A. Tonomura and M. S. Sasaki, Chromosome aberrations and DNA repair synthesis in cultured human cells exposed to nitrofurans, *Japan. J. Genet.*, 1973, **48**, 338–340.

906. D. Anderson and B. J. Phillips, Nitrofurazone – genotoxicity studies in mammalian cells *in vitro* and *in vivo*, *Food Chem. Toxicol.*, 1985, **23**, 1091–1098.

907. A. J. Baars, W. G. H. Blijleven, G. R. Mohn, A. T. Natarajan and D. D. Breimer, Preliminary studies on the ability of *Drosophila* microsomal preparations to activate mutagens and carcinogens, *Mutat. Res.*, 1980, **72**, 257–264.

908. M. Bignami, A. Carere, G. Conti, R. Crebelli and M. Fabrizi, Evaluation of 2 different genetic markers for the detection of frameshift mutagens in *A. nidulans*, *Mutat. Res.*, 1982, **97**, 293–302.

909. A. D. Chandler and R. R. Parent, Isolation and characterisation of a nitrofurazone resistant strain of *Salmonella* TA98, *Environ. Mutagen.*, 1982, **4**, 319–320.

910. H. Chess, T. McLaughlin, Z. Mroczkowski, W. D. Rupp and K. B. Low, Radiosensitization, mutagenicity, and toxicity of *Escherichia coli* by several nitrofurans and nitroimidazoles, *Radiat. Res.*, 1978, **75**, 424–431.

911. J. Gajewska, M. Szczypka, B. Tudek and T. Szymczyk, Studies on the effect of ascorbic acid and selenium on the genotoxicity of nitrofurans: nitrofurazone and furazolidone, *Mutat. Res.*, 1990, **232**, 191–197.

912. M. H. L. Green and A. M. Rogers, W. J. Muriel, A. C. Ward and D. R. McCalla, Use of a simplified fluctuation test to detect and characterize mutagenesis by nitrofurans, *Mutat. Res.*, 1977, **44**, 139–143.

913. P. Maier, R. M. Philpot, G. R. Mohn and H. V. Malling, Influence of subcellular fractions of mammalian testes on the mutagenic activity of nitrofurans towards *Escherichia coli*, *Mutat. Res.*, 1979, **63**, 233–243.

914. A. Matsuoka, M. Hayashi and M. J. Ishidate, Chromosomal aberration tests on 29 chemicals with S9 mix *in vitro*, *Mutat. Res.*, 1979, **66**, 277–290.

915. D. R. McCalla, Mutagenicity of nitrofurans derivatives. Review, *Environ. Mutagen.*, 1983, **5**, 745–765.

916. H. Morie, S. Sugie, M. Yoshimi, T. Kinouchi and Y. Ohnishi, Genotoxicity of a variety of nitroarenes and other compounds in DNA-repair tests with rat and mouse hepatocytes, *Mutat. Res.*, 1987, **190**, 159–167.

917. E. E. Obaseiki-Ebor and J. O. Akerele, Nitrofuran mutagenicity: induction of frameshift mutations, *Mutat. Res.*, 1986, **175**, 149–152.

918. P. L. Olive and D. R. McCalla, Damage to mammalian cell DNA by nitrofurans, *Cancer Res.*, 1975, **35**, 781–784.

919. P. L. Olive, Nitrofurazone-induced DNA damage to tissues of mice, *Chem. Biol. Interact.*, 1978, **20**, 323–331.

920. P. L. Olive, Macromolecular, antineoplastic and radiosensitization effects of nitrofurans, *Carcinogenesis*, 1978, **4**, 131–169.

921. P. L. Olive, Influence of cellular environment on toxicity of nitro-heterocycles, *Chem. Biol. Interact.*, 1979, **27**, 281–290.

922. P. L. Olive, Correlation between the half-wave reduction potential of nitroheterocycles and their mutagenicity in Chinese hamster V79 spheroids, *Mutat. Res.*, 1981, **82**, 137–145.

923. T.-M. Ong, Mutagenic activities of nitrofurans in *Neurospora crassa*, *Mutat. Res.*, 1977, **56**, 13–20.

924. T. Yahagi, T. Matsushima, M. Nagoa, Y. Seino, T. Sugimura and G. T. Bryan, Mutagenicities of nitrofuran derivatives on a bacterial tester strain with a R factor plasmid, *Mutat. Res.*, 1976, **40**, 9–14.

925. A. Zampieri and J. Greenberg, Nitrofurazone as a mutagen in *Escherichia coli*, *Biochem. Biophys. Res. Commun.*, 1964, **14**, 172–176.

926. Joint FAO/WHO Expert Committee on Food Additives, Toxicological Evaluation of Certain Veterinary Drug Residues in Food, The Fortieth Meeting of the Joint FAO/WHO Expert Committee on Food Additives (JECFA), International Programme on Chemical Safety, World Health Organization, Geneva, 1993, pp. 85–123 and 125–145.

927. F. W. Kari, J. E. Huff, J. Leininger, J. K. Haseman and S. L. Eustis, Toxicity and carcinogenicity of nitrofurazone in F344/N rats and B6C3F₁ mice, *Food Chem. Toxicol.*, 1989, **27**, 129–137.

928. National Toxicology Program, Toxicology and carcinogenesis studies of nitrofurazone (CAS No. 59-87-0) in F344/N rats and B6C3F₁ mice, Technical Report Series No. 337, US Department of Health and Human Services, Public Health Service/National Institutes of Health, National Toxicology Program, 1989. Available from: http://ntp-server.niehs.nih.gov/.

929. T. Nomura, S. Kimura, T. Kanzaki, H. Tanaka, K. Shibak, H. Nakajima, Y. Isa, N. Kurokawa, T. Hatanaka, M. Kinuta, K. Masada and Y. Sakamoto, Induction of tumours and malformations in mice after prenatal treatment with some antibiotic drugs, *Med. J. Osaka Univ.*, 1984, **35**, 13–17.

930. J. E. Morris, J. M. Price, J. J. Lalich and R. J. Stein, The carcinogenic activity of some 5-nitrofuran derivatives in the rat, *Cancer Res.*, 1969, **29**, 2145–2156.

931. R. R. Maronpot, Ovarian toxicity and carcinogenicity in eight recent National Toxicology Program studies, *Environ. Health Perspect.*, 1987, **73**, 125–130.

932. J. E. Huff, S. L. Eustis and J. K. Haseman, Occurrence and relevance of chemically-induced benign neoplasms in long-term carcinogenicity studies, *Cancer Metastasis Rev.*, 1989, **8**, 1–22.

933. S. M. Cohen, F. Eturk, A. M. Von Esch, A. J. Crovetti and G. T. Bryan, Carcinogenicity of 5-nitrofurans, 5-nitroimidazoles, 4-nitrobenzenes and related compounds, *J. Natl. Cancer Inst.*, 1973, **51**, 403–417.

934. S. M. Cohen, Toxicity and carcinogenesis of nitrofurans, *Carcinogenesis*, 1978, **4**, 171–231.

935. International Agency for Research on Cancer, Nitrofural (nitrofurazone), IARC Monographs on the Evaluation of Carcinogenic Risks to Humans, *Pharmaceutical Drugs*, IARC, Lyon, 1990, vol. 50, pp. 195–209.

936. International Agency for Research on Cancer, Nitrofurantoin, IARC Monographs on the Evaluation of Carcinogenic Risks to Humans, *Pharmaceutical Drugs*, IARC, Lyon, 1990, vol. 50, pp. 211–231.

937. L. H. M. Vroomen, M. C. J. Berghmans, P. J. van Bladeren, J. P. Groten, C. J. Wissink and H. A. Kuiper, *In vivo* and *in vitro* metabolic studies of furazolidone: A risk evaluation, *Drug Metab. Rev.*, 1990, **22**, 663–676.

938. L. H. M. Vroomen, M. C. J. Berghmans, P. J. van Bladeren, J. P. Groten, C. J. Wissink and H. A. Kuiper, Bound residues of furazolidone, a potential risk for the consumer in *Veterinary Pharmacology and Therapy in Food Producing Animals*, ed. F. Simon, P. Lees and G. Semjen, Unipharma, Budapest, 1990, pp. 257–266.

939. L. A. P. Hoogenboom, The use of pig hepatocytes for biotransformation and toxicity studies, Thesis, Landbouwuniversiteit te Wageningen, Netherlands, 1991.

940. L. A. Hoogenboom, M. C. Berghmans, T. H. Polman, R. Parker and I. C. Shaw, Depletion of protein-bound furazolidone metabolise

containing the 3-amino-2-oxazolidinone side-chain from liver, kidney and muscle tissues from pigs, *Food Addit. Contam.*, 1992, **9**, 623–630.

941. L. A. Hoogenboom, T. H. Polman, A. Lommen, M. B. Huveneers and J. van Rhijn, Biotransformation of furaltadone by pig hepatocytes and *Salmonella typhimurium* TA 100 bacteria, and the formation of protein bound metabolites, *Xenobiotica*, 1994, **24**, 713–727.

942. I. De Angelis, L. Rossi, J. L. Pedersen, A. L. Vignoli, O. Vincentini, L. A. Hoogenboom, T. H. Polman, A. Stammati and F. Zucco, Metabolism of furazolidone: alternative pathways and modes of toxicity in different cell lines, *Xenobiotica*, 1999, **29**, 1157–1169.

943. K. Christiansen, Fusidic acid adverse drug reactions, *Int. J. Antimicrob. Agents.*, 1999, **12**(2), S3–S9.

944. J. F. Westphal, D. Vetter and J. M. Brogard, Hepatic side-effects of antibiotics, *J. Antimicrob. Chemother.*, 1994, **33**, 387–401.

945. K. Bendtzen, M. Diamant and V. Faber, Fusidic acid, an immunosuppressant drug with functions similar to cyclosporine A, *Cytokine*, 1990, **2**, 423–429.

946. A. Bellahsène and A. Forsgren, Effects of fusidic acid on the immune response in mice, *Infect. Immun.*, 1980, **29**, 873–878.

947. S. Teckchandani, S. Robertson, A. Almond, K. Donaldson and C. Isles, Rhabdomyolysis following co-prescription of fusidic acid and atorvastatin, *J. R. Coll. Physicians Edinb.*, 2010, **40**, 33–36.

948. H. Hoeksma, J. L. Johnson and J. W. Hinman, Structural studies on streptonivicin, a new antibiotic, *J. Am. Chem. Soc.*, 1955, **77**, 6710–6711.

949. A. Maxwell, The interaction between coumarin drugs and DNA gyrase, *Mol. Microbiol.*, 1993, **9**, 681–686.

950. R. J. Lewis, F. T. F. Tsai and D. B. Wigley, Molecular targets of drug inhibition of DNA gyrase, *Bioessays*, 1996, **18**, 661–671.

951. A. Maxwell and D. M. Lawson, The ATP-binding site of type II topoisomerases as a target for antibacterial drugs, *Curr. Top. Med Chem.*, 2003, **3**, 283–303.

952. A. Maxwell, DNA gyrase as a drug target, *Biochem. Soc. Trans.*, 1999, **27**, 48–53.

953. G. Rappa, A. Lorico and A. C. Sartorelli, Reversal of etoposide resistance in non-P-glycoprotein expressing multidrug resistant tumor cell lines by novobiocin, *Cancer Res.*, 1993, **53**, 5487–5493.

954. M. J. Kennedy, D. K. Armstrong, A. M. Huelskamp, K. Ohly, B. V. Clarke, O. M. Colvin, L. B. Grochow, T. L. Chen and N. E. Davidson, Phase I and pharmacologic study of the alkylating agent modulator novobiocin in combination with high-dose chemotherapy for the treatment of metastatic breast cancer, *J. Clin. Oncol.*, 1995, **13**, 1136–1143.

955. J. Nordenberg, J. Kornfeld, L. Wasserman, M. Shafran, E. Halabe, E. Beery, O. Landau, A. Novogrodsky and Y. Sidi, Novobiocin modulates colchicine sensitivity in parental and multidrug resistant B16 melanoma cells, *J. Cancer Res. Clin. Oncol.*, 1994, **120**, 599–604.

956. D. J. Stewart, R. Goel, M. C. Cripps, S. Huan, J. Yau and S. Verma, Multiple resistance modulators combined with carboplatin for resistant malignancies: a pilot study, *Invest. New Drugs*, 1997, **15**, 267–277.

957. J. P. Eder, C. A. Wheeler, B. A. Teicher and L. E. Schnipper, A phase I clinical trial of novobiocin, a modulator of alkylating agent cytotoxicity, *Cancer Res.*, 1991, **51**, 510–513.

958. P. J. Smith and S. M. Bell, A DNA topoisomerase II-independent route for novobiocin-mediated resistance to DNA binding agents, *Cancer Chemother. Pharmacol.*, 1990, **26**, 257–262.

959. P. Duan and G. You, Novobiocin is a potent inhibitor for human organic anion transporters, *Drug Metab. Disp.*, 2009, **37**, 1203–1210.

960. Committee for Veterinary Medicinal Products, Novobiocin, EMEA/MRL/610/99-FINAL CORRIGENDUM. Available from: http://ema.europa.eu.

961. M. E. Conrad, J. P. Knochel and W. H. Crosby, Novobiocin jaundice: demonstration of a haemolytic state, *Antibiotic Med. Clin. Ther.*, 1960, **7**, 382–385.

962. A. Aznar Reigh, A. Lopex, M. Gutirrez Rodriguez and A. Lallemand Carpio, Yellow pigmentation (pseudojaundice) in brucellosis treated with novobiocin, *Medicina (Madrid)*, 1959, **27**, 460–474.

963. T. Hargreaves and J. B. Holton, Jaundice of the newborn due to novobiocin, *Lancet*, 1962, **i**, 839.

964. S. B. Meness, M. Maneerattannaporn, H. M. Kim and W. D. Chen, The efficacy and safety of rifaximin for the irritable bowel syndrome: a systematic review and meta-analysis, *Am. J. Gastroenterol.*, 2012, **107**, 28–35.

965. F. Cremonini and A. Lembo, Rifaximin for the treatment of irritable bowel syndrome, *Expert Opin. Pharmacother.*, 2012, **13**, 433–440.

966. K. M. Eltawil, M. Laryea, K. Peltekian and M. Molinari, Rifaximin vs. conventional oral therapy for hepatic encephalopathy: a meta-analysis, *World J. Gastroenterol.*, 2012, **18**, 767–777.

967. L. M. Hynika and K. N. Silva, Probable rifaximin-induced neutropenia, *Am. J. Health Syst. Pharm.*, 2012, **69**, 583–586.

968. D. Bertoli and G. Borelli, Fertility study of rifaximin (L/105) in rats, *Chemoterapia*, 1986, **5**, 204–207.

969. G. Borelli and D. Bertoli, Acute, subacute, chronic toxicity and mutagenicity studies of rifaximin (L/105) in rats, *Chemoterapia*, 1986, **5**, 263–267.

970. D. Bertoli and G. Borelli, Teratogenic action of rifaximin in the rat and rabbit and its effect on perinatal development in the rat, *Boll. Soc. Ital. Biol. Sper.*, 1984, **60**, 1079–1085.

971. Committee for Veterinary Medicinal Products, Rifaximin, EMEA/MRL/309/97-FINAL. Available from: http://ema.europa.eu.

972. G. L. Mandell and W. A. Petri, Drugs used in the chemotherapy of tuberculosis, *Mycobacterium avium* complex disease, and leprosy in *Goodman and Gilman's The Pharmacological Basis of Therapeutics*, ed. J.

G. Hardman, L. E. Limbird, P. B. Molinoff, R. W. Ruddon and A. G. Goodman, McGraw-Hill, London, 9th edn, 1996, pp. 1155–1174.

973. A. Ibn Sellam, M. Soualhi, R. Zahraoui, K. Marc, J. Benamor, J. E. Bourkadi and G. Iraqi, A rare form of rifampicin-induced skin toxicity: bullous pemphigoid, *Rev. Mal. Respir.*, 2011, **28**, 365–371.

974. M. D. Katz and E. Lor, Acute interstitial nephritis associated with intermittent rifampin use, *Drug Intell. Clin. Pharm.*, 1986, **20**, 789–792.

975. M. A. Rajan, R. Soundararajan, V. Krishnamuthy and G. Ramu, Acute renal failure following rifampicin, *Indian J. Lepr.*, 1987, **59**, 286–292.

976. V. V. Rekha, T. Santha and M. S. Jawahar, Rifampicin-induced renal toxicity during retreatment of patients with pulmonary tuberculosis, *J. Assoc. Physicians India*, 2005, **53**, 811–813.

977. J. Grosset and S. Leventis, Adverse effects of rifampin, *Rev. Infect. Dis.*, 1983, **5**(3), S440–S450.

978. L. A. Ozick, L. Jacob, G. M. Comer, T. P. Lee, J. Ben-Zvi, S. S. Donelson and C. P. Felton, Hepatotoxicity from isoniazid and rifampin in inner-city AIDS patients, *Am. J. Gastroenterol.*, 1995, **90**, 1978–1980.

979. M. Sabaté, L. Ibáñez, E. Pèrez, X. Vidal, M. Buti, X. Xiol, A. Mas, M. Forné, R. Solà, J. Castellote, J. Rigau and J. R. Laporte, Risk of acute liver injury associated with the use of drugs: a multicentre population survey, *Aliment. Pharmacol. Ther.*, 2007, **25**, 1401–1409.

980. F. F. Fountain, E. A. Tolley, A. R. Jacobs and T. H. Self, Rifampin hepatotoxicity associated with treatment of latent tuberculosis infection, *Am. J. Med. Sci.*, 2009, **337**, 317–320.

981. J. Yue and R. Peng, Does CYP2E1 play a major role in the aggravation of isoniazid toxicity by rifampicin in human hepatocytes? *Br. J. Pharmacol.*, 2009, **157**, 331–333.

982. C. Shen, Q. Meng, G. Zhang and W. Hu, Rifampicin exacerbates isoniazid-induced toxicity in human but not in rat hepatocytes in tissue-like cultures, *Br. J. Pharmacol.*, 2008, **153**, 784–791.

983. C. Shen, X. Cheng, D. Li and Q. Meng, Investigation of rifampicin-induced hepatotoxicity in rat hepatocytes maintained in gel entrapment culture, *Cell Biol. Toxicol.*, 2009, **25**, 265–274.

984. S. Attri, S. V. Rana, K. Vaiphei, C. P. Sodhi, R. C. Goel, C. K. Nain and K. Singh, Isoniazid and rifampicin-induced oxidative hepatic injury – protection by N-acetylcysteine, *Hum. Exp. Toxicol.*, 2000, **19**, 517–522.

985. C. P. Sodhi, S. F. Rana, S. Attri, S. Mehta, K. Yaiphei and S. K. Mehta, Oxidative-hepatic injury of isoniazid-rifampicin in young rats subjected to protein and energy malnutrition, *Drug Chem. Toxicol.*, 1998, **21**, 305–317.

986. S. V. Rana, S. Attri, R. Vaiphei, R. Pal, A. Attri and K. Singh, Role of acetylcysteine in rifampicin-induced hepatic injury of young rats, *World J. Gastroenterol.*, 2006, **12**, 287–291.

987. D. M. Boothe, Dermatologic therapy in *Small Animal Clinical Pharmacology and Therapeutics*, ed. D. M. Boothe, W. B. Saunders Company, London, pp. 654–675.

988. Committee for Veterinary Medicinal Products, Dapsone (1). Available from: http://ema/europa.eu.

989. S. G. Kosseifi, B. Guha, D. M. Nassour, D. S. Chi and G. Krishnaswamy, The dapsone hypersensitivity syndrome revisited: a potentially fatal multisystem disorder with prominent hepatopulmonary manifestations, *J. Occup. Med. Toxicol.*, 2006, **1**, 9.

990. A. Chao, A. Tan, C. Theng and L. Y. Hian, Dapsone syndrome – a severe drug hypersensitivity reaction, *National Skin Centre (Singapore)*, 1995. Available from: http://www.nsc.gov.sg/showpage.asp?id-210.

991. S. Itha, A. Kumar, S. Dhingra and G. Choudhuri, Dapsone induced cholangitis as a part of dapsone syndrome: a case, *BMC Gastroenterol.*, 2003, **3**, 21.

992. K. S. Leslie, K. Gaffney, C. N. Ross, S. Ridley, T. H. Barker and J. J. Garioch, A near fatal case of the dapsone hypersensitivity syndrome in a patient with urticarial vasculitis, *Clin. Exp. Dermatol.*, 2003, **28**, 496–498.

993. P. N. Rao and T. S. Lakshmi, Increase in the incidence of dapsone hypersensitivity syndrome – an appraisal, *Lepr. Rev.*, 2001, **72**, 57–62.

994. E. N. Alves-Rodrigues, L. C. Ribeiro, M. D. Silva, A. Takiuchi and C. J. F. Fontes, Dapsone syndrome with acute renal failure during leprosy treatment: case report, *Braz. J. Infect. Dis.*, 2005, **9**, 84–86.

995. A. Subramaniam, C. Corallo and R. Nagappan, Dapsone-associated methaemoglobinaemia in patients with a haematologic malignancy, *Anaesth. Intensive Care*, 2010, **38**, 1070–1076.

996. J. G. Walker, T. Kadia, L. Brown, H. S. Juneja and J. F. de Groot, Dapsone induced methaemoglobinemia in a patient with glioblastoma, *J. Neurooncol.*, 2009, **94**, 149–152.

997. P. M. Naik, G. M. Lyon, A. Ramirez, E. C. Lawrence, D. C. Neujahr, S. Force and A. Pelaez, Dapsone-induced haemolytic anemia in lung allograft recipients, *J. Heart Lung Transplant.*, 2008, **27**, 1198–1202.

998. W. B. Shelley and M. I. Goldwein, High dose dapsone toxicity, *Br. J. Dermatol.*, 1976, **95**, 79–82.

999. G. A. Luzzi and T. E. Peto, Adverse effects of antimalarials, *Drug Saf.*, 1993, **8**, 295–311.

1000. H. O. AlKadi, Antimalarial drug toxicity: a review, *Chemotherapy*, 2007, **53**, 385–391.

1001. M. D. Coleman, Dapsone toxicity: some current perspectives, *Gen. Pharmacol.*, 1995, **26**, 1461–1467.

1002. M. D. Coleman, Dapsone-mediated agranulocytosis: risks, possible mechanisms and prevention, *Toxicology*, 2001, **162**, 53–60.

1003. M. D. Tingle, R. Mahmud, M. Maggs, M. Pirmohamed and B. K. Park, Comparison of the metabolism and toxicity of dapsone in rat, mouse and man, *J. Pharmacol. Exp. Ther.*, 1997, **283**, 817–823.

1004. R. E. Bluhm, A. Adedoyin, D. G. McCarver and R. A. Branch, Development of dapsone toxicity in patients with inflammatory dermatoses: activity of acetylation and hydroxylation of dapsone as risk factors, *Clin. Pharmacol. Ther.*, 1999, **65**, 598–605.

1005. S. J. Grossman, J. Simon and D. J. Jollow, Dapsone-induced haemolytic anemia: effect of N-hydroxy dapsone on the sulfhydryl status and membrane proteins of rat erythrocytes, *Toxicol. Appl. Pharmacol.*, 1992, **117**, 208–217.

1006. D. J. Jollow, T. P. Bradshaw and D. C. McMillan, Dapsone-induced hemolytic anemia, *Drug Metab. Rev.*, 1995, **27**, 107–124.

1007. S. J. Grossman and D. J. Jollow, The role of dapsone hydroxylamine in dapsone-induced haemolytic anemia, *J. Pharmacol. Exp. Ther.*, 1988, **244**, 118–125.

1008. M. D. Coleman, M. J. Winn, A. M. Breckenridge and B. K. Park, Sex-dependent sensitivity to dapsone-induced methaemoglobinaemia in the rat, *Biochem. Pharmacol.*, 1990, **39**, 805–809.

1009. R. J. Riley, P. Roberts, M. D. Coleman, N. R. Kitteringham and B. K. Park, Bioactivation of dapsone to a cytotoxic metabolite: *in vitro* use of a novel two compartment system which contains human tissues, *Br. J. Clin. Pharmacol.*, 1990, **30**, 417–426.

1010. R. Mahmud, M. D. Tingle, J. L. Maggs, M. T. Cronin, J. C. Dearden and B. K. Park, Structural basis for the haemotoxicity of dapsone: the importance of the sulphinyl group, *Toxicology*, 1997, **117**, 1–11.

1011. K. N. Woodward, Veterinary pesticides in *Mammalian Toxicology of Insecticides*, ed. T. C. Marrs, RSC Publishing, Cambridge, 2012, pp. 348–426.

1012. L. Griciute and L. Tomatis, Carcinogenicity of dapsone in mice and rats, *Int. J. Cancer*, 1980, **25**, 123–129.

1013. Committee for Veterinary Medicinal Products, Dapsone (2). Available from: http://www.ema.europa.eu.

1014. I. R. Sanchez, S. F. Swaim, K. E. Nusbaum, A. S. Hale, R. A. Henderson and J. A. McGuire, Effects of chlorhexidine diacetate and povidone-iodine on wound healing in dogs, *Vet. Surg.*, 1988, **17**, 291–295.

1015. L. K. M. Evans, T. G. Knowles, G. Werrett and P. E. Holt, The efficacy of Chlorhexidine gluconate in canine skin survey and clinical trials, *J. Small Anim. Pract.*, 2009, **50**, 458–465.

1016. W. P. Stubbs, J. R. Bellah, D. Vermaas-Hekman, B. Purich and P. S. Kubilis, Chlorhexidine gluconate versus chloroxylenol for preoperative skin preparation in dogs, *Vet. Surg.*, 1996, **25**, 487–494.

1017. J. Kennedy, J. Kek and D. Griffin, Selection and use of disinfectants, *NebGuide*, University of Nebraska, Lincoln. Available at: http://www.triton-vet.com.

1018. F. K. Neave, R. G. Dodd, R. G. Kingwill and D. R. Westgarth, Control of mastitis in the dairy herd by hygiene and management, *J. Dairy Sci.*, 1969, **52**, 696–707.

1019. S. P. Oliver, S. H. King, M. J. Lewis, P. M. Torre, K. R. Matthews and H. H. Dowlen, Efficacy of chlorhexidine as a postmilking prevention of bovine mastitis during lactation, *J. Dairy Sci.*, 1990, **73**, 2230–2235.

1020. R. E. W. Halliwell, Rational use of shampoos in veterinary dermatology, *J. Small Anim. Pract.*, 1991, **32**, 401–407.

1021. D. M. Foulkes, Some toxicological observations on chlorhexidine, *J. Periodont. Res.*, 1973, **8**(12), 55–57.

1022. D. E. Case, Safety of hibitane. I. Laboratory experiments, *J. Clin. Periodontol.*, 1977, **4**, 66–62.

1023. D. A. Ribeiro, C. Scolastici, P. L. De Lima, M. E. Marques and D. M. Salvadori, Genotoxicity of antimicrobial endodontic compounds by single cell gel (comet) assay in Chinese hamster ovary (CHO) cells, *Oral Surg. Oral Med. Oral Pathol. Oral Radiol. Endod.*, 2005, **99**, 637–640.

1024. F. Rodrigues, M. Lehmann, V. S. do Amaral, M. L. Reguly and H. H. de Andrade, Genotoxicity of three mouthwash products, Vepacol, Periogard, and Plax, in the Drosphila wing-spot test, *Environ. Mol. Mutagen.*, 2007, **48**, 644–649.

1025. J. Kolahi, P. Ghalayani and J. Varshosaz, Systemic toxicity following ingestion of the chlorhexidine gluconate solution: a case report, *J. Int. Acad. Periodontal.*, 2006, **8**, 45–46.

1026. C. R. Balit, A. M. Lynch, S. P. Gilmore, L. Murray and G. K. Ibister, Lignocaine and chlorhexidine toxicity in children resulting from mouth paint ingestion: a bottling problem, *J. Paediatr. Child Health*, 2006, **42**, 350–353.

1027. Y. Xue, S. Zhang, Y. Yang, M. Lu, Y. Wang, T. Zhang, M. Tang and H. Takeshita, Acute pulmonary toxic effects of chlorhexidine (CHX) following an intratracheal instillation in rats, *Hum. Exp. Toxicol.*, 2011, **30**, 1795–1803.

1028. Y. Igarashi and J. Suzuki, Cochlear ototoxicity of chlorhexidine gluconate in cats, *Arch. Otolaryngol.*, 1985, **242**, 167–176.

1029. S. M. Merchant, T. M. Neer, B. L. Tedford, A. C. Twedt, P. M. Cheramie and G. M. Strain, Ototoxicity assessment of a chlorhexidine otic preparation in dogs, *Prog. Vet. Neurol.*, 1993, **4**, 72–75.

1030. J. Aursnes, Vestibular damage from chlorhexidine in guinea pigs, *Acta Otolaryngol.*, 1981, **92**, 89–100.

1031. J. Aursnes, Cochlear damage from chlorhexidine in guinea pigs, *Acta Otolaryngol.*, 1981, **92**, 259–271.

1032. P. Lai, C. Coulson, D. D. Pothier and J. Rutka, Chlorhexidine ototoxicity in ear surgery, part I: review of the literature, *J. Otolaryngol. Head Neck Surg.*, 2011, **40**, 437–440.

1033. P. Lai, C. Coulson, D. D. Pothier and J. Rutka, Chlorhexidine ototoxicity in ear surgery, part 1I: Survey of preparation solution used by otolaryngologists in Canada: Is there cause for concern? *J. Otolaryngol. Head Neck Surg.*, 2011, **40**, 441–445.

1034. K. Sata, Y. Kusaka, N. Suganuma, S. Nagasawa and Y. Deguchi, Occupational allergy in medical doctors, *J. Occup. Health*, 2004, **46**, 165–170.

1035. B. Lasthein, L. Anderson and F. Brandrup, Contact dermatitis from chlorhexidine, *Contact Dermatitis*, 1985, **13**, 307–309.

1036. A. Barbaux, M. Vigan, J. L. Delrous, H. Assier, M. Avenel-Audran, E. Collett, A. Dehlemmes, H. Dutarte, C. Géaut, C. Le Coz, B. Milpied-Homsi, A. Nassif, A. Pons-Guiraud and N. Raison-Peyron, and Membres du Groupe du REVIDA. Contact allergy to antiseptics: 75 cases analysed by dermato-allergovigilance network (Revidal), *Ann. Dermatol. Venereol.*, 2005, **132**, 962–965.
1037. K. Aalto-Korte and S. Mäkinen-Kiljunen, Symptoms of immediate chlorhexidine hypersensitivity in patients with a positive prick test, *Contact Dermatitis*, 2005, **55**, 173–177.
1038. K. S. Lim and P. C. Kam, Chlorhexidine – pharmacology and clinical applications, *Anaesth. Intensive Care*, 2008, **36**, 502–512.
1039. T. Aida, T. Kimura, N. Ishikawa and K. Shinkai, Evaluation of allergic potential of low-molecular compounds by mouse popliteal lymph node assay, *J. Toxicol. Sci.*, 1998, **23**, 425–432.
1040. S. M. MacRae, B. Brown and H. F. Edelhauser, The corneal toxicity of presurgical skin antiseptics, *Am. J. Ophthalmol.*, 1984, **97**, 221–232.
1041. L. M. Hamed, F. D. Ellis, G. Boudreault, F. M. Wilson and E. M. Helveston, Hibiclens keratitis, *Am. J. Ophthalmol.*, 1987, **104**, 50–56.
1042. Committee for Veterinary Medicinal Products, Chlorhexidine, EMEA/MRL/107/96-FINAL. Available from: http://www.ema.europa.eu.

Subject Index

Note: entries are prefixed by the volume number.